KU-272-496

OXFORD MEDICAL PUBLICATIONS

Oxford Handbook for the

Foundation
Programme

Published and forthcoming Oxford Handbooks

Oxford Handbook for the Foundation Programme 4e
Oxford Handbook of Acute Medicine 3e
Oxford Handbook of Anaesthesia 3e
Oxford Handbook of Applied Dental Sciences
Oxford Handbook of Cardiology 2e
Oxford Handbook of Clinical and Laboratory Investigation 3e
Oxford Handbook of Clinical Dentistry 5e
Oxford Handbook of Clinical Diagnosis 2e
Oxford Handbook of Clinical Examination and Practical Skills 2e
Oxford Handbook of Clinical Haematology 3e
Oxford Handbook of Clinical Immunology and Allergy 3e
Oxford Handbook of Clinical Medicine – Mini Edition 8e
Oxford Handbook of Clinical Medicine 9e
Oxford Handbook of Clinical Pathology
Oxford Handbook of Clinical Pharmacy 2e
Oxford Handbook of Clinical Rehabilitation 2e
Oxford Handbook of Clinical Specialties 9e
Oxford Handbook of Clinical Surgery 4e
Oxford Handbook of Complementary Medicine
Oxford Handbook of Critical Care 3e
Oxford Handbook of Dental Patient Care
Oxford Handbook of Dialysis 3e
Oxford Handbook of Emergency Medicine 4e
Oxford Handbook of Endocrinology and Diabetes 3e
Oxford Handbook of ENT and Head and Neck Surgery 2e
Oxford Handbook of Epidemiology for Clinicians
Oxford Handbook of Expedition and Wilderness Medicine
Oxford Handbook of Forensic Medicine
Oxford Handbook of Gastroenterology & Hepatology 2e
Oxford Handbook of General Practice 4e
Oxford Handbook of Genetics
Oxford Handbook of Genitourinary Medicine, HIV and AIDS 2e
Oxford Handbook of Geriatric Medicine 2e
Oxford Handbook of Infectious Diseases and Microbiology
Oxford Handbook of Key Clinical Evidence
Oxford Handbook of Medical Dermatology
Oxford Handbook of Medical Imaging
Oxford Handbook of Medical Sciences 2e
Oxford Handbook of Medical Statistics
Oxford Handbook of Neonatology
Oxford Handbook of Nephrology and Hypertension 2e
Oxford Handbook of Neurology 2e
Oxford Handbook of Nutrition and Dietetics 2e
Oxford Handbook of Obstetrics and Gynaecology 3e
Oxford Handbook of Occupational Health 2e
Oxford Handbook of Oncology 3e
Oxford Handbook of Ophthalmology 2e
Oxford Handbook of Oral and Maxillofacial Surgery
Oxford Handbook of Orthopaedics and Trauma
Oxford Handbook of Paediatrics 2e
Oxford Handbook of Pain Management
Oxford Handbook of Palliative Care 2e
Oxford Handbook of Practical Drug Therapy 2e
Oxford Handbook of Pre-Hospital Care
Oxford Handbook of Psychiatry 3e
Oxford Handbook of Public Health Practice 3e
Oxford Handbook of Reproductive Medicine & Family Planning 2e
Oxford Handbook of Respiratory Medicine 3e
Oxford Handbook of Rheumatology 3e
Oxford Handbook of Sport and Exercise Medicine 2e
Handbook of Surgical Consent
Oxford Handbook of Tropical Medicine 4e
Oxford Handbook of Urology 3e

Oxford Handbook for the
Foundation
Programme

Fourth edition

Tim Raine

Clinical Fellow, Wellcome Trust
Clinical Lecturer, Gastroenterology, University of Cambridge,
Honorary Registrar, Addenbrooke's Hospital, Cambridge

James Dawson

Consultant Anaesthetist, Nottingham

Stephan Sanders

Assistant Specialist at University of California, San Francisco

Simon Eccles

Consultant in Emergency Medicine, St Thomas Hospital, London

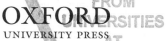

OXFORD
UNIVERSITY PRESS

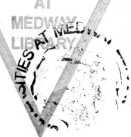

OXFORD
UNIVERSITY PRESS

Great Clarendon Street, Oxford, OX2 6DP,
United Kingdom

Oxford University Press is a department of the University of Oxford.
It furthers the University's objective of excellence in research, scholarship,
and education by publishing worldwide. Oxford is a registered trade mark of
Oxford University Press in the UK and in certain other countries

© Oxford University Press 2014

The moral rights of the authors have been asserted

First edition published 2005
Second edition published 2008
Third edition published 2011
Fourth edition published 2014, Reprinted 2015, 2016

Impression: 4

Published in the United States of America by Oxford University Press
198 Madison Avenue, New York, NY 10016, United States of America

British Library Cataloguing in Publication Data

Data available

Library of Congress Control Number: 2014931114

ISBN 978-0-19-968381-9

Typeset by GreenGate Publishing Services, Tonbridge, UK
Printed in China
on acid-free paper by
C&C Offset Printing Co., Ltd

Contents

To every doctor who's ever stood there thinking:
'What on earth do I do now?'

Detailed contents

Preface

Since this book was first written the training of doctors has altered dramatically. The Foundation Programme, Specialty Training and the rise and fall of MTAS have all affected the role, careers, and morale of junior doctors. This new edition emerges into a landscape of medical training, which is set to be restructured yet again, creating yet more uncertainty for those starting out. And yet, through all of this turbulence, the fact remains that the leap from being a final year medical student to a junior doctor remains immense. No matter what elements may be introduced to final year curricula, or to Foundation Programme inductions, the psychological and professional gear-shift is a change that many feel unprepared for.

Overnight the new doctor inherits huge responsibility, an incessantly active bleep, and an inflexible working rota. They also become a valued member of the medical team, someone who patients look to for help, someone with the capacity to offer the care that patients and their relatives need, and a new doctor with the potential and flexibility to learn and shape a career in just about any area of medicine they wish to pursue.

While nothing can make this transition easy we hope that this book can act as a guide. Based on feedback from foundation doctors we feel that this fourth edition builds on the strengths of previous editions whilst improving on their weaknesses. The clinical chapters have been completely updated to reflect all the latest developments, the prescribing pages given an overhaul to keep them current, and the front of the book reworked to reflect the challenges and environment facing the foundation doctor for 2014 and beyond.

Please continue to help us to improve this book by sending comments and suggestions to: ohfp.uk@oup.com.

Acknowledgements

The authors would like to say a huge 'thank you' to many people for their wisdom, knowledge and support:

Tim thanks Dr Roger Lewis, who taught him much he once knew, and Prof. Arthur Kaser who has indulged his efforts to try to retain it. And, as always, Lucy, the constant, and now Beatrice, the ever changing.

James would like to thank, in no particular order: Simon Denning, Tobias Long, Will Tomlinson, John Gell, and my beautiful fellow authors.

Stephan thanks Imogen Hart and Xanthe Sanders for making life wonderful.

Simon would like to dedicate this to Amy and Arthur.

To everyone who helped with the first three editions: our job was so much easier for all your hard work and we've not forgotten you. In particular, our ongoing thanks to Nat Hurley, Shreelata Datta and Katherine McGinn.

We would also like to thank all the staff at Oxford University Press for their help and for making our writing into a book. In particular, Liz Reeve and Hannah Lloyd for their terrific efforts and support in making the OHFP4e such a pleasure to work on, along with the rest of the OUP team:

- Michael Hawkes
- Richard Martin
- Mark Knowles
- Kate Wilson
- Catherine Barnes
- Kelly Hewinson
- Fiona Chippendale
- Abigail Stanley
- Anna Winstanley
- Eloise Moir-Ford
- Tracey Mills
- Jamie Hartmann-Boyce
- David Gardner

Symbols and abbreviations

🔲	Cross-reference
▶▶	Don't dawdle
🖱	Website
↑	Increased
↓	Decreased
→	Leading to
±	Plus/minus
>	Greater than
<	Less than
♀	Female
♂	Male
A+E	Accident and emergency (now the emergency department)
AAA	Abdominal aortic aneurysm
ABG	Arterial blood gas
ABPI	Ankle brachial pressure index
ABx	Antibiotics
ACCS	Acute care common stem
ACEi	Angiotensin-converting enzyme inhibitor
ACF	Academic Clinical Fellowship
ACS	Acute coronary syndrome
ACTH	Adrenocorticotrophic hormone
ADH	Antidiuretic hormone
ADL	Activities of daily living
AED	Automated external defibrillator
AF	Atrial fibrillation
AFB	Acid-fast bacilli
αFP (AFP)	α-fetoprotein
AIDS	Acquired immunodeficiency syndrome
AKI	Acute kidney injury
ALL	Acute lymphoblastic leukaemia
ALP	Alkaline phosphatase
ALS	Advanced Life Support®
ALT	Alanine aminotransferase
AML	Acute myeloid leukaemia

AMPLE	Allergies; Medications; Past medical history; Last meal; Events leading to presentation
ANA	Antinuclear antibody
ANCA	Antineutrophil cytoplasmic antibody
AP	Anteroposterior
APH	Antepartum haemorrhage
APLS	Advanced Paediatric Life Support
APTT	Activated partial thromboplastin time
APTTr	Activated partial thromboplastin time ratio
AR	Aortic regurgitation
ARB	Angiotensin receptor blocker
ARDS	Acute respiratory distress syndrome
ARF	Acute renal failure
AS	Aortic stenosis
ASA	American Society of Anesthesiologists
ASAP	As soon as possible
ASD	Atrial septal defect
AST	Aspartate transaminase
ATLS	Advanced Trauma Life Support
ATN	Acute tubular necrosis
AV	Atrio-ventricular
AVR	Aortic valve replacement
AXR	Abdominal X-ray
Ba	Barium
BAL	Bronchoalveolar lavage
BCG	Bacille Calmette–Guérin (TB vaccination)
bd	Bis die (twice daily)
BE	Base excess
BFG	Big friendly giant
β-hCG	β-human chorionic gonadotrophin
BIH	Benign intracranial hypertension
BiPAP	Biphasic positive airways pressure
BKA	Below knee amputation
BLS	Basic Life Support
BM	Boehringer Mannhein meter (capillary blood glucose) or Bone marrow
BMA	British Medical Association
BMI	Body mass index
BNF	*British National Formulary*
BP	Blood pressure
BPH	Benign prostatic hypertrophy

BX	Biopsy
C+S	Culture and sensitivity
Ca^{2+}	Calcium
Ca	Carcinoma
CABG	Coronary artery bypass graft
CAH	Congenital adrenal hyperplasia
CAPD	Continuous ambulatory peritoneal dialysis
CBD	Case-based discussion/Common bile duct
CBT	Cognitive-behavioural therapy
CCF	Congestive cardiac failure
CCST	Certificate of Completion of Specialist Training
CCT	Certificate of Completion of Training
CCU	Coronary care unit
CD	Controlled drugs
CDT	*Clostridium difficile* toxin
CEA	Carcinoembryonic antigen
CEPOD	Confidential Enquiry into Perioperative Deaths
CEX	Clinical Evaluation Exercise
cf	Compared with
CHD	Coronary heart disease
CI	Contraindication
CJD	Creutzfeldt–Jakob disease
CK	Creatine kinase
CK-MB	Heart-specific creatine kinase (MB-isoenzyme)
CLL	Chronic lymphocytic leukaemia
CLO	Campylobacter-like organism
CML	Chronic myeloid leukaemia
CMV	Cytomegalovirus
CNS	Central nervous system
CO	Carbon monoxide
CO_2	Carbon dioxide
COAD	Chronic obstructive airway disease
COC	Combined oral contraceptive
COPD	Chronic obstructive pulmonary disease
CPAP	Continuous positive airway pressure
CPK	Creatine phosphokinase
CPN	Community psychiatric nurse
CPR	Cardiopulmonary resuscitation
CRB	Criminal Records Bureau
CRF	Chronic renal failure

CRP	C-reactive protein
CRT	Capillary-refill time
CSF	Cerebrospinal fluid
CSU	Catheter specimen of urine
CT	Computer tomography/Core training
CTG	Cardiotocograph
CTPA	CT pulmonary angiogram
CVA	Cerebrovascular accident
CVP	Central venous pressure
CVS	Cardiovascular system
CXR	Chest X-ray
d	Day(s)
D+C	Dilatation and curettage
D+V	Diarrhoea and vomiting
DEXA	Dual-energy X-ray absorptiometry (DXA)
DH	Drug history
DH	Department of Health
DHS	Dynamic hip screw
DI	Diabetes insipidus
DIB	Difficulty in breathing
DIC	Disseminated intravascular coagulation
DIPJ	Distal interphalangeal joint
DKA	Diabetic ketoacidosis
DM	Diabetes mellitus
DMARD	Disease modifying anti-rheumatic drug
DNA	Deoxyribonucleic acid/Did not attend
DNR	Do not resuscitate
DoB	Date of birth
DOPS	Direct Observation of Procedural Skills
DRE	Digital rectal examination
DSM-5	*The Diagnostic and Statistical Manual of Mental Disorders* 5th revision
DTP	Diphtheria, tetanus and pertussis
DU	Duodenal ulcer
DVLA	Driver and Vehicle Licensing Agency
DVT	Deep vein thrombosis
d/w	Discuss(ed) with
Dx	Diagnosis
DXA	Dual-energy X-Ray absorptiometry (DEXA)
EBM	Evidence-based medicine
EBV	Epstein–Barr virus

ECG	Electrocardiogram
ECHO	Echocardiogram
ECV	External cephalic version
ED	Emergency department (formerly A+E)
EDD	Expected due date (pregnancy)
EEG	Electroencephalogram
EMD	Electromechanical dissociation or pulseless electrical activity (PEA)
EMG	Electromyogram
ENP	Emergency nurse practitioner
ENT	Ear, nose, and throat
EØ	Eosinophil
EPO	Erythropoietin
ERCP	Endoscopic retrograde cholangiopancreatography
ERPC	Evacuation of retained products of conception
ESM	Ejection systolic murmur
ESR	Erythrocyte sedimentation rate
ESRF	End-stage renal failure
ET	Endotracheal
EtOH	Ethanol (alcohol)
ETT	Endotracheal tube
EUA	Examination under anaesthetic
EVD	Extra-ventricular drain
EWTD	European Working Time Directive
F1/F2	Foundation year one/two
FAST	Focused assessment with sonography in trauma
FB	Foreign body
FBC	Full blood count
FDP	Fibrin degradation product
FEV_1	Forced expiratory volume in one second
FFP	Fresh frozen plasma
FH	Family history/Foetal heart
FiO_2	Fraction of inspired oxygen
FNA	Fine needle aspiration
FOB	Faecal occult blood
FOOSH	Fall on outstretched hand
FRC	Functional residual capacity
FSH	Follicle stimulating hormone
FTSTA	Fixed-term specialty training appointment
FVC	Forced vital capacity
G+S	Group and save

G6PD	Glucose-6-phosphate dehydrogenase
GA	General anaesthetic
GB	Gall bladder
GBS	Group B *Streptococcus*/Guillain–Barré syndrome
GCS	Glasgow Coma Scale
GFR	Glomerular filtration rate
γGT (GGT)	γ-glutamyl transpeptidase
GH	Growth hormone/Gynae history
GI	Gastrointestinal
GMC	General Medical Council
GN	Glomerulonephritis
GORD	Gastro-oesophageal reflux disease
GP	General practitioner
GTN	Glyceryl trinitrate
GTT	Glucose tolerance test
GU(M)	Genitourinary (medicine)
h	Hour(s)
H@N	Hospital at night
HAART	Highly active antiretroviral therapy
HAI	Hospital acquired infection
HAV	Hepatitis A virus
Hb	Haemoglobin
HbA_{1c}	Glycosylated haemoglobin
HBV	Hepatitis B virus
HCA	Healthcare assistant
HCC	Hepatocellular carcinoma
hCG	Human chorionic gonadotrophin
HCT	Haematocrit
HCV	Hepatitis C virus
HDL	High-density lipoprotein
HDU	High dependency unit
HELLP	Haemolysis, elevated liver enzymes, low platelets (syndrome)
HIV	Human immunodeficiency virus
HLA	Human leucocyte antigen
HMMA	4-hydroxy-3-methoxymandelic acid (phaeochromocytoma)
HOCM	Hypertrophic obstructive cardiomyopathy
HONK	Hyperosmolar non-ketotic state
HPA	Health Protection Agency
HR	Heart rate
HR	Human resources

HRT	Hormone replacement therapy
HSP	Henoch–Schönlein purpura
HSV	Herpes simplex virus
HTN	Hypertension
HUS	Haemolytic uraemic syndrome
HVS	High vaginal swab
I+D	Incision and drainage
IBD	Inflammatory bowel disease
IBS	Irritable bowel syndrome
ICD-10	*International Classification of Diseases* 10th revision
ICP	Intracranial pressure
ICU	Intensive care unit
ID	Identification
ID	Infectious diseases
IDDM	Insulin-dependent diabetes mellitus (outdated term)
IE	Infective endocarditis
IFG	Impaired fasting glucose
Ig	Immunoglobulin
IGT	Impaired glucose tolerance
IHD	Ischaemic heart disease
ILS	Immediate Life Support
IM	Intramuscular
Imp	Impression (clinical)
IN	Intranasal
INH	By inhalation
INR	International normalised ratio
ITP	Idiopathic thrombocytopenic purpura
ITU	Intensive care unit
iu	International unit
IUCD	Intrauterine contraceptive device
IUP	Intrauterine pregnancy
IV	Intravenous
IVDU	Intravenous drug user
IVI	Intravenous infusion
IVP	Intravenous pyelogram
IVU	Intravenous urogram
Ix	Investigation(s)
JACCOL	Jaundice, anaemia, clubbing, cyanosis, oedema, lymphadenopathy
JDC	Junior Doctors' Committee of BMA
JVP	Jugular venous pressure

K-nail	Küntscher nail
kPa	Kilopascal
KUB	Kidneys, ureter, bladder (X-ray)
K-wire	Kirschner wire
l	Litre(s)
LA	Local anaesthetic
LACS	Lacunar circulation stroke
LAD	Left axis deviation/Left anterior descending
LBBB	Left bundle branch block
LDH	Lactate dehydrogenase
LDL	Low-density lipoprotein
LFT	Liver function test
LH	Luteinising hormone
LHRH	Luteinising hormone releasing hormone
LIF	Left iliac fossa
LMA	Laryngeal mask airway
LMN	Lower motor neuron
LMP	Last menstrual period
LMWH	Low-molecular-weight heparin
LN	Lymph node
LOC	Loss of consciousness
LØ	Lymphocyte
LP	Lumbar puncture
LSCS	Lower segment Caesarean section
LTOT	Long-term oxygen therapy
LUQ	Left upper quadrant
LVF	Left ventricular failure
LVH	Left ventricular hypertrophy
MAOI	Monoamine oxidase inhibitor
mane	In the morning
MAP	Mean arterial pressure
M,C+S	Microscopy, culture, and sensitivity
MCPJ	Metacarpal phalangeal joint
MCV	Mean cell volume
MDDUS	Medical and Dental Defence Union of Scotland
MDR	Multi-drug resistant
MDU	Medical Defence Union
ME	Myalgic encephalitis
MEWS	Modified Early Warning Score
mg	Milligram(s)
MI	Myocardial infarction

min	Minute(s)
ml	Millilitre(s)
MMC	Modernising Medical Careers
mmH$_2$O	Millimetres of water
mmHg	Millimetres of mercury
MMR	Measles, mumps, and rubella
MMSE	Mini-mental State Examination
MND	Motor neuron disease
MPS	Medical Protection Society
MR	Mitral regurgitation/modified release
MRCP	Magnetic resonance cholangiopancreatography
MRI	Magnetic resonance imaging
MRSA	Meticillin-resistant *Staphylococcus aureus*
MS	Multiple sclerosis/Mitral stenosis
MSF	Multisource feedback
MSSA	Meticillin-sensitive *Staphylococcus aureus*
MST	Morphine sulfate
MSU	Mid-stream urine
MTPJ	Metatarsal phalangeal joint
mth	Month(s)
MVR	Mitral valve replacement
N+V	Nausea and vomiting
NAD	Nothing abnormal detected
NAI	Non-accidental injury
NBM	Nil by mouth
NEB	By nebuliser
NG	Nasogastric
NHS	National Health Service
NICE	National Institute for Health and Care Excellence
NICU	Neonatal intensive care unit
NIDDM	Non-insulin dependent diabetes mellitus (outdated term)
NJ	Nasojejunal
NNU	Neonatal unit
NØ	Neutrophil
nocte	At night
NPA	Nasopharyngeal aspirate
NSAID	Non-steroidal anti-inflammatory drug
NSTEMI	Non-ST-elevation myocardial infarction
NTN	National training number
NVD	Normal vaginal delivery
NYHA	New York Heart Association

OA	Osteoarthritis
Obs	Observations
OCD	Obsessive-compulsive disorder
OCP	Oral contraceptive pill/Ova, cysts and parasites
od	Omni die (once daily)
OD	Overdose
OGD	Oesophagogastroduodenoscopy
OHA	*Oxford Handbook of Anaesthesia*
OHEM	*Oxford Handbook of Emergency Medicine*
OHAM	*Oxford Handbook of Acute Medicine*
OHCC	*Oxford Handbook of Critical Care*
OHCLI	*Oxford Handbook of Clinical and Laboratory Investigation*
OHCM	*Oxford Handbook of Clinical Medicine*
OHCS	*Oxford Handbook of Clinical Specialties*
OHFP	*Oxford Handbook for the Foundation Programme*
OHGP	*Oxford Handbook of General Practice*
OHOG	*Oxford Handbook of Obstetrics and Gynaecology*
om	Omni mane (in the morning)
on	Omni nocte (at night)
ORIF	Open reduction and internal fixation
OSCE	Objective structured clinical examination
OT	Occupational therapy
P	Pulse
PA	Posteroanterior
$PaCO_2$	Partial pressure of arterial carbon dioxide
PACS	Partial anterior circulation stroke/Picture archiving and communication systems
PAD	Peripheral arterial disease
PAN	Polyarteritis nodosa
PaO_2	Partial pressure of arterial oxygen
PAT	Peer Assessment Tool
PBC	Primary biliary cirrhosis
PCA	Patient-controlled analgesia
pCO_2	Partial pressure of carbon dioxide
PCOS	Polycystic ovary syndrome
PCR	Polymerase chain reaction
PCT	Primary care trust
PCV	Packed cell volume
PDA	Patent ductus arteriosus/Personal digital assistant
PE	Pulmonary embolism
PEA	Pulseless electrical activity

PEEP	Positive end expiratory pressure
PEFR	Peak expiratory flow rate
PERLA	Pupils equal and reactive to light and accommodation
PET	Positron emission tomography
PICU	Paediatric intensive care unit
PID	Pelvic inflammatory disease
PIP	Peak inspiratory pressure
PIPJ	Proximal interphalangeal joint
PMETB	Postgraduate Medical Education and Training Board
PMH	Past medical history
PMT	Pre-menstrual tension
PND	Paroxysmal nocturnal dyspnoea
PNS	Peripheral nervous system
PO	Per os (by mouth)
pO_2	Partial pressure of oxygen
PoC	Products of conception
POCS	Posterior circulation stroke
PONV	Post-operative nausea and vomiting
POP	Plaster of Paris/Progesterone only pill
PPH	Postpartum haemorrhage
PPI	Proton pump inhibitor
PR	Per rectum
PRHO	Pre-registration house officer (old training system but still widely used)
PRN	Pro re nata (as required)
PROM	Premature rupture of membranes (pregnancy)
PRV	Polycythaemia rubra vera
PSA	Prostate specific antigen
PSH	Past surgical history
PT	Prothrombin time
PTH	Parathyroid hormone
PU	Passed urine/Peptic ulcer
PUD	Peptic ulcer disease
PUO	Pyrexia of unknown origin
PV	Plasma viscosity/Per vagina
PVD	Peripheral vascular disease
qds	Quarter die sumendus (four times daily)
RA	Rheumatoid arthritis
RAST	Radioallergosorbant test
RBBB	Right bundle branch block
RBC	Red blood cell

RDW	Red cell distribution width
RF	Rheumatic fever
Rh	Rhesus
RhF	Rheumatoid factor
RIF	Right iliac fossa
ROM	Range of movement
ROS	Review of systems
RR	Respiratory rate
RS	Respiratory system
RSI	Rapid sequence induction
RTA	Road traffic accident
RTI	Road traffic incident
RUQ	Right upper quadrant
RVH	Right ventricular hypertrophy
Rx	Prescription
s	Second(s)
SAH	Sub-arachnoid haemorrhage
SALT	Speech and language therapy
SARS	Severe acute respiratory syndrome
Sats	O_2 saturation
SBE	Sub-acute bacterial endocarditis
SBP	Systolic blood pressure
SC	Subcutaneous
SCBU	Special care baby unit
SCC	Squamous cell carcinoma
SE	Side effects
SH	Social history
SHDU	Surgical high dependency unit
SHO	Senior house officer (old training system but still widely used)
SIADH	Syndrome of inappropriate antidiuretic hormone secretion
SIRS	Systemic inflammatory response syndrome
SL	Sublingual
SLE	Systemic lupus erythematosus
SOA	Swelling of ankles
SOB	Short of breath
SOBAR	Short of breath at rest
SOBOE	Short of breath on exertion
SOL	Space occupying lesion
SpO_2	Oxygen saturation in peripheral blood

SpR	Specialist registrar (old training system but still widely used)
SR	Slow release/Sinus rhythm
SSRI	Selective serotonin re-uptake inhibitor
STAT	Statim (immediately)
ST	Specialty Training/Trainee
STD	Sexually transmitted disease
STEMI	ST-elevation myocardial infarction
STI	Sexually transmitted infection
STOP	Surgical termination of pregnancy
StR	Specialty Training Registrar
SVC	Superior vena cava
SVR	Systemic vascular resistance
SVT	Supraventricular tachycardia
Sx	Symptoms
Temp	Temperature
T_3	Tri-iodothyronine
T_4	Thyroxine
TAB	Team Assessment of Behaviour
TACS	Total anterior circulation stroke
TB	Tuberculosis
TBG	Thyroxine-binding globulin
TCA	Tricyclic antidepressant
tds	Ter die sumendus (three times daily)
Teds	Thromboembolism deterrent stockings
Temp	Temperature
TENS	Transcutaneous electrical nerve stimulation
TFT	Thyroid function test
THR	Total hip replacement
TIA	Transient ischaemic attack
TIBC	Total iron binding capacity
TIMI	Thrombolysis in myocardial infarction
TIPS	Transjugular intrahepatic porto-systemic shunting
TKR	Total knee replacement
TLC	Total lung capacity/Tender loving care
TMJ	Temporomandibular joint
TNM	Tumour, nodes, metastases – cancer staging
TOE	Transoesophageal echocardiogram
TPHA	*Treponema pallidum* haemagglutination assay
TPN	Total parenteral nutrition
TPR	Total peripheral resistance

TSH	Thyroid stimulating hormone
TTA	To take away
TTO	To take out
TTP	Thrombotic thrombocytopenic purpura
TURP	Transurethral resection of prostate
TWOC	Trial without catheter
Tx	Treatment
u/U	Units (write out 'units' when prescribing)
U+E	Urea and electrolytes
UA	Unstable angina
UC	Ulcerative colitis
UMN	Upper motor neuron
UO	Urine output
URTI	Upper respiratory tract infection
US(S)	Ultrasound scan
UTI	Urinary tract infection
UV	Ultraviolet
V/Q	Ventilation/perfusion scan
VA	Visual acuity
VC	Vital capacity
VDRL	Venereal disease research laboratory (test)
VE	Vaginal examination/Ventricular ectopic
VF	Ventricular fibrillation
VMA	Vanillylmandelic acid
VP shunt	Ventriculoperitoneal shunt
VSD	Ventriculoseptal defect
VT	Ventricular tachycardia
VZV	Varicella-zoster virus
WB	Weight bear(ing)
WBC	White blood cell
WCC	White cell count
WHO	World Health Organization
wk	Week(s)
WPW	Wolff–Parkinson–White syndrome
wt	Weight
X-match	Crossmatch
yr	year(s)
ZN	Ziehl–Neelsen

Introduction

Welcome to the 4th edition of the *Oxford Handbook for the Foundation Programme* – the ultimate FP doctor's survival book. It is set out differently from other books; please take 2 minutes to read how it works:

Being a doctor (📖 p1) covers the non-clinical side of being a junior doctor:
- *The FP* (📖 p2) how to get a place, what it's all about, the ePortfolio
- *Starting as an F1* (📖 p11) essential kit, efficiency, being organised
- *Communication* (📖 p19) breaking bad news, translators, languages
- *Quality and ethics* (📖 p25) confidentiality, consent, capacity
- *When things go wrong* (📖 p30) errors, incident forms, hating your job
- *Boring but important stuff* (📖 p36) NHS structure, money, benefits
- *Your career* (📖 p43) exams, CVs, getting ST posts, audits, research.

Life on the wards (📖 p65) is the definitive guide to ward jobs; it includes advice on ward rounds, being on-call, night shifts, making referrals and writing in the notes. A section on common forms includes TTOs and 'fit' notes. There's a whole new section on death – covering attitudes, palliative care, certifying, death certificates and cremation forms. Ward dilemmas including nutrition, pain, death, and aggression are covered in detail, along with a section designed to help surgical juniors pick their way through the hazards of the operating theatre and manage their patients peri-operatively.

History and examination (📖 p123) covers these old medical school favourites, from a 'real-world' perspective, to help you rapidly identify pathology and integrate your findings into a diagnosis.

Prescribing (📖 p167) and **Pharmacopoeia** (📖 p181) cover how to prescribe, best practice, complex patients, interactions, and specific groups of drugs; commonly prescribed drugs are described in detail, with indications, contraindications, side effects, and dosing advice.

Clinical chapters (📖 p223) These chapters cover common clinical and ward cover problems. They are described by symptoms because you are called to see a breathless patient, not someone having a PE:
- *Emergencies* The inside front cover has a list of emergencies according to symptom (cardiac arrest, chest pain, seizures) with page references. These pages give step-by-step instructions to help you resuscitate and stabilise an acutely ill patient whilst waiting for senior help to arrive
- *Symptoms* The clinical pages are arranged by symptom; causes are shown for each symptom, along with what to ask and look for, relevant investigations and a table showing the distinguishing features of each disease. Relevant diseases are described in the pages following each symptom
- *Diseases* If you know the disease you can look it up in the index to find the symptoms, signs, results, and correct management.

Procedures (📖 p509) contains instructions on how to perform specific procedures, along with the equipment needed and contraindications.

Interpreting results (📖 p565) gives a guide to understanding investigations including common patterns, the important features to note and possible causes of abnormalities.

Appendices (📖 p599) are several pages of useful information including contact numbers, growth charts, unit conversion charts, driving regulations, blank timetables, and telephone number lists.

10 tips on being a safe junior doctor

These tips are taken from or the **N**ational **C**onfidential **E**nquiry into **P**atient **O**utcome and **D**eath (NCEPOD) report *An Acute Problem?*[1] NCEPOD is an independent body which aims to improve the quality and safety of patient care. The report summarises a survey over one month of admissions to UK Intensive Care Units.

1) More attention should be paid to patients exhibiting physiological abnormalities. This is a marker of increased mortality risk (📖 p224)

2) The importance of respiratory rate monitoring should be highlighted. This parameter should be recorded at any point that other observations are being made (📖 p224)

3) Education and training should be provided for staff that use pulse oximeters to allow proper interpretation and understanding of the limitations of this monitor. It should be emphasised that pulse oximetry does not replace respiratory rate monitoring (📖 p224)

4) It is inappropriate for referral and acceptance to ICU to happen at junior doctor (<ST3) level

5) Training must be provided for junior doctors in the recognition of critical illness and the immediate management of fluid and oxygen therapy in these patients (📖 p226)

6) Consultants must supervise junior doctors more closely and should actively support juniors in the management of patients rather than only reacting to requests for help

7) Junior doctors must seek advice more readily. This may be from specialised teams such as outreach services or from the supervising consultant

8) Each hospital should have a track and trigger system that allows rapid detection of the signs of early clinical deterioration and an early and appropriate response (📖 p224)

9) All entries in the notes should be dated and timed and should end with a legible name, status and contact number (bleep or telephone) (📖 p74)

10) Each entry in the notes should clearly identify the name and grade of the most senior doctor involved in the patient episode (📖 p74).

The full report and several other NCEPOD reports are available online[1] and are well worth reading; there are many learning points for doctors of all grades and specialties.

[1] *An Acute Problem?* NCEPOD (2005) at ⁀**www.ncepod.org.uk/2005aap.htm** See also *Emergency Admissions: A journey in the right direction?* (2007) at ⁀**www.ncepod.org.uk/2007ea.htm** and *Deaths in Acute Hospitals: Caring to the End?* (2009) at ⁀**www.ncepod.org.uk/2009dah.htm**

10 tips on being a happy doctor

1) **Book your annual leave** Time off is essential. Spend it doing something you really enjoy with people you really like. If you have fixed leave, at least you'll get what you're owed (hopefully), but swaps can be a pain and take a lot of persistence. If you have to book time off, it will be your responsibility to swap on-calls. You usually need to book your leave 6wk in advance and summer is always popular. Sit down early with your team and discuss your leave plans

2) **Be organised** This is important but difficult when you first start as a doctor. Come in early, keep a list of useful names and numbers (there are pages in the appendix to help you with this, 📖 p608), and pick up hints and tips from your predecessor

3) **Smile** You cannot cure most diseases, you cannot make procedures pleasant, you cannot help the fact that you, ward staff, and patients are in the hospital, but smiling and being friendly can make all the difference

4) **Never shout at anyone** Shouting or being insulting is unprofessional. If you have a problem it should be addressed in private. The job rapidly becomes unpleasant if you get a reputation for being rude and reputations (good and bad) travel quickly

5) **Ask for senior help** Never feel you cannot ask for help, even for something you feel you 'should' know. It is always better to speak to someone senior rather than guess, even if it is in the middle of the night

6) **Check in the *BNF*** If you are not familiar with a drug then always check in the *BNF* before you give it. Trust nobody: it will be your name next to the prescription

7) **Look at the obs** Acutely ill patients nearly always have abnormal observations. Always remember to look at the respiratory rate as this is the observation most commonly ignored by junior doctors.

8) **Stay calm** It is easy to panic the first time you are called to an acutely ill patient, but staying calm is important to help you think clearly about how to manage the situation. Take a deep breath, work through the 'ABC' whilst performing initial investigations and resuscitation (the emergency pages will guide you through this) and call someone senior

9) **Be reliable** If you say you are going to do something then do it. If you are unable to do so then let someone know – nursing staff in particular also have many things to remember and constantly reminding doctors of outstanding jobs is frustrating

10) **Prepare for the future** Medicine is competitive, you need to give yourself the best chance. Over the first 2 years you should:

- Think about your career
- Create a CV and portfolio
- Get good referees and mentors
- Participate in audit
- Present interesting cases
- Organise specialty taster sessions
- Consider sitting examinations
- Enjoy being a 'proper' doctor.

10 tips on being a happy doctor

Being a doctor

The Foundation Programme

'Training is patient safety for the next 30 years'[1]

The concept

The UK Foundation Programme (FP) was established in 2005 as part of a series of reforms to UK medical training, known collectively as Modernising Medical Careers (MMC). The intention of the FP was to provide a uniform, 2-year structured training for all newly qualified doctors working in the UK, to build upon medical school education and form the basis for subsequent training. Sadly, much of the introduction of MMC was a shambles. In relative terms the FP fared well, although the early days were not without problems with a lack of flexibility and an ideologically driven focus on competence rather than excellence, and as late as 2010 Professor John Collins reported to Medical Education England that the programme still lacked a clearly articulated purpose. His report[2] identified a number of areas for improvement to the FP, that led to key changes in the selection procedures and the assessment process, amongst others. As such, the programme continues to evolve. At a national level, a new curriculum was introduced in 2012, scheduled for review in 2015. Just as importantly, at a local level the reconfigurations and adjustments necessary to deliver effective training are filtering through – an iterative process that all FP doctors can contribute to.

The structure

The FP consists of 2 years, and in >90% of programmes, each year involves rotation through 3 different 4-month placements, which may be in hospital or community-based medicine. About a quarter of programmes involve a placement in a 'shortage specialty' (where the number of current trainees is likely to fall short of future consultant needs), and despite a shift towards the management of chronic disease in the community, much of the FP emphasis remains on the acute care of adult patients in a hospital setting.

At the start of the FP, you will be required to hold 'provisional registration' with the General Medical Council (GMC)(Table 1.1). Strictly, the first FP year (F1) represents the final year of basic medical education and remains the responsibility of the medical school from which you graduated – this responsibility may be delegated for those doctors completing F1 in a different geographical region from their medical school. After successfully completing F1, you will be issued with a Certificate of Experience, which entitles you to apply for full GMC registration and start F2. Successful completion of F2 results in the awarding of a foundation achievement of competence document (FACD) which opens the door to higher specialty training (see 📖 p43).

The Foundation Programme Office

All aspects of the administration of the FP are overseen by the UK Foundation Programme Office (UKFPO) which provides several important documents at ⏛www.foundationprogramme.nhs.uk These include the application handbooks, the FP reference guide (the 'rules'), the Curriculum (full list of educational objectives), careers advice and advice for applicants from overseas.

---

[1] Professor Sir John Temple, 'Time for Training', 2010 Crown Copyright available free at ⏛www.mee.nhs.uk/pdf/JCEWTD_Final%20report.pdf

[2] Professor John Collins, 'Foundation for Excellence An Evaluation of the Foundation Programme' available at ⏛www.mee.nhs.uk/pdf/401339_MEE_FoundationExcellence_acc.pdf

Table 1.1 *The FP hierarchy*

The GMC	Overall responsibility for all aspects of medical practice and training in the UK
The UK FPO	Manages applications to and delivery of the FP
Local Education Training Boards (LETB) (formerly: Deaneries)	Responsible for ensuring that local delivery of the FP is in accordance with GMC standards. The LETB support financial costs of training and provide the acute employing trust with salary costs for 'basic' contract hours (additional out of hours 'banding' is paid by the acute trust 📖 p36)
Foundation school	Deliver the FP locally. May overlap with the LETB. Headed by Foundation school director
Foundation training programme director (FTPD)	Responsible for the management and quality control of a specific training programme. Your FTPD will oversee the panel that reviews your annual progress and is responsible for signing off on successful completion of each foundation year
Acute Trust/Local Education Provider	Acute trusts provide the employment contract, salary and HR for foundation doctors. For community placements (eg GP practice), the responsibility for education passes to this 'Local Education Provider' but the contract of employment remains with the acute trust. There can be conflicts between the needs of the acute trusts (doctors on the wards delivering services to patients) and some of the educational requirements of the FP (📖 p57)
Educational supervisor	Doctor with responsibility for training of individual foundation doctor – ideally for a whole year but occasionally for just a single attachment. Will meet and review your progress on a regular basis, check that your assessments are up to date, and help you plan your career
Clinical supervisor	Senior doctor who supervises your day-to-day learning and training for each attachment. In some posts, the roles of educational supervisor and clinical supervisor may be merged
Academic supervisor	Those undertaking an academic foundation programme (that includes a designated period of research) will be assigned an individual responsible for overseeing academic work and providing feedback
Local administrator	Individuals in each trust and Foundation school who help with FP registration and administration
The Foundation Doctor	Responsible for own learning and becoming fully involved in the educational, supervised learning and assessment processes of their foundation training. A key part of this is providing constructive feedback through local routes (clinical and educational supervisors) as well as local and national training surveys

Applying to the Foundation Programme

All applications to the FP are through the on-line FP Application System (FPAS) at ⊕www.foundationprogramme.nhs.uk. There are several stages.

Registration for FPAS You will need to be nominated to apply. For final year students in UK medical schools, your medical school will do this on your behalf. Those applying from outside the UK will need to contact the UKFPO Eligibility Office in good time to allow checks to take place.[1] You can register for an account before nomination, but you will be unable to access the application form until your nomination is confirmed.

Completing the application form Within a designated window each year (usually in early October) nominated applicants will be able to access the application form. This has a number of parts:

- *Personal* Name, contact details, DOB etc.
- *Qualifications* Educational qualifications
- *Clinical Skills* You will be asked to self-assess against a list of practical skills – this does not form part of the assessment process but will be used by Foundation schools for coordinating training
- *Equal Opportunities* Monitoring information
- *Referees* Details of 2 referees: 1 academic and 1 clinical. Seniority is not important: References are not part of the assessment process but are only used once an offer has been made as part of pre-employment checks, and the only requirement is to tick a series of boxes indicating no significant concerns about your suitability
- *Educational achievements* You will be asked to list any additional degrees for scoring against a very specific system and to upload a copy of your certificate; 5 total percentage points are available for your degree, with 2 further points for publications (proof is required and will be assessed)
- *UoA Preferences* Foundation schools are grouped into Units of Application (UoA) that process applications jointly. You will be asked to rank all UoA in order of preference, with successful applicants allocated to UoA in score order (you will be allocated to your highest preference UoA that still has places when your turn comes). Tables showing vacancies and competition ratios for previous years are available on the UKFPO website but these do tend to vary between years (see box)
- *Academic selection* If applying to the academic FP (see 📖 p5)
- *Declaration* You are required to sign various declarations of probity.

Scoring Your application will be scored based upon 2 components:

- *Educational Performance Measure (50 points)* This comprises a score between 34-43 based upon which decile your medical school decides your performance falls in, relative to your peers (this is locally determined) with 7 further points for education achievements detailed on the application form as above
- *Situational Judgement Tests (50 points)* See box.

[1] These include: evidence of the right to work in the UK; of having undertaken medical training solely in English or having IELTS scores of ≥7.5 in all domains; of complying with GMC requirements for provisional registration which may include passing PLAB; a statement of support from your medical school dean; academic transcripts and proof of medical qualifications. You should allow sufficient time for this complex process of verification.

Units of Application and 2013 competition data

- Coventry and Warwick 91 (87%)
- East Anglia 286 (57%)
- LNR 140 (63%)
- Mersey 306 (80%)
- North Central Thames 315 (156%)
- North East Thames 331 (89%)
- North West Thames 263 (424%)
- North Western 511 (86%)
- Northern 386 (83%)
- Northern Ireland 244 (98%)
- Oxford 223 (148%)
- Peninsula 198 (94%)
- Scotland 787 (81%)
- Severn 273 (162%)
- South Thames 798 (117%)
- Staffordshire 108 (31%)
- Trent 311 (63%)
- Wales 361 (66%)
- Wessex 296 (75%)
- West Midlands Central 430 (88%)
- Yorkshire and Humber 584 (80%)

The 21 UoA shown represent the 25 UK Foundation schools. The number of F1 vacancies for appointments in 2013 are shown, with figures in brackets representing the number of applicants ranking the UoA as their first preference, expressed as a percentage of this number of jobs.

Situational Judgement Tests (SJT)

These computer marked tests of 70 questions sat under examination conditions over 2h 20min confront you with situations in which you might be placed as an F1 doctor, and ask how you would respond. There are 2 basic response formats: (i) rank five possible responses in order and (ii) choose three from eight possible responses. Marks are assigned according to how close to an 'ideal' answer you come, with marks for near misses and no negative marking. Raw scores are subject to statistical normalisation and scaling to generate a final mark out of 50.

Officially, you cannot 'revise' for the test, since it is an assessment of your attitudes, but there is a strong weighting on medical ethics which certainly can be revised, and you can also familiarise yourself with what is expected of you and try to understand model answers.[1]

When introduced into FP selection for 2013 appointments, problems with SJT marking led to hundreds of altered appointment offers. Ongoing controversy surrounds SJTs as a means of selection into the FP, the thin evidence base behind them and the heavy weighting they receive. One prominent researcher closely involved in the pilots and advocating their use is also a director of a company that provides SJTs, as well as being a key figure behind the selection process that so spectacularly failed as part of the 2007 MMC reforms. Nonetheless, it is difficult to argue that previous systems based upon answering generic questions or students competing to get references from a few blessed Professors were any better. Our advice for now: 'Get studying!'

[1] Practice paper available on UKFPO website. Mock questions available as *Situational Judgement Test* (Oxford Assess and Progress) 2nd edition Metcalfe and Dev 2013 019968815X OUP

The Academic Foundation Programme For those interested approximately 450 programmes offer a research period alongside the same FP curriculum and outcomes. This may take the form of a dedicated academic rotation, or time set aside throughout the year. You may select up to 2 'Academic' UoAs (these differ slightly from standard UoAs) during the application process, and you will be asked to provide additional information on your academic suitability. Shortlisted candidates are interviewed and offers made in advance of the main FP selection process so that unsuccessful applicants can still compete for a regular FP position.

Results Your total score will be used to determine your place in the queue for matching to a FP, and you will be offered a place in your highest preference UoA which still has FP vacancies when your turn comes. Results will be communicated by email and you will have a limited window to accept this. Depending on the UoA, you will either be able to review the individual programmes available and asked to rank these, or (in larger UoAs) you will be asked to rank groups of programmes clustered by, eg acute trusts. Methods of allocation will vary between UoAs, with some using crude FPAS scores, and others adding local scoring variables. Further information should be available on each UoA website.

Posts A typical F1 year usually consists of three placements of 4mth: one in a general medical specialty, one in a general surgical specialty; options for the third specialty vary widely in just about all areas of medicine. F2 posts also typically consist of three 4mth jobs; for 80% of F2s one of these will be a GP placement. Allocation to F2 posts varies between UoAs, with some assigning all F1 and F2 posts at the outset, whilst others may invite you to select F2 posts during your F1 year. Once you are appointed to the FP, you are guaranteed an F2 post in the same Foundation school, but often in a different acute trust. If you do not get an F2 post in a specialty you are particularly interested in, most will allow individual FP doctors to swap rotations, providing they have the support of their educational supervisors. Some Foundation schools will organise 'swap shops' to facilitate this process. You can also arrange week-long 'tasters' in another specialty to help plan your career; to arrange these talk to your educational supervisor and a consultant in the relevant specialty.

If you are unsuccessful In recent years, the supply of applicants has threatened to exceed places on the FP. Those whose FPAS scores place them below the cutoff to be guaranteed a FP post will be placed on a reserve list and are often able to gain a training post when an unexpected event befalls another candidate. If you are not successful in securing a post first time round do not give up hope! If you feel you have been unfairly marked you may be able to appeal; discuss this with your medical school dean. Try to seek feedback from the application process in order to identify weaknesses that you may be able to amend in case you have to wait to reapply the next year. Should you still be without a post after you know you have qualified from medical school, contact LETBs and hospitals directly; some of your peers may not be able to take up their posts due to exam failure so you may be able to apply directly to these posts.

Finally, consider taking a year out to either strengthen your application by doing research, further study, or other activities that add to your skills. Also consider applying overseas; it has been possible in previous years to do some or all of foundation training in Australia or New Zealand with prior approval of posts from a UK LETB. Alternatively, it is possible to apply to any post within the EU or to consider equivalency exams for other countries.

Finally, there is always the option of a career outside of medicine. Advice on this and other options will be available from your university careers office, or from websites such as Prospects (⌂www.prospects.ac.uk).

Linked applications During the FPAS application process, it is possible for any two individuals to link their applications. In this case, you must both supply each other's email addresses in the relevant section of the application form, and rank all UoAs in identical order. The score of the *lower* scoring applicant will then be used to allocate both applicants to the same UoA. Although policies vary between UoAs, linking does not necessarily guarantee appointment to the same trust or town – check individual UoA websites for their policies. Note also that if one of you accepts a place on an Academic Foundation Programme, the link is broken.

Special circumstance For those who meet specific criteria, it may be possible to be allocated to a specific Foundation school, regardless of your FPAS score. These cases include if:
• You are a parent or legal guardian of a child <18, who lives with you
• You are a primary carer for someone who is disabled (defined by the Equality Act 2010)
• You have a medical condition or disability for which ongoing follow-up in the specified location is an absolute requirement.

If any of these apply to you, discuss with your medical school dean or tutor well in advance of the application process opening.

Less than full-time training Those wishing to train less than full-time should apply through the FPAS alongside other candidates; upon successful appointment, they should contact their new Foundation school to discuss training opportunities and plans.

The FP curriculum and assessment

The Foundation Programme Curriculum acts as a guide for what you will be expected to achieve over the 2 years of the FP, how you will get there, and how you will be assessed. Core to the curriculum is a syllabus that lists a large number of core 'competences' that you will be expected to achieve, divided into subsections. Each subsection is headed by outcome descriptors indicating the broad levels of performance that you must achieve in each year, and the subsections grouped into principal sections with core themes.

Principal sections of the FP curriculum (2012 version)	
1 Professionalism	7 Good clinical care
2 Relationship and communication with patients	8 Recognition and management of the acutely ill patient
3 Safety and clinical governance	9 Resuscitation and end of life care
4 Ethical and legal issues	10 Patients with long-term conditions
5 Teaching and training	11 Investigations
6 Maintaining good medical practice	12 Procedures

ePortfolio The ePortfolio tool forms an electronic personal record of your progress through the FP. At the core is a copy of the syllabus to which you can link evidence of achievement of competences using a variety of tools. Alongside this sits a record of all meetings that you have with your supervisors and your end of year reports. It may also be used in interviews for specialty training programmes to demonstrate competence and highlight your achievements. You can also upload a wide range of supporting material (see box 🕮 p10). It is absolutely vital that you engage with your ePortfolio early on and continue to keep it up to date since this forms a measure by which you will be judged. The effort required is not minimal, but nor should you underestimate the burden placed on your supervisors who will also be required to access and inspect your ePortfolio. You can certainly help them by keeping your ePortfolio current and complete.

Assessment It would be impossible to document evidence of achievement of every one of the competences in the curriculum. Instead, you need to provide evidence that you have achieved the outcome descriptors for each subsection appropriate to F1, and subsequently F2. In order to do this, a variety of tools are available (see Table 1.2). For some subsections, the descriptors for F1 and F2 are the same, in which case in your F2 year no further evidence may be required, or you may wish to document evidence of ongoing achievement. In previous years the burden of documentation was overwhelming, both for FP doctors and their seniors, whilst the curriculum used forms designed to allow for formative feedback as a means of summative evaluation. This risked creating a 'tickbox' mentality amongst many concerned. Sense has (partially) prevailed in the 2012 curriculum, with the number of assessments significantly reduced and a shift towards use of assessments for formative feedback.

Meetings There are a number of meetings you need to record in your ePortfolio. These are detailed in the box 🕮 p10.

Table 1.2 *Supervised learning events (SLEs) and assessments*

SLEs provide a means to record evidence of clinical learning. They offer a framework for feedback from a senior colleague whenever a learning opportunity presents itself, and for you to reflect on the experience. A number of different formats are available and you will be required to document a minimum number each year – though you may record far more. You should cover a spread of acute and long-term conditions in a range of clinical settings. SLEs do not always need to be planned in advance and can be used to record a useful educational experience after it has occurred. You can generate a form for each SLE through your ePortfolio – this can be filled out at the time by your assessor, or you can send them an email link to the form, in which case you should include as much information as possible to remind them of the event.

Direct observation of doctor/patient encounter:	≥9 per year – including
• *Mini-clinical evaluation exercise (mini-CEX)*	≥6 mini-CEX (≥2 per
• *Direct observation of procedural skills (DOPS)*	attachment)[1]

For mini-CEX, you will be observed speaking to and/or examining a patient and receive feedback on your performance. For DOPS, you will be observed performing a clinical skill and receive feedback on your interaction with the patient.

• *Case-based discussion (CbD)*	≥6 per year (≥2 per attachment)

You will present and discuss a case (or an aspect of a complex case) you have been closely involved in and discuss the clinical reasoning and rationale.

• *Developing the clinical teacher*	≥1 per year

This requires you to deliver an observed teaching session – you will receive feedback according to the very latest in educational jargon.

Assessments differ from SLEs in that they are *summative* – they evaluate your progress and achievements. In addition to your end of placement and end of year assessments with your supervisors, you will also complete two other assessments:

• *Core procedure assessment forms*	1 per procedure during F1

By the end of F1 you need to be signed off as competent in 15 core procedures:

- Venepuncture
- IV cannulation
- Giving IV medication and fluids
- ABG
- Blood culture (peripheral)
- IV infusion including the prescription of fluids
- IV infusion of blood and blood products

- Injection of local anaesthetic to skin
- SC injection
- IM injection
- Perform and interpret an ECG
- Perform and interpret peak flow
- Urethral catheterisation (♀)
- Urethral catheterisation (♂)
- Airway care including simple adjuncts

• *Team assessment of behaviour (TAB)*	1 per year

You will be required to engage in a Maoist process of self-criticism, then select up to 15 colleagues who will be invited to feedback anonymously to your educational supervisor who will collate the results and share them with you. Your assessors must include ≥2 individuals from the following groups: doctors (more senior than F2, including at least 1 consultant or GP principal); nurses (band 5 or above); allied healthcare professionals; any other team members (eg ward clerks, secretaries).

---

[1] There is no minimum number of DOPS required per year.

Keeping the ePortfolio

As well as recording your structured learning events, you can upload a wide range of other documents to your ePortfolio to serve as evidence of your progress. Some suggestions include:

Clinical work

- Copies of discharge/referral letters (anonymised)[1]
- Copies of clerkings (anonymised)[1]
- Attendance at clinic (date, consultant, learning points)
- Procedures (list of type, when, observing, performing, or teaching)
- Details of any complaints made against you and their resolution
- Incident forms you have been involved in (useful for reflective practice and demonstrating that you have learned from mistakes)
- 'Triumphs' – difficult patients you've diagnosed/treated
- Praise – all thank you letters/cards/emails.

Presentations, teaching, audit, and research

- Copies of presentations given
- Details of teaching you've done (with feedback if possible)
- Copies of audit or research you've been involved in
- Copies of your publications.

Training

- Details of courses you've attended (with certificates of attendance)
- Online course modules completed
- Reflective practice notes on key learning experiences
- Study leave and associated forms (F2 only).

[1] Remember that all data you upload is subject to the Data Protection Act. This means that you should avoid recording patient identifiable information within your ePortfolio, since this is not the purpose for which it was collected. Using hospital numbers rather than names, or completely obscuring personal details is considered acceptable.

Meetings during the FP

There are a number of required meetings which you should record in your ePortfolio. The onus is on you to schedule and prepare for these meetings: you and your supervisors are all busy clinicians, and it can sometimes be difficult to arrange these in a timely manner. Be flexible but persistent!

Induction At the start of each placement you should meet with both your educational and clinical supervisors[2] to agree learning objectives and review what opportunities are available during the placement.

Midpoint Meetings in the middle of each placement with your supervisors to review progress are encouraged, particularly where you or they have concerns, but are not compulsory. You may also decide to have a mid-year review with your educational supervisor.

End of placement Both your supervisors should meet with you separately to review your achievements, feedback the observations of the team, provide advice and listen to your feedback.

End of year You should meet your educational supervisor to discuss your total progress. Your supervisor will complete a report for the panel performing your annual review and inform their decision to sign you off.

[2] Separate meetings: your clinical supervisor should address what is expected of you and what is available to you; your educational supervisor should take an overview of your progress and goals. In reality, for some placements they will be the same person.

Before you start

Important organisations

The prices quoted change frequently; they are intended as a guide.

General Medical Council (GMC) To work as a doctor in the UK you need GMC registration with a licence to practice; £90 for F1 (provisional registration), £185 for F2 (full registration), £390 thereafter.

NHS indemnity insurance This covers the financial consequences of mistakes you make at work, providing you abide by guidelines and protocols. It automatically covers all doctors in the NHS free of charge.

Indemnity insurance This is essential; do not work without it. These organisations will support and advise you in any complaints or legal matters that arise from your work. They also insure you against work outside the hospital. There are three main organisations, all offer 24h helplines (📖 p600):
- Medical Protection Society (MPS) – £10 for F1, £40 for F2
- Medical Defence Union (MDU) – £10 for F1, £40 for F2
- Medical and Dental Defence Union of Scotland (MDDUS) – £10 for F1, £35 for F2.

British Medical Association (BMA) Political voice of doctors; campaigns for better conditions, hours, pay, and comments on health issues. Membership includes a weekly subscription to the *BMJ*. Costs £113 as an F1 then £222 as an F2.

Income protection Pays a proportion of your basic salary ± a lump sum (rates vary) until retirement age if you are unable to work for health reasons. Check if it covers mental health problems, and if it still pays if you are capable of doing a less demanding job. NHS sickness benefits are not comprehensive (and only provide 1mth as an F1 and 4mth the next year):
- Available from various providers, typically starting at £24/mth as an F1, rising according to age, pay, illness, and risks.

NHS pension scheme Despite various changes afoot, this remains the best pension available, do not opt out; a percentage of your pay will be diverted to the pension.

Important documents for your first day[1]

P45/P60 tax form When you leave a job you will receive a P45; if you continue in the same job you will receive a P60 every April. These need to be shown when starting a new job.

Bank details Account number, sort code, and address.

Hepatitis B You need proof of hep B immunity and vaccinations. You should keep validated records of your immunisations and test results.

GMC registration certificate Proves you are a registered doctor.

Disclosure and Barring service (DBS) certificate (formerly CRB checks) It is the employer's responsibility to perform these checks. You must complete all paperwork in good time, but payment is the responsibility of the trust.

Induction pack and contract Sent by the trust before you start[2]; otherwise contact human resources to find out where and when to meet.

---

[1] In theory, the medical staffing department of your acute trust should sort a lot of this out in advance of your first day; in reality, do not underestimate their ability to mislay your paperwork and request multiple copies – keep plenty of photocopies and do not part with originals.

[2] There has been a trend towards online induction. Unfortunately, some trusts occasionally attempt to force new starters to complete this prior to starting work for the trust with threats of loss of employment. There is a clear BMA position on this: induction is work, and should be undertaken during work time or, if undertaken outside work time, should receive additional payment.

Your first day

Leave plenty of time to find the hospital and your accommodation on your first day. Many hospitals organise a session for new doctors to speed up the signing-in process. The following are the essentials:

House If you are living on site this is your top priority. Phone the accommodation office before you start to check their opening hours. It may cost up to £700/month. Avoid leaving your car filled with all your possessions.

Pay roll It can take over a month to adjust pay arrangements so it is vital to give the finance dept your bank details on or before the first day if you want to be paid that month. Hand in a copy of your P45/P60 too.

Parking Check with other staff about the best places to park and 'parking deals'; you will probably need to get several people to sign a form.

ID badge This may also be used to access secure sections of the hospital. If so, insist on getting access to all clinical areas since you will be on the crash team. If the card doesn't give access to all wards return it and get it fixed.

Computer access This allows you to get results, access the internet and your NHS email. Memorise all the passwords, usernames, etc and keep any documents handed out. Ask for the IT helpdesk phone number in case of difficulty.

Work rota This should have arrived before the job starts. If it hasn't, you should contact the medical staffing department to request it.

Colleagues' mobile numbers This will probably be the last time you are all gathered in one place. Getting numbers makes social activities and rota swaps much easier. Arranging swaps on the first day is also easier.

Important places in the hospital

Try to get hold of a map; many hospitals have evolved rather than been designed. There are often shortcuts.

Wards Write down any access codes and find out where you can put your bag. Ask to be shown where things are kept including the crash trolley and blood-taking equipment.

Canteen Establish where the best food options are at various times of day. Note the opening hours – this will be invaluable for breaks on-call.

Cash and food dispensers Hospitals are required to provide hot food 24h a day. This may be from a machine.

Doctors' mess Clearly essential. Write down the access code and establish if there is a freezer. Microwave meals are infinitely preferable to the food from machines.

Radiology Find out which consultants deal with different imaging. You will spend a lot of time chasing investigations so make friends early, including with their secretaries!

Occupational health

Most hospitals have an occupational health department that is responsible for ensuring that the hospital is a safe environment for you and your patients. This includes making sure that doctors work in a safe manner. You can find your local unit at 🖰www.nhshealthatwork.co.uk

Common visits

During the Foundation Programme your contact with occupational health is likely to be one of the following:

- *Initial check* you will have a blood test to show you do not have hepatitis C ± HIV; they will need to see photographic proof of identity, eg a passport
- *Hepatitis B booster* depends on local policies and your antibody levels
- *Needle-stick/sharps injury/splashes* (📖 p106)
- *Illness* that affects your ability to work may require a consultation.

Infection control

Patients are commonly infected by pathogens from the hospital and ward staff. The infections are more likely to be resistant to antibiotics and can be fatal. It is important to reduce the risk you pose to your patients:

- If you are ill stay at home, especially if you have gastroenteritis
- Keep your clothes clean and roll up long sleeves to be bare below the elbows in clinical areas
- White coats, ties, and long sleeves are generally discouraged
- Avoid jewellery (plain metal rings are acceptable) and wrist watches
- Clean your stethoscope with a chlorhexidine swab after each use
- Wash your hands or use alcohol gel after every patient contact, even when wearing gloves; rinsing all the soap off reduces irritation. *Clostridium difficile* spores are resistant to alcohol, so always wash your hands after dealing with affected patients
- Be rigorous in your use of aseptic technique
- Use antibiotics appropriately and follow local prescribing policies.

Sharps and bodily fluids

As a doctor you will come into contact with bodily fluids daily. It is important to develop good habits so that you are safe on the wards:

- Wear gloves for all procedures that could involve bodily fluids or sharps. Gloves reduce disease transmission when penetrated with a needle – consider wearing two pairs for high-risk patients
- Dispose of all sharps immediately; take the sharps bin to where you are using the sharps and **always dispose of your own sharps**
- Vacutainers are safer than a needle and syringe. Most hospitals now stock safety cannulas and needles for phlebotomy, use of which decreases the risk of needle-stick injuries yet further
- Mark bodily fluid samples from HIV and hepatitis B+C patients as 'High Risk' and arrange a porter to take them safely to the lab
- Consider wearing goggles if bodily fluids might spray
- Cover cuts in your skin
- Avoid wearing open-toed shoes or sandals
- Make sure your hepatitis B boosters are up to date.

What to carry

Essentials

Pens These are the most essential piece of equipment. Remember you need a biro for writing on blood bottles; all writing must be in black (better for photocopying – allegedly).

Stethoscope A Littmann® Classic II or equivalent is perfectly adequate, however, better models offer clearer sound.

Money Out-of-hours, loose change is useful for food dispensers.

ID badge This should be supplied on your first day.

Bleep This will be on the ward, at switchboard or with a colleague.

Optional extras

Clipboard folder See 📖 p17.

Smartphone/PDA There is a wealth of medical apps available for these devices allowing you to carry vast amounts of information in your pocket. Always check who has written the program and whether they are a reliable source. Many of the books in the Oxford Handbook Series, including this one, have been made available in this format by a 3rd party developer.

Pen-torch Useful for looking in mouths and eyes; very small LED torches are available in 'outdoors' shops or over the internet and can fit onto a keyring or attached to stethoscopes to prevent colleagues borrowing and not returning them.

Tendon hammer These are rarely found on wards. Collapsible pocket-sized versions can be bought for £12–15.

Ward dress

Patients and staff have more respect for well-dressed doctors, however it is important to be yourself; be guided by comments from patients or staff.

Hair & piercings Long hair should be tied back. Facial metal can be easily removed while at work; while ears are OK, other piercings draw comments.

Shoes A pair of smart comfy shoes is essential – you will be on your feet for hours and may need to move fast.

Scrubs Ideal for on-calls, especially in surgery. Generally they should not be worn for everyday work. Check local protocol.

Mobiles Almost all doctors carry a mobile phone in hospital and it is often the best way to contact other members of your team. Previous rules restricting their use have largely been eased, though it remains the case that they can interfere with monitoring equipment in use in ICU, CCU and theatres.

How to be an F1

Being an F1 involves teamwork, organisation, and communication – qualities that are not easily assessed during finals. As well as settling into a new work environment, you have to integrate with your colleagues and the rest of the hospital team. You are not expected to know everything at the start of your post; you should always ask someone more senior if you are in doubt.

As an F1, your role includes:
- Clerking patients (ED, pre-op clinic, on-call, or on the ward)
- Updating patient lists and knowing where patients are (📖 p17)
- Participating in ward rounds to review patient management
- Requesting investigations and chasing their results
- Liaising with other specialties/healthcare professionals
- Practical procedures, eg taking blood (📖 p514), cannulation (📖 p518)
- Administrative tasks, eg theatre lists (📖 p112), TTOs (📖 p78), rewriting drug charts (📖 p169), death certificates (📖 p96)
- Speaking to the patient and relatives about progress/results.

Breaks
Missing breaks does not make you appear hard-working – it reduces your efficiency and alertness. Give yourself time to rest and eat (chocolates from the ward do not count); you are entitled to 30min for every 4h worked. Use the time to meet other doctors in the mess; referring is much easier if you know the team you are making the referral to.

Know your limits
If you are unsure of something, don't feel embarrassed to ask your seniors – particularly if a patient is deteriorating. If you are stuck on simple tasks (eg difficult cannulation) take a break (the patient will welcome this) and try later or ask a colleague to try.

Responsibility
As an F1 you will make many difficult decisions, some with potentially serious consequences. Always consider the worst case scenario and how to avoid it. Ensure you can justify your actions; carefully document events and discussions with relatives.

Expectations
Seniors will expect you to know Mrs Jones' current medication dose, the details of the operation they performed yesterday, and the blood results from 5d ago. Initially this seems impossible, but with time your memory for such details will improve.

Your bleep

What at first seems like a badge of having 'made it' quickly becomes the bane of your existence. When the bleep goes off repeatedly, write down the numbers then answer them in turn. Try to deal with queries over the phone; if not, make a list of jobs and prioritise them, tell the nurses how long you will be and be realistic. Ask nurses to get useful material ready for when you arrive (eg an ECG, urine dipstick, the obs chart and notes). Encourage ward staff to make a list of routine jobs instead of bleeping you repeatedly. The bleep should only be for sick patients and urgent tasks. Learn the number of switchboard since this is likely to be an outside caller waiting on the line. Crash calls are usually announced to all bleepholders via switchboard. If your bleep is unusually quiet, check the batteries. Consider handing over your bleep to a colleague when breaking bad news, speaking to relatives or performing a practical procedure.

- *Dropping the bleep in the toilet* This is not uncommon; recover the bleep using non-sterile gloves. Wash thoroughly in running water (the damage has already been done) and inform switchboard that you dropped it into your drink.
- *Other forms of bleep destruction* You should not have to pay for a damaged bleep, no matter how dire the threats from switchboard; consider asking for a clip-on safety strap.

Learning

You need to be proactive to learn interpretation and management skills as an F1. This is especially true when most of the decisions you make will be reviewed by a senior almost immediately. Despite this, 'Bloods, CXR, senior r/v' is not an adequate plan and represents a failure to engage with a potential learning opportunity. Formulate a management plan for each patient you see and compare this with your senior's version; ask about the reasons for any significant differences.

Service provision vs training?

Acute trusts need doctors to see patients so that they can be treated, discharged and the trust reimbursed. Behind this simple fact lies an important point of tension between the aims of the trust and those of the individual doctor who will want to develop and acquire new skills. As a foundation doctor, you are in an educationally approved post, for which the LETB releases funds to the trust. It is therefore important that you should be given the opportunities to train and develop, and that you should be released from routine ward work to attend all dedicated training sessions. At the same time, the discharge summaries need to be typed, the drug charts rewritten and a seemingly endless number of venflons resited. The challenge for all involved is to achieve educationally useful outcomes within these constraints. This situation is not unique to the foundation programme – all doctors within the NHS have to balance these demands and some of those tasks you aspire to be able to perform will be the same tasks that have become routine and even frustrating for your seniors. There are no magic answers, but a preparedness to work hard, a keenness to seize educational opportunities whenever they present and a supportive educational supervisor will all go a long way.

Getting organised

Your organisational abilities may be valued above your clinical acumen. While this is not why you became a doctor, being organised will make you more efficient and ensure you are soon going home on time most days.

Folders and clipboards These are an excellent way to hold patient lists, job lists, and spare paperwork along with a portable writing surface. Imaginative improvements can be constructed with bulldog clips, plastic wallets, and dividers.

- *Contents:* spare paper, drug charts, TTOs, blood forms, radiology forms, phone/bleep numbers, job lists, patient lists, theatre lists, spare pen, computer and ward access codes.

Patient lists Juniors are often entrusted with keeping a record of the team's patients (including those on different wards, called 'outliers') along with their background details, investigation results and management plans. With practice most people become good at recalling this information, but writing it down reduces errors.

One means of keeping track is updating an electronic patient list; this also allows every member of the team to carry a copy. It can be invaluable for discussing/referring a patient whilst away from the ward (📖 p81). **These must be kept confidential and disposed of securely**.

Job lists During the ward round make a note of all the jobs that need doing on a separate piece of paper. At the end of the round these jobs can be allocated amongst the team members.

Serial results Instead of simply writing blood results in the notes try writing them on serial results sheets (with a column for each day's results). This makes patterns easier to spot and saves time.

Timetables Along with ward rounds and clinical jobs there will be numerous extra meetings, teaching sessions, and clinics to attend. There are three blank timetables at the end of this book.

Important numbers It can take ages to get through to switchboard so carrying a list of common numbers will save you hours (eventually you will remember them). At the end of this book there are three blank phone number lists for you to fill in. Blank stickers on the back of ID badges can hold several numbers.

Ward cover equipment Finding equipment on unfamiliar wards wastes time and is frustrating. You can speed up your visits by keeping a supply of equipment in a box. Try to fill them with equipment from storerooms instead of clinical areas. Alternatively if you are bleeped by a nurse to put in a cannula, you could try asking them nicely to prepare the equipment ready for you for when you arrive (it works occasionally).

Being efficient

Despite the many years spent at medical school preparing for finals and becoming a doctor, being efficient is one of the most important skills you can learn as a house officer.

Working hours When you first start as an F1, you will always work longer hours than those you are paid for, especially towards the beginning of your career. The best way to make your day run as smoothly as possible is to come in early to prepare for the ward round – you will be expected to have the latest bloods, investigation results, and any overnight interventions at hand, before your seniors arrive.

Time management You will nearly always seem pressed for time, so it is important to organise your day efficiently. Prioritise tasks in such a way that things such as blood tests can be in progress while you chase other jobs. Requesting radiology investigations early in the day is important as lists get filled quickly, whereas writing blood forms for the next day and prescribing warfarin can wait till later on. TTOs should also be written as soon as the team decides a patient is almost ready for discharge – this will save any unnecessary delays on the day they go home.

On-call It will seem like your bleep never stops going off, especially when you are at your busiest. Always write down every job, otherwise you run the risk of forgetting what you were asked to do. Consider whether there is anyone else you could delegate simple tasks to, such as nurse practitioners or ward staff whilst you attend to more urgent tasks.

How to be efficient
- Make a list of common bleeps/extensions (see 📖 p608)
- Establish a timetable of your firm's activities (see 📖 p609)
- Make a folder/clipboard (see 📖 p17)
- Prioritise your workload rather than working through jobs in order. Try to group jobs into areas of the hospital. If you're unsure of the urgency of a job or why you are requesting an investigation, ask your seniors
- If you are working with another house officer split the jobs at the end of the ward round so that you share the workload
- Submit phlebotomy requests at the start/end of each day (find out what time the phlebotomists come); if a patient will need bloods for the next 3 days then fill them all out together with clear dates
- Be aware of your limitations, eg consent should only be done by the surgeon doing the procedure or one trained in taking consent for that particular procedure
- Bookmark online or get a copy of your hospital guidelines/protocols, eg pre-op investigations, anticoagulation, DKA, pneumonia etc
- Get a map of the hospital if you haven't got your bearings.

Patient-centred care

The traditional medical model made the patient a passive recipient of care. Healthcare was done *to* people rather than *with* them. Many patients were happy with this, but the patient should be able to be in charge of their own healthcare should they so wish.

Our task as clinicians is to find out our patients' expectations of their relationship with their doctors and then try to fulfil these. From 'whatever you feel is best doc' to reams of printouts and self-diagnoses from the internet, neither extreme is wrong and our task is to help.

Patient expectations Find out whether your patient wants guidance regarding what treatment may be best.

Respect their right to make a decision you believe may be wrong. If you feel that they are doing so because they do not fully understand the situation or because of flawed logic, then alert your team to this so that things can be explained again.

Find out their other influences, these can be very powerful. Examples include: religious beliefs, friends, the internet, and death/illness of relatives with similar conditions.

Treatment expectations Patients may have clear expectations of their treatment (eg an operation or being given a prescription). These expectations are important sources of discontentment when not fulfilled. Find out what their expectations are and why. Useful questions may include: 'What do you think is wrong with you?' 'What are you worried about?' 'What were you expecting we'd do about this?'

Yourself in their shoes Make time to imagine yourself in your patient's place. Isolation or communication difficulties will heighten fear at an already frightening time. Long waits without explanation are sadly common. Aggression from friends or relatives is often simply a manifestation of anxiety that not enough is being done. Ask yourself 'How would I want my family treated under these circumstances?' then do this for every patient.

Ensuring dignity Hospitals can rob people of their dignity. Wherever and whenever possible help restore this:
- Keep your patients covered (including during resuscitation)
- Ensure the curtains are around the bed on the ward round
- Make sure they have their false teeth in to talk and glasses/wigs on whenever possible
- Help them self-care when possible.

Over-examination Patients are often clerked over four times for a single admission. This is frustrating for them and often seen as indicative of a lack of coordination within the hospital. Patients may need to be clerked and examined more than once, but the context of this should be explained carefully – is this to gain more insight about their condition or to allow a training doctor to learn? People rarely mind when they understand the reasons. Keep examinations which are invasive or cause discomfort to an absolute minimum.

Communication and conduct

Good communication with patients and colleagues is a vital part of the job.

All communication

Whenever you are communicating with another health professional you should include the following details:

- Your name and role (eg Dr Charles Flint, F1 on Mercury Ward)
- The patient's name, location, and primary problem (eg Eleanor Rigby who has suspected appendicitis in bed B4 on Neptune Ward)
- What you wish them to do (eg please keep her nil by mouth)
- Urgency (eg immediately)
- How to contact you if there are any problems (eg I'm on bleep 3366).

Handover[1]

Reductions in working hours, a move towards shift-based rotas and the increased cross-cover between specialties mean that the number of doctors caring for a patient during their hospital stay has increased, making the effective transfer of critical information more important than ever. Handover occurs at the beginning and end of every shift and it is vital that sufficient time is set aside to allow for this. Some hospitals will have formal handover meetings with a senior doctor chairing and a standardised approach to the discussion of sick patients. However, very often the handover process may just involve you sitting down with a colleague to discuss a list of jobs and patients. Whatever the setting, it is important that the incoming doctor receives a clear overview of the situation within the area that they are covering, including the names, locations and clinical details of acutely unwell patients and those patients requiring review, as well as outstanding tasks requiring completion and their order of priority. Giving and receiving a good handover is a key skill and one you should pride yourself on perfecting.

[1] 'Safe handover: Safe patients.' Junior Doctors Committee, BMA (2004) available at ⁀bma.org.uk

---

Written communication

Clinical notes see 📖 p74   *Referral letters* see 📖 p82
Sick notes see 📖 p80   *TTOs* see 📖 p78

Self-discharge If your patient decides to discharge themselves, try to explain why they need hospital management and what could happen if they leave. If you think the patient lacks capacity to make this decision (📖 p28), consult your seniors urgently. If they are capable to make the decision then ask them to sign a 'self-discharge form' to indicate they are taking their own discharge against medical advice. You, the patient, and a second witness (eg nurse) should sign it, recording the time, date, and the patient's decision. Keep it in the notes and inform the GP if relevant. Arrange follow-up and TTOs as usual.

Professional conduct

As a doctor you are a respected member of the community and a representative of the medical profession. People will expect you to act in a professional manner; this does not mean you cannot be yourself, but you must be aware of expectations:

- Always introduce yourself, especially over the telephone or when answering a bleep; 'Hello' is not enough
- Wear your ID badge at all times in hospital

- Never be rude to colleagues/ward staff; you will get a bad reputation
- Never be rude to patients, no matter how they treat you
- Never: shout, swear, scream, hit things, or wear socks with sandals
- Do not gossip about your work colleagues; address any problems you have with a colleague directly and in private
- When you do something wrong, apologise and learn from your mistake; it's a natural part of the learning curve
- If you are going to be late, let the person know in advance especially for handover or ward rounds
- If you think it is not appropriate for you to do a job then run it by the ward staff or your seniors. Ask for help if you feel overrun with tasks.

Patients' relatives

Communication with relatives can be difficult if done badly, or rewarding when things go well. They may be scared, assuming the worst and be in the frustrating position of not knowing what is going on. They could have a full time job that prevents them coming in during the day:
- If you are on-call and do not know the patient well then be honest about this, but attempt to answer simple questions as best possible using the notes; explain what times the usual ward staff will be present
- Try to arrange a time when you can discuss the patient's progress in a quiet room (ask a colleague to hold your bleep)
- To avoid repeating yourself, speak to the family collectively or ask them to appoint a representative
- Check the patient is happy to have their confidential medical details discussed (📖 p27) and encourage them to be present if possible
- Address concerns and answer each question in turn
- Be honest and aware of your limitations; if necessary ask them to arrange a time to meet with a senior
- Document the date, time, what was discussed, and who was present in the notes.

Patient communication

A patient's perception of your abilities as a doctor depends largely on your communication skills. Remember that patients are in an alien environment and are often worried about their health.

Introductions Always introduce yourself to patients and clearly state your name and position. Ask your patient how they wish to be addressed (eg Denis or Mr Smith). Patients meet many staff members daily so reintroduce yourself each time you see them.

General advice Try to avoid using medical jargon. Be honest with your replies to them, and give direct answers when asked a direct question. If you do not know the answer, be honest about this too.

Results Explain why the investigation was performed, what it shows and what this means.

Diagnosis Try to give the everyday name rather than a medical one (heart attack instead of MI). Explain why this has happened. A patient who understands their condition is more likely to comply with treatment.

Prognosis Along with the obvious questions about life expectancy (📖 p22), patients are most interested in how their life will be affected. Pitch your explanation in terms of activities of daily living (ADLs), walking, driving (📖 p605) and working. Bear in mind that patients may want to know about having sex, but are often too embarrassed to ask.

Breaking bad news

Ideally, breaking bad news should always be done by a senior at a pre-determined time when relatives and friends ± specialist nurses can be present. In reality you are likely to be involved in breaking bad news, often whilst on-call. It can be a positive experience if done well.

Preparation Read the patient's notes carefully and ensure that all results are up to date and for the right patient. Be clear in your mind about the sequence of events and the meaning of the results. Consider the further management and likely prognosis – discuss with a senior.

Consent and confidentiality (📖 p29 and 📖 p27) A patient has a right to know what is going on or to choose not to know. Ask before the investigations are done and document their response. If a patient does not want their relatives to know about their diagnosis you must respect this. Always ask, do not assume – many families have complex dynamics.

Warning shot Give a suggestion that bad news is imminent so it is not completely out of the blue, eg 'I have the results from … would you like anyone else here when I tell you them/shall we go to a quiet room?'.

How to do it The SPIKES model is often used:

Setting Ask a colleague to hold your bleep and set aside suitable time (at least 30min); use a quiet room and invite a nurse who has been involved in the patient's care. Arrange the seats so you can make eye contact and remove distractions. Introduce yourself and find out who everyone is.

Perception Find out what the patient already knows by asking them directly; this will give you an idea of how much of a shock this will be and their level of understanding to help you give appropriate information.

Invitation Explain that you have results to give them and ask if they are ready to hear them. It helps to give a very brief summary of events so they understand what results you are talking about.

Knowledge Break the bad news, eg 'A doctor has looked at the sample and I'm sorry to say it shows a cancer'. Give the information time to sink in and all present to react (shock, anger, tears, denial). Once the patient is ready, give further information about what this means and the expected management. Give the information in small segments and check understanding repeatedly. Prognosis can be difficult; never give an exact time ('months' rather than '4 months'). Be honest and realistic. Try to offer hope even if it is just symptom improvement or leaving hospital.

Empathy Acknowledge the feelings caused by the news; offer sympathy. This will take place alongside the 'Knowledge' step. Listen to their concerns, fears, worries. This will guide what further information you give and help you to understand their reactions.

Summary Repeat the main points of the discussion and arrange a time for further questions, ideally with a senior and yourself present. Give a clear plan of what will happen over the next 48h.

Remember to document the discussion in the patient's notes (diagnosis, prognosis, expectations) with your name and contact details.

Cross-cultural communication

For patients who can't understand or speak the same language as you, the consultation can leave them feeling isolated, frustrated and anxious. You may have to rely on a third party to translate for you.

Professional interpreters

Professional interpreters can be arranged before the appointment – ask ward staff or phone switchboard:

- Allow extra time for the consultation and check the interpreter is acceptable to the patient
- Address both the patient and the interpreter and look at the patient's non-verbal response to gauge their level of understanding
- Ask simple, direct questions in short sentences to avoid overloading or confusing the interpreter; avoid jargon
- Use pictures or diagrams to explain things wherever possible; provide written/audiovisual material in the patient's own language to take away
- If you cannot organise an interpreter, you may be able to contact a telephone interpreting service who translate for you and the patient directly over the phone (ask nurses or switchboard)
- Document that a trained interpreter has been used with their name and contact details so that the same interpreter can accompany the patient for future appointments.

Never assume you know what the patient wants without asking them.

Family members as interpreters

There are many reasons why family members and friends should *not* be used as interpreters. Nevertheless, in emergency situations, this may prove necessary. Address the patient directly and look carefully at the patient's response to gauge their understanding. Record the fact that a family member was used for interpretation in the notes.

Friends and relatives are commonly used as informal interpreters. The main drawbacks are the lack of confidentiality and the bias the relative may have on the patient's decision-making – particularly when underlying family issues are present (you may be unaware of these).

Children can interpret for their parents from an early age, but again their views can bias the consultation and its outcome (eg sexual health and vulnerable adults) and even routine clinical questions can be very frightening or inappropriate for children. Use only as a point of last resort.

Conflict of interests if you think the relative is biasing the conversation or it is an important issue then explain that you are professionally obliged to request a trained interpreter.

Consent relatives cannot consent on behalf of adults, see 📖 p29.

Who can interpret

- Hospital interpreters
- Local interpreting agencies
- Hospital staff (switchboard may have a list)
- Telephone service with which the hospital has a contract
- Family and friends – as a last resort – see above.

Outside agencies

Outside agencies who could enquire about your patients include: police, media, solicitors, fire brigade, paramedics, general practitioner, researchers, and the patient's employer. Patient confidentiality must be respected.

The rules
- Do you really know who you are talking to?
- Check and arrange to call them back unless certain
- Do they have any right to the information they are seeking?
  - GPs, healthcare professionals and ambulance staff may well do, police have limited rights (see below), many others do not
- Should you be the one discussing this or should a more senior member of the team?
- Do not talk to the media about a patient/your hospital unless:
  - You have the patient's permission *and:*
  - You have permission from your consultant/management (for trust issues) *and:*
  - You are accompanied by the trust public relations officer
- Do not 'chat' to a police/prison officer about a patient, no matter what the alleged circumstances; all patients have an equal right to privacy
- Breaching a patient's confidentiality without good cause is treated as misconduct by the GMC.

Confidentiality and the police
Immediate investigation of assaults The police may well ask the clinical condition of an assault victim. 'Is it life-threatening, doctor?' The purpose of this question is to know how thoroughly to investigate the crime scene. It is reasonable to give them an assessment of severity.

In the public interest In situations where someone may be at risk of serious injury, disclosure is permitted by the GMC. This should be a consultant-level decision.

The Road Traffic Act Everyone has a duty to provide the police with information which may lead to the identification of a driver who is alleged to have committed a driving offence. You are obliged to supply the name and address, not clinical details. Discuss with your seniors first.

Being a witness in court
Inform your clinical supervisor; they should accompany you to court. Remember you are a professional witness to the court so your evidence should be an impartial statement of the facts. Do not get rattled by the barristers – stick to the facts, do not give opinions, explain the limits of your knowledge/experience. Address your remarks to the judge. Wear your best suit. Get an expenses form from the witness unit to claim your costs back.

Medical research
You may be asked to provide patient details for research. Ask the researcher to provide you with ID and if they have consent from the patient. It is reasonable to direct researchers towards appropriate patients to get consent.

Clinical governance/quality

DH definition: 'Clinical governance is the system through which NHS organisations are accountable for continuously improving the quality of their services and safeguarding high standards of care, by creating an environment in which clinical excellence will flourish.'

What this means for you as an individual

- You are responsible for your clinical practice which you should be aiming to improve continuously
- You need a mechanism for assessing the standard of your practice
- Whilst in training this is done for you by your consultant/trainer as part of your regular appraisal process. Additionally you may have audits and regular departmental meetings
- You should be aiming to continuously learn and improve your care for patients. Again, whilst still in training, this almost goes without saying; revising for endless examinations and diplomas helps too.

What this means for you as part of a team

- You should ensure you stick to departmental or hospital protocols and don't undertake procedures for which you have not been trained
- You will be asked to participate in regular departmental audits, usually of morbidity and mortality. These are used to ensure consistency of practice and to pick up problems early
- You should attend departmental and hospital-wide audit meetings and grand rounds to keep up to date with changes
- You should answer any responses to complaints promptly.

Clinical governance/quality mechanisms

The clinical governance structure in every hospital includes:
- Audit of practice (eg reattendances within 1wk or wound infections)
- Appraisal and revalidation structures
- Regular departmental meetings (eg morbidity and mortality) to allow clinicians to compare their care and highlight common concerns
- Clear routes of accountability for all staff. It can be obvious when these have broken down, leading to problems which everyone can identify but seemingly no one is responsible for fixing
- A risk management structure to identify practices which jeopardise high-quality patient care (critical incident reporting, 📖 p32)
- A complaints department to respond to complaints and ensure lessons are learned from them; may be part of the risk management department
- A clinical governance/quality committee structure which oversees and ensures compliance with all of the above.

Compliance with clinical governance/quality mechanisms are measured both regionally and nationally through quality boards.

Medical ethics

What is medical ethics?

Ethics are moral values, and in the context of medicine are supported by four main underlying principles:

Autonomy is the right for the individual to make decisions for themselves, and not be overtly pressurised or swayed by others (namely doctors, nurses, relatives, etc). Patients should be allowed to contribute when decisions are made about their care. If an individual lacks capacity (📖 p28) then it might not be appropriate to let them make important autonomous decisions.

Beneficence is concerned with doing what is right for the patient and what is in their best interests. This does not necessarily mean we should do everything to keep a 90-year-old patient alive who has widespread metastatic disease. There will be times when it is *beneficent* to keep a patient comfortable, and allow them to die naturally.

Non-maleficence ensures care-givers refrain from doing harm to the patient, whether physical or psychological. An example of a breach in non-maleficence would be if a patient came to harm as a result of a doctor performing a procedure in which they had inadequate training or supervision.

Justice requires that all individuals are treated equally and that both the benefits and burdens of care are distributed without bias. *Justice* also covers openness within medical practice and the acknowledgement that some activities may have certain consequences – specifically legal action.

Two further principles are important to consider:

Dignity should be retained for both the patient and the people delivering their healthcare.

Honesty is a fundamental quality which doctors (as well as other care-givers) and patients should be expected to exhibit in order to strengthen the doctor–patient relationship.

Ethical conflict

Ethical dilemmas frequently arise in clinical practice and while the principles listed do not necessarily provide an immediate answer, they do create a framework on which the various components of the conflict can be teased out and addressed individually, which often allows a harmonious solution to be identified.

Ethics and communication

It is quite common that apparently complex ethical issues arise because of a failure in communication between the patient or their loved ones and healthcare professionals. The solution to most of these conflicts is the establishment of effective and transparent lines of communication.

Patient confidentiality

To breach patient confidentiality is unlawful and unprofessional; several doctors are disciplined and even struck off the medical register each year for this. You should be careful when talking about patients in public places, including within the hospital environment, and only disclose patient information to recognised healthcare staff as appropriate. Pieces of paper with patient information on must never leave the hospital and should be shredded if they are no longer required. **Do not leave patient lists lying around**. Personal electronic databases of patients should be disguised so individual patients cannot be identified. Electronic devices on which patient information is stored outside of the hospital should be encrypted and registered under the Data Protection Act. You avoid giving any information (names or nature of injuries) to the police, press, or other enquirers; ask your seniors for advice when dealing with these (see 📖 p24).

Publications Medical journals will often insist that any article which involves a patient must be accompanied by written consent from the patient for the publication of the material, irrespective of how difficult it would be to track down and identify that patient.

Presentations and images If you are talking about a patient to a group of healthcare workers in your own hospital you do not need to obtain consent, but doing so is courteous. If you are talking to an audience from outside your hospital it is advisable you seek the patient's consent unless the patient is fully anonymised. Equally, if you want to keep copies of radiographs or digital images, ensure these are made anonymous and if this isn't possible obtain the patient's written consent. Bear in mind that presentations can easily end up online and be accessed by those other than your original audience.[1]

Relatives Your duty lies with your patient and if a relative asks you a question about the patient, it is essential you obtain verbal consent from the patient to talk to the relative; alternatively offer to talk to the relative in the presence of the patient. Relatives do not have any rights to know medical information. If the patient lacks capacity then seek senior advice before talking to the relatives. Document all conversations in the notes.

Children As described for adults, if the child has capacity to give consent (see 'Gillick competence'/Fraser guidelines, 📖 p28), you must seek verbal consent from the patient to tell the relatives (parents) about their health. If the patient refuses, then offer to talk to the patient about their condition in the presence of their relatives. If you sense the situation will be difficult, seek senior advice/support.

Telephone calls Wards receive many telephone calls asking how patients are and if they have had tests or operations yet. The potential to break patient confidentiality here is great. Often there is a telephone by each bed, so encourage callers to speak to the patient directly. Otherwise, inform the patient who the caller is and relay a message from the patient to the caller. Apologise to the caller for not being able to offer any further information and suggest that you could talk things over with both themselves and the patient when they visit. See 'Outside agencies', 📖 p24.

[1] For a good discussion of the ethical issues, see Draper, H. and Rogers, W. *APT* 2005 **11**:115 available free at 🖰 apt.rcpsych.org/content/11/2/115.full.pdf

Capacity

Someone who has capacity can comprehend and retain information material relevant to the decision, especially as to the consequences of not having the intervention in question, and must be able to use and weigh this information in the decision-making process.

For a patient to have capacity they must:
- Be able to understand the information relevant to making the decision and consequences of refusal
- Retain the information long enough to allow for decision-making
- Weigh up the information to arrive at a decision
- Be able to communicate the decision they have made.

Remember that:
- Patients may have the capacity to make certain decisions and not others
- Capacity in the same patient may fluctuate over time.

Capacity is most often impaired by chronic neurological pathology such as dementia, learning difficulties, and psychiatric illness, but is also impaired by acute states such as delirium, acute severe pain, alcohol and drug intoxication (both recreational and iatrogenic – eg morphine).

Children and capacity Children under 16yr of age were once regarded as lacking capacity to give consent, but now if the child meets the criteria then they are regarded as having 'Gillick' competence (Fraser guidelines[1]), and may give consent. It is always advisable, however, to involve the parent or guardian in discussions about the patient's care if the patient allows (see also 📖 p403).

No capacity When the patient does not have capacity and is over 18, family and friends are not able to make a decision on the patient's behalf; their views should, however, be listened to. Where the patient lacks capacity and there is no next of kin to consult an Independent Mental Capacity Advocate (IMCA)[2] may need to be appointed who advises clinicians in making decisions on behalf of the patient in their best interests. In an emergency situation, the patient is treated under the 'doctrine of necessity', that is, doing what is in the patient's best interests until they attain capacity to make the decisions themselves.

Gillick competence/Fraser guidelines

Although 16 is the usual age at which people are automatically allowed to give their own consent, younger people can consent to most treatments or operations if they are capable. This follows a famous case in 1986 when Victoria Gillick went to the courts to get authority to be informed if her daughters sought contraceptive treatments. The law disagreed and decided that if a child was competent, he/she could consent to treatment without parental knowledge – this is often referred to as being 'Gillick' competent when a child meets the criteria in that case.

---

[1] Gillick or Fraser? A plea for consistency over competence in children. *BMJ* 2006; **332**:807.
[2] Mental Capacity Act (2005); 🔗**www.legislation.gov.uk/ukpga/2005/9/section/35**

Consent

Understanding consent and obtaining it satisfactorily can be difficult. If you are ever unsure seek senior help.

Obtaining consent The individual who obtains consent from the patient should be aware of the risks and benefits and be able to communicate the procedure in a language that the patient will understand. **If you do not regularly perform the procedure yourself or are not trained to take consent for the procedure then you must not obtain consent for it**. Obtaining consent satisfactorily is a skill that can be learned from senior colleagues, so initially shadow your seniors when they are taking consent from a patient to learn how to do it properly, then have a senior colleague supervise you the first few times to ensure you include all the relevant information.

Informed consent In order to give informed consent, patients must first be deemed to have capacity to consent under the specific circumstances (📖 p28). Consent should reflect the fact that the patient is aware of what is going to happen and why. They should be aware of the consequences of not undergoing the procedure, the potential benefits, and any alternatives, and be free from any coercion. The common risks and side effects should be discussed, as should the potentially rare but serious consequences of the procedure. As a rule, any risks which might affect the decision of a normal person should be discussed – plus any risks that might be of specific importance for the individual patient, such as where the profession of the patient makes a normal trivial risk of special importance (eg a tiny risk of post-operative vertigo might be of particular importance for a window cleaner). The patient should be provided with information well in advance of the procedure to allow them to think it over and prepare any questions they may wish to ask.

Types of consent There are three main types of consent:
- *Implied* The patient offers you their arm as you approach them with a needle and syringe to take blood
- *Expressed – **verbal*** You explain that you are going to perform a lumbar puncture, by describing the procedure and potential complications and the patient agrees to have it done
- *Expressed – **written*** The patient is given an extensive explanation of the procedure and complications and informed of the alternatives. A record of the consultation is made which both patient and doctor sign. This document should be completed prior to the planned treatment or procedure, and consent verified at the time of the procedure.

Difficult situations There are many situations where problems arise with consent issues. If in doubt seek senior advice or consult one of the medical defence unions (📖 p600) which have 24h telephone support.

If a patient has capacity to give or withhold consent, and chooses not to receive treatment even in the face of death, then treating that patient against their will is potentially a criminal offence. This includes patients with psychiatric illness. Note that this situation is distinct from that of a patient with a psychiatric illness who may lack capacity to make decisions regarding psychiatric treatment, and may be detained and given psychiatric (but not medical treatment) under the Mental Health Act (📖 p364).

Medical errors

Every doctor makes mistakes varying from the trivial and correctable to the severe and avoidable.

What to do at once/within an hour

- Stabilise the patient, call for senior help early
- Do not compound the error by trying to cover it up or ignoring it
- Correct where possible, apologising to the patient as appropriate
- Don't underestimate the seriousness of the situation; have a low threshold for asking for help to ensure things do not get any worse
- If serious and you have time, start documenting events, including times
- If, sometime after an error, you realise you wish to add further details to the notes then do so but make it clear when these additions have been written by timing and dating them. This is perfectly acceptable
- Amending notes, without making it clear that your entry was made retrospectively and with a clear date and time, is serious misconduct.

Serious untoward incidents – rare

- An apology is not an admission of guilt, so apologise and explain to the patient early. Apologise that the event has taken place, it is not necessary to 'give confession' at this stage
- Inform your senior/consultant immediately
- If you believe your error has caused the patient significant harm then you should speak to your defence organisation (📖 p600) as soon as practical.

Disciplinary procedures

If you have made a really serious error the hospital may choose to exclude you from working. That is, to send you home at once and ask you not to return until they have carried out preliminary enquiries. It is not a judgemental act but is designed to allow a calm and quick investigation. You must be informed why you have been excluded. You may be asked not to talk to others involved. If this happens to you, ring your defence organisation at once. You should be given a named person to contact in the hospital. You cannot be excluded for more than 2wk without a review. Go and stay with friends or family, don't be on your own. Let the hospital and others know how to get hold of you.

Less serious errors should be treated as a training issue and dealt with by your consultant initially or the trust clinical tutor/postgraduate dean. A period of close supervision or retraining may be appropriate.

Sources of help

- *Clinical events* Your consultant, your educational and clinical supervisors, the postgraduate dean, your defence organisation
- *Non-clinical events* Your consultant, the postgraduate dean, the BMA.

Don't forget friends, and family and remember that these events resolve extremely slowly, taking years in the big cases, so don't expect large numbers of answers in the first week.

Complaints

Every doctor has complaints made about them. These can be about your clinical ability, conduct, or communication skills. They may be justified or spurious but they are inevitable, therefore do not feel your world has fallen apart when you are told a complaint has been made about you.

How the system handles complaints

There are two types of complaints – formal and informal. If a patient complains to you informally it is in everyone's best interest, and will save many hours of clinical time, if you are able to resolve the situation to the patient's satisfaction there and then. If you are unable to do so, but feel the problem may be solvable by more senior input, then call for help. Don't agree to do something which you are unable to carry out.

How to respond to a complaint

- All formal complaints are collated centrally in the hospital. In the rare event you are sent a complaint personally, do not respond but pass it to the complaints department. In most trusts the department that handles complaints is known as PALS (Patient Advice and Liaison Service). They also provide more general advice and support for patients
- If a patient makes a complaint to you about care they have received from a colleague (doctor, nurse or other) then listen to them but try to avoid appearing to agree or support their position, no matter how much you may share their opinions. Depending on the seriousness of their allegations, either offer to feedback the comments or advise them to discuss matters further with PALS
- If a complaint has been made about the care of a patient you saw, you may be asked for a statement. This is an internal document and should be written as a letter, but bear in mind if the case goes to court this document could be requested by the patient's lawyers
- Simply state the facts as you see them, do not try to apportion blame. You may be able to expand on your notes, particularly the details of conversations which may not have been documented
- **Do not take it personally**
- If you feel it is clear how any error could be avoided in future then state this as well. Patients are often satisfied by knowing that any mistake they suffered will not be repeated for others
- All the statements made by the staff involved are then collated and a letter is written on behalf of the chief executive (and usually signed by them) to the patient. This usually ends the matter
- There are further steps, both with the trust and then regionally, if this is not enough.

Serious errors

- Preventable death of a patient
- Significant harm to a patient, in a predictable way
- Disciplinary offences including:
  - substance abuse
  - being drunk on duty
  - sexual/racial harassment.

Incident reporting

Clinical incidents are defined as:
- Anything which harms patients' care or disrupts critical treatment
- An event which could potentially lead to harm if allowed to progress ('near misses'). They range from minor incidents, eg incorrect results, to life-threatening, eg wrong blood group in a blood transfusion.

Non-clinical incidents include:
- Incidents which involve staff, relatives, or visitors
- Incidents which involve non-clinical equipment or property.

The aim of incident reporting is to highlight adverse incidents or 'near misses', assess them, and review clinical practice as a result. Ultimately it is designed to reduce clinical risks and improve overall quality of patient care.

When a clinical incident/near miss occurs
- Make sure the patient is safe
- Complete a trust critical incident reporting form (usually online)
- Forward the form to the clinical risk coordinator (usually automatic if form is electronic)
- Ensure your seniors are aware of what has happened
- Consider completing some formal reflective practice in your ePortfolio.

Examples of all too common clinical incidents[1]
- Blood samples from two different patients being confused
- Failure to report or follow-up abnormal results
- Equipment failure
- Drugs prescribed to patients who have a documented allergy
- Delay in treatment/management.

Completing incident forms
- Fill in an incident form as soon as you can after the event so that you don't forget any relevant information
- Check you are filling in the correct form. All NHS trusts now use online incident reporting systems though there may be paper backups
- Include the time, date, staff involved, as well as the issues being reported
- Check if the named consultant needs to fill in/sign the form
- If you are reporting an incident involving your colleagues, inform them and explain the situation. Learn from their mistakes without judging them.

The critical incident form is copied to clinical risk directors for evaluation at panel meetings, where changes to clinical practice are discussed.

Hints and tips
- If a critical incident form is filed involving yourself, don't assume you're a bad doctor; use it as a learning experience
- Find out the reason and circumstances and clarify the situation with the person filing the report
- Go over the incident and review your actions, asking if there is anything you would change; if it helps, discuss it with a colleague.

[1] See ⫶**https://www.gov.uk/government/news/never-events-list-update-for-2012-13** for a list of events that should *never* happen (but sadly, still sometimes do).

Colleagues and problems

Many of us may have worked with a colleague who worried us professionally – 'I wouldn't want to be treated by Dr X'. When does this become enough to do something? And what do you do?

Clinical incompetence

- The GMC is quite clear that we all have a clinical duty to report colleagues who we believe to be incompetent. This does not equate to pointing out every fault of every other doctor but it does mean that you cannot ignore serious concerns if you believe patients are at risk of harm
- Serious concerns about a trainee should be passed to the relevant consultant. Ask to see them in private. It may be easiest to open the conversation with a question, to ask them to put your mind at rest: *'I don't know if you are aware that Dr X does not use chaperones? I've always been told we should use them for intimate examinations. I'm here because two women told me that they had felt uncomfortable with Dr X.'*
- If the problem is with a consultant then you should either talk to another consultant or, if it is very serious, the medical director
- If you are unsure whether a problem exists, or how serious it is, then talk to a friendly consultant informally (eg your supervisor or a clinical lecturer you got on with at medical school).

Recreational drugs/alcohol

- There is a clear difference between a doctor occasionally drinking too much whilst off-duty and one who helps themselves to controlled drugs or who has developed an alcohol problem
- Likewise, regardless of substance, there is a difference between what someone does that only affects themselves and actions which affect quality of care. Any colleague who appears on duty whilst badly hungover is a potential risk to patient care and should be removed from clinical duties (and should be encouraged to recover in the mess or go home). Repetitive behaviour of this kind should be discussed with the colleague, and/or their educational supervisor
- Drinking during working hours, arriving drunk, or use of controlled drugs are totally unacceptable and you have a duty to alert your consultants to any such problem. They will consider the GMC guidance and following a meeting with the individual involved will decide if GMC referral is appropriate or if a local warning and period of 'probation' is needed These problems are better tackled early whilst solvable than left until they cause patient harm and ruin a career.

Psychological problems

- Every year doctors develop serious psychological illnesses just like the rest of the population and doctors are just as bad at self-diagnosis
- The more common problems include frank depression and hypomania, the rare include psychosis and schizophrenia (📖 p365); the symptoms often come on gradually such that even close colleagues may not notice the transition from mildly eccentric to frankly pathological
- Depression is commonly masked well whilst at work
- Talk to an individual directly, or their consultant, if you are concerned about their health.

Hating your job

Experiencing problems at work is common and usually transient. If you find things do not improve try to identify the problem. However difficult things are at work, you should always remain polite, punctual, and helpful. If you don't you may be the one perceived to be the problem.

Stress at the workplace

The responsibility that comes with being a doctor, the demands of your job, fear of litigation, and high expectations from peers and patients can leave you physically and mentally exhausted. If you feel things are getting on top of you reassess your workload. Speak to colleagues to find out if there are easier ways of doing things. Take annual leave and upon your return approach your work schedule differently to help regain control of things. Ensure you have time to relax away from work and keep up your outside interests. If things don't improve, talk to a friend, contact the BMA (📖 p600) for advice, or discuss the situation with a trusted senior or mentor.

Handing in your resignation

If you can find no other option and you are clear medicine isn't for you, you can always leave your job. Find out how much notice you are required to give and who to direct your letter of resignation to. During your last weeks, stay an active member of the team rather than taking a short-timer's attitude. Complete any outstanding work and tidy up loose ends before leaving.

Bullying at work

Bullying can be from your seniors, peers, other healthcare professionals, patients or their relatives. If you feel you are being bullied, discuss it with someone, either at work or independently (eg the BMA). Speak to your predecessors to find out if they had similar difficulties and how they handled the problem. Keep a diary of relevant events, together with witnesses, and approach your consultant. If it is your consultant who is the problem, approach another consultant you trust or contact BMA counselling (📖 p600).

Sexual harassment

This may start very innocently and gradually escalate into intimidating behaviour which may affect your work, social life, and confidence. In the first instance make it clear that their advances are not welcome and confide in someone you trust. Find out if other colleagues are also being harassed and report the harassment to your educational supervisor. Again, the BMA can be a useful source of advice.

Discrimination

All employers must abide by an equal opportunities policy that includes standards on treating all employees. Before deciding to take things further confide in a trusted senior colleague. Keep a record of any events that stand out as being discriminatory, documenting dates, times, and witnesses. Contact the BMA for advice. You may have to submit a formal letter outlining your concerns, so make sure you are prepared to pursue a formal complaint before committing yourself on paper.

Relaxation

Have a break There are few problems that must be solved immediately. Leave the ward, ask someone to hold your bleep, and take 5min to unwind. Try taking deep breaths and concentrating on the feeling of the air rushing in and out of your lungs. Count the breaths and try to clear your mind. Try squeezing the muscles in your feet then feeling them relax; do this with all the muscle groups from your legs to your neck. Think about something you are looking forward to.

Do not let medicine take over your life. It doesn't take much to make life seem massively better; try the following:

- Go for a walk
- Watch a film
- Go shopping
- Exercise
- Watch a comedy
- Take a long bath
- Go out for a meal
- Talk to friends
- Watch sport
- Play a game
- Have a good cry
- Go to the pub
- Have a massage
- Cook
- Plan a holiday
- Talk to parents
- Have a lie in
- Listen to music
- Have an early night
- Join a class/club
- Read (another) book.

Try to avoid the following:

- Smoking
- Excessive alcohol
- Drugs/sleeping tablets
- Excessive caffeine.

Causes of stress

Attitude

There is no point worrying about things you have no control over; it is natural to feel concerned about future events but almost everything will turn out well in the end, even if it is not as you have planned it.

The job

See 📖 p18 on being efficient. The job gets much easier with time; these skills become second nature and you perform individual tasks quicker.

Yourself

Be honest with yourself: Are you tired? Everything is harder, slower, and more stressful when you have not had enough sleep.

Think about what makes you stressed and whether this is a problem with your attitude, the way you do the job, other people or the nature of the job. Try to accept, change or avoid these stressors.

Other people

If someone is annoying you then consider telling them so. Plan how you will tell them, do it in private and do not blame them; just explain how it makes you feel. Most people will be apologetic and try to change.

If you feel it is all getting too much and/or nobody cares try speaking to:	
BMA counselling (you don't need to be a member)	08459 200 169
Samaritans	08457 90 90 90

Pay and contracts

The number of hours you are allowed to work in a shift and the total for a given week are determined by two sets of rules:

- *'New Deal'* on junior doctors' hours and pay, which was an agreement between the BMA and all the UK Departments of Health to improve the working conditions of junior doctors.
- *European Working Time Directive* (EWTD) – this sets limits on working hours and minimum rest periods that are more stringent than those in the New Deal. Junior doctors across Europe were initially excluded from the EWTD, but there has been a staggered process of hours reduction and all posts must now be EWTD compliant.

EWTD

- Maximum of 48h of work a week
- Maximum shift length of 13h
- 11h of continuous rest every 24h or compensatory rest must be given
- 24h continuous rest each week or 48h in a fortnight
- All time when you are required to be on site counts as work, whether you are actively working or resting.

New deal

- Set limits on working hours now superseded by the EWTD
- 30 min of uninterrupted break after approximately 4 hours of work
- Detailed requirements about the requirements for different working patterns. These affect the maximum length of any on-call period; most foundation doctors will work a 'full shift' rota.

Monitoring and rebanding

- Monitoring actual hours worked by junior doctors is done to check they mirror the theoretical hours of the rota. All training posts have to be monitored for at least 2wk by all participants every 6mth. This is a contractual requirement for employer and employee
- Accurate hours monitoring is a matter of probity and is important to ensure that you, your colleagues and future post holders are not put in a position where patient safety may be compromised. You should monitor your hours honestly – this includes resisting pressure to *under*-report hours. Sadly, this pressure may come from your own consultants and can be difficult to deal with. Discuss with your colleagues, your educational supervisor and your local BMA representative if this happens
- If your post turns out to be monitored as a different band to the one you're paid then your pay can go up but is protected against going down. Your rota cannot be changed in such a way as to affect your salary without the agreement of the majority of the doctors on the rota
- The guidance for 'rebanding' and pay protection is complex. It is available from the NHS Employers website, where the latest basic salary rates can also be found: ⏁www.nhsemployers.org
- If you are a BMA member, they have several further resources on-line regarding pay, contracts and hours: ⏁bma.org.uk

Pay and banding contracts

Junior doctors in the NHS receive a set 'basic' rate of pay, according to the grade and the number of years they have worked. Those whose posts involve more than 40h/wk and/or out-of-hours working, receive an additional sum, known as a 'banding supplement', based on a multiple of their basic salary (Table 1.3). This supplement should reflect the overall workload and the extent of out-of-hours working required in the post.

- *Band 1* average total hours of actual work under 48h/wk
- *Band 2* average total hours of actual work <56h but >48h/wk
- *Band 3* average total hours of actual work over 56h/wk.

Bands 2 and 3 are not compliant with the EWTD and should no longer be in use. Bands 1 and 2 are subdivided according to the number of hours worked at antisocial times (weekends, evenings and nights), with 'A' representing more out-of-hours working than 'B' and 'C'.

Table 1.3 *Banding multiplier*

These rates are subject to annual review as part of the doctors' annual pay award. Posts with <40h/wk worked exclusively between 8am–7pm Mon–Fri are 'unbanded' and receive no supplement.

Band 1A	+50%	Band 2A	+80%	Band 3	+100%
Band 1B	+40%	Band 2B	+50%		
Band 1C	+20%				

For more information on pay and pay slips, see Fig. 1.1 (p39).

Making more money

There are several ways to make money in addition to your basic income. You must keep records of all additional income and declare these in your self-assessment to the Inland Revenue at the end of each tax year.[1]

Research There are usually several research projects being undertaken in most hospitals which require volunteers to have experiments performed on them. These range from a 5min interview to a week-long study and in most circumstances the volunteers are rewarded financially (eg £5 to over £500). These may carry a risk of harm.

Locums Most hospitals employ locum doctors to cover staff sickness or at busy times. Locum doctors often already work for the hospital, but work additional shifts for extra money; alternatively they may be from outside the hospital. It is important to remember that the hours you work as a locum should be added to your basic or regular hours and should not exceed the limits of the New Deal[2] or European Working Time Directive; some contracts may stipulate that you cannot work locum shifts in other hospitals or departments. There are many locum agencies that you can register with; they are often advertised in *BMJ Careers*. Rates of pay vary, but an F1 can expect pre-tax rates of £20–30 per hour, and F2s £25–35. If your own hospital is employing you as a locum, you may be able to negotiate a better rate.

Cremation certificates The cremation form has two parts (📖 p94). The first is completed by a ward doctor (usually the F1) and the second by a senior doctor, often from another department. Under arrangements prior to 2014, junior doctors were paid around £70 for the form; this fee is under review as part of the 2014 reforms (see 📖 p98). The bereavement office handles the forms and issues any cheques. Make sure you see the body, checking identity and that there is no implantable device that needs removing (📖 p94); they do really explode. However, this system and the associated fee is under review as part of the 2014 reforms to death certification.

Published articles A small number of journals and medical newspapers pay authors for articles which appear in print. The amount varies from between £25 to £250 depending on the length and importance. The journals' websites often outline payment and the types of articles they are after.

Gifts The GMC are quite clear in their message that you should not encourage patients or their families to give, lend, or bequeath gifts to yourself, others, or to organisations.[3] If you are given a gift then it is acceptable to take it as long as it has negligible financial value. If you are given money then it is sensible to pass this onto the ward sister who can put it in the ward fund account.

---

[1] www.hmrc.gov.uk/sa/index.htm
[2] *Junior Doctors' Handbook 2012*. British Medical Association.
[3] www.gmc-uk.org/guidance/good_medical_practice.asp

Fig. 1.1 A sample pay slip.

Always check your payslips carefully, before storing them safely: make backups of electronic payslips and never throw paper copies away. They can be a useful record of tax, pension, and loan payments long after you have enjoyed spending the money. If you think a mistake has been made, contact the salaries and wages division of the HR office for your trust, quoting your assignment number (employee number). In the event of significant underpayment, you can request an interim payment be made pending the resolution.

Department	Employee name	Location	
Gen Med	Dr Tertius Lydgate	Middlemarch Hospital	
NHS	**Job Title** Foundation House Officer 1	**Payscale description** Foundation House Officer 1	
	Sal/wage 22636.00 ①	**Inc. date** 5 Aug 2015 ②	**Standard hours** 48	**PT sal/wage** 22636.00
	Tax office ref 199/C2		**Tax code** 1000L ③	**NI number** JD354523D

Description	Amount	Description	Amount
Basic pay	1886.33 ④	Tax	494.22 ⑥
Banding supplement	754.53 ⑤	NI	219.05 ⑦
		NHS Pension	169.77 ⑧
		Mess fee	6.00
		Student loan	119.23 ⑨

Gross pay ⑩	Taxable pay	This period summary
	Tax paid	Pensionable pay 1886.33 ⑫
NI letter	Pension conts	Pay date 26 March 2015 ⑬
D ⑪	Employee number	Pay method BACS ⑭
		Taxable pay 2471.09 ⑮
		Total payments 2640.86 ⑯
		Total deductions 1008.27 ⑰
		NET PAY 1632.59 ⑱

1 This is the total annual basic salary for your pay point. Latest updates are released as 'Pay Circulars' on the NHS Employers website ⏏ www.nhsemployers.org
2 This is the date when you are next due to go a point up the pay scale, usually 12 months of full time employment after your previous date (or date of first starting working as a doctor). When changing trusts mistakes can be made so always check this date is correct.
3 Your tax code shows the amount of income you are entitled to earn in the current tax year that you do not pay any tax on. This figure should be multiplied by 10 to give your total allowance. This will be the basic personal allowance for the tax year, as set by the government, adjusted to take account of any under- or over-payments you may have made in previous years. Each tax year runs from April to April. After your first tax year in paid employment, you will receive a P60 summarising your tax paid during that year with the code that should apply to you in the next tax year. A copy should also be sent to your trust, but if you move trusts around this time, the new trust may not receive the correct information unless you show them your copy of the P60. If your new trust does not know the correct code for you, they will use an 'emergency' code, set as the basic personal allowance, which may or may not be correct. The letter after the code should be an 'L' unless very specific circumstances apply to you. See also ⏏ www.hmrc.gov.uk
4 This will be approximately 1/12 of your annual salary.
5 If you receive a banding supplement, it will appear here (see Table 1.6).
6 Under the 'Pay as you earn' scheme (PAYE), your trust will automatically deduct your tax from your income each month. Both your basic pay and your banding supplement are taxable. In your first few months of employment, you may not pay any tax until your income has risen above the personal allowance for that year. Enjoy this while it lasts!
7 National Insurance contributions pay for certain state benefits, including your state pension. These are not optional, and will be deducted automatically, according to thresholds. The current rate is 9% of income over £149/week, though this is subject to annual review.
8 The NHS pension scheme remains a very good deal, although terms and conditions have been changed significantly in recent years and are subject to further negotiations. Your pension contributions are not taxed and will also be deducted automatically according to various earnings thresholds, unless you opt out of the scheme. Pension contributions are calculated from your basic pay - your banding supplement is not subject to any deductions.
See also ⏏ www.nhsbsa.nhs.uk/pensions
9 Any loan you have taken from the Student Loans Company will enter repayment in the April of the first year after you graduate in which your gross pre-tax income rises above a threshold (currently £16,365). Any earnings should be deducted automatically at 9% of earnings above this threshold. You can choose to repay faster if you wish. Keep a record of all repayments you make and check them against your annual statement - errors are common when changing trusts. Payments that appear to have gone missing can be credited to your account easily if you can provide a copy of your payslips.
See ⏏ www.studentloanrepayment.co.uk
10 The numbers in this section will keep a tally of your total payments from that employer during the current tax year. If you change trusts, the numbers will be reset, but your tax thresholds should not be.
11 Your NI letter reflects the contribution group you fall into. For almost all of those in the NHS pension scheme, this will be 'D'.
12 Pensionable pay does not include any banding supplement.
13 Pay dates will vary between trusts but are generally around the last Thursday in the month. It can be difficult to get paid on time at the start of employment with a new trust.
14 Trusts will transfer the money into your bank account by BACS transfer. These can take up to 3 working days.
15 Your taxable pay includes your basic pay and your banding supplement, less any pension contributions.
16 Don't get too excited by this number…
17 …and try not to get too sad about this one…
18 …because this is what you're going to have to spend until next month comes around.

Money and debt

As the average medical graduate debt now exceeds £24,000, and rising fast, financial management priorities have changed. This section is not comprehensive but aims to give some important pointers and warnings.

Debt clearance

Most graduates have three different types of debt:

(1) *Short-term* high-interest debts (eg credit cards ±overdraft, if at full charge). Pay these back first and as fast as possible. Try not to extend them just because you have an income

(2) *Medium-term* commercial loans (eg a high street bank graduate studies loan). These should be paid back next, as spare funds allow

(3) *Student-loans* at very low rates of interest – pay these back last.

Pay close attention to the annual percentage rate (APR) and charges attached to any loan arrangement. Interest-free loans or credit cards can help in the short term but ensure you don't get saddled with a high APR later. Loans are a competitive market so shop around – especially for something like a car loan where the car dealer rarely offers the best rate. Think 'total cost' not just 'monthly repayments'.

Some basic rules for financial planning

- *Short term* Clear debts with the highest interest as soon as possible
- *Medium term* Try to accumulate about one month's salary as 'emergency' savings
- *Long term* The NHS pension scheme remains the best available at present and you will be automatically enrolled in it unless you opt out. With this taken care of, you could think about trying to save for the deposit on a property (even if just £100/mth). With interest rates currently low, home ownership is an attractive option if you can raise a deposit. Bear in mind that there are large up-front costs to house buying (eg legal fees, stamp duty), you will be responsible for all maintenance and will not be able to take the property with you when you move to another part of the country.

Financial advice

Since you now have a salary increasing every year and virtually guaranteed for life, finance companies will swarm round you like wasps round jam. Beware of some very slick sharks – their aim is only to get you to buy their products. There is no altruism here:

- Truly independent financial advice is hard to obtain – ask how independent they really are
- Firms must now show what commission will be received for any product you choose, both to the individual who sold it to you as well as to their company
- Do not buy from the first or most persuasive salesperson, but take your time to consider what you really want and need.

Financial and other products

Critical illness cover and income protection See 📖 p11. Check if it still pays if you are capable of doing a less demanding job. Check if it pays for all conditions you may get at work.

Life insurance Pays out a lump sum if you die; only really makes sense if you have dependants.

Pension The NHS scheme is getting more expensive but still better than commercial alternatives. You should revisit your retirement planning at regular intervals through your career. You will also receive a state pension through your NI payments. You will also receive a state pension through your NI payments.

BMA Protection for non-clinical matters, eg wrong salary or poor accommodation; the trade union for doctors.

Tax

Now that you are earning a salary you will be paying tax. Most will be collected by PAYE (Pay As You Earn). If you have no other sources of income then you can leave it at that. If you have any other income then you should ask for a tax return and complete it.

Tax codes See 📖 p39.

Tax deductible It is possible to claim back the income tax you paid on:
• Job-related expenses (eg stethoscope); make sure you keep receipts
• Professional subscriptions eg GMC, BMA, MDU/MPS, Royal College
• Examination fees and course fees (previously not deductible, but HMRC has relented on this since 2012).

Tax reclaims may be made through full self-assessment, but this is not essential. If you pay tax through PAYE, simply send a letter to HM Revenue & Customs, Pay As You Earn, PO Box 1970 stating your name, NI number and detailing your professional expenses as listed above. You **must** also **include details of any additional, undeclared income, including cremation forms.** Your tax code for subsequent years will be adjusted accordingly.

Tax returns A tax return is an online form asking for details of all the money you have received which may have tax owing on it. This includes your salary and other income whether earned (eg locum shifts or cremation fees) or unearned (eg lodger/flatmate, bank interest and dividend yields).
• If you are asked to complete one then obtain a Government Gateway ID (www.gov.uk) and password. This takes time, don't leave it until January
• Fill it in on-line and the maths is done automatically
• Return it after 1st February you will be fined £100/6mth plus interest
• Claim your deductible allowances but also list your additional income.

The Inland Revenue has been known to ask an undertaker to list all payments to doctors and then cross-check. If your tax is simple then tax returns are not hard to do, otherwise pay a company/accountant to do it for you.

Documents to keep safe for at least 7 years

• P60 – sent every April to all employees
• P45 – sent to you every time you change trust
• Pay slips – issued every month – if electronic, then save copies
• Record of additional income – eg locums
• Annual interest statements from bank, savings/shares – issued annually.

NHS entitlements

As a doctor working in the NHS you have certain entitlements, defined under your 'Terms and Conditions of Service'. Those relating to salary are discussed in 'Pay and contracts' (📖 p36). Others are listed here. Your first point of contact for any questions is your local medical staffing department and the Foundation school. Always ask for copies of their written policies.

Accommodation
- Doctors in their first year after graduation are no longer entitled to free accommodation at their employing trust, except in Wales
- Rooms may well be available on site at a market rate and can be useful when attached to a trust for a short period that would otherwise make finding local accommodation difficult.

Leave entitlement
- You are entitled to a total of 27d/yr of paid leave or 9d/4mth. You are also entitled to all bank holidays in addition – or compensatory days off if you are scheduled to work on any part of a bank holiday
- If a compensatory day off eg after working nights, or pre-allocated annual leave falls on a bank holiday, you are entitled to an extra day off
- You are rarely allowed to carry leave over between jobs/years
- You will usually need to give 6wk notice for leave not pre-assigned; arrange this in good time and have your form signed by your consultant
- Many posts have 'fixed leave' instead of allowing you to choose when to take it. Swaps are often difficult; ask your consultant or colleagues
- If you need leave in a forthcoming post (eg getting married), write to let them know. Ask for the rota position which is off for those dates
- Study leave entitlements vary between Foundation schools, with some counting mandatory teaching sessions as taking place during study leave. Check local policy and discuss requests with your educational supervisor.

Maternity/paternity leave
- All women are entitled to up to 52wk of maternity leave and must be allowed to return to work after this. Those who have worked for the NHS for 26wk by the 15th wk before their due date are entitled to statutory maternity pay (SMP) of 90% of full pay for 6wk, and at £136.78 for 33wk (39wk total). In addition, if you have worked for the NHS for 12 continuous mth by the 11th wk before your due date, you receive occupational maternity pay for 8wk at your full time salary (during which you don't receive SMP) and 18wk at half pay (alongside SMP payments)
- Fathers are currently entitled to up to 2wk paid paternity leave if they have worked for over 6mth. New regulations relating to the transfer of parental leave between parents are due to come into force and you should consult local policies
- If you are absent from your F1 or F2 post for any reason for >4wk, you are unlikely to be signed off and will need to arrange to complete your training on your return. For practical reasons, your foundation school may ask you to repeat the whole year – ask your educational supervisor.

Less than full-time/flexible training
- Foundation Programme doctors are entitled to train less than full-time if they have a valid reason
- A comprehensive list of valid reasons (eg having a baby or ill health) and advice on how to apply is available from your Foundation school.

Specialty training

After the FP you need to apply for specialty training. You have three main choices:

- *Specialty training* (ST) or *Core-training* (CT), the majority of junior doctors will choose this route
- *Academic clinical fellowship* (ACF) for those interested in research (📖 p64 and www.nihrtcc.nhs.uk) The recruitment process takes place earlier in the year than for other posts so that those who are unsuccessful are not disadvantaged from applying to regular ST/CT posts
- *Locum appointment for Training/for Service* (LAT/LAS) single-year posts for specialty training for those who cannot commit to, or are unable to secure, a formal training rotation. LAT posts can count towards formal training requirements whereas LAS will offer experience but no formal training recognition. Posts are advertised and appointed locally, and may only be available in a highly restricted number of specialties.

Routes to CCT

The ultimate goal of all training programmes is the awarding of a Certificate of Completion of Training (CCT). This qualifies the doctor for entry to the Specialist or GP Register held by the GMC and entitles them to work as a consultant or GP. After leaving the foundation programme, there are two distinct paths to CCT:

Run-through training In certain specialties (eg paediatrics, GP, neurosurgery) competitive entry at ST1 leads to a 4–8yr **'run-through'** programme in one region (up to ST8 in some specialties), with no further competition points.

Core training In other specialties (eg medical training, most surgical specialties) competitive entry for 'core training' leads to a 2–3yr **'core training'**. Successful completion of this entitles the doctor to apply on a competitive basis for higher training (ST3/4 and above) in a related subspecialty, leading to CCT. Such specialties are said to be **'uncoupled'**.

The job titles for core-training are CT1, CT2 (and CT3 where used) depending on the year of training. If you apply to an uncoupled specialty, you will initially train via one of these routes:

- Acute Care Common Stem programmes (ACCS 📖 p46 – 3 years)
- Anaesthesia
- Core Medical Training (2 years)
- Core Psychiatry Training (3 years)
- Core Surgical Training (2 years)
- Broad Based Training (2 years) – a structured, core training programme newly introduced in 2013 and only available in a few regions; placements in medicine, GP, psychiatry and paediatrics lead to entry at CT2/ST2 level into 1 of these programmes, without further competition and in the same region.

CESR For those who do not follow a straightforward career path through to CCT, periods of time spent in training posts and experience gained may all be taken into consideration as part of an application to the GMC for a 'certificate of eligibility for specialist registration' (CESR). This route is especially useful for those who have spent considerable time overseas.

Specialty training applications

Recruitment process

The application process varies between specialties and is rapidly evolving. Most recruitment is organised nationally by the appropriate Royal College or a 'lead' LETB using a web-based application system. A small number of specialties still recruit through local applications. There is no limit to the number of specialties you can apply to, providing you fulfil the eligibility criteria set out in the 'person specification'. Begin preparing well in advance.

- *Choose a specialty/specialties* (🕮 p51) considering person specifications and competition rates available at specialtytraining.hee.nhs.uk
- *Check your eligibility* for applying to a training programme eg GMC registration, right to work in the UK, language skills, prior experience
- *Find suitable jobs* (🕮 p50) These will be advertised by recruitment offices according to a nationally agreed timetable
- *Complete the application form* paying close attention to deadlines. For several specialties, a single online application portal called Oriel is being developed
- *Wait* As applications are reviewed applicants are shortlisted for interview; in certain specialties (eg GP) a further assessment is used in shortlisting
- *Interview/selection centre* (🕮 p56) You should receive at least 5d notice, but this is not always adhered to; you need to bring a long list of supporting documentation, including your portfolio (🕮 p18). Formats will vary between a traditional panel based interview (eg core training programmes) or performing a number of exercises in front of assessors (eg GP)
- *Offers* are made electronically through the UK offers system according to a coordinated timetable. You will be asked to rank all LETBs where you would accept a job; successful applicants are then allocated to LETBs in score order (you will be allocated to your highest preference that still has places when your turn comes). You then have 48h to review offers and decide whether to accept, hold, or reject. You may also elect to receive automatic 'upgrades' if a higher ranking choice becomes available
- *Re-advertisement* to unfilled posts will take place in a 2nd application round. If you accept a job in round 1, you may still apply for a different post in round 2, but you need to inform all those concerned
- *Employment checks* and contract signing – remarkably NHS employers claim to need up to 2 months *after* you start work to get around to issuing a contract and some manage to miss even this. Speak to your BMA representative in the event of contract problems.

Unsuccessful applications

'If you can trust yourself when all men doubt you, But make allowance for their doubting too ... If you can dream – and not make dreams your master ... If you can meet with Triumph and Disaster And treat those two impostors just the same ... Yours is the Earth and everything that's in it, And – which is more – you'll be a Man, my son!'[1]

The nature of a competitive jobs field, is that not everyone will get their first choice post on first application. In this instance, a miss and a mile are very different entities and it is important that you ask for feedback to establish how far wide of the mark you were and whether you need to consider an application to a less competitive specialty. Discuss your options with your clinical and educational supervisors. Look and ask around for LAT and LAS posts advertised locally, and consider how else you may enhance your CV.

[1] Rudyard Kipling (1865–1936) 'If', first published in 'Rewards and Fairies' (1910).

Career structure

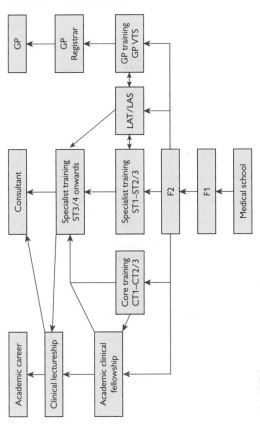

Fig. 1.2 Career structure for NHS doctors.

Specialty training options

There are 23 different training schemes that an F2 can apply to (shown in Table 1.4). On top of these there are:

- **Academic clinical fellowships** in most specialties with separate nationwide application procedures that take place in advance of the main recruitment process, so that unsuccessful candidates can still apply for a regular training post. Most ACFs allow for run-through training, even in specialties where uncoupling is the norm
- **LAT/LAS posts** in many specialties (generally just in run-through specialties). Applications may take place alongside or after the main application process at any point through the year.

Acute care common stem (ACCS)

For trainees with an interest in acute specialties ACCS provides a core 2yr experience in acute medicine, anaesthetics, emergency medicine, and critical care, with a further training year spent in one of three streams (acute medicine, anaesthetics, emergency medicine). Choice of stream is determined at the point of application to ACCS. Although the curricula and competences gained are transferable between ACCS streams, it is not possible to move between career paths without further competitive selection.

- *Acute medicine* CT1 and CT2 in ACCS specialties then a CT3 year spent in acute medicine. At the end of CT3 it is theoretically possible to switch specialties from acute medicine to a General Internal Medicine specialty
- *Anaesthetics* CT1 and CT2 in ACCS specialties then an extra CT2 year of anaesthetics; competitive entry to ST3 anaesthetics requires having passed the Primary FRCA (💷 p57). Anaesthetics can also be applied for directly as a 2yr core-training programme
- *Emergency medicine* CT1 and CT2 in ACCS specialties then a CT3 year of emergency medicine; competitive entry to ST4 emergency medicine requires having passed the MCEM (💷 p57).

General Practice Specialty Training

General practice has run-through training coordinated through a nationwide application. The application consists of four stages:

- Application form (establish eligibility)
- Computer-based testing (clinical problems and professional dilemmas)
- Assessment centre selection (communication and written exercises)
- Job allocation and offer.

Successful applicants undertake 18mth spent in hospital specialties, followed by 18mth as a GP registrar during which the MRCGP must be completed to join the GP register and get a job.

Core Surgery/Core Medical Training

These are popular uncoupled training schemes. You apply for core-training, with most deaneries allowing a choice of specific rotations only after successful appointment into post. After 2yr of core-training (CT1–CT2) there is a competitive application for ST3 in a specific surgical or medical specialty. To apply for ST3 in surgery you need full MRCS; for medical ST3 posts you need Part 1 of MRCP to apply, but need full MRCP by the date of starting your ST3 post. It should be possible to apply for specialties other than those in which you did your core-training if you can demonstrate appropriate competences; it helps if you can arrange taster weeks, audit or research in the subspecialty you are applying for.

Table 1.4 *Specialty training programmes at CT1/ST1 (2014)[1]*

Specialty	Recruitment contact details
Run-through specialties	
Academic clinical fellowships	National Institute for Health Research Trainees Coordinating Centre (NIHRTCC) www.nihrtcc.nhs.uk
Cardiothoracic surgery	Health Education Wessex wessex.hee.nhs.uk
Chemical pathology	Local recruitment – see individual deanery websites
Emergency medicine[2]	Health Education Yorkshire & the Humber yh.hee.nhs.uk
General practice	National Recruitment Office for GP Training gprecruitment.hee.nhs.uk
Histopathology	London Shared Services www.londondeanery.ac.uk
Medical microbiology	NHS Education for Scotland www.nes.scot.nhs.uk
Medical virology	NHS Education for Scotland www.nes.scot.nhs.uk
Neurosurgery	Health Education Yorkshire & the Humber yh.hee.nhs.uk
Obstetrics and gynaecology	Royal College of Obstetricians and Gynaecologists obsjobs.rcog.org.uk
Ophthalmology	Health Education South West southwest.hee.nhs.uk
MaxFax surgery[2]	Health Education South West southwest.hee.nhs.uk
Paediatrics and child health	Royal College of Paediatrics and Child Health www.rcpch.ac.uk
Public health	Health Education East Midlands em.hee.nhs.uk
Clinical radiology	London Shared Services www.londondeanery.ac.uk
Sexual health	Health Education East of England eoe.hee.nhs.uk
Uncoupled specialties	
ACCS – Acute medicine	Royal College of Physicians www.ct1recruitment.org.uk
ACCS – Anaesthetics	Health Education West Midlands wm.hee.nhs.uk
ACCS – Emergency medicine	London Shared Services www.londondeanery.ac.uk
Anaesthetics	Health Education West Midlands wm.hee.nhs.uk
Broad-based training	Health Education North West nw.hee.nhs.uk
Core medical training	Royal College of Physicians www.ct1recruitment.org.uk
Core surgical training	Health Education Kent, Surrey and Sussex kss.hee.nhs. uk and www.surgeryrecruitment.nhs.uk
Core psychiatry training	Health Education North West nw.hee.nhs.uk

[1] From **specialtytraining.hee.nhs.uk** – this website is the best starting point.
[2] New programmes being piloted in 2014.

Person specifications These list the required competences for that specialty. In making an application, you will need to provide evidence to prove that you have achieved the specified competences. Consult these as soon as you anticipate an application to a scheme so that you can see what you need to do. Full details are available at specialtytraining.hee.nhs.uk

If you are applying for an Academic Clinical Fellowship (ACF), you will need to meet the criteria in both the clinical person specification for your chosen specialty and level and the ACF person specification.

Specialty training competition

Competition for different specialties varies, as does competition for the same specialty in different parts of the country.

Competition ratios are published annually to allow applicants to view the previous year's ratios. These typically show the number of applications received for each specialty and the number of posts available; a competition ratio is derived by dividing the former (number of applications) by the latter (number of posts). This ratio roughly represents the number of people applying for each available post (see Table 1.5).

Only the highest scoring candidates will stand a chance at getting a job in specialties with a high competition ratio; for specialties with a lower competition ratio the applicant must still meet the minimum requirements for the job to be offered it. Remember that applicants can apply for multiple posts so the actual chances of getting a job are higher than the ratio shown.

In previous years, applicants have had to factor in not only competition ratios by specialty, but also by deanery. The move to national recruitment has removed this element – you can rank all deaneries/LETBs where you would be prepared to accept a job without disadvantaging your chances in any one region. After completion of the assessment process you will be ranked nationally, and assigned to your highest choice deanery that still has a vacancy when your turn in the queue comes.

That said, it is important to consider what your own priorities are. If you are adamant that you want to stay in one particular area of the country, you may need to recognise that the area may be very popular (eg London). Are you happy to pick a less popular specialty to increase your chances? Equally, if you are determined that you want to enter a highly competitive specialty, are you willing to pick a region potentially miles away from your current home as the competition there is much less? These are decisions which should be talked through with friends, family, mentors and your educational supervisor.

Specialty training in the UK

Although applications to specialty training are coordinated throughout the UK, within each of the four countries a degree of local structure remains.

- *England* specialtytraining.hee.nhs.uk
- *Northern Ireland* www.nimdta.gov.uk
- *Scotland* www.scotmt.scot.nhs.uk/
- *Wales* www.walesdeanery.org

Table 1.5 Competition ratios for CT1/ST1 applications (2013)[1]

Specialty	Applications	Posts	Competition Ratio	Fill rate
ACCS – Emergency medicine	534	203	2.6	100%
Anaesthetics	1189	478	2.5	100%
Broad-based training	429	52	8.3	82%
Cardiothoracics	68	6	11.3	100%
Radiology	751	185	4.1	100%
Core medical training	3088	1209	2.6	100%
Core psychiatric training	650	437	1.5	89%
Core surgical training	1296	676	1.9	99%
GP	6447	2787	2.3	99%
Histopathology	154	120	1.3	61%
Microbiology and virology	108	21	5.1	90%
Neurosurgery	183	37	4.9	89%
O&G	591	204	2.9	100%
Ophthalmology	323	71	4.5	100%
Paediatrics	793	360	2.2	100%
Public health	602	70	8.6	97%

[1] From **specialtytraining.hee.nhs.uk** – visit website for most recent data. Data is not available for all training programmes. Applications and posts are for Round 1 only and do not count subsequent re-advertisements. Competition ratio represents the number of applicants per post – bear in mind that candidates may apply for multiple training posts. Fill rate is the final number of posts in each specialty that were filled – including appointments made in additional rounds of re-advertisement.

Choosing a job

Once you have secured a training rotation, you still need to choose which specific jobs to do. There are also jobs outside of specialty training rotations (such as LAT/LAS posts) that have a local application process. This page gives ideas about how to find and choose jobs.

Priorities Before looking for a job, write a list of factors that matter to you in making this potentially life-changing decision. Important considerations include:

- *Partner/spouse* Can they get a job nearby?
- *Location* Could you move? How far would you commute?
- *Family/friends* How far away are you willing to go?
- *Career* Is the job in the right specialty/specialties?
- *Duration* Can you commit to several years in the same area?
- *Rota/pay* What banding and rota do you want or need?
- *Type of hospital* Large teaching hospital vs. district general.

If you have no firm career intentions then choose by location and rota since these will affect your life most over the next few months. Look for suitable jobs on www.jobs.nhs.uk, specialtytraining.hee.nhs.uk, deanery websites, or the *BMJ*.

Job offers A national timescale for FP and ST/CT job applications exists whereby all job offers are made at the same time. This allows you to accept the highest ranked job that you applied for. Bear in mind that you cannot change your job rankings after submitting your application.

Competition Medical jobs are competitive; it is important to maximise your chances of getting a job. Apply for several specialties; rank as many regions as possible; check competition ratios and person specifications (p49, specialtytraining.hee.nhs.uk); consider a back-up choice, eg a less competitive specialty or region. A good CV also helps (p54).

Researching a job Adverts rarely give a true reflection of a job. Phone up hospitals within the region and ask to speak to the person doing the job at the moment. Quiz them on the types of placements available, hours, support, teaching, conditions, and what their interview was like. Would they accept the job again?

Contacts With human resource departments and structured interviews, the days of jobs being just a consultant phone call away have gone. There is no doubt that some networking still occurs, with mixed results. Senior contacts are useful for tailored career guidance, CV advice, and giving realistic views of where your CV can get you.

Accepting a job With a move towards unified, online application processes, strict and automated rules are essential to ensure a rapid and fair allocation to posts. In order to allow for choice, under certain circumstances it may be possible to accept, or hold, an offer, and later upgrade, or apply to a different post, providing you notify all those concerned. Outside of this formal process, it is unacceptable to turn down a post you have already accepted unless you have an extremely good reason. The GMC take a clear position on your obligation to protect patient care by not compromising the recruitment process in this way, though notice periods vary by seniority.

Specialties in medicine

The Certificate of Completion of Training (CCT) can be awarded in numerous specialties shown as follows. A selection of subspecialties are also shown with bullet points:

Allergy

Anaesthesia
- Paediatric anaesthesia
- Obstetric anaesthesia
- Pain management

Acute medicine

Audiological medicine

Cardiology

Cardiothoracic surgery

Chemical pathology

Child and adolescent psychiatry

Clinical genetics

Clinical neurophysiology

Clinical oncology

Clinical pharmacology

Clinical radiology
- Interventional radiology

Dermatology

Emergency medicine (EM)

Endocrinology and diabetes

Forensic psychiatry

Gastroenterology
- Hepatology

General adult psychiatry
- Addictions psychiatry
- Liaison psychiatry
- Rehabilitation psychiatry

General internal medicine

General practice

General surgery
- Breast surgery
- Colorectal surgery
- Upper GI surgery
- Vascular surgery

Genitourinary medicine

Geriatric medicine
- Stroke
- Orthogeriatrics

Haematology

Histopathology
- Forensic pathology

Immunology

Infectious diseases

Intensive care medicine

Medical microbiology and virology

Medical oncology

Medical ophthalmology

Medical psychotherapy

Neurology

Neurosurgery

Nuclear medicine

Obstetrics and gynaecology
- Materno-foetal medicine
- Gynaecological oncology
- Urogynaecology

Occupational medicine

Old age psychiatry

Ophthalmology

Oral and maxillo-facial surgery

Otolaryngology (ENT surgery)

Paediatric surgery

Paediatrics
- Community paediatrics
- Neonatology
- Oncology

Palliative medicine

Pharmaceutical medicine

Plastic surgery

Psychiatry of learning disability

Public health medicine

Rehabilitation medicine

Renal medicine

Respiratory medicine

Rheumatology

Sport and exercise medicine

Sexual health and reproductive medicine

Trauma and orthopaedic surgery
- Hand surgery
- Spinal surgery

Tropical medicine

Urology.

For more details on the career options available to doctors, including all of the above, see So You Want To Be A Brain Surgeon? (Eccles and Sanders, OUP, 2008).

Your curriculum vitae

What is a CV? This is a Latin phrase which means 'course of life'. In modern days it means a document by which you advertise yourself to a potential employer: a summary of you.

When will I use a CV? You will need a CV for many of the jobs you will apply for after graduating. If you join a locum agency, they will use your CV when finding you work. You should also upload your current CV to your ePortfolio in advance of every annual review.

What is included in a CV? The most important information to include are your contact details, a list of your qualifications (those already acquired and those you are studying for), any outstanding achievements, a summary of your employment to date, and the details of your referees. Other information can be included, but do not overcrowd your CV.

CV philosophy Your CV should not be a static piece of work, it should evolve with you and reflect your changing skills and attitudes. It is important to keep your CV up to date, and from time to time reformat it to freshen it up. Use your CV to demonstrate how you have learnt from your experiences rather than just listing them; a potential employer will be much more impressed if you indicate you learnt about the importance of clear communication whilst working at a holiday resort, than by the actual job itself.

Getting help Human resource departments and educational supervisors can give advice on writing a CV, and often you can find people's CVs or templates on the internet by searching for 'CV'. Try to keep your CV individualised, so do not simply copy someone else's template.

Before writing your CV Ascertain what a potential employer is looking for when sending in your CV; check the essential and desirable criteria and try to echo these. You need to alter the emphasis in your CV to match the position you are applying for, eg highlighting your communication skills or leadership experience.

Layout Your CV should look impressive; for many jobs hundreds of CVs are received and yours must stand out. It needs to be clearly laid out and easy to follow. The key information and your most important attributes should stand out prominently. Think about the layout before you start writing.

Length Two sides of A4 paper are ideal for a basic CV (and an optional front page); add more as your career progresses.

Remember For most jobs, the candidates applying will have very similar qualifications and so the only way you may stand out to be short-listed for interview is via your CV. Make it as interesting as possible, without it looking ludicrous.

Personal details Name, address which you use for correspondence, contact telephone numbers (home, work, mobile) and email address are essential. You must state your type of GMC membership (full/provisional) and number. Stating gender, date of birth, marital status, nationality, and other information is optional.

Personal statement This is very much an optional section. Some feel it gives you an opportunity to outline a little about yourself and where you see yourself in 10yr; others feel it is an irritating waste of space.

Education List your qualifications in date order, starting with the most recent or current and progressing backwards in time. Indicate where each was undertaken, the dates you were there, and grade. Highlight specific courses or modules of interest. GCSE and A-level results are less important once you have graduated.

Employment and work experience List the placements you have undertaken during the F1 and F2 years starting with the most recent. Include the dates, specialty, your supervising consultant, and address of the employer; consider adding key skills that you attained.

Interests An optional section which gives you a chance to outline what you like to do outside of medicine. A well-written paragraph here can show potential employers that you are interesting as well as intelligent.

Publications If you have not yet got your name in print try to get a letter in a medical journal (📖 p58). If you have got publications put the most recent first; ensure they are referenced in a conventional style (see www.pubmed.com for examples).

Referees Your referees should know your academic record as well as your ability to interact with others. State their relationship to you (such as personal tutor) and give contact address, telephone number, and email address. Ensure they are happy to provide a reference, give them a copy of your CV, and tell them when you are applying for jobs.

Headers and footers Having the month and year in either a header or footer shows the reader you keep it up to date.

Photographs Some people include a small passport-sized photograph of themselves near the start of their CV; this is optional but not necessarily recommended. Why should your physical appearance be of relevance for selection for any job outside fashion and media?

The finished CV Use the spell-checker and get a tutor or friend to read over it to identify mistakes and make constructive criticism; be prepared to make numerous alterations to get it right.

Technical points Use just one clear font throughout. To highlight text of importance use the <u>underline</u>, **bold** or *italic* features. When printing your CV use good quality white paper and a laser printer if possible.

The covering letter Whenever you apply for a job, you must send a covering letter with your CV and application form. This should be short and to the point. Indicate the position you are applying for and briefly say why the job appeals to you, and highlight why you are suitable for the job.

Post-Foundation Programme CV

Name:	Charles J Flint
Address:	14 Abbeyvale Crescent
	McBurney's Point
	McBurney
	McB1 7RH
Home:	0111 442 985
Mobile:	0968 270 250
Work:	0111 924 9924 bleep 1066
Email:	charles.flint@mcburney.ac.uk
Date of birth:	12 June 1991
GMC:	0121231 (full)

Personal statement

I am an outgoing doctor with an enthusiastic yet mature outlook. I have strong communication skills and experience of working independently, both as a team member and leader. I am conscientious, trustworthy, quick to learn, and to employ new skills. My long-term aim is to practise an acute specialty within the hospital environment.

Education

2008–2013
University of McBurney, McBurney's Point, McB1 8PQ
MBChB: 2013
BMedSci (Hons):   Upper Second Class, 2011

Employment history

3 Apr 15–to date	F2 to Miss Broom, Emergency Medicine
	McBurney Royal Infirmary
5 Dec 14–2 Apr 15	F2 to Dr Fungi, Microbiology
	McBurney Royal Infirmary
31 Jul 14–4 Dec 14	F2 to Dr Golfer, General Practice
	Feelgood Health Centre, Speakertown
3 Apr 14–30 Jul 14	F1 to Mr Grimshaw, General Surgery
	McBurney City Hospital
5 Dec 13–2 Apr 14	F1 to Dr Mallory, Gastroenterology
	McBurney City Hospital
31 Jul 13–4 Dec 13	F1 to Dr Haler, Respiratory Medicine
	McBurney City Hospital

Postgraduate clinical experience

During my F1 year I developed my clinical and practical skills and became confident with the day-to-day organisation of emergency and elective admissions in both medicine and surgery.

Since commencing F2 I have built upon these skills and now appreciate the wider role of the doctor in the smooth running of acute admissions and liaison with the community teams prior to, and after, hospital discharge.

Formal skills I have include:
- ALS provider (2013)
- Basic surgical skills, including suturing and fracture management.

Research and audit

- I am currently involved in a research project comparing capillary blood gas analysis with arterial blood gases in acute asthmatics
- I undertook an audit of antibiotic prescribing on surgical wards to investigate whether patients were being managed in accordance with trust guidelines. I presented the data at a departmental meeting and repeated the audit after 2 months, demonstrating increased compliance
- During my SSM I was involved in research investigating the role of caffeine upon platelet aggregation.

Interests

I am a keen rock and ice climber and have continued to improve my grade since leaving university. I have organised several climbing trips to Scotland and one to the Alps. I am interested in medical journalism and have spent a week in the editorial office of the *International Journal of Thrombophlebitis*.

Publications

- **Flint CJ**. Letter: Student debt. *Medical Students' Journal* 2013; **35**(2): 101
- **Flint CJ** and West DJ. Multiple Sclerosis in social class three. *Journal of Social Medicine* 2013; **12**(9): 118
- Lee S, **Flint CJ** and West DJ. Caffeine as an activator of platelet aggregation. *International Journal of Thrombophlebitis* 2011; **54**(3): 99.

References

- Dr Ian Haler, Educational Supervisor, Department of Respiratory Medicine, McBurney's Medical Centre, McBurney's Point, McBurney, McB1 7TS Tel 0111 924 9924 ext 2370. ian.haler@mcburney.ac.uk
- Mr Ivor Grimshaw, Educational Supervisor, Department of General Surgery, McBurney's Medical Centre, McBurney's Point, McBurney, McB1 7TS Tel 0111 924 9924 ext 4637. ivor.grimshaw@mcburney.ac.uk

Interviews

Interview preparation Employers must allow you time off to attend the interview itself; try to give them as much notice as possible. Look at the recruitment website for information about interview format, questions and what to bring; try to talk to previous applicants.

Interview day Arrive at the interview with plenty of time, allow for all sorts of delays on the roads or train, even if this means you have to read the newspaper for an hour. Relax and be yourself with the other candidates before you are called in; most of them will have similar qualifications and experience as yourself and will be just as nervous. Dress smartly in a simple suit and tie for men and suit for women (trouser or skirt). You will normally receive specific instructions as to what documentation to bring, which you should follow exactly; as a minimum, bring a copy of your CV (📖 p52) and a summary printout from your ePortfolio (📖 p8).

The interview Relax. The worst that can happen is that you are not offered the job, which is not the end of the world. The format of interviews varies, but there are usually 2–3 interviewers; introduce yourself to all the panel and wait to be offered a seat. For some posts there will be a series of panels, each with a different brief (eg CV verification, clinical scenarios, personal skills), and you will rotate between panels. Take a few moments to think about the questions before answering and ask for a question to be rephrased if you don't understand it. Always make good eye contact with all members of the panel and be aware of your own body language.

Common questions It is impossible to predict the questions you will be asked, but they are likely to include questions about your portfolio, relevant clinical scenarios, and current medical news/issues. Many questions have no correct answer and test your communication skills, common sense, and ability to think under pressure:
- Talk us through your portfolio; what are you most proud of on it?
- What is missing from your portfolio?
- What qualities can you offer our training programme?
- Why have you chosen a career in …?
- What do you understand by 'clinical governance'?
- Tell us about your audit. Why is audit important?
- If you were the Secretary for Health, where would your priorities lie?
- How would you manage … (specific clinical scenario)?
- Where do you see yourself in 5, 10 years time?
- If you were the CT1 in the hospital alone at night and you were struggling with a clinical problem, what would you do?
- Tell us about your teaching experiences. What makes a good teacher?

Clinical scenarios Interviewers should not ask you specific medical questions (eg what is the dose of …); they can pose scenarios to discuss your management of a situation. These often focus on key issues like communication, prioritisation, calling for senior help when appropriate, multidisciplinary teams, clinical safety. For some specialties, a few formal OSCE-style stations may be included – you should be told about this in advance.

Results and feedback If you are unsuccessful, try to obtain some verbal or written feedback about how you could improve your CV or your interview skills. Remember there are always medical jobs so you will find something.

Membership exams

To progress beyond through the ST years you will need to complete the membership exams of your chosen specialty and meet the appropriate level of competency. The exams are difficult (often only ~30% of candidates pass per exam) and expensive (though often tax deductible 📖 p41). Most membership exams take place 2–3 times a year. You need to apply about 2–4mth before each exam. In the past, Foundation doctors have received advice *not* to sit membership examinations – this may well allow focus on other areas of development but you may then miss early opportunities to start building this aspect of your CV.

Medicine Regional examination centres throughout UK and overseas; all centres use the same exams. The MRCP has three sections:
- *Part 1 Written* basic science, £419, ≥12mth after graduation
- *Part 2 Written* clinical, £419, <7yr since Part 1
- *PACES* clinical skills, £657, <7yr since Part 1.

You need to have already passed Part 1 to *apply* for a medical ST3 post, and pass all parts of MRCP in order to *commence* such a post.

Surgery Regional examination centres throughout UK and overseas; all centres use the same exams. The MRCS has two parts, you are permitted 6 attempts to pass Part A, and 4 attempts to pass part B:
- *Part A MCQ (Basic sciences and Principles of Surgery in General)*, £493, eligible from graduation
- *Part B OSCE* £894, eligible after part A.

To apply for an ST3 position in surgery you need to have completed the entire MRCS.

General practice You need to be a GP registrar to take the MRCGP exams. There are three parts and no time limits though the GP registrar post is a year long; 10% fee reductions apply to associate RCGP members:
- *AKT* (written exam) £517
- *CSA* (clinical skills) OSCE stations, £1737
- *ePortfolio* similar to the FP portfolio. Access costs £611, but is free amongst other benefits for RCGP members (£163 registration, plus £369 annual cost).

You need to complete the MRCGP to become a GP.

Other membership exams in the Foundation years
Emergency medicine (MCEM) Three-part exam (two written and one clinical) required to apply for ST4. Part A may be sat as early as F1, but all parts must be passed within 4 years of first *sitting* Part A (not passing)
Anaesthetics (FRCA) Full primary (MCQ and OSCE) exam only open to anaesthetic trainees, though F1 and F2 doctors can attempt MCQ component. Applications to ST3 are only permitted when all parts of the primary FRCA are passed
Obstetrics and Gynaecology (MRCOG) Part 1 (written) eligible after graduation; part 2 (written + OSCE) after further 2yr O+G experience
Pathology MRCPath normally completed during ST
Paediatrics (MRCPCH) 3 written papers (attempted in any order after graduation); clinical exam after 12mth paeds experience and passing all written
Radiology (FRCR) Can only be attempted after gaining training post
Psychiatry (MRCPsych) Can only be attempted after gaining training post.

Continuing your education

Educational requirements You will be assessed throughout the FP to ensure that you are developing as a doctor and learning new skills. This will be done by Foundation assessments (📖 p8), your ePortfolio (📖 p8), meetings with your clinical supervisor, informal feedback from ward staff, presentations and attendance at teaching sessions. These assessments should not be difficult but it is essential that you complete them.

Study leave There is no formal provision for study leave for the F1 year; in the F2 year you will be offered the chance to spend taster weeks in specialties of your choice. You may be allowed study leave for specific courses but this will be at the discretion of your clinical supervisor and policies vary widely between Foundation schools.

Study expenses F2s may get a study leave budget of £300–400 per 12mth though again this varies by Foundation school. Check with your postgraduate centre. You can only use the money for recognised courses and revision courses; never for sitting membership examinations.

Postgraduate courses There are hundreds of these and the costs range from free to >£1000 per day, most are about £100–150 per day. During the FP years Advanced Life Support (ALS) is important and may be compulsory. Check the BMJ advert section for potential courses and try to speak to other people who have done the course.

Exam planning Once you have decided on a career plan (📖 p51), you will need to consider taking the appropriate membership examination. Membership exams are difficult and expensive but essential for career progression, so start early. See 📖 p57 or the relevant Royal College website (📖 p600) for more detail.

Getting published

Having publications on your CV will give you a huge advantage when applying for jobs. It will be far easier to understand what sort of thing journals are looking for if you read a few regularly. There are many ways to get your name in print and you don't have to write a book (which is not great for the social life).

- *Book reviews* Get in touch with a journal and express interest in reviewing books for them; you don't have to be a professor to give an opinion on whether a book reads well or is useful
- *Case reports* If you see something interesting, rare, or just very classical then try writing it up. Include images if possible; get a senior co-author and ensure you obtain patient consent in line with the journal's policy
- *Fillers* Some journals have short stories or funny/moving one-liners submitted by their readers. Write up anything you see which others might be interested in; ensure you obtain patient consent
- *Letters* If an article is incorrect, fails to mention a key point or has relevance in another field then write to the journal and mention this; it might be worthwhile asking a senior colleague to co-author it with you
- *Research papers* If you have participated in research make sure you get your name on any resulting publications. If your audit project had particularly interesting results you may be able to publish it.

Audit

Audit is simply comparing practice in your hospital with best practice or clinical guidelines. There are six main stages to the 'audit cycle':
(1) Define standards (eg replace cannulas every 72h)
(2) Collect data (duration of placement for 50 consecutive cannulas)
(3) Compare data to standards (87% of cannulas replaced in 72h)
(4) Change practice (present data to colleagues and propose new approaches, eg date of placement written on cannula dressings)
(5) Review standards (replace cannulas every 72h unless final dose in 2h)
(6) Reaudit (repeat data collection after 3mth – has anything changed?).
Without reaudit the cycle is not complete and those assessing your audit will look for evidence of this.

Why does audit matter? The aim of audit is to improve the quality of patient care; it allows a unit to applaud areas of strength and improve areas of weakness. Audits will also benefit you as an FP doctor since they are important in job applications and interviews and without at least one it will be hard to get an ST job. Try to do ≥2 during your FP.

Choosing an audit Almost any aspect of hospital/ward life can be audited. Choose something simple that interests you; alternatively look at relevant guidelines and choose one that is simple to measure.

Defining standards Try searching the National Library for Guidelines (accessible via www.library.nhs.uk); alternatively define best practice yourself by asking seniors and supervisors about what is expected.

Collecting data The simpler your audit the quicker and easier this will be. There are many ways of doing this including checking clinical notes, questionnaires, and monitoring activities yourself. Try to make your methods objective so that you do the same for every set of notes/subject.

Compare data to standards The method for doing this depends on the type of data you have collected; it is easy to do some simple statistical tests on data – seek advice from your educational supervisor or other seniors.

Change practice Try to present your audit to relevant clinicians, eg an FP teaching session or a ward meeting; use your findings to propose feasible changes to practice and discuss these with the audience.

Review standards You may feel that the original standards you defined are still suitable; alternatively the process of auditing may have shown you that these standards need updating.

Close the loop Repeat the data collection to see if the changes to practice have made a difference; it is a good way to stay in touch with old wards and looks fantastic on a CV.

Example audits A few ideas:
- Are ECGs performed within 20min in ED patients with chest pain?
- Are drugs prescribed in accordance with local guidelines?
- Do all patients have appropriate thromboprophylaxis prescribed?
- Do patients admitted with chest pain have their cholesterol measured?

Presentations and teaching

The thought of having to give an oral presentation provokes anxiety in most of us. Being able to relay information to an audience is a valuable skill and one which gets easier with time and experience, though it is helped by a logical approach.

Types of presentation There are four main types of presentation: audit/research, journal club (critical appraisal of research), case presentation, and a teaching session.

When is the presentation? If you have months to prepare then you can really go to town, whilst if you have only a few hours you need to concentrate on the essentials.

How long should it last? A 5min presentation will still need to be thorough, but less detailed than that lasting an hour. The length of the presentation will also aid you in choosing the topic.

What is the topic? Clarify as early as possible the topic you are to present and any specific aspect of the topic you should be discussing. If you can choose the topic, select something you either know about or are interested in researching.

Audience Are you presenting to your peers, your seniors or juniors? Are they ignorant of the topic or world experts? This information will determine the level of depth you need to go into.

Venue and means of delivery How far away is the audience, how big is the screen? (so all your text and diagrams are clear). Will you use your laptop or their computer? Back up on memory stick in current as well as 2003 version of PowerPoint.

Sources of information Do you already have books on the subject? Read about the topic on the internet by undertaking a search with a website such as www.bmj.com. Search *PubMed* using keywords; recent review articles are a good place to start.

If there is no information If you cannot find enough information then it is likely you are not searching correctly; ask library staff for help. If there really is a lack of information then consider changing the topic, or choose an easier approach to it.

How many slides? This depends on how much detail is present on each slide. On average 20–25 slides will last about 30min.

Slide format Don't get too clever. Slides should be simple; avoid borders and complex animation. PowerPoint has numerous pre-set designs, though remember it is the content of your talk the audience needs to be focused upon. Consider using a remote slide advance device (<£15).

Presentation format The presentation is in essence an essay which the speaker delivers orally. It should comprise a title page with the topic, speaker's name and an introduction which states the objectives. The bulk of the presentation should then follow and be closed with either a summary or conclusion. Consider ending with a slide acknowledging thanks and a final slide with simply 'Questions?' written on it to invite discussion.

Titles Give each slide a title to make the story easy to follow.

Font Should be at least size 24. Ensure the text colour contrasts with the background colour (eg yellow text on blue background). Avoid using lots of effects; stick to one or two colours, **bold**, *italics*, or <u>underline</u> features.

Graphics Use graphics to support the presentation; do not simply have graphics adorning the slide to make it look pretty.

How much information Avoid overcrowding slides; it is better to use three short slides than one hectic one. Each slide should deliver one message and this should be in six bullet points or less.

Bullet points Use to highlight key words, not full sentences.

PowerPoint effects Keep slides simple. Avoid text flying in from all directions and don't use sound effects as these distract the audience.

Rehearsing Go through the presentation a few times on your own so you know the sequence and what you are going to say. Then practise it in front of a friend to check timing and flow.

Specific types of presentation

Audit/research Ensure you give a good reason why the audit or research was chosen and what existing research has already been undertaken. State your objectives, your method, and its limitations. Use graphs to show numerical data and clearly summarise your findings. Discuss limitations and how your audit/research may have been improved. Draw your conclusions and indicate where further research may be directed. Thank the appropriate parties and invite questions/discussion. See audit/research section, 📖 p59/64.

Journal club Begin with a brief explanation of why you have chosen to discuss the particular clinical topic and list the articles which you have appraised. Aim to include why the study was undertaken, the appropriateness of the study, the methods and statistics used, the validity of the study, and make comparisons between different studies. Include latest guidelines and invite discussion regarding how the research may affect current clinical practice. Finish with a summary of the studies undertaken, their results, and where they were published for future reference.

Case presentation The presentation should tell a story about a patient and let the audience try and work out the diagnosis as though they are clerking the patient for the first time. Name the talk something cryptic, eg 'Headache in the traveller'. Refer to your patient by initials only and make sure patient details are blanked on all images and test results. Present the history and physical examination. Invite audience suggestions for the diagnosis and management. Give the results of investigations and again invite the audience to comment. Give the diagnosis and discuss subsequent management. Summarise with an outline of the topic and management; end with a question/discussion session.

Teaching session It is helpful to base a topic around a patient if this is appropriate. Keep the session interactive; have question slides where the audience can discuss answers. Summarise with learning points; it is helpful to provide a hand-out of your slides for people to take away (📖 p63).

Giving the presentation

Equipment Ensure that the projector/computer you need will be available well in advance. Ideally check it works and leave enough time to find new equipment if there is a problem.

Timing Arrive early and check your slides project correctly. Leave the title page projected so the correct audience attends.

Speaking You need to talk loudly enough to be heard at the back of the room. This can be daunting, but a good presentation given inaudibly is more disappointing than a poor presentation delivered audibly.

Body language Stand at the front of the audience and avoid walking into the projected image. Direct your talk at the audience, not the screen. This makes you appear more confident and also allows you to gauge if people are confused or bored. Try to make eye contact with everyone in the room.

Beginning Introduce yourself and your position, outline the topic you are going to talk about, and explain why you chose the topic. This is a good time to interact with the audience; ask if people at the back can hear you.

To use notes or not You should not need notes to prompt you but have them available; points on the slides should be enough.

Style Keep it professional, but show you are human; it is acceptable to be light-hearted and make the audience laugh.

Pacing You probably speak quicker than you think; take your time, pause and allow the audience to read all your points.

Questions Decide in advance if you would like questions to be asked during your presentation or at the end. Anticipate what questions may be asked and prepare for these. Do not be afraid to say you do not know the answer, though offer to find out.

Feedback

Whenever possible ask for constructive criticism from someone who saw your presentation and try to learn from their comments. Consider using the presentation for a formal 'Developing the clinical teacher' assessment (📖 p9).

Summary of points for a good presentation
• Plan well in advance
• Keep slides simple, avoid unnecessary graphics
• Rehearse your talk
• Try to stay calm and speak clearly
• Look at the audience, not the screen
• Thank the audience for attending.

Teaching medical students

Teaching will benefit you as much as the recipient; it will challenge you to fill any gaps in your knowledge and organise your thinking on the subject. You may not feel that you know enough to teach medical students but you are probably the best teacher on the ward for them, for two reasons:

- You have recently passed the finals exam that they are trying pass, often at the same medical school
- Finals are meant to test core medical knowledge; this is what you do every day when you clerk and manage a patient.

Portfolio Keep a record of teaching sessions, ideally with feedback (consider using a simple online survey tool). At least once a year you will need to complete a 'Developing the clinical teacher' form assessment (📖 p9).

Teaching principles

Whatever information you are trying to convey it is important to follow a few simple guidelines:

- Be clear about your objectives
- Plan what you are going to teach to give it structure
- Be interactive; this means that the students do some of the work and also are more likely to remember it
- Try not to use too much medical jargon
- Give relevant examples
- Check the students' understanding throughout and invite questions.

Suitable patients

One of the worst parts of being a medical student is finding suitable patients to take a history from or examine. You can use your patient lists (📖 p17) and first-hand experience of the patients to guide medical students to conscious, orientated, and friendly folk or those with clinical signs. Better still, offer to introduce the student.

Clinical examination

Offer to watch the student examine a patient and give feedback on their technique. You are likely to examine more patients in your first month as a doctor than in all your years as a medical student so your clinical skills will have advanced very quickly.

FP applications

With all the recent changes to medical training many students feel bewildered about what lies ahead. Once again you are in the ideal position to advise since you have already successfully applied for the FP. Simple advice about which are the best jobs, how to fill in the application form, or even showing a copy of your own form can be a great help.

Clinical approach

You can also teach 'how to be a doctor' type skills that are rarely passed on. The trick is to choose a simple subject you know lots about, eg:

- Managing chest pain/breathlessness
- Fluid management and volume assessment
- Writing in notes.

Research and academia

Research Whatever direction you see your future career heading in, the opportunity to undertake a period of research will help you gain insight into this vital area that underpins all of medical practice as well as to develop the skills necessary to understand research output. You don't need to cure cancer – often the most successful projects are those that set out to answer a simple, well formulated question.

Academia is not turning your back on clinical medicine, but rather adding a new dimension to your clinical experience: most academic doctors do research alongside clinical work. There are many advantages (interest, worldwide conferences, really understanding your subject, making a difference) but pay is not one of them. There are various training routes for academics detailed as follows – there is no one single way in; if at any stage you want to do research or a PhD there are always opportunities if you look and ask.

Foundation years There are small numbers of 2yr academic Foundation Programmes (📖 p5). These are often a normal F1 year with a 4mth academic attachment in F2 (eg academic rheumatology); a few have academic components scattered throughout F2 ± F1.

ST years There are also academic ST positions called Academic Clinical Fellowships. Most of these are available for entry either at ST1 or ST3 level and are 2–3yr long, including clinical rotations alongside 25% of working time set aside for academia. The first year will be almost entirely clinical; the purpose of the second and third years is to give you the opportunity to design a PhD/MD research project, generate preliminary data and apply for funding. Once you successfully get funding you enter the Training Fellowship.

Training fellowship This is a 3yr research project designed by yourself with the aim of getting a PhD (or alternatively a 1–2yr MD) with small amounts of protected clinical time to maintain your skills.

Clinical lectureship With a PhD/MD under your belt you can apply for a 3–4yr lectureship post. This will give you clinical experience whilst training to consultant level, and allow you to pursue postdoctoral research interests. You will again need to apply for funding, eg a Clinician Scientist Fellowship. Once you have completed this post you will be eligible for consultant or senior lecturer positions.

Finding a project Although some academic posts will come with funding already tied to a specific laboratory or project, the most rewarding projects are often those that you design yourself, together with a senior academic mentor. It is important to speak to a range of people and read and discuss broadly. Keep three things in mind: (1) Do I get on with the supervisor and have other clinicians had good experiences in the group? (2) Does the project interest me? (3) Where will the project lead? (eg will you be able to apply for the career or subspecialty that you want?).

Funding One of the challenges of academic medicine is that you often need to raise funding to pay for yourself and your research. The process can take time (eg >6mth) and involves filling in multiple forms. Always talk to your potential supervisor for advice on best options.

Life on the wards

The medical team

The changes to medical training have caused widespread confusion about the names and roles of different trainees. The medical team or 'firm' usually consists of four grades: (1) consultant-level, (2) registrar-level, (3) SHO-level, (4) F1 (house officer). Many firms have more than one doctor at each level so you may work alongside other F1s under two or more consultants.

Consultant-level

These are the most senior doctors on the team; there are several posts at this level:

- *Academic* Doctors who split their time between research and clinical medicine. They are often called 'honorary consultants' alongside an academic grade (eg senior lecturer, reader, professor)
- *Consultant* The most common post at this level is reached by obtaining the CCT (📖 p43), formerly known as the CCST, or via proof of equivalent training known as the CESR.
- *Associate specialist* A doctor with consultant-level ability and experience who has not got a CCST/CCT/CESR. They do not have the accountability or management commitments of consultants.

> *Consultant role* Consultants are responsible for everything that happens on the ward including the actions of junior doctors. They may lead ward rounds, work in clinics, supervise a laboratory, or spend time in theatre; their level of involvement in the day-to-day running of the ward varies between specialties and management styles. They will perform your FP appraisals (📖 p25) and are a good source of advice for careers, audits, and presentations. If ever you need help and only the consultant is available then do not hesitate to contact them.

Registrar-level If you describe yourself as 'a registrar' most people will assume that you are at this grade. All of these doctors will share an on-call rota that is usually separate from the SHO-level on-call rota. The posts have a natural hierarchy according to experience:

- *Specialist registrar (SpR)* Doctors training under the old system; virtually none of these remain, but you will still hear the term
- *Staff grade/specialty doctor* A non-training post with equivalent experience to an SpR but not working towards a CCT award
- *Clinical fellow* A specialty doctor who is undertaking research; they may need to secure an ST3/4 post afterwards
- *Clinical lectureship* The academic equivalent of ≥ST3/4 they will split their time between clinical and research
- *Senior specialty training registrar (StR, ≥ST3/4)* In most specialties this grade starts at ST3; however it is ST4 in emergency medicine, paediatrics, and psychiatry. These are posts that work towards the CCT award and a consultant post.

> *Registrar role* These doctors supervise the day-to-day running of the ward; they perform similar jobs to consultants (ward rounds, clinics, theatre) but without the management responsibilities. Registrars usually receive referrals from other teams and will spend time reviewing these patients. Their presence on the ward varies between specialties.

SHO-level Like the registrar-level position there are a range of posts performing similar roles with a hierarchy of experience:

- *Academic clinical fellow (ACF)* The academic equivalent of ST1–2/3 and CT1–2/3 at this level they will perform a similar role except that they have 25% of their time set aside for research. The situation can be confused in certain posts where the ACFs are appointed at ST3 level
- *Junior specialty training registrar (StR, ST1–2/3)* Doctors in specialties with run-through training (📖 p43) who will progress to registrar-level specialist training unless they fail to attain competencies or exams. Despite the title it is misleading to call them 'a registrar'
- *Core-training (CT1–2/3)* Doctors in specialties with uncoupled training (📖 p43) who can apply for registrar-level specialist training posts if they attain the relevant competencies and exams. The difference between ST and CT posts is the specialty, not experience
- *Fixed-term specialty training appointment (FTSTA)* A post for doctors who were unwilling or unable to secure an ST/CT post. The post lasts 1 year and will be at ST1, ST2, or ST3 level; at the end of the year they can apply for an ST or FTSTA post at the next level if they have attained the relevant competencies
- *F2* doctors in the second year of the Foundation Programme; this will often be their first experience in the specialty and at SHO level. At the end of the year they will apply for ST/CT/FTSTA posts.

> **SHO role** These doctors are your first port of call for help. They can advise on patient management, ward jobs, and supervise practical procedures; they often work alongside F1s on the ward though they may have clinic and theatre commitments too. They are an excellent source of advice on careers, applications, exams, and training courses.

F1-level These are doctors in their first year with limited registration. They are still often called house officers or PRHOs from the old system.

> **F1 role** F1s manage the day-to-day running of the ward including ward rounds, ward jobs, procedures, and reviewing unwell patients; see 📖 p69 for more detail.

The multidisciplinary team

Nurses have a 'hands-on' role, ranging from administering medications to attending doctors' rounds. Don't be afraid to ask their advice – their experience means they can often help you out. Most can take blood and perform ECGs, some can cannulate and insert male urinary catheters (all female nurses should be able to insert female catheters).

Bed managers are highly stressed people who are in charge of managing the hospital beds and arranging transfers and admissions. They will frequently ask you when patients are likely to be ready for discharge so they can plan ahead for routine admissions.

Discharge coordinators work in conjunction with social workers, physiotherapists, and occupational therapists to expedite patients' discharges. They often assist in finding intermediate care placements.

Healthcare assistants (HCAs) perform more basic nursing tasks eg help with personal care and recording observations including finger-prick glucose. They cannot dispense medication or give injections, but many can take blood.

Nurse practitioners are specially trained senior nurses who can assess acutely unwell patients, perform practical procedures (eg cannulation), and assist in theatre. Most cannot prescribe, although there are some who are qualified to use the nurses' formulary.

Nurse specialists include stoma, respiratory, pain, cardiac, diabetes, tissue viability, and Macmillan nurses. They are excellent for giving advice and are an important first port of call for the junior doctor.

Occupational therapists work with patients to restore, develop, or maintain practical skills such as personal care. Assess patient ± home for adaptations required to help with activities. Many elderly patients require OT assessment before discharge – nurses usually make the referral. OTs work in primary and secondary care.

Pharmacists dispense drugs and advise you on medication. They check the accuracy of every prescription that is written. Most hospitals have a drugs information-line which you can call for prescribing advice.

Phlebotomists are professional vampires who appear on the wards with the specific aim of taking blood. They often appear at unpredictable times and they may not come at all at weekends, so leave your blood forms out well in advance. Some can take blood from central lines and perform blood cultures.

Physiotherapists use physical exercises and manipulation to treat injuries and relieve pain. Chest physios are commonly found on respiratory and surgical wards to help improve respiratory function and sputum expectoration by teaching specific breathing exercises. Involve them early in patient management – nurses usually make the referral, but do not hesitate to discuss your patient's needs or progress directly with them.

Social workers support patients' needs in the community. They assess patients and help organise care packages (invaluable for elderly patients). Where residential care is required they help guide family and patient through the decision-making process and financial issues. They are also involved in child protection and vulnerable adult safeguarding work.

Daily ward duties

First thing

- Handover from night team about any overnight events
- Submit any missing or extra blood/CXR/ECG requests
- Review new patients, consider writing a brief summary.

Ward round

- See 📖 p70 for ward round duties, try to keep a jobs list
- Attempt to start simple jobs (eg TTOs) during ward round.

After the ward round

- Spend a few minutes comparing and allocating jobs with the other team members; try to group jobs by location and urgency
- Radiology requests (USS, CT, MRI)
- Referrals to other teams, eg surgery/cardiology/psychiatry
- Complete TTOs and other forms
- Take blood from patients whom the phlebotomists have been unable to bleed or that have been requested during the ward round.

Lunch

- Do you need to do anything for yourself, eg book holidays, pay bills?
- You may have teaching/grand round/journal clubs.

After lunch

- Review patients you are worried about. Liaise with nurses re any problems they have identified and attend to routine tasks they may have
- Check and record blood results; serial results sheets help
- Check other results; chase outstanding requests or results
- Spend time talking to patients ± relatives
- Submit blood and other investigation requests for the next day
- Check the patients' drug cards – do any need rewriting?

Before you go home

- Review results and outstanding jobs with other team members; make a note of anything that needs doing the next day
- Check that all warfarin and insulin doses have been written up
- Prescribe sufficient IV fluids for patients overnight where safe to do so
- Handover patients who are sick or need results chasing to the on-call doctor (📖 p72); write down their ward, name, DoB and hospital number and exactly what you want the doctor to do (ie not just 'check bloods').

Before weekends

- Only submit blood requests for patients who really need them
- Try to prescribe 3 days of warfarin doses where safe to do so
- Make sure that no drug cards will run out over the next 2 days, rewrite them if they will (this is infuriating to do as an on-call job)
- Ensure notes contain a brief and easy to find summary of each patient for the on-call team (especially for those who are unwell); include presenting complaint, relevant investigations, and plan for the weekend.

Ward rounds

A smooth ward round requires preparation of notes, investigations, and results. Try to predict requests and start the ward round armed with the appropriate answers. See Fig. 2.1 for guidance on recording rounds in patient notes.

Before the ward round

- Update the patient list with patient details, location, summary of clinical problems, key investigations/results, referrals made, and jobs
- Ask the nurses if any patients have changed condition overnight and try to avoid any nasty surprises on the round; briefly review individual patients where appropriate
- Check notes, drug cards, obs charts, X-rays, and blood results are present
- Clearly document all relevant investigation results and reports in the notes with a brief summary on your patient list
- Check all notes have continuation sheets headed with the patient's name, DoB, and hospital number/address (use a hospital sticker)
- Consider writing out the patient's problem list/summary
- If your patients have moved, find out where they have been transferred to and plot an efficient route through the hospital to visit all your outlying patients
- Check or chase the dates/times for outstanding investigations
- Learn your consultant's favourite questions from your predecessor (eg patient occupation)
- Consider multidisciplinary issues which may alter further management or delay discharge for the patient (eg home circumstances)
- Think about management dilemmas you want/need answers to.

During the ward round

- Ask a nurse to join you on the ward round
- If there are two junior doctors then one can prepare the notes, obs, drug cards, and X-rays for the next patient whilst the other presents
- When presenting a patient, always begin in the same logical way, eg 'Mrs Smith is a 64-year-old lady who presented with a 4-day history of worsening shortness of breath' then proceed to past medical history, investigation, and blood results, then your management plan
- If you have a spare moment start filling in forms or doing the jobs generated on the ward round (eg prescribing fluids)
- If you have any queries about the next step of management or investigation results, ask during the ward round. Also ask about rationale for imaging if unsure as this makes requesting imaging easier for you (🔲 p85)!
- Referrals made in the presence of your consultant are often more readily accepted and queries can be discussed directly
- If you have not done something or cannot recall details, be honest; never make up results.

After the ward round

- Sit down with the rest of the team and go through the jobs generated from the ward round over a cup of tea
- Prioritise the jobs and group by location, eg outlying wards, radiology
- Allocate the jobs between your team as appropriate
- If you are unsure of how to approach any of the jobs, ask your seniors
- Clarify any gaps in your understanding of the patients' management.

Mr Johnston/Miss Jain's patient list 16/09/14

Patients, Details	Problem list	Investigation/Detail	Jobs
Angel Ward			
Eleanor Rigby W876470 26/06/1933	Chest pain COPD Hiatus hernia	LBBB on ECG	Cardiac Marker TTO
Seabright Ward			
Annie Popple T589124 08/09/1945	Dysphagia Haematemesis Anaemia	3u Bld 15/09/14 OGD - Ca stomach	Macmillan referral Gastro r/v

Sample patient list

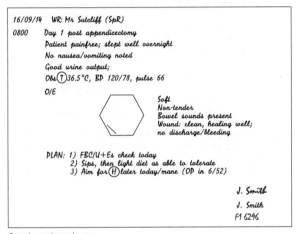

16/09/14   WR: Mr Sutcliff (SpR)

0800   Day 1 post appendicectomy
       Patient painfree; slept well overnight
       No nausea/vomiting noted
       Good urine output;
       Obs Ⓣ 36.5°C, BP 120/78, pulse 66

       O/E

                          Soft
                          Non-tender
                          Bowel sounds present
                          Wound: clean, healing well;
                          no discharge/bleeding

       PLAN: 1) FBC/U+Es check today
             2) Sips, then light diet as able to tolerate
             3) Aim for Ⓗ later today/mane (OP in 6/52)

                                          J. Smith
                                          J. Smith
                                          F1 6296

Sample ward round entry

Fig. 2.1 Sample of a ward round entry in the patient's notes.

Being on-call

Being 'on-call' will occupy a large amount of your time and may involve care of a different group of patients and a greater range of specialties than during the day. Requirements, expectations and priorities are different.

What's important
- Ensure you have a clear handover about which patients are waiting to be seen, how urgently they need seeing, and where they are
- Know who you are on call with and how best to contact them
- Identify the sick and get help early
- Prioritise effectively and stay organised
- Eat and stay well hydrated – there is always time for a cup of water and you will be much less efficient if you don't look after yourself.

How to handle the bleep when tired
- Always try to answer promptly; when you don't it will be the boss or someone really unwell
- Write down who called and the job required
- Learn common extension numbers so you can spot the call from switchboard, the mess, or your consultant's office.

Being organised on-call
- Document every task, otherwise you **will** forget something – do not use scraps of paper; use a notepad or PDA
- Have a means of identifying when you've done it (drawing a box to tick when complete helps)
- Visit all the areas you cover in order and tell the wards this is what you'll be doing; ask them to compile a list of non-urgent tasks for when you arrive
- When you order a test on-call, make a note to check the result as it's easy to forget.

Prioritising
- Sick patients need seeing first; if you have more than one really sick patient then tell your senior
- If the patient's condition is clearly life threatening then consider asking the ward to bleep your senior while you're on your way there
- Check if a task has a deadline (eg before pharmacy closes)
- If you see an abnormal blood result check the patient/notes/previous blood results (see 📖 p566–571)
- Ask if a task can wait until you're next in that area; tell the staff when this will be and try to stick to it.

Taking breaks

You are entitled to a 30min paid break for every 4h work. Whilst you must not ignore a sick patient, there will be a constant supply of work that can usually wait. Breaks are not just about food, they keep you alert and reduce stress and tension headaches. It is in your patients' interests that you recharge. Drink plenty of water. Where possible, arrange to take breaks with the other members of the team on-call – it allows you to catch up and stops you feeling isolated.

Night shifts

Few doctors look forward to their night shifts, especially if they are doing several in a row. That said, on nights you will gain a lot of experience.

Things to take with you
- Food, both a main meal and several quick snacks
- Toothbrush, toothpaste, comb/hairbrush, and deodorant
- Stuff for gaps in workload – eg books for private study.

Things to check (on the first night)
- What areas and specialties are you responsible for?
- Who are your seniors and what are their bleep/mobile numbers?
- When and where is handover?

What is expected of you
- Turn up on time; your colleague will be late home if you don't
- Prioritise work according to urgency – when bleeped to a sick patient ask for obs ± ECG to be done while you get there
- Tour the wards you are covering regularly and delegate simple tasks
- Document all interventions in the notes.

Hospital at night (H@N)
This system is now in place in many hospitals to improve efficiency and the standard of care provided by the limited number of doctors on duty at night. Generally all bleeps should go via the Night Sister, who then filters them appropriately, eg assessing which jobs could be done by a nurse (eg cannula) and which patients need urgent review by a doctor.

Learning at night
Nights can be a good learning opportunity. Ensure the other doctors on at night know if you have particular skills you wish to learn at that time (eg lumbar punctures). They can then call you to observe or be supervised.

Pitfalls
The potential to make mistakes during night shifts is greater than during the day. If you are unsure, check. The following are some of the common problem areas:
- Poor handover; ensure you know who needs review (📖 p20)
- Failing to appreciate a sick patient and not calling for help
- Fluid prescriptions (eg failing to note renal/heart failure, DM, electrolyte imbalance)
- Warfarin prescriptions with INRs coming back out of hours.

How to cope when not at work
- Try to sleep (or at least lie down) for a few hours during the day before your first night shift
- Go to bed for at least 7h each day, even if you don't sleep you'll rest
- Make your room dark and quiet – eye masks/earplugs help; ensure anyone else in the house knows you are working nights
- Eat enough; have a meal when you get up and before going in
- Travel home safely; if you feel too tired take a 20–30min nap first.

Writing in the notes

See Fig. 2.2. Most new F1s are unsure about writing in medical notes since this is rarely practised as a medical student. There are a few rules which everyone, irrespective of grade, should conform to (Fig. 2.2):

Notepaper The patient's name, DoB, and hospital number or address should identify every sheet (using a hospital sticker is preferable).

Documentation Each entry should have the date and time. It is useful to have a heading such as 'WR ST2 (Smith)' or 'Discussion with patient and family'. Sign every entry and print your surname and bleep number clearly.

What to write Document the condition of the patient, relevant changes to the history, obs, examination findings, the results of any new investigations, and end with a clear plan. The notes should contain enough information so that in your absence someone else can learn what has happened and what is planned for the patient. Always allow yourself plenty of space when writing in the notes, especially if documenting a ward round – your seniors may mention a point of the plan early on (which needs to go at the end of the entry) but then perform a detailed examination which you should document in the space you have left. Try to document everything that is discussed or observed – it is extremely frustrating for a senior to ask a series of detailed questions with medicolegal implications and then to find nothing documented.

Problem lists It is helpful to write a problem list in the notes either every day if there are frequent changes (eg new admissions or in ICU/HDU), or less frequently for chronic conditions. This should include both medical and social problems. Having problem lists also makes it easier for on-call doctors to understand the patient's condition if they are asked to review them, as well as refreshing your memory at the start of the next ward round. See Fig. 2.3.

What not to write Patients can apply to read their medical notes and notes are always used in legal cases. Never write anything that you do not wish the patient to read or that would be frowned upon in court. Documenting facts is accepted (eg obese lady) but not subjective material (eg annoying time-waster). Never doodle in the notes and do not write humorous comments.

How to write Write clearly in black; poorly legible notes result in errors and are indefensible in court. Use only well recognised abbreviations and don't worry about length as long as sufficient information is documented. Always write in the notes at the time of the consultation, even if it means asking the ward round to wait a few moments.

Making changes If you wish to cross something out simply put a single line through the error and initial the mistake. Never cross it out so it cannot be read as this looks suspicious. Previous entries should not be altered, instead make a new entry indicating the change or difference.

Notes and the law It is unlikely that your notes will be used in court. If they are, you want them to show you as a caring and clear-thinking individual; make that clear from how you write. As far as a court is concerned, if it's not documented then it didn't happen.

Hints and tips Bullet points are a useful and clear means of documentation. It is acceptable to write about a patient's mood and it is useful to document if you have cheered them up or discussed some bad news (📖 p22). It is also acceptable to document 'no change' if this is the case.

16.9.14	WR ST4 (Ackerman)
10:20	<u>Problem:</u> Admitted last night with central chest pain ?ACS
	<u>Progress:</u>
	Pt comfortable. No further chest pain.
	P70 reg, BP 132/81, RR 15, Sats 99% on room air.
	~~CXR shows bilateral pleural effusions~~ (Wrong patient CJF)
	Rpt ECG Ⓝ, no new changes.
	Imp
	• Atypical chest pain, unlikely to be cardiac.
	Ⓟ
	• Await cardiac markers—if Ⓝ, Ⓗ o– no f/u.
	• Pt wants to discuss risk factors when family
	arrive.
	Dr C J Flint F1
	Bleep 3294

16.9.14	d/w with pt and wife
11:12	Pt wanted to talk about cardiac risk factors.
	Given British Heart Foundation leaflet on risk factors and talked about
	lifestyle changes.
	Cardiac nurse will see pt before discharge.
	Rpt cardiac markers Ⓝ. Pt much relieved.
	Ⓗ later.
	Dr C J Flint F1
	Bleep 3294

16.9.14	Review, F1 (Flint)
15:34	No change. TTO completed. Ⓗ.
	Dr C J Flint F1
	Bleep 3294

Fig. 2.2 Example of entries in medical notes.

16/9/14	Mrs Jones' current problems:
09:00	1 Left lower lobe pneumonia – on day 2 IV co-amoxiclav
	2 Atrial fibrillation (2009) – on digoxin and warfarin
	3 Hypertension – well controlled on ramipril
	4 Previous CVA (2009) with right sided weakness
	5 Previous left knee replacement (2002)
	6 Not able to manage at home – needs increased package of care prior to D/C

Fig. 2.3 Example of a problem list.

Common symbols in the notes

Ⓗ	Home
Ⓝ	Normal
Ⓟ	Plan
Ⓛ	Left
Ⓡ	Right
Ⓣ	Temperature
dd/DD/δδ/ΔΔ	Differential diagnosis
x/Dx/Δ	Diagnosis
Imp	Impression
Rx	Prescription or drugs
Sx	Symptoms
Tx	Treatment
Ix	Investigations
O/E	On examination
–ve	Negative
+ve	Positive
+/–	Equivocal
+	Presence noted
++	Present significantly
+++	Present in excess
h/o	History of
d/w	Discussed with or discussion with
WR	Ward round
r/v	Review
f/u	Follow-up
ATSP	Asked to see patient
IP	In-patient
OP	Out-patient
c/o	Complains of or complaining of
Pt	Patient
c̄	With
@	At
E+D	Eating and drinking
N+V	Nausea and vomiting
D+V	Diarrhoea and vomiting
BO	Bowels open
PUing	Passing urine
blds	Bloods
°	No/negative (as in °previous MI)
1°	Primary
2°	Secondary
mane	Tomorrow morning
N/S	Nursing Staff

Anatomical terms and planes

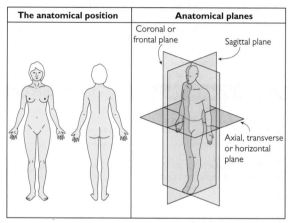

Fig. 2.4 The anatomical position and anatomical planes.

Commonly used anatomical terms and their meanings

Anterior/ventral	Front of the body
Contralateral	On the opposite side
Coronal/frontal plane	Divides anterior from posterior
Distal	Away from the trunk
Inferior/caudal	Away from the head
Ipsilateral	On the same side
Lateral	Away from the midline
Medial	Towards the midline
Palmar	Pertaining to the palm of the hand
Plantar	Pertaining to the sole of the foot
Posterior/dorsal	Back of the body
Prone	Face down position
Proximal	Close to the trunk
Radial	The lateral (thumb) aspect of the forearm
Sagittal plane	Divides left side from right side
Superior/cephalic	Towards the head
Supine	Face up position
Transverse/horizontal/axial plane	Divides upper and lower sections
Ulnar	The medial (little finger) aspect of the forearm

Discharge summaries (TTOs/TTAs)

'TTOs' or 'TTAs' (to take out or away) are summaries of the patient's admission from the ward doctors sent to the patient's GP and are often the most complete summary written. TTOs are written on a computer (very occasionally by hand with carbon copies); you should receive training on the local system as part of induction. They form a point of reference at future clinic visits or admissions. They also provide clinical coding information with which the hospital bills primary care for care provided.

TTOs should contain the following information

- Patient details: name, DoB, hospital number, address
- Consultant and hospital ward
- Presenting complaint, clinical findings, and diagnosis
- Investigations/procedures/operations/treatment, including any complications
- Treatment on discharge and instructions to the GP, including medications stopped and reasons why
- Follow-up arrangements
- Your name, position, and bleep number.

When to write TTOs

TTOs should be written as soon as you know the patient is likely to be discharged. This allows the drugs to be dispensed from pharmacy as soon as possible so that the patient's discharge is not delayed. See Fig. 2.5.

- Begin to enter information on the TTO at the earliest opportunity; check any queries with your team, particularly regarding the principal diagnosis
- Check the duration of the medication for discharge (eg ABx) and stop any unnecessary drugs (eg prophylactic low-molecular-weight heparin)
- Check drug doses and frequencies with the *BNF*, your seniors, a pharmacist or by calling your hospital's drug information-line
- Check required follow-up appointments, give details and be clear on who will arrange them(eg the ward clerk or the clinic administrators)
- Phone the GP if the patient needs an early check-up, has a poor social situation, or self-discharges. It may take several days for a TTO to reach the GP: written instructions such as 'check K^+ in 3/7' are unsafe
- Hand the TTO and the patient's drug chart to the patient's nurse or inform them that you have completed it to avoid unnecessary bleeps
- If you are unsure whether the TTO has been done check the drug chart; there is often a tick in a box showing if TTOs have been dispensed
- Discuss the diagnosis, results, and discharge plan with your patient; if they understand the management plan they are more likely to comply.

Controlled drugs for TTOs

These are slightly more complex, but can still be written by F1 doctors in most trusts. They must include all the information in Table 2.1. CD prescriptions are only valid for 28d from the date of signing and only 30d of CDs can be dispensed on a single prescription. See also Fig. 2.6.

Examples of controlled drugs

Morphine, diamorphine, pethidine, fentanyl, alfentanil, remifentanil, methadone, methylphenidate (ie Ritalin®), cocaine.

Table 2.1 *Controlled drug TTOs must meet the following requirements*

Content rules	• The prescriber's name and work address • Signed and dated by the prescriber • All the information included in a regular TTO.
Drug rules	• The drug name, dose, frequency and route • If the drug is a 'preparation' (ie liquid) state the concentration • The total volume (ml) or weight (mg) of the preparation or the total number of tablets/capsules/patches in words and figures.

Discharge form McBurney City Hospital

Name: *Eleanor Rigby*   Consultant: *Dr Singh*

DOB: *26/06/1932*   Date of admission: *15/09/2014*

Hospital number: *W876470*   Date of discharge: *16/09/2014*

Ward: *E4*

NHS/~~Private~~   In-patient/~~Out-patient/Day~~case

Presenting complaint: *Chest pain*

Diagnosis: *Musculoskeletal chest pain*   Co-morbidities: *Anxiety, L THR 2001*

Investigations: *ECG shows LBBB, cardiac markers Ⓝ*

Discharge Plan/Additional notes to GP: *Has had some toothache recently, advised her to see a dentist*

Discharge Medications:

Drug	Dose	Frequency	Route	Duration	GP to continue?
Co-amoxiclav	625mg	TDS	PO	5d	No
Paracetamol	1g	QDS	PO	7d	No
Morphine oral solution (10mg/5ml)	10ml	BD	PO	5d	No
	Total = 100ml (one hundred millilitres)				

Follow up? *None required*   Date: *16-09-2014*

Print name ... *Flint* ...   Signature *C J Flint*

Fig. 2.5 Sample TTO.

Morphine oral solution (10mg/5ml); dose: 10ml/12h PO for 5 days. Total = 100ml (one hundred millilitres)

Morphine sulfate MR 10mg capsules; dose: 10mg/12h PO for 14 days. Total = 280mg (two hundred and eighty milligrams)

Fentanyl 50 patch; dose: one patch every 72 hours for 14 days. Total = 5 (five) patches

Fig. 2.6 Sample TTOs for controlled drugs excluding the patient and prescriber's details.

Fitness to work notes[1]

As the most junior member of the team, the writing of 'fit notes' (Statement of fitness for work, Form Med 3) will usually fall to you. These notes provide evidence that your patient has a condition that will impact upon their fitness to work and enables statutory sick pay and social security payments. You can advise that a patient is 'not fit for work' or 'may be fit for work' under restricted conditions. A separate form (Form Med 10) may be required for periods of time spent as a hospital inpatient. These forms are available in both electronic and paper formats from the Department for Work and Pensions – ask the ward clerk for advice. A sample is shown below in Fig. 2.7.

Usage

Typical uses include surgical patients who have been admitted routinely for a procedure and require time off work to recover post-operatively. Medical patients may also require time to convalesce, whilst patients with wounds or injuries may require workplace adjustments during their recovery period on return to work. Patients can self-certify for the first week of any illness so do not require a note if they will be able to return to work within this time. Never instruct a patient to 'see your GP for a sick note' where the need for this can be anticipated at the time of discharge – the duty to provide a Med 3 rests with the doctor with clinical responsibility for the patient.

Format

You should fill in the patient's name, a brief explanation of their needs (sickness absence, adjustments to the workplace, or modified duties), and accurate clinical diagnosis (without mentioning intimate details that might be damaging to the wellbeing of patient for their employer to discover). Sign and date the form. You need to give an appropriate amount of time for the patient to recover from their illness as reasonably anticipated at the time of discharge, up to a maximum of 3mths. If recovery takes longer than you anticipate, the patient can then see their GP for a further note.

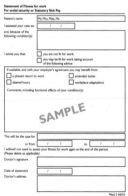

Fig. 2.7 Example of Statement of Fitness for Work (Med 3). Reproduced with permission from the Department of Work and Pensions. ᐟwww.dwp.gov.uk/healthcare-professional/news/statement-of-fitness-for-work.shtml

[1] Useful guidance available at ᐟwww.rcplondon.ac.uk/sites/default/files/completion-statement-fitness-for-work.pdf

Referrals

Referring a patient to another medical team can be one of the most difficult parts of the job. The other doctor is often very busy and will inevitably know more about the patient's condition than you (hence the referral). At times it can feel like they are trying to make you feel stupid – this is rarely the case. Consider this from the point of view of the other doctor: They need to establish:

• How unwell the patient is
• How urgently they need to be seen
• What investigations have already been done and what still need to be done to assist them in their review
• If they are the right person to see them.

You will often be asked to refer a patient by your senior: Ask them directly:
• Why does the patient need referring?
• What do they want the other team to do (advise over the phone, formal review, take over care, see in clinic, procedure/operation)?
• How urgent is the referral?

Next, think about what information the other doctor will want. Many specialties have additional components to history and examination that you will need to be able to describe, see the pages in the history and examination chapter; if necessary, go and examine the patient yourself:

Breast surgery	📖 p141	Haematology	📖 p140	Psychiatry	📖 p160
Cardiology	📖 p128	Neurology	📖 p132	Renal	📖 p373
Dermatology	📖 p138	Obstetrics	📖 p158	Respiratory	📖 p130
Endocrine	📖 p137	Oncology	📖 p140	Rheumatology	📖 p146
ENT	📖 p144	Ophthalmology	📖 p142	Urology	📖 p154
Gastro	📖 p131	Orthopaedics	📖 p146	Vascular surgery	📖 p128
Gynaecology	📖 p156	Paediatrics	📖 p164		

Before referring make sure you have the following in front of you:
• Hospital notes with patient's name, DoB, hospital number and ward
• Obs chart (including latest set and trends) and the patient's drug card
• Most recent results or serial results sheet.

Phone the relevant specialist, introduce yourself and say, 'My consultant has requested that I refer one of our patients who has [medical condition] with the view to [taking over care, advising on treatment, etc]'.

Offer a brief summary of their condition and management; look up the relevant condition or referral page (above) before calling so that you know what you are talking about. ***It is never acceptable to make a referral for a patient you know little about just because it's on the jobs list.***

Always know what investigations have been performed so far, and what the results were – sit at a computer with these already called up when you make the call.

Before you put the phone down determine exactly what action the specialist will do and when this will take place. Write the referral and outcome in the notes along with the specialist's name and bleep number.

Referral letters

The basics

These may be used for within hospital referrals (using a specific referral slip) or for referral to outpatient clinics or other hospitals (use hospital headed notepaper).[1] Try to make referral letters as professional as possible. It is essential that the referral contains the following information:

- Who you are and how to contact you
- Who the patient is (full name, DoB, hospital number, ± address)
- Why you want them to be seen.

Fig. 2.8 is an example of an referral letter for you to follow.

Diagnoses

List all the patient's active diagnoses and relevant past diagnoses; try to put the ones most relevant to the specialty you are referring to near the top.

Presenting complaint

Start with a statement telling the other doctor what you would like them to do (eg see on the ward, in clinic, or give written advice). Give a brief description of the patient's presentation and management during this admission as if you were writing a discharge summary.

Medical information

This will form the bulk of the referral. Think carefully about what information will help the other doctor in deciding when to see the patient and how to manage them; see the relevant history and examination page (📖 p123). Try to set the referral out like a brief medical clerking and make sure you include:

- Relevant investigation results
- Latest medications
- Relevant social history (particularly if this will affect how they are seen in clinic, eg poor mobility, language difficulties).

Finishing the referral

You should write your name, post and consultant's name. If sending an outpatient or inter-hospital referral, you should also include who the letter is copied to ('cc' stands for carbon copy) which will include the notes and GP. It is recommended practice to send a copy to the patient though this varies between trusts and doctors.

Sending the letter

Ask your ward clerk for assistance. Print off several copies, sign them and ensure it is clear where each copy should be sent.

Faxing a letter

If you need to fax a copy then include a header sheet. This is simply a piece of paper saying who the fax is to, who it is from and the number of pages (and whether this includes the header sheet). You may need to add a number to the fax number to get an outside line, eg '9'. File the faxed letter and the sent message confirmation (with date and time sent) in the patient's notes.

---

[1] Non-urgent outpatient referrals to other specialties should go through the patient's GP, since payment comes from their budget. If this is required, a note should be made on the discharge summary with specific details of why this referral is being recommended. Urgent referrals (especially for suspected malignancies) can still be made directly. Check with the consultant recommending the referral.

Dr Charles Flint
McBurney City Hospital
McBurney
McB1 4CT

Dr I N Haler
Respiratory Consultant
McBurney City Hospital
McBurney
McB1 4CT

17th September 2014

Dear Dr Haler,
Re: Eleanor Rigby, DoB 26/06/32, Hospital No. W876470

Diagnoses:
(1) COPD
(2) Musculoskeletal chest pain
(3) LBBB
(4) Hiatus hernia

Please review Mrs Rigby in your respiratory clinic to treat her deterioration in respiratory function with COPD.

Mrs Rigby is an 82-year-old lady who presented with chest pain. She was admitted overnight and diagnosed with musculoskeletal chest pain following normal repeat cardiac markers. She was discharged on 16/9/2014. During her admission she was noted to have reduced exercise tolerance (from 200m to 50m). Her latest ABG on air is:

$$PaO_2 \quad 9.3kPa$$
$$PaCO_2 \quad 6kPa$$

We feel that her COPD is the likely cause of her limited mobility and she has been referred for repeat respiratory function tests.

PMH She was diagnosed with COPD by you 3 years ago following respiratory function tests which showed an FEV_1 of 65% predicted. She has not had any acute exacerbations in the last year.

DH She is currently on:

Salbutamol inhaler	2 puffs	PRN
Tiotropium inhaler	18mcg	OM
Symbicort inhaler (200/6)	2 puffs	BD
Bendroflumethiazide	5 mg	OM

SH She lives alone but gets home help for cleaning. She can walk about 50m with a stick. She stopped smoking 30 years ago after 50 pack years.

Yours sincerely,

Dr Charles Flint
F1 to Dr N Stemi
cc   GP
         Eleanor Rigby
         Notes

Fig. 2.8 Example of a referral letter.

Investigation requests

Increasingly, these are handled electronically. For paper forms, complete:
- Full name and at least one other patient identification detail (ie DoB, hospital number or address); G+S/X-match requires at least two more
- Status (in-patient/out-patient) and location (ward or home address)
- Name, position, and contact details of doctor ordering the test
- Date, test(s) requested and reason for request

Clinical information

Appropriate information on request forms affects how the test is performed and reported; too much information is better than too little. Justify the investigation requested, even if a simple blood test. Always consider if a test is *really* required, no matter how trivial – daily 'routine' bloods are often unnecessary, waste resources and cause patient discomfort.

- *Blood tests* Brief clinical details may be acceptable, eg 'chest pain', 'suspected PE'. Some tests require more information, eg blood films, antibodies, hormones, drug levels (doses and timing of doses), genetics
- *Histology* Describe the macroscopic appearance of the tissue as well as the clinical suspicions, radiology findings and any specific questions
- *Microbiology* As a bare minimum include the sample type (eg urine) and current/recent antibiotics; the more information you include the better the microbiologist will be able to interpret laboratory results
- *Radiology* see 📖 p85.

'Chasing' results

As a junior doctor, a large proportion of your time will be spent checking results. This used to involve 'chasing' endless pieces of paper which were prone to going astray. With the move to full computerisation, most reports are now easily available: Simply keep track of the investigations you have requested then check the results systems regularly. Nonetheless, there are a few tips to consider:

- For urgent results, particularly where there might be a delay in transcription (eg radiology reports) or uploading onto the system (eg biochemistry/ haematology) you can call the lab, or reporting room (or attend in person). You will be interrupting a colleague doing their job, so do not abuse this privilege
- Blood samples reaching the lab early in the day will be processed first; it can help to beat the rush that will hit the labs after the phlebotomists do their rounds
- Rarer tests may only be run on samples reaching the lab by a certain time, or on certain days of the week, or may even need to be send to an outside lab – find out local policies and, if in doubt, call the lab before taking the sample
- Bloods requiring urgent processing should be marked as such; indiscriminate use of this facility will delay genuinely critical results. Arrange an urgent porter (or take to the lab yourself). At top speed, biochemistry results take around 20–30min and haematology results around 30min.
- For microbiology results, preliminary evidence of positive cultures is usually reported at 48h; otherwise consider telephoning the lab at this stage to see if there is any preliminary growth. Positive results will be further cultured and tested over subsequent days to give a more detailed analysis
- For histology, all biopsies taken with a provisional diagnosis of malignancy should be processed urgently, but this depends upon sample being correctly marked at the time; call the pathology secretaries if there is any doubt or delay.

Be careful not to make important decisions on preliminary results – if there is an urgent clinical situation in which you are unsure whether to act on a specific result, ask your seniors.

Radiology

Since Wilhelm Röntgen's first hazy images of the bones of his wife's hand in 1895, radiological imaging has revolutionised the approach of physician and surgeon alike in diagnosis and treatment.

Imaging modalities

- *X-rays* exploit the different absorbance of a pulse of X-ray radiation by different anatomical structures and foreign bodies. This allows the visualisation and distinction of metal, bone, soft tissue, fat, fluid and air
- *Fluoroscopy* uses X-ray images acquired in real time, often with addition of a contrast material, eg coronary angiogram or barium swallow
- *CT* uses a series of 2D X-ray images acquired in different planes to construct cross-sectional 3D images. IV or PO contrast can be used to accentuate, eg blood vessels or the GI tract
- *MRI* uses strong magnetic fields to align hydrogen nuclei (protons) within tissues. Disturbance of the axis of these protons by radiowaves allows the recording of radiowaves emitted as the protons return to baseline. MRI offers excellent soft tissue imaging and does not require ionising radiation exposure. Image acquisition can be slow and require multiple different 'sequences' whilst the patient lies in a cramped space
- *Ultrasound* exploits the differential reflection of high-frequency sound waves to visualise structures, including soft tissues in real time. Overlying air and fat compromise signal quality, and bone penetration is poor
- *Nuclear medicine* depends upon the detection of radiation emitted by the decay of radiolabels attached to substances with affinity for certain body tissues. **Positron emission tomography (PET)** is a specific form of nuclear medicine that typically uses radiolabelled glucose analogues to detect regions of metabolic activity, eg in cancer. These techniques are especially powerful when combined with anatomical imaging approaches such as CT to increase localisation (eg **PET/CT**).

Requesting

Selecting, performing, interpreting and managing medical imaging resources falls to the specialty of radiology. These doctors often have little direct contact with your patient and depend upon effective communication from you to select and prioritise imaging modalities (including appropriate use of contrast agents and imaging sequences), as well as inform their image interpretation; always include specific clinical questions on request forms.

Radiologists have a vital duty to limit unnecessary exposure to ionising radiation. Doses involved can range from minimal (eg CXR: <1% annual background radiation exposure) to substantial (eg contrast CT C/A/P: ~10yr background radiation). Even a trivial radiation exposure will be associated with an appreciable cancer risk to a population if performed often enough.[1] Always ensure you know why any investigation you are asked to request is needed, how urgent it is, and how it will change the patient's management. For less urgent investigations or simple X-rays, it is usually enough to submit a request giving sufficient clinical information. For more urgent or specialist imaging, request the scan or fill in the form, then phone or go to the radiology department, and speak to the duty radiologist. Be polite, explain why the test has been requested (and by whom), and ask if there is any way it could be performed today if necessary. If this fails and the test is very urgent, your registrar should discuss with the radiologist directly.

---

[1] Converting low-dose radiation exposure to cancer risk is fraught with difficulty; attempts to extrapolate from cancer rates in those exposed to very high dose radiation are unsound. The general principle must be to keep exposure **A**s **L**ow **A**s **R**easonably **P**ossible (ALARP).

Pain

Worrying features ↓↑HR, ↓↑BP, ↓↑RR, ↓GCS, sweating, vomiting, chest pain.

Think about Headache (📖 p358), chest pain (📖 p241), abdominal pain (📖 p289), back pain (📖 p356), limb pain (📖 p448), infection (📖 p482; ***common*** post-operative, musculoskeletal, chronic pain.

Ward round Assess daily the effectiveness of analgesia (whether pain hinders activity (coughing, getting out of bed etc)) and about side effects (drowsiness, nausea, vomiting and constipation).

Ask about (SOCRATES) **S**ite, **O**nset, **C**haracter, **R**adiation, **A**lleviating factors, **T**iming (duration, frequency), **E**xacerbating factors, **S**everity, associated features (sweating, nausea, vomiting); ***PMH*** stomach problems (acid reflux, ulcers), asthma, cardiac problems; ***DH*** allergies, tolerance of NSAIDs, analgesia already taken and perceived benefit; ***SH***?drug abuse.

Obs ↑HR and ↑BP suggests pain; RR, pupil size and GCS if on opioids.

Look for source/cause of pain.

Investigations These should be guided by your history and examination; none are specifically required for pain.

Treatment No patient should be left in severe pain, consider titrating an IV opioid after an antiemetic (📖 p304). Use the steps of the WHO pain ladder (Table 2.4). Ensure regular analgesia is prescribed, with adequate PRN analgesia for breakthrough pain. If a patient has moderate or severe pain start at step 3 or 4; using paracetamol and NSAIDs reduces opioid requirement and consequently side effects.

Table 2.4 *WHO pain ladder*

	Step 1	Step 2	Step 3	Step 4
Strong opioids				✓
Weak opioids			✓	
NSAIDs		✓	✓	✓
Paracetamol	✓	✓	✓	✓

Paracetamol **contraindications** moderate liver failure; ***side effects*** rare.
● **Paracetamol** 1g/4h, max 4g/24h PO/PR/IV.

NSAIDS good for inflammatory pain, renal or biliary colic and bone pain; **contraindications** (BARS) **B**leeding (pre-op, coagulopathy), **A**sthma, **R**enal disease, **S**tomach (peptic ulcer or gastritis). 10% of asthmatics are NSAID-sensitive, try a low dose if they have never used them before. Avoid use in the elderly. Increased risk of CVA/MI; ***side effects*** worsen renal function, GI bleeding (upper and lower – co-prescribe a PPI or high-dose H₂-blocker for those at risk: ≥65 yrs, previous peptic ulcer, use of other medicines with GI side effects, or major comorbidity). Both NSAIDs and COX-2 inhibitors are associated with increased risk of MI and CVA; use with ***caution*** in those at risk.
● **Ibuprofen** 400mg/6h, max 2.4g/24h PO, weaker anti-inflammatory action, but less risk of GI ulceration
● **Diclofenac** 50mg/8h, max 150mg/24h PO/PR (also IM/IV, see *BNF*).

COX-2 inhibitors are similar to NSAIDs and share an increased risk of MI and CVA, but with less risk of gastroduodenal ulceration.

Weak opioids Dependence and tolerance to opioids do not occur with short-term use for acute pain. Consider prescribing regular laxatives and PRN antiemetics, use with **caution** if head injury, ↑ICP, respiratory depression, alcohol intoxication; **side effects** N+V, constipation, drowsiness, hypotension; **toxicity** ↓RR, ↓GCS, pinpoint pupils (see Table 2.5).
- **Codeine** 30–60mg/4h, max 240mg/24h PO/IM, constipating
- **Dihydrocodeine** 30–60mg/4h, max 240mg/24h PO, constipating
- **Tramadol** 50–100mg/4h, max 400–600mg/24h PO/IM, stronger than others and less constipating for long-term use.

Table 2.5 *Weak opioid to oral morphine converter*

Drug and dose (oral route)	Equivalent to oral morphine
Codeine 8mg	0.7mg oral morphine
Codeine 30mg/6h	10mg oral morphine/24h
Dihydrocodeine 10mg	1mg oral morphine
Dihydrocodeine 30mg/6h	12mg oral morphine/24h
Tramadol 50mg	5mg oral morphine
Tramadol 100mg/6h	40mg oral morphine/24h

Paracetamol and weak opioid combinations useful for TTO analgesia; it is better to prescribe the components separately in hospital:
- **Co-codamol** 30mg codeine and 500mg paracetamol; two tablets/6h PO, nurses must give 8/500 dose if 30/500 not specified
- **Co-dydramol** 10mg dihydrocodeine and 500mg paracetamol; two tablets/6h PO
- **Co-proxamol** contained dextropropoxyphene and has been withdrawn owing to its potential toxicity and poor analgesic properties. Some patients may still be taking this, but it is not prescribed to new patients.

Strong opioids morphine is used for severe pain. Use regular fast-acting opioids for acute pain with regular laxatives and PRN or regular antiemetics. See 'weak opioids' for **cautions**, **side effects** and **toxicity**. Use only one method of administration (ie PO, SC, IM, or IV) to avoid overdose:
- **Oral** eg Sevredol® or Oramorph® 10mg/2–4h
- **SC/IM** morphine 10mg/2–4h or diamorphine 5mg/2–4h
- **IV** titrate to pain; dilute 10mg morphine into 10ml H_2O for injections (1mg/ml), give 2mg initially and wait 2min for response. Give 1mg/2min until pain settled observing RR and responsiveness.

Long-acting opioids are used after major surgery or in chronic pain. Use standard opioids initially until morphine requirements known (🕮 p93) then prescribe a regular long-acting dose along with PRN fast-acting opioids to cover breakthrough pain (equivalent to 15% or one-sixth of daily requirements). Laxatives will be needed.
- **Oral** MST® dose = half total daily oral morphine requirement (🕮 p93) given every 12h, usually 10–30mg/12h, max 400mg/24h
- **Topical** fentanyl patch lasts 72h, available in 12–100micrograms/h doses.

Naloxone given orally antagonises the constipating effects of opioids, but is metabolised on 'first pass' through the liver and does not interfere with analgesic effects. Compound preparations oxycodone/naloxone preparations (eg Targinact®) may be of benefit for chronic pain relief in those who develop painful constipation despite regular laxatives.

Other analgesic options/adjuncts

Nefopam a non-opioid analgesia that can be given with paracetamol, NSAIDs, and opioids; ***contraindications*** epilepsy and convulsions; ***side effects*** urinary retention, pink urine, dry mouth, light-headedness.
- **Nefopam** 30–90mg/8h PO.

Hyoscine butylbromide gives good analgesia in colicky abdo pain; ***contraindications*** paralytic ileus, prostatism, glaucoma, myasthenia gravis, porphyria; ***side effects*** constipation, dry mouth, confusion, urine retention.
- **Buscopan**® (hyoscine butylbromide) 20mg/6h PO/IM/IV.

Diazepam acts as a muscle relaxant, eg spasm with back pain ***contraindications*** respiratory compromise/failure, sleep apnoea ***side effects*** drowsiness, confusion, physical dependence (use for short-term only).
- **Diazepam** 2mg/8h PO.

Quinine used for nocturnal leg cramps; ***contraindications*** haemoglobinuria, optic neuritis, arrhythmias; ***side effects*** abdo pain, tinnitus, confusion.
- **Quinine** 200mg/24h PO—at night.

Patient-controlled analgesia (PCA) a syringe driver that gives a bolus of IV opioid (usually morphine, but occasionally tramadol or fentanyl) when the patient activates a button. A background infusion rate, bolus dose and maximum bolus frequency can be adjusted to prevent overdose/pain; changes to the PCA are usually undertaken by the pain team (see box). The patient must be alert, cooperative, have IV access and their pain under control before starting. Check hospital protocols.

Epidurals are inserted by the anaesthetist in theatre usually prior to surgery. A local anaesthetic infusion (±opioid) anaesthetises the spinal nerves, and usually produces a sensory level below which the patient has little or no feeling; if this level rises too high (higher than T4 (nipples)) there is risk of respiratory failure. The anaesthetist or pain team (see box) usually look after epidurals and their dosing post-op. Complications include local haematoma, abscess (causes cord compression, 📖 p357) or local infection; if there are concerns about an epidural speak to the anaesthetist covering acute pain immediately.

Syringe driver These are used mainly for palliative analgesia and symptom control (📖 p93).

Pain team

Most hospitals have pain teams, often sub-divided into acute and chronic services. These comprise of nurses and a pain specialist (usually an anaesthetist). The acute pain service is sometimes run by the Outreach Team.

In-patients with pain issues can be referred to the teams for assessment, though ensure all simple measures have been undertaken to address the patient's pain first, namely identify and treat cause of pain, and ensure the patient is receiving adequate simple analgesia (regular paracetamol, NSAIDs (if not contraindicated), and an opioid, if appropriate).

Neuropathic and chronic pain

Neuropathic pain is caused by damage to or chronic stimulation of nerve fibres, eg radiculopathy (nerve root pain), peripheral neuropathy, and phantom limb pain. The pain tends to be difficult to describe or pinpoint and is often aching, burning, throbbing, or shooting in nature. Chronic conditions can cause significant pain, eg chronic pancreatitis, arthritis, post-traumatic, DM, trigeminal neuralgia; there is frequently a psychogenic component. Standard analgesia is often ineffective and the services of a chronic pain specialist should be sought. Commoner chronic pain therapies include:

Tricyclic antidepressants given at a low dose; **contraindications** recent MI, arrhythmias; **side effects** dry mouth, constipation, sedation. This is the first-line treatment for neuropathic pain according to NICE guidance.[1]
- **Amitriptyline** 10–75mg/24h PO.

Pregabalin **Contraindications** hypersensitivity, pregnancy, lactation; **side effects** dizziness, tiredness, cerebellar signs. Can be used instead of amitriptyline as first-line treatment for neuropathic pain.
- **Pregabalin** 75–300mg/12h PO.

Duloxetine **Contraindications** uncontrolled hypertension, pregnancy, seizures; **side effects** nausea, dizziness, somnolence, dry mouth. First line for painful diabetic neuropathy. Avoid abrupt discontinuation.
- **Duloxetine** 60–120mg/24h PO.

If first-line drugs are unsuccessful, combination therapy with two or more agents can be considered. If this is unsuccessful then referral for a specialist opinion should be considered. The following are examples of more advanced therapies a pain specialist may prescribe.

TENS **T**ranscutaneous **E**lectrical **N**erve **S**timulation is believed to affect the gate mechanism of pain fibres in the spine and/or to stimulate the production of endorphins. Use at a high frequency for acute pain or slow frequency for chronic/neuropathic pain.

Steroids and nerve blocks Injections of steroids combined with local anaesthetic into joints or around nerves can reduce pain for long periods. This needs to be done by a specialist.

Sympathectomy and nerve ablation The ablation of sensory and sympathetic nerves by surgery or injection; used as a last resort in some forms of chronic pain.

Acupuncture Effective in some trials and with a greater evidence base than most complementary therapies.

Counselling and cognitive–behavioural therapy (CBT) to develop coping strategies are widely studied in chronic pain and may be considered by appropriately skilled specialists. Concern remains that it make things worse for some patients.

Some terms in chronic pain

Allodynia	Seemingly harmless stimuli such as light touch can provoke pain
Hyperpathia	A short episode of discomfort causes prolonged, severe pain
Hyperalgesia	Discomfort which would otherwise be mild is felt as severe pain

[1] NICE guidelines available at guidance.nice.org.uk/CG173

Thinking about death

The best medicine in the world can only delay death; it is an inevitable outcome for us all. Patients often die in hospital and as a junior doctor you will have a vital role in supporting the individual and their loved ones through this process. As with everything else in medicine, playing this role well requires knowledge, skills and compassion. Getting things right can be enormously challenging, but equally rewarding. The following pages act as a guide to help you in these regards.

Fears

It is natural for patients to have a fear of death and dying. It is common to most of us. It should also be noted that many patients, especially the elderly, may be entirely at ease with the prospect of their own death.

If your patient is afraid, it is important to establish exactly what they are afraid of; this may be different from your assumptions:
• Loss of dignity and control
• Symptoms, eg suffocating/pain
• Their relatives seeing them suffering
• The unpleasant death of a relative years ago.

Many of these can now be carefully managed or avoided. When death is not expected or deterioration sudden, then your role in talking to the patient and allaying their fear cannot be overstated. This will be emotionally difficult and you must never hesitate to seek support yourself.

Breaking bad news (🕮 p22)
Other sources of help
Even with sudden deteriorations there are many other sources of help:
• Macmillan nurses and the palliative care team (🕮 p91)
• The acute pain team (usually part of anaesthetics)
• The chaplaincy.
Do not forget you're working with nursing staff who may know the patient much better than you, so discuss their care with them.

Sorting arrangements
Needless to say, marching in and offering a priest and solicitor will be insensitive, but the hospital will be able to provide legal support or an appropriate religious official if asked. Many patients' strongest wish is to die in comfort, often in their own home. Get the Macmillan and/or palliative care team involved early and this can frequently be arranged.

Do not resuscitate orders
This decision should be initiated at consultant or registrar level, and requires ratification by a consultant at the earliest opportunity. It should be clearly written in the notes, on a DNAR form, signed and dated. As the patient's condition changes, further review may be appropriate. It should be discussed with the patients and/or their relatives. Always inform nursing staff.

Requests for euthanasia
Deliberately quickening a patient's death is illegal. Relieving suffering so that you allow someone to die naturally, and free from pain, is not.
• Explain you will always aim to minimise suffering
• Explain to relatives that relieving pain may hasten an inevitable death, before giving opioids (relieving pain removes the adrenergic stimulus which may appropriately lead to a natural death within a few minutes)
• Ensure you could justify actions in court; if in doubt, ask a senior colleague.

Palliative care

Palliative care is the non-curative treatment of a disease; originally focused on terminal cancer, but now covers other disorders. In practice, cancer patients are still able to access more services, including the excellent Macmillan nurses who should be involved as early as possible. The aim is to provide the best quality of life for as long as possible – this may include admission to a hospice (often temporarily).

Pain (📖 p86) This is a common problem in palliative care; opioids are often used. It is important to use all modalities of treatment. Consider:
- Treating the source (urinary retention, bowel spasm, bony mets)
- Non-opioid analgesia (nerve blocks, TENS, neuropathic pain)
- Alternative routes (intranasal, PR, transdermal, SC, IM, IV).

Table 2.6 is a guide to converting between opioids, it is not an exact science and changes need to be monitored for over- or under-dosing.

Table 2.6 *Opioids and their relative potency*

Opioid	Route	Typical dose	24h max	Relative
Codeine	PO	60mg/4h	240mg	0.1
Dihydrocodeine	PO	30mg/4-6h	240mg	0.1
Tramadol	PO	50mg/4h	600mg	0.2
Oral morphine	PO	10mg/1–4h	N/A	1
Oxycodone	PO	5mg/4-6h	400mg	2
Morphine	SC/IM/IV	5mg/1–4h	N/A	2
Diamorphine	SC	2.5mg/1–4h	N/A	3
Fentanyl	Topical	25micrograms/h	2400micrograms	100–150

Other symptoms Many of the treatments listed in Table 2.7 can be used in non-palliative patients. For further information on prescribing in palliative problems see *BNF* and OHCM9 📖 p532.

Table 2.7 *Symptom management in palliative care*

Symptom	Treatments
Breathlessness	O_2, open windows, fans, diamorphine, benzodiazepines, steroids, heliox (helium and oxygen for stridor)
Constipation	See 📖 p310, also bisacodyl
Cough	Saline nebs, antihistamines, simple/codeine linctus, morphine
Dry mouth	Chlorhexidine, sucking ice or pineapple chunks, consider Candida (thrush) infection, synthetic saliva
Hiccups	Antacids, eg Maalox®, Gaviscon®, chlorpromazine, haloperidol
Itching	Emollients, chlorphenamine, cetirizine, colestyramine (obstructive jaundice), ondansetron
Nausea/vomiting	See 📖 p304, also levomepromazine and haloperidol

The dying patient

'...it seems still to be the case that, in practice, the discussion of death as an inevitable and, in some cases, imminent aspect of life is regarded as morbid and thus avoided. Even with patients suffering from terminal conditions, it is common for there to have been no discussion with patients, their consultants or GPs, relatives, and carers, about preparing for dying.'[1]

For those patients who have reached the final stage of their illness and are not expected to survive, the decision may be taken by a senior doctor to withdraw active treatment and focus on keeping the patient comfortable. These decisions and discussions are highly emotive and should be handled with consideration and skill (📖 p90). Much emphasis has been placed on achieving better deaths for hospital patients, but outcomes have been mixed (see box).

Identifying the dying The patient will often (but not always) be bed-bound with minimal oral intake and reduced GCS. This simple definition has poor specificity, with potential for recovery, whilst timescales can be difficult to predict. Since considerable uncertainty will always persist, effective and honest communication is vital, along with regular review of treatment decisions by the senior responsible clinician.

Communication Wherever possible, discussions should happen with the patient and their relatives well in advance; all views should be documented and used to draw up a care plan. Even where an illness progresses rapidly, the withdrawal of active treatment needs to be carefully considered and every effort made to discuss with the relatives; withdrawal of care by junior staff during out-of-hours periods should be avoided.

Stopping medications Administering drugs may cause unnecessary distress, particularly those aimed at prophylaxis of long-term conditions. Review all medications with a senior and stop those deemed to be unnecessary. The decision to stop antibiotics can be a particularly difficult one, but again, this is made easier by documented prior conversations.

Stairway to Heaven or Conveyor Belt to Death?

The Liverpool Care Pathway for the Dying Patient (LCP) was originally developed in the 1990s by the Royal Liverpool University Hospital and the Marie Curie Hospice in Liverpool and aimed to introduce some of the best principles of hospice care into the care of dying patients in other settings, particularly hospitals. Wide dissemination and uptake was not always accompanied by necessary training, in some instances leading the 'pathway' to become little more than a series of protocols for death, with complex paperwork delegated to junior doctors or nursing staff, or left incomplete. Worse was to come, when in some areas the percentage of dying patients placed on the LCP was deemed to be a measure of quality of care, and financial incentives attached. Widespread public concern about the 'Death Pathway' and associated media pressure led the Department of Health to commission an independent review of the LCP,[1] which identified multiple instances of poor practice and concluded that the LCP should be phased out and replaced with more patient-centred end-of-life care plans. More guidance is sure to follow, but protocols, pathways and tick boxes will have no place.

'More Care, less pathway: a review of the Liverpool Care Pathway' Independent Review of the Liverpool Care Pathway, July, 2013. Available free at 🖰www.gov.uk/government/publications/review-of-liverpool-care-pathway-for-dying-patients

Resuscitation Attempts at cardiopulmonary resuscitation in patients with end stage disease are inappropriate. Although the decision rests with the senior responsible clinician, patients and their relatives should be involved in the discussion and informed of decisions where possible prior to signing a 'DNAR' form (📖 p90).

Investigations These may be unnecessary. This includes routine blood tests, where the outcome will not influence clinical management, but will also extend to the taking of nursing observations in the final stages of illness.

Food and fluid A loss of appetite in the terminal stages of disease is common and at this stage nutrition should not be forced. The intake of oral fluids should be supported as long as tolerated, even if this incurs a risk of aspiration. Beyond this stage, artificial hydration (IV or SC) should be used only where it increases comfort, although regular mouth care may continue. Bear in mind that studies have shown no clear benefit to length or quality of life in a palliative setting.[1]

Analgesia Not all dying patients are in pain, and overuse of syringe drivers is inappropriate. However, where present, it is vital to control pain whilst avoiding oversedation (📖 p91). Always exclude a treatable causes eg urinary retention, constipation. If the patient is currently in pain give an immediate diamorphine bolus (2.5–5mg SC max 1hrly if not currently on diamorphine or give 1/6th of 24h dose 1hrly if already on diamorphine). Where pain is regular and predictable, discuss starting a syringe driver with a SC diamorphine infusion giving a total 24h dose equivalent to current cumulative opioid requirements (use Table 2.6 to convert between opioids).

Agitation This may be a sign of pain. Try PRN doses initially; add a syringe driver (with additional PRN dose) if regular doses are required:
- *PRN* levomepromazine 12.5–25mg SC 6–12hrly **or:**
- *PRN* midazolam 2.5–5mg/4h SC max 4hrly
- *Syringe driver* levomepromazine 50–150mg/24h and/or midazolam 10–20mg/24h SC (higher doses up to 60mg/24h may be required).

Nausea + vomiting Continue existing antiemetics in a syringe driver if they are controlling the symptoms; if there is no nausea then prescribe PRN cyclizine and add a syringe driver if it is needed regularly. If further antiemetics are required use a $5HT_3$ antagonist (eg ondansetron).
- *PRN* cyclizine 50mg/8h SC
- *Syringe driver* levomepromazine 5–12.5mg/24h SC.

Secretions The patient's breathing may become rattly due to the build-up of secretions with a poor cough/swallow reflex. Sitting the patient up slightly may help; medication improves the symptoms if started promptly. Start with a PRN dose and add a syringe driver if regular doses are required:
- *PRN* glycopyrronium 200–400micrograms SC 6hrly or hyoscine butylbromide 20mg SC 6hrly
- *Syringe driver* glycopyrronium 1.2–2mg/24h SC or hyoscine butylbromide 90–120mg/24h SC.

Further care Review the patient regularly. Ask the patient and/or relatives if there are any new symptoms and adjust medications accordingly. If you are unable to control symptoms ask for palliative care review.

[1] Good, P. *et al. Cochrane Database of Systemic Reviews*, 2008 available at 🔗onlinelibrary.wiley.com/doi/10.1002/14651858.CD006273.pub2/full

Death

Declaring death

You will often be asked to declare that a patient has died. This is not an urgent request, but the patient cannot be transferred to the mortuary until it is done. There may be other members of staff who can do this if you are busy and unable to attend in a timely fashion. If you are uncomfortable doing this alone, or are doing it for the first time, ask another member of staff to accompany you.

The Academy of Medical Royal Colleges have guidance on the diagnosis and confirmation of death from which the following advice is adapted,[1] but your hospital may have specific guidelines which you should follow.

1. Confirming cardiorespiratory arrest

You should observe the patient for a **minimum of five minutes** to confirm irreversible cardiorespiratory arrest has occurred:
- Listen for heart sounds in two places, for one minute in each place (total two minutes), *then*
- Palpate over a central artery (carotid/femoral) for one minute, *then*
- Listen for breath sounds in two places, for one minute in each place (total two minutes).

It is common to hear transmitted gastrointestinal sounds when auscultating the chest, which should be ignored. However, in a very recently deceased patient it is also not uncommon for a lone complex to appear on the ECG, or for them to take a 'last' (agonal) breath: This or any other spontaneous return of cardiac or respiratory activity during your period of observation should prompt a further five minute observation from the next point of cardiorespiratory arrest, unless the patient is for active resuscitation.

2. Confirming the absence of motor response

After five minutes of continued cardiorespiratory arrest confirm the absence of motor response in the patient:
- Absence of the pupillary response to light; the pupils will often be dilated and they should not change when exposed to a bright light source (eg pen torch)
- Absence of the corneal reflex; passing rolled up cotton wool over the edge of the cornea should not elicit a blinking response
- Absence of any motor response to supra-orbital pressure; applying firm supra-orbital pressure should not elicit any motor response.

3. Documentation

The time of death is recorded as the time at which these criteria are fulfilled (Fig. 2.9). Remember to sign and print your name and bleep number.

---

[1] Academy of Medical Royal Colleges 'A code of practice for the diagnosis and confirmation of death', 2010. Available at www.aomrc.org.uk/publications/statements/doc_view/42-a-code-of-practice-for-the-diagnosis-and-confirmation-of-death.html

16/09/14   Asked to verify death.
03:30

No heart sounds for 2 minutes
No carotid pulse for 1 minute
No breath sounds for 2 minutes
Pupils unreactive to light
No corneal reflex
No response to supra-orbital stimulation

Death confirmed at 03.25 on 16/09/2014

Dr CJ Flint
FLINT, F1
Bleep 3294

Fig. 2.9 Example of what to write in the notes when a patient dies.

What happens to the patient after death

When a patient dies the nurses prepare the body,[1] including: closing the curtains, lying them flat with one pillow, closing their eyes and closing the jaw (this may need to be propped closed with a rolled towel under the chin), washing the body, using pads to absorb any leakage from the urethra, vagina or rectum, and removing attachments (eg fluids, pumps). Lines and tubes are not removed since these will be inspected if a post-mortem examination is undertaken. The patient is completely covered with a sheet.

Once they have been declared dead and the body has been prepared, they are taken to the mortuary in a portable coffin. Curtains and portable partitions are used to try and screen this from other patients.

Communication around death

On occasion, it will be your duty to inform others of the death of a loved one. This will produce strong emotions, even when the news is expected, and calls for skilful and sensitive communication (📖 p22). Ensure you are mentally ready to break this news (ask a nurse to accompany you wherever possible), know the identity of everyone in the room and that the environment is appropriate. Study the notes beforehand so that you can answer questions relating to events leading up to the death – if you are still unsure of details, be honest and offer to check. Ask if they would like to see the body at that time, and be clear that there will be later opportunities too. The most important element is to give those receiving the news time – both silence and emotion are completely acceptable and to be expected and should not be talked over or hurried. You will not be able to remove sorrow, but your empathy and professionalism may just help to soften a painful memory that will be mentally revisited many times in the coming months and years.

Always remember to inform the GP of the patient's death, especially if it was unexpected. This is both courteous and prevents any unfortunate phone calls from the GP enquiring about the patient's health.

[1] Henry C, Wilson J. Personal care at the end of life and after death, *Nursing Times* 8 May 2012, available free online at: **www.nursingtimes.net/Journals/2012/05/08/h/i/z/120805-Innov-endoflife.pdf**

Medical Certificate of Cause of Death

All deaths in the United Kingdom must be registered with a local registrar's office. In order for this to happen, a doctor may issue a 'medical certificate of cause of death' (MCCD), confusingly often referred to as a 'death certificate'. Alternatively, where the cause of death is not clear or there are any circumstances requiring clarification, the coroner's office must be informed (📖 p100). In Scotland, different legislation applies and a slightly different MCCD is used and the procurator fiscal takes the coroner's role.

Eligibility In hospital, it is ultimately the consultant's responsibility to ensure the MCCD is properly completed but it can be delegated to a member of the team who 'attended' the patient in the last 14d of life (28d in Northern Ireland). This applies to those involved in the patient's care and who reliably know the history and course of in-patient stay. Where circumstances require involvement of the coroner's office/procurator fiscal (📖 p100), do not complete the MCCD unless they instruct you to do so.

Completing the MCCD Most of the entries are self-explanatory:
- *Name of deceased:* full name of the deceased
- *Date of death as stated to me:* eg fifteenth day of August 2014
- *Age as stated to me:* eg 92 years
- *Place of death:* ward, hospital, and city where they died
- *Last seen alive by me:* eg fourteenth day of August 2014

Then circle just **one** of these (most commonly option '3'):
1. *The certified cause of death takes account of information obtained from post-mortem.*
2. *Information from post-mortem may be available later.*
3. *Post-mortem not being held.*
4. *I have reported this death to the Coroner for further action.*

Then circle just **one** of these (most commonly option 'a'):
a. *Seen after death by me.*
b. *Seen after death by another medical practitioner but not by me.*
c. *Not seen after death by a medical practitioner.*

Cause of death This can be difficult: It is important to take advice from the consultant the patient was under.[1] It is important to think of this as a sequence of events leading up to the death of the patient. The pathology listed in I(a) is whatever ultimately resulted in the patient dying (eg intraventricular haemorrhage, myocardial infarction, meningococcal septicaemia); avoid using modes of death (Table 2.8) as this may lead to delays later in the process. The I(b) and I(c) entries should be the pathology/sequence of events which led up to I(a). Include pathology in II which likely contributed to death but might not have necessarily been part of the main sequence of events leading up to the death. It is not compulsory to have entries in I(b), I(c) or II and these can be left blank. Avoid abbreviations.

Approximate interval between onset and death This gives the sequence of events a time frame.

An example

I(a)	Pulmonary embolism	6 hours
(b)	Fractured femur	7 days
(c)	Osteoporosis	30 years
II	Ischaemic heart disease	30 years

[1] As part of the reforms to death certification proposed for introduction in 2014, the new role of Medical Examiner (Medical Reviewer in Scotland) will provide an additional source of advice (📖 p100).

The death might have been due to or contributed to by the employment followed at some time by the deceased If you think the death was in any way related to their employment or an industrial disease you should refer the case to the coroner/procurator fiscal for their consideration.

Signing the certificate requires your signature and medical qualifications, alongside which your local office will usually ask you to print your name and often your GMC number. For *Residence* it is acceptable to enter the name of the hospital and the city. *For deaths in hospital:* you also need to enter the name of the patient's consultant at the time of death.

Completing the sides Make sure you complete the stubs on either side of the main form, copying exactly your entries off the main form.

Completing the back If you have spoken to the coroner's or procurator fiscal's office, and they have decided it is appropriate for you to complete the MCCD, they may ask you to circle one of the options and initial in box A on the reverse of the MCCD.

Post-mortem There are two types of post-mortem (PM): Those mandated by the coroner or procurator fiscal, and those undertaken after a medical request (a 'hospital PM').

The coroner's PM (or procurator fiscal in Scotland) is undertaken to find out how someone died and to inform the decision on whether an inquest is needed or not. The next of kin is informed, but not asked for permission, as the law requires a PM to be performed.

A hospital PM is usually undertaken at a doctor's request to provide more information about an illness or the cause of death. Consent must be given by the patient before they died, or by the next of kin after their death. The hospital bereavement office can assist with this should you be asked to gain consent.

Table 2.8 *Causes and modes of death*

Causes of death (use these terms)	Modes of death (avoid these terms)
Myocardial infarction, cardiac arrhythmia	Cardiac arrest, syncope
Sepsis, hypovolaemia, haemorrhage, anaphylaxis	Hypotension, shock, off-legs
Congestive cardiac failure, pulmonary oedema	Heart failure, cardiac failure, ventricular failure
Bronchopneumonia, pulmonary embolism, asthma, chronic obstructive pulmonary disease	Respiratory failure, respiratory arrest
Cerebrovascular accident	Collapse
Cirrhosis, glomerulonephritis, diabetic nephropathy	Liver failure, renal failure, uraemia
Carcinomatosis, carcinoma of the ...	Cachexia, exhaustion

Cremation forms[1]

Statute While individual crematoria or regions may have slightly different looking cremation forms, they all follow a similar pattern and ask very similar questions. Guidance on how to complete cremation forms is freely available online,[2] though the bereavement office will also be able to guide you and answer your questions.

Cremation form nomenclature The main form to be completed for adult cremation is 'Cremation 4' (Form B in Northern Ireland) – see box. The senior doctor (who must be fully registered for more than 5 years) who checks and verifies the details in Cremation 4 subsequently completes 'Cremation 5' (Form C in Northern Ireland). Other cremation forms are available for stillbirths, and for the cremation of body parts.[1]

Eligibility For deaths in hospital, it is expected that the person completing Cremation 4 treated the deceased during their last illness and to have seen the deceased within 14 days of death. Medical practitioners completing Cremation 4 must hold a licence to practise with the GMC, which includes temporary or provisional registration.

Examining the body If you are completing a cremation form you were previously required to see the body to check the patient's identity (wrist band and physical appearance) and examine them to see if they have any implant which may cause a problem during cremation (see Table 2.9). Under the proposed 2014 reforms, this responsibility will transfer to the Medical Examiners. If you are required to view the body, check the notes, ECGs and X-rays for possible implants, but also examine the patient for scars or palpable implants (pacemakers are usually, but not always, on the anterior chest wall). If you believe there is an implant talk to the mortuary staff who will be able to remove it.

Remuneration Under arrangements prior to 2014, junior doctors were paid around £70 for completing the form (see 📖 p38); this fee is under review as part of the 2014 reforms. Any fee comes from the patient's relatives via the funeral director who keeps the money if you fail to take it. The reason you are paid is because this is not a standard NHS service and you are taking responsibility for the fact the body will not be able to be exhumed for evidence if there is any doubt in the future as to the cause of death.

Table 2.9 *Problematic implants for the cremation of human remains*

Pacemakers; implantable cardioverter defibrillators; cardiac resynchronisation therapy devices; implantable loop recorder

Ventricular assist devices

Implantable drug pumps including intrathecal pumps

Neurostimulators and bone growth stimulators

Hydrocephalus programmable shunts

Any other battery powered implant

Fixion nails (intramedullary nails for fixing long bone fractures)

Brachytherapy implants

[1] In Scotland, the information previously contained on the cremation form will be included on the revised MCCD from 2014 onwards. Arrangements in the rest of the UK are under review.
[2] eg For England and Wales: 🔗 www.justice.gov.uk/downloads/burials-and-coroners/cremations/cremation-doctors-guidance.pdf

Completing Cremation 4

Most of the questions are self-explanatory:

- Details of the deceased: Name, address, occupation
- Date and time of death, place of death
- Are you a relative of the deceased?
- Have you, so far as you are aware, any pecuniary interest in the death of the deceased?
- Were you the deceased's usual medical practitioner? Generally it is the patient's GP who is regarded as the usual medical practitioner.
- Please state for how long you attended the deceased during their last illness? eg 5 days
- Please state the number of days and hours before the deceased's death that you last saw them alive? eg 1 day, 12 hours
- Please state the date and time that you saw the body of the deceased and the examination that you made of the body? eg date, time, external examination to confirm identify and check for implantable devices
- From your medical notes, and the observations of yourself and others immediately before and at the time of the deceased's death, please describe the symptoms and other conditions which led to your conclusions about the cause of death. Outline the symptoms in the period leading up to the patient's death; include the date of admission to hospital
- Has a post-mortem examination been made? Usually the answer to this is no, but if it has, tick yes and give details
- Please give the cause of death. Copy what appears on the MCCD
- Did the deceased undergo any operation in the year before their death? If yes, give brief details
- Do you have any reasons to believe that the operation(s) shortened the life of the deceased? If yes, the case should be discussed with your seniors/Medical Examiner/coroner's office/procurator fiscal
- Please give the name and address of any person who nursed the deceased during their last illness. Usually enter the name of the sister responsible for the ward where the patient died, eg Sister Jayne Smith, Ward 26
- Were there any persons present at the moment of death? If yes, give details, as above
- If there were persons present at the moment of death, did those persons have any concerns regarding the cause of death? If yes, give details
- In view of your knowledge of the deceased's habits and constitution do you have any doubts whether about the character of the disease or condition which led to the death? Yes or no
- Have you any reason to suspect the death of the deceased was: violent (yes or no) or unnatural (yes or no)?
- Have you any reason at all to suppose a further examination of the body is desirable? If yes, give details
- Has the coroner been informed about the death? If yes, give details
- Has there been any discussion with a coroner's office about the death of the deceased? If yes, give details
- Have you given the certificate required for the registration of death? If no, give the details of who has completed the MCCD
- Was any hazardous implant placed in the body? See Table 2.9.
- If yes, has it been removed? Yes or no
- Sign, date and enter your contact details.

Death certification, registrars, examiners and the coroner[1]

Steps involved in registering a death If a medical practitioner completes the MCCD, this is given to the next of kin, usually by the bereavement office; if the doctor cannot complete a MCCD, the coroner sends the relevant paperwork directly to the registrar after establishing a cause of death to the best of his/her satisfaction, through a post-mortem and/or investigation and/or inquest. Only once the registrar has the relevant paperwork can the death be entered into the register and a death certificate issued to the next of kin, permitting a burial or cremation to take place.

Death Certification Reforms In response to the Shipman Inquiry and more recently the Francis Inquiry, a new system is being introduced. All MCCDs will be scrutinised by a **_Medical Examiner_**, who will be able to make certain changes to the MCCD after examining the case notes or talking to staff involved in the patients care and to the individual who initially completed the MCCD, if the cause of death is inaccurate. Junior doctors may speak to their local Medical Examiner before completing the MCCD for guidance. Any case which would normally have been referred to the coroner will still be referred to the coroner, but if not accepted by the coroner will then be subsequently scrutinised by the Medical Examiner. The purpose of the Medical Examiner system is to: ensure more accurate reporting of disease processes; to better identify unusual patterns of death which may have public health or local clinical governance implications; to ensure the individual completing the MCCD understands the cause of death, and to provide an opportunity to raise other matters which might require the death to be reported to the coroner.

Medical Examiner These are medical practitioners from any speciality background who are licensed to practise by the GMC and with at least 5 years' experience. As well as scrutinising MCCD and guiding doctors to complete these, they will also discuss the cause of death with the family and act on any additional information the family provides. They will work closely with the coroner's service and registrations services, and feed information back to clinical governance structures to aid in future healthcare planning and provision.

The Coroner The coroner is a government official and is usually a lawyer but may have joint degrees in law and medicine; their job is to investigate a death when the cause of death is unknown or cannot readily be certified as being due to natural causes (see box 🕮 p101).

The Coroner's Office This is staffed by Coroner's Officers. They are not usually medically or legally qualified and are often serving, or ex-police officers. They take the majority of enquiries, and will filter which cases are escalated to the coroner.

---

[1] The term 'coroner' as used here applies to the coronial service in use in England and Wales and Northern Ireland, as well as the role of the Procurator Fiscal in Scotland. Although these are all covered by different legislation, the same basic roles and rules apply. Likewise the new role of 'Medical Examiner' in England and Wales is equivalent to 'Medical Reviewer' in Scotland.

Making a referral to the coroner Any case which meets the criteria in the box should be referred to the coroner's office for their consideration; after discussing the case, the coroner's officer may suggest it is appropriate for the referring doctor to complete the MCCD. Occasionally the coroner's officer will either take over the case, or wish to discuss it directly with the coroner first, and in these situations the MCCD should not be completed by the referring doctor unless instructed to do so.

To refer, or not to refer? If you are in any doubt about whether to refer to the coroner or not, speak first to your seniors, or the local Medical Examiner for advice.

A death should be referred to HM Coroner if either:[1]

- the cause of death is unknown;
- it cannot be readily certified as being due to natural causes;
- the deceased was not attended by the doctor during his last illness or was not seen within the last 14 days or viewed after death;
- there are any suspicious circumstances or history of violence;
- the death may be linked to an accident (whenever it occurred);
- there is any question of self-neglect or neglect by others;
- the death has occurred or the illness arisen during or shortly after detention in police or prison custody (including voluntary attendance at a police station);
- the deceased was detained under the Mental Health Act;
- the death is linked with an abortion;
- the death might have been contributed to by the actions of the deceased (such as a history of drug or solvent abuse, self injury or overdose);
- the death could be due to industrial disease or related in any way to the deceased's employment;
- the death occurred during an operation or before full recovery from the effects of an anaesthetic or was in any way related to the anaesthetic (in any event a death within 24 hours should normally be referred);
- the death may be related to a medical procedure or treatment whether invasive or not;
- the death may be due to lack of medical care;
- there are any other unusual or disturbing features to the case;
- the death occurred within 24 hours of admission to hospital (unless the admission was purely for terminal care);
- it may be wise to report any death where there is an allegation of medical mismanagement.

This note is for guidance only, it is not exhaustive and in part may represent desired local practice rather than the statutory requirements. If in any doubt contact the coroner's office for further advice.

[1] Taken from: Dorries, C. *Coroners' Courts: a guide to law and practice*, 2nd edition, Oxford University Press, 2004.

Nutrition

A patient's nutritional state has a huge effect on their well-being, mood, compliance with treatment, and ability to heal. You should consider alternative nutrition for all patients without a normal oral diet for over 48h. IV fluids are only for hydration, they are not nutrition. See Table 2.10 for nutritional requirements.

Enteral feeding (via the gut)

Oral Most patients manage to consume sufficient quantities of hospital food to stay healthy. If not (eg due to inability to feed self, increased demand due to malnutrition) consider simple remedies, eg assisted feeding, favourite foods from home, medications for reflux/heartburn (📖 p294) or nausea (📖 p185). If they are still not consuming adequate nutrition then discuss with the dietician who can advise on nutritional supplements and high-energy drinks.

Nasogastric (NG) See 📖 p549 for insertion procedure. This is a good short-term measure, however placing the tube may be uncomfortable and some people find the sensation of the tube uncomfortable once it is in. Liquid foods and most oral medicines (except slow release and enteric coated preparations) can be given via NG tube; advice regarding medications via this route may be required from a pharmacist. Tubes can also be endoscopically placed naso-jejunally if required, eg gastric outlet obstruction.

Gastrostomy Often called 'PEGs' (percutaneous endoscopic gastrostomy) these are a good long-term method of feeding in patients who cannot feed orally. They are typically sited endoscopically, though surgical and radiological approaches are possible (a radiologically inserted gastrostomy is referred to as a RIG). It is also possible to place a jejunostomy if required.

Parenteral feeding (via the blood)

Parenteral nutrition (PN) or total parenteral nutrition (TPN) requires central access because extravasation of the feed causes severe skin irritation. Central access can be via a long-line (eg PiCC) or central line (eg Hickman). It is used when the patient cannot tolerate sufficient enteral feeds, eg short gut syndrome or when gut rest is required.

There is significant risk associated with PN use including line insertion, line infection, embolism/thrombosis, and electrolyte abnormalities. It is essential to monitor blood electrolytes regularly including Ca^{2+}, PO_4^{3-}, Mg^{2+}, zinc, and trace elements, particularly in those starting PN after a period of malnutrition (see below).

Refeeding syndrome

After a prolonged period of malnutrition or parenteral nutrition, feeds must be reintroduced slowly (over a few days) to prevent electrolyte imbalance, particularly ↓PO_4^{3-}. It can be fatal but is entirely avoidable if blood tests are checked daily during the at risk period (for 3–5d, until full feeding rate established) and any electrolyte abnormalities are corrected promptly.

Nutritional requirements

Table 2.10 *Nutritional requirements*

Name	Sources	Daily requirement	Deficiency
Carbohydrate	Almost all foods	300g	Malnutrition
Protein	Meat, dairy, vegetables, grain	50g	Kwashiorkor
Fat	Nuts, meat, dairy, oily foods	56g	Malnutrition
Calcium	Dairy, leafy vegetables	1g	Osteoporosis
Iodine	Fish, seafood, enriched salt	150micrograms	Hypothyroid
Iron	Meat, vegetables, grains	15mg	Anaemia
Magnesium	Dairy, leafy vegetables, meat	420mg	Cramps
Potassium	Fruits, vegetables	3.5g	Hypokalaemia
Selenium	Meat, fish, vegetables	55micrograms	Keshan disease
Sodium	Processed foods, salt	2.4g	Hyponatraemia
Zinc	Cereals, meat	11mg	Hair/skin problems
Vitamin A (retinoid)	Dairy, yellow or green leafy vegetables, liver, fish	900micrograms	Night blindness
Vitamin B_1 (thiamine)	Bread, cereals	1.2mg	Beri Beri
Vitamin B_2 (riboflavin)	Meat, dairy, bread	1.3mg	Ariboflavinosis
Vitamin B_3 (niacin)	Meat, fish, bread	16mg	Pellagra
Vitamin B_5 (pantothenic acid)	Meat, egg, grains, potato, vegetables	5mg	Neurological problems, paraesthesia
Vitamin B_6 (pyridoxine)	Meat, fortified cereals	1.7mg	Anaemia
Vitamin B_7 (biotin)	Liver, fruit, meat	30micrograms	Dermatitis
Vitamin B_9 (folate)	Bread, leafy vegetables, cereals	400micrograms	Anaemia
Vitamin B_{12} (cobalamin)	Meat, fish, fortified cereals	2.4micrograms	Anaemia
Vitamin C (ascorbic acid)	Citrus fruits, tomato, green vegetables	200mg	Scurvy
Vitamin D	Fish, liver, fortified cereals	5–15micrograms	Rickets/osteomalacia
Vitamin E	Vegetables, nuts, fruits, cereals	15mg	None
Vitamin K	Green vegetables, cereals	120micrograms	↑PT

Difficult patients

Alcoholism[1] Many patients will drink over the recommend limits (3-4 units/d for ♂ and 2–3 units/d for ♀), but not all of these will be 'alcoholics'. Defining alcoholism is hard, but if drinking, or the effects of drinking, repeatedly harms work or social life it is clearly a problem. Answering 'yes' to three out of four of the **CAGE** questions suggests alcoholism: Ever felt you should **C**ut down on your drinking? Have people **A**nnoyed you by criticising your drinking? Ever felt **G**uilty about your drinking? Ever had an **E**ye-opener in the morning?

The medical aspects of alcohol excess and withdrawal are covered on 📖 p348. Excessive drinking can be a psychiatric issue in its own right but can also complicate many psychiatric diseases. Modifying drinking behaviour is difficult and only of benefit in patients who want to change.

- **Abuse** Excessive drinking despite mental or physical harm
- **Dependence** Alcohol tolerance, withdrawal symptoms if not drinking.

Alcoholism management Have a low threshold for commencing benzodiazepine therapy to avoid alcohol withdrawal (see suggested regimen in Table 2.11 or your trust's own protocol). In addition, start vitamin B₁ supplementation with either IV preparations (Pabrinex® 2 pairs/8h IV for 2d) or oral thiamine 200mg/24h PO and multi-vitamins (1–2 tablets/24h PO).

Table 2.11 *Chlordiazepoxide regimen for alcohol withdrawal*

Day 1	20mg/6h PO	Day 5	5mg/6h PO
Day 2	20mg/8h PO	Day 6	5mg/8h PO
Day 3	10mg/6h PO	Day 7	5mg/12h PO
Day 4	10mg/8h PO	Day 8	STOP

If not treated, thiamine deficiency can lead to Wernicke's encephalopathy (see 📖 p363). This is characterised by a triad of nystagmus, ophthalmoplegia, and ataxia, but can also present with confusion, altered consciousness, vomiting, and headache. Untreated it can progress to Korsakoff's syndrome characterised by an irreversible inability to acquire new memories associated with a tendency to confabulate to fill in the gaps. Both are treated with Pabrinex® or oral thiamine, but the memory loss in Korsakoff's is usually permanent.

Other management Alcohol diaries, reduced intake or abstinence plans, individual and group counselling, eg Alcoholics Anonymous, pharmacological assistance, eg disulfiram, address underlying social and psychiatric problems.

Elderly patients often take many medications, making interactions and side effects more common. Declining renal function means lower doses may be needed for renally excreted drugs. Likewise, elderly patients are more prone to heart failure from fluid boluses/excessive IV fluids. Other problems include: increased susceptibility to infections; higher pain threshold (can mask fractures or other acute pathology); atypical disease presentations; poor thermoregulation (easily develop hypothermia); malnourishment (if unable to obtain/prepare food); history taking can be difficult if hard of hearing. Elderly patients can suffer with depression and other psychiatric illness (📖 p367) and social circumstances must always be considered prior to discharge – liaise with OT, physiotherapy, and social services.

---

[1] NICE guidelines available at ⏁guidance.nice.org.uk/CG115

Aggression and violence

The majority of patients have respect for NHS staff; however under certain circumstances anyone can become aggressive:

- Pain (🕮 p86)
- Reversible confusion or delirium, eg hypoglycaemia (🕮 p341)
- Dementia (🕮 p342)
- Inadequate communication/fear/frustration (🕮 p19)
- Intoxication (medications, alcohol, recreational drugs)
- Mental illness or personality disorder (🕮 p364–369).

The aggressive patient Ask a nurse to accompany you when assessing aggressive patients. Position yourselves between the exit and the patient and ensure that other staff know where you are. The majority of patients can be calmed simply by talking; try to elicit why they are angry and ask specifically about pain and worry. Be calm but firm and do not shout or make threats. If this does not help, offer an oral sedative or give emergency IV sedation (see 🕮 p364) or call hospital security.

The aggressive relative Relatives may be aggressive through fear, frustration, and/or intoxication. They usually respond to talking, though make sure you obtain consent from the patient before discussing their medical details. Consider offering to arrange a meeting with a senior doctor. If the relative continues to be aggressive, remember that your duty of care to patients does not extend to their relatives; you do not have to tell them anything or listen to threats/abuse. In extreme cases you can ask security or police to remove the relative from the hospital.

Violence Assault (the attempt or threat of causing harm) and battery (physical contact without consent) by a patient or relative is a criminal offence. If you witness an assault or are assaulted yourself, inform your seniors and fill in an incident form including the name and contact details of any witnesses. If no action is taken on your behalf inform the police yourself.

Abuse Abuse is a violation of an individual's human and civil rights and may consist of a single act or repeated actions. It may be physical, sexual, financial, psychological or through neglect. Patients of any age can be abused. Do not be afraid of asking patients how they sustained injuries or asking directly if someone caused them. Inform a senior if you suspect a patient has been abused (see box).

Safeguarding and protection

As a doctor you will often meet your patients at their most vulnerable moments. In most instances, the forces of nature will have conspired to weaken the individual to bring them to this point. But in sad and rare cases, vulnerable individuals are not afforded the protection they need, and a presentation to acute healthcare services may be a manifestation of abuse. Two groups are particularly at risk: vulnerable adults (those in need of community services because of mental or other illness, disability or age) and children. Whilst government policy on protecting these groups continues to evolve, and new statutory regulations are likely to be introduced, your local healthcare organisation should have clear policies on child protection and adult safeguarding. In all instances, your first and most important action if you believe a patient may be subject to any form of abuse is to bring your concerns to the attention of your consultant.

Needle-stick injuries

Many doctors have received needle-stick injuries without serious consequences (see Table 2.12). However, if you have just been exposed get advice as soon as possible.

Immediately

Stop what you are doing. If it is urgent, phone your senior/colleague to do it. Your future health is your top priority.

- *Percutaneous exposure* (needle or sharp) squeeze around the wound so that blood comes out and wash with soap and water; avoid scrubbing or pressing the wound directly
- *Mucocutaneous exposure* (eyes, nose, mouth) rinse with water (or 1l of 0.9% saline through a giving set for eyes/nose).

Within an hour

A colleague should:

- *Talk* to the patient alone, explain what has happened and ask about risk factors:
  - injecting drugs, blood transfusions, tattoos or piercings in foreign countries, unprotected sex (particularly in last 3mth, in a developing country or, if male, with a man), prior testing for hepatitis B+C or HIV and the results
- *Ask* to take a blood sample for testing for hepatitis B+C and HIV.

You should:

- *Phone* occupational health if during office hours or go to the ED and follow their advice exactly
- *Document* the event in the patient's notes and complete an incident form.

Post-exposure prophylaxis

You may be prescribed antiretrovirals (triple therapy, within 1h), hepatitis B immunoglobulin (within 24h), or hepatitis B booster (within 24h) according to the significance of the exposure. There is currently no post-exposure prophylaxis for hepatitis C.

Table 2.12 *Viruses associated with needle-stick injuries*

	Hepatitis B	**Hepatitis C**	**HIV**
UK prevalence	<0.5%	<0.5%	<0.1%
Transmission risk	1 in 3 (without vaccine)	1 in 50	1 in 300
Vaccination	Vaccines at 1, 2, + 12mth	None	None
Post-exposure	Immunoglobulin or booster	None	Triple therapy

Over the next few weeks

The patient's blood tests should take <2d for HIV and hepatitis B+C results. Following high-risk exposure you may be advised to have a blood test in the future (2–6mth); during this time you should practise safe sex (condoms) and not donate blood. **You cannot be forced to have an HIV test**. Discuss with occupational health about involvement in surgery.

Pre-op assessment

Elective patients generally attend pre-admission clinics a few weeks before their operation. This enables you to:

- Assess the patient's problem (ie do they still need the operation?)
- Gauge their medical fitness for an anaesthetic and surgery
- Request any pre-op investigations (see NICE guidelines, Table 2.13)
- Check consent (this should only be obtained by the surgeon performing the procedure or a person competent to undertake it, see 🕮 p129)
- Answer any questions the patient may have.

Pre-op investigations

Table 2.13 *Pre-operative investigations[1]*

Investigation	Indication
FBC	To exclude infection or anaemia
Sickle-cell screen	African/Mediterranean patients, +ve family history
U+E	Age >60yr, cardiac/renal disease, patients on steroids, diuretics, ACEi
LFT	Previous/suspected abnormal liver function, biliary surgery
Clotting	Established/suspected abnormal liver function or clotting disorder
Urine β-hCG	Women of child-bearing age
CXR	Age >60yr, cardiorespiratory disease, malignancy, major thoracic and upper abdominal surgery, unexplained SOB
ECG	Age >50yr, cardiovascular disease, DM, smokers

[1] NICE guidelines: 🖰guidance.nice.org.uk/CG3

Requesting blood pre-op

Each hospital will have guidelines on the transfusion requirements for most elective operations; become familiar with these. Blood for transfusion is in limited supply and should only be cross-matched when necessary. Table 2.14 shows common blood requirements for elective surgery.

Table 2.14 *Summary of operations and blood requirements*

Blood request	Operation
No request	Minor day-case surgery (carpal tunnel release, peripheral lipoma excision, etc)
Group and save	Laparoscopy, appendicectomy, cholecystectomy, hernia repair, simple hysterectomy, liver biopsy, mastectomy, varicose veins, thyroidectomy
X-match 2units	Colectomy, hemiarthroplasty, laparotomy, TURP, total hip replacement
X-match 4units	Abdominoperineal resection, hepatic/pancreatic surgery
X-match 6units	Aneurysm repair (book ICU bed post-op)

Patients with medical problems
- *DM* See 📖 p328, put the patient first on the operating list
- *CVS* Inform the anaesthetist if patients have had recent chest pain, an undiagnosed murmur, or symptoms of heart failure. The anaesthetist may want you to request an echo or may see the patient personally
- *Rheumatoid arthritis/ankylosing spondylitis* Inform the anaesthetist as these patients may be difficult to intubate or have an unstable C-spine – the anaesthetist may want to see the patient or request radiological imaging.

Contacting the anaesthetist/ICU
Find out who the anaesthetist is for your list and inform them as soon as possible about any patients who may need further investigations or review prior to surgery. If a patient needs an ICU bed post-op, inform ICU well in advance with the date the bed is required (contact details should be available from the anaesthetic department office). Phone to confirm that the bed is still available on the day of the operation; if it is not the operation may be cancelled.

Special circumstances
- *Steroids* (📖 p177) Patients taking regular steroids must have extra steroid cover during surgery and be converted to IV preparations if NBM. Discuss each patient's needs with your team and the anaesthetist
- *Warfarin* should be stopped at least 5d pre-operatively. The INR should be <1.5 for most operations and lower if spinal or epidural anaesthetic techniques are to be used; warn the anaesthetist. Patients with prosthetic heart valves may need IV or SC heparin whilst warfarin is omitted (📖 p406)
- *Clopidogrel* must be stopped 7–10d prior to surgery, aspirin is usually continued unless otherwise instructed by senior surgeon (if in doubt check with the operating surgeon/named consultant)
- *Oestrogens and progestogens* HRT can be continued as long as DVT/PE prophylaxis is undertaken. Progestogen-only contraceptives can be continued, but combined oral contraceptives should be stopped 4wk prior to surgery and alternative means of contraception used
- *Bowel preparation* see table 2.15 📖 p109.

Writing the drug chart
Try and do this at pre-admission clinic to save yourself time later. Document any allergies. Things to check include:
- *Prophylactic anticoagulation* (📖 p406)
- *Antibiotics* Consider pre-op antibiotics (check local guidelines)
- *Bowel preparation and IV fluid* (📖 p109)
- *Regular drugs* Review these and write up those which should be continued in hospital (stop COCP, clopidogrel as above, etc)
- *TED stockings* Prescribe these under regular medications for all patients
- *Analgesia and anti-emetics* (📖 p86 and 📖 p304) The anaesthetist will usually write these up during the operation

Instructions for the patient
- Where and when to go for admission (write this down for them)
- If they are to have bowel prep, they should usually be on clear fluids at least 24h before the operation (see 📖 p111)
- Tell the patient about any drains, NG tubes or catheters which may be inserted during the operation
- Tell them if they are being admitted to ICU post-op.

Bowel preparation

Before endoscopy and some GI surgery procedures patients are given laxatives to clear the bowel (Table 2.15). For surgery the aim is to reduce the risk of post-op anastomotic leak and infections. Accumulating evidence suggests that it does not improve complication rates and may even be harmful,[1] hence use of bowel preparation prior to surgery is declining. Check your local policy for guidance. Where bowel preparation is required, it is vital that patients are instructed properly and the importance of good compliance is stressed. For example, during colonoscopy inadequate bowel preparation can lead to pathology being missed or the procedure being aborted.

Table 2.15 *Procedures and the potential need for bowel preparation*

Bowel preparation	Procedure
None	OGD, ERCP, closure (reversal) ileostomy
Phosphate enema (on day of surgery)	Anal fissure, haemorrhoidectomy, examination under anaesthetic (sigmoid colon/rectum/perianal area), flexible sigmoidoscopy
Full bowel prep (see below)	Colonoscopy, rectopexy, right hemi-/left hemi-/sigmoid/pancolectomy, anterior resection, abdominoperineal resection, Hartmann's reversal

Full bowel preparation

A variety of oral bowel cleansing products are available in the UK. In 2009 the National Patient Safety Agency issued an alert in response to safety incidents including a reported death following bowel preparation. In particular, patients at risk of renal impairment and electrolyte imbalance need careful identification and prescribing.
- Sodium picosulfate/Magnesium citrate combinations (eg Picolax®) give excellent bowel preparation and are relatively acceptable to patients; they are relatively contraindicated in those with stage 4 or 5 CKD or those at risk of electrolyte imbalance, cardiac or liver failure
- Polyethylene glycols/macrogols (eg Klean-Prep®, MoviPrep®) require large volumes of liquid to be drunk, but are safer in at-risk groups.

Consider admitting elderly patients and those with comorbidities for IV fluids and monitoring during bowel preparation. Oral medications should not be taken 1 h before or after administration of bowel cleansing preparations; where reduced absorption could prove catastrophic (eg immunosuppressives post-transplant) consider admission for IV administration. Advise patients taking the OCP to take alternative precautions during the week following taking the bowel preparation.

Offer patients written dietary advice on *low-residue foods* for the 2d prior to their procedure (local documents should be available); those taking insulin will require specific advice and guidance for management.

[1] Guenaga, K. *et al.* Mechanical bowel preparation for elective colorectal surgery. *Cochrane Database of Systematic Reviews* 2005, Issue 1. Art. No.: CD001544.

Surgical terminology

Prefix/suffix	Meaning and example
Angio-	Relating to a vessel Angioplasty – reconstruction of a blood vessel
Chol-	Relating to the biliary system Cholecystitis – inflammation of the gallbladder
Hemi-	Meaning half of something Hemicolectomy – excising half the colon
Hystero-	Relating to the uterus Hysterectomy – removal of the uterus
Lapar-	Relating to the abdomen Laparotomy – opening the abdomen
Nephr-	Relating to the kidney Nephrotoxic – damaging to the kidney
Pan-	Total/every Pancolectomy – complete removal of the colon
Per-	Going through a structure Percutaneous – going through the skin
Peri-	Near or around a structure Perianal – near the anus/around the anus
Proct-	Relating to the rectum Proctoscopy – examination of the rectum
Pyelo-	Relating to the renal pelvis Pyelonephritis – inflammation of the renal pelvis
Thoraco-	Relating to the thorax Thoracotomy – opening the thorax
Trans-	Going across a structure Transoesophageal – across the oesophagus
-ectomy	Surgical excision Nephrectomy – removal of a kidney
-gram	A radiological image often using contrast medium Angiogram – contrast study of arteries
-itis	Inflammation of an organ Pyelonephritis – inflammation of the renal pelvis
-olith	Stone-like Faecolith – solid, stone-like stool
-oscope	A device for looking inside the body Sigmoidoscope – device for looking into the distal colon
-ostomy	An artificial opening between two cavities or to the outside Colostomy – opening of the colon to the skin
-otomy	Cutting something open Craniotomy – opening the cranium (skull)
-plasty	Reconstruction of a structure Myringoplasty – repair of the tympanic membrane

Preparing in-patients for surgery

Checklist

Before your patient goes to theatre, you have a responsibility to check the following have been done:

- The consent form has been signed by the patient and surgeon
- The patient has been seen by the anaesthetist
- The operation site has been marked by the surgeon (imperative if the operation could be bilateral, eg inguinal hernia repair)
- The pre-operative blood results are in the notes
- The pre-operative ECG and/or CXR are available
- Prophylactic LMWH, TED stockings and antibiotics have been prescribed where relevant (do not give heparin <12h pre-op if having spinal/epidural)
- The patient has received bowel preparation if necessary
- The patient has been adequately fasted (see next section)
- Blood has been crossmatched and is available if required (📖 p398)
- Check if the patient has any last minute questions or concerns and is still happy to proceed with the operation.

Oral fluids pre- and post-op

In general, patients should not eat for at least 6h before going to theatre but can have clear fluids until 2h. In emergencies this rule may be over-ruled, but the risk of aspiration of gastric contents will be increased.

If patients are having an operation which requires bowel preparation, check local guidelines as to what oral intake the patient is allowed whilst taking the laxatives, usually it is either clear fluids only or a low-residue diet (see 📖 p109).

Nil by mouth (NBM) Patients cannot have any oral food or significant fluid intake; hydration must be maintained with IV fluids. However, oral medication (eg anti-arrhythmics) may be taken with a sip of water, if not taking them would put the patient at more risk. Non-essential medication such as vitamin supplements may be omitted; check with your seniors.

Clear fluids Include non-carbonated drinks such as black tea, black coffee, water, squash drinks (not milk or fruit juice).

Sips 30ml water/hour orally, usually given for the first day after major abdominal surgery involving bowel anastomoses.

Soft diet This includes food such as soup and jelly. Once patients have been tolerating clear fluids post-operatively for at least 24h, they may be allowed to start a soft diet.

Most patients can safely drink clear fluids up to 2h before surgery. The following increase the risk of aspiration:
- Pregnancy
- Being elderly
- Obesity
- Stomach disorders, eg hiatus hernia, reflux
- Pain (+opioids).

Booking theatre lists

Elective lists

In some centres this is done by the surgeon or their secretary, however in many places this task may fall to the surgical house officer. If you are required to book elective lists this will likely be electronically using a local system which you should receive training for (very occasionally paper systems are still in place). You should find out about your local procedures for booking elective lists.

Discuss the order of the list with your consultant/registrar (you may need to obtain the operating list from your consultant's secretary or direct from theatre).

The list usually must be submitted by the afternoon before the operating day. You should include:
• Theatre number
• Name of the consultant surgeon
• Name, sex, age, hospital number, and location of each patient
• Special patient requirements (eg DM, blood requested, ICU bed booked)
• Operation and side in full (eg open repair left inguinal hernia)
• Sign and leave your bleep number
• If the order of the list needs to be changed, contact theatres and inform them as soon as possible.

Booking the order of operations

In general, surgeons tend to prefer a specific order of patients:
• Older patients before younger (except children)
• Patients with comorbidities (eg DM) before healthy
• Clean operations before dirty (eg bowel resection)
• Longer, more complex operations before shorter.

▶▶Booking emergency operations

• Ensure you discuss the case with the ST1/2 and registrar on-call and that they have agreed to put the patient on the list
• Enter the patient's details as outlined above, noting the time at which the patient last ate
• Inform the anaesthetist covering the emergency theatre about the patient (usually the on-call anaesthetic registrar)
• Check the patient has been consented and make sure the results of any relevant investigations are available (including a G+S sample and a pregnancy test in women of child-bearing age)
• You also need to inform the theatre coordinator.

Surgical instruments

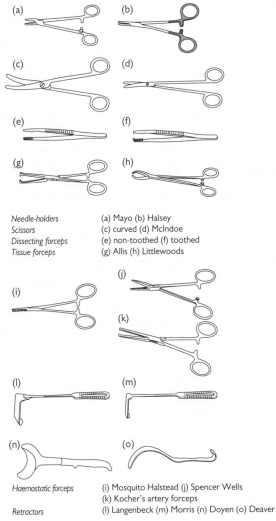

Needle-holders
Scissors
Dissecting forceps
Tissue forceps

(a) Mayo (b) Halsey
(c) curved (d) McIndoe
(e) non-toothed (f) toothed
(g) Allis (h) Littlewoods

Haemostatic forceps

Retractors

(i) Mosquito Halstead (j) Spencer Wells
(k) Kocher's artery forceps
(l) Langenbeck (m) Morris (n) Doyen (o) Deaver

Fig. 2.10 Surgical instruments.

The operating theatre

Theatre design

Operating theatres include an operating area, a scrubbing-up area, a preparation room, a sluice (area for dirty equipment and dirty laundry), and an anaesthetic room. There will also be a whiteboard (to document date, operation and number of swabs/blades/sutures used), a display system for viewing radiology and an area to write up the operation notes and histopathology forms. Above the operating table, there are usually main sets of lights, as well as smaller, more mobile units (satellites).

Theatre staff

Each operating theatre has a team of assistants who clean and maintain the theatre. The 'scrub nurse' scrubs for each operation to select instruments as requested by the surgical team. One other trained nurse and an auxiliary nurse act as 'runners' to fetch equipment for the scrub nurse and to monitor the number of swabs and sutures used (displayed on the whiteboard). An operating departmental assistant (ODA) maintains the anaesthetic equipment and assists the anaesthetist. Each operation is logged, with details of the patient, name of the operating surgeon, patient's consultant, and anaesthetist.

Theatre clothing

Fresh scrubs should be worn for each operating list and should be changed between lists, or between cases if they become dirty or potentially infected with MRSA. Theatre shoes are essential for safety purposes and you will not be allowed to enter without them. Theatre scrubs and shoes should not be worn uncovered outside of theatres except in an emergency.

Scrubbing up

Scrubbing up is an art and a key part of minimising infection risk to the patient. If in doubt, a theatre nurse can show you how to do it.
- Prior to scrubbing, remove jewellery and put your mask and a theatre hat on
- Open a gown pack and drop a pair of sterile gloves on top
- When scrubbing up for the first patient, scrub under your nails using a brush with iodine or chlorhexidine. Wash hands for a further 5min
- Unravel your gown; ensure that it does not touch the floor
- Touching its inner aspects only, put it on with the end of the sleeves covering your hands
- Put on your gloves. Do not touch the outside of your gloves with your bare hands
- For high-risk operations (eg Caesarean, HIV +ve) double-glove and protect your eyes with a visor or safety spectacles
- Wait for an assistant to tie your scrub gown from behind
- If your hand becomes non-sterile, change your glove. If your gown becomes non-sterile you need to rescrub; change your gown and gloves.

Theatre etiquette

- If you are scrubbed up:
  - ask someone not scrubbed to adjust the lights for you
  - do not pick up instruments which fall to the ground
  - if you are handed an instrument by someone who is not scrubbed, check that you can touch it before accepting it
- In operations involving the abdomen and the perineum, if you are asked to move from the perineum to the abdomen you must rescrub. This is not necessary when swapping from abdomen to perineum
- If you sustain a needle-stick injury, leave the operation and report to occupational health (📖 p106)
- Always eat/drink and go to the toilet before going to an operating list.

Watching an operation

Make sure you can see; get a stool or stand at the patient's head if the anaesthetist allows. Although you are not actively participating in the operation, use the time to learn surgical techniques. If you can't follow what's going on, ask. As the operation finishes, fill in any histology forms or TTOs if appropriate. Check histology samples are labelled accurately.

WHO Surgical Safety Checklist

In 2009 NHS Patient Safety Agency (NPSA) released guidance on the WHO Surgical Safety Checklist, a process by which all members of the theatre team have a discussion about the operation and the patient in advance of undertaking the procedure. The aim of this is to improve patient safety and prevent errors such as wrong-site surgery, retained throat-packs, avoidable delays in obtaining blood products or senior help should an unexpected incident arise. Most Trusts have devised their own checklist so these vary between hospitals, but are all based on the NPSA guidance.[1]

The checklist is read out loud before the anaesthetic is given, before the operation starts, and after the operation is completed. Before the operation everyone in theatre introduces themselves, the patient's details, the procedure about to take place and the site are confirmed, relevant equipment is checked to be present, and VTE prophylaxis measures are declared. At the checkout after the operation swab counts, instrument and sharps counts are checked, the operation note is confirmed, and specimens labelled. Plans for post-operative management are also confirmed.

---

[1] www.nrls.npsa.nhs.uk/resources/clinical-specialty/surgery/?entryid45=59860

Post-op care

As well as seeing patients pre-operatively, you should review them after the operation. This means you can review and discharge day cases with your team, as well as making sure the in-patients are stable after the operation.

Discharging day cases (this may be done by nursing staff).

Before sending day surgery patients home, you should make sure they are alert, have eaten and had fluids without vomiting, have passed urine, are mobilising without fainting, and have adequate pain relief. Inspect the operation site and check their observations. Go through the operation procedure, findings, and follow-up with the patient.

Organise appropriate follow-up care and clarify if they need dressing changes, suture removal dates and where this can be done (GP surgery, the ED or ward). If the patient develops any post-operative temperatures, pain or bleeding, they should contact their GP or come to the ED.

Common questions about discharge
- Patients can self-certify as unfit for work for up to a total of 7d (including time spent as in-patient); if you anticipate required time off work will routinely be longer than this, issue a Fitness to Work/Med 3 note (📖 p80) for the total expected time; this is the responsibility of the hospital team, not the patient's GP. *Unanticipated* extensions to the recovery period can be handled by the GP
- Patients requiring proof of hospital admission (for sick pay or social security payments) should be issued with a Form Med 10 (📖 p80)
- Tell the patient if their sutures are dissolvable or if they need to return to have them removed (give dates; often GP practice nurses will do this)
- Patients can shower and commence driving again 48h after minor surgery (as long they can perform an emergency stop; see 📖 p605)
- Advise patients not to fly for 6wk following major surgery.

In-patient post-op care

Post-op patients are at risk of complications associated with the operation, either directly (eg haemorrhage) or indirectly (eg PE).

When reviewing post-operative patients, document the number of days since the operation and the operation they underwent (eg 2d post left mastectomy).

Ask about pain, ability to eat and drink, nausea/vomiting, urinary output and colour, bowel movements/flatus, mobilisation.

Examine wound site, chest, abdomen, legs, drains, stoma bags, IV cannulae, catheter bag, drain entry site, amount drained, colour of any fluid being drained.

Look at the observations pyrexia, HR, BP, RR, 24h fluid balance (total input and output (including drains) and net balance); document all findings.

Review the drug chart for analgesia, antibiotics, fluids.

Check post-operative Hb; transfuse if necessary (📖 p398).

Involve other members of the multidisciplinary team if necessary, eg stoma nurse, pain team, physiotherapists, social worker, occupational therapist.

Post-op problems

Hypotension (📖 p473)

Ask about pre-op BP, fluid input, epidural, drugs, pain.

Look for repeat BP, HR, fluid input/urine output, temperature, GCS, orientation, skin temp, cap-refill, signs of hypovolaemia/sepsis, wounds, drain, abdomen, any signs of active bleeding.

Management Hypotension is common post-op and does not always require intervention. Tachycardia is a worrying feature suggesting shock. If this or other adverse features are present do 15min obs and monitor hourly urine output (catheterise bladder). Lie the patient flat, and give oxygen. Get IV access, consider fluid challenge (eg 500ml crystalloid STAT, 📖 p476). Send bloods for FBC and crossmatch (blood cultures if you suspect sepsis). Apply pressure to any obvious bleeding points. Call for senior review early.

Pyrexia
Temp 37.5°C, investigate if this persists/increases after the first 24h post-op (📖 p482).

Ask about cough/SOB, wound, dysuria/frequency, abdo pain, diarrhoea.

Look for BP, HR, temp, wound, catheter, IV cannulae, chest, abdomen.

Management **Urine** M,C+S; **blds** FBC, U+E, CRP, blood cultures; **imaging** CXR, consider abdominal USS or CT, echo if new onset murmur.

Possible causes of post-op pyrexia by day post-surgery

- **Day 1–2** atelectasis; treat with salbutamol/saline nebs and chest physio
- **Day 3–4** pneumonia; treat with antibiotics and chest physio
- **Day 5–6** anastomotic leak; need to take back to theatre
- **Day 7–8** wound infection; treat by opening up wound, antibiotics, may need to return to theatre
- **Day 9–10** DVT/PE; treat with heparin/LMWH then warfarin.

Shortness of breath/↓O₂ sats (📖 p271)

Ask about chronic lung/CVS disease, previous PE, chest pain, ankle swelling, new onset cough.

Look for BP, HR, temp, pallor, lungs (consolidation, crackles, air entry), signs of fluid overload, leg oedema/calf swelling.

Management Sit up and give O₂; **blds** FBC, ABG; **CXR**, **ECG**. Consider 0.9% saline nebs, antibiotics and regular chest physiotherapy. If you suspect a PE (📖 p278) call for senior help and specialist advice (medical registrar on-call).

Post-op problems covered elsewhere	
Pain	📖 p86
Nausea and vomiting	📖 p304
Low urine output	📖 p378

Wound management

Types of wound healing

- *Primary closure* This is most common in surgery, where wound edges are opposed soon after the time of injury and held in place by sutures, steristrips™ or staples. The aim is to minimise the risk of wound infection with minimal scar tissue formation (Table 2.16)
- *Delayed primary closure* This is more commonly used in 'dirty' or traumatic wounds. The wound is cleaned, debrided and then initially left open for 2–5d. Antibiotic cover may be given until the wound is reviewed for closure
- *Secondary closure* This is much less commonly encountered in surgery. Healing by secondary intention happens when the wound is left open and heals slowly by granulation. This is used in the presence of large areas of excised tissue, infection or significant trauma, where closing the wound would be impossible or would give rise to significant complications.

Table 2.16 *Abdominal wound complications*

	Ask about	Examine	Management
Superficial dehiscence	Pink serous discharge, burst sutures	Skin and fat cavity exposed (rectus sheath closed)	Not an emergency but ask for senior review – wound may need packing ± antibiotics
Deep dehiscence	Pink serous discharge, haematoma, bowel protrusion	Separation of wound edges with bowel exposed	Call for senior help urgently. Cover the bowel with a large sterile swab soaked in 0.9% saline. Check analgesia and fluid replacement, give antibiotics
Infection	Pyrexia, pain, erythema, white, yellow or bloody exudate from wound site	Tenderness, odorous discharge, swelling	Wound swab, broad-spectrum antibiotics initially (see 🕮 p179), discuss with your senior

Common elective operations

Laparoscopic cholecystectomy

Operation to remove the gallbladder.

Indications Symptomatic gallbladder stones, asymptomatic patients at risk of complications (diabetics, history of pancreatitis, immunosuppressed).

Pre-op No bowel prep required, 6h fasting pre-anaesthetic (see 📖 p109).

Procedure Involves insufflating the abdomen with CO_2, inserting 3 or 4 ports through the anterior abdominal wall to enable laparoscopy and the use of operating instruments to remove the gallbladder.

Post-op Patients can eat as soon as they recover from the anaesthetic, can usually go home later in the day or the following morning. Not all patients are followed up; some consultants like to review patients in clinic after 6–8wk.

Complications Haemorrhage, wound infections, bile leakage, bile duct stricture, retained stones; may require conversion to more major open surgery.

Colectomy

Operation to remove part or all of the colon (Fig. 2.11).

Indications Malignancy, perforation, IBD which can no longer be managed medically.

Pre-op Full bowel prep rarely required, 6h fasting pre-anaesthetic (see 📖 p109).

Procedure Involves a midline longitudinal laparotomy incision and resection of the diseased bowel if done open, can be done laparoscopically. A stoma may or may not be formed.

Post-op Sips of fluid orally for 24h post-op, gradually built up to free fluids and then light diet. Hospital stay 3–7d ('enhanced recovery pathways' used to streamline post-operative recovery). All patients followed up in clinic.

Complications Haemorrhage, wound infection, wound dehiscence, anastomotic leak.

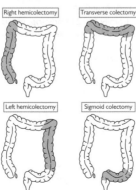

Fig. 2.11 Common large bowel resections (the shaded area represents the section of colon removed during the operation).

Anterior resection

Operation to resect the rectum with a sufficient margin (usually 5cm) and anastomose the left side of the colon with the rectal stump. See Fig. 2.12.

Indications Rectal carcinoma.

Pre-op Full bowel prep rarely required, phosphate enema 1h pre-op, 6h fasting pre-anaesthetic (see 📖 p109).

Procedure Involves a midline longitudinal laparotomy incision and resection of the diseased rectum if done open. Can be done laparoscopically.

Post-op Sips of fluid orally for 24h post-op, gradually built up to free fluids and then light diet. Hospital stay 4–10d. All patients followed up in clinic.

Complications Haemorrhage, wound infection, wound dehiscence, anastomotic leak.

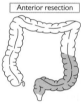

Fig. 2.12 Anterior resection.

Abdominoperineal resection (AP resection)

Operation to resect the rectum/anus and form a permanent colostomy. See Fig 2.13.

Indications Low rectal carcinoma where it would be impossible to resect the tumour without removing the anus, can also be performed as part of a panproctocolectomy for ulcerative colitis.

Pre-op Full bowel prep rarely required, phosphate enema 1h pre-op, 6h fasting pre-anaesthetic (see 📖 p109), stoma nurses to be involved.

Procedure Involves a midline longitudinal laparotomy incision and resection of the diseased rectum and anus.

Post-op Sips of fluid orally for 24h post-op, gradually built up to free fluids and then light diet. Hospital stay 4–10d. All patients followed up in clinic.

Complications Haemorrhage, wound infection, wound dehiscence, stoma retraction.

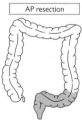

Fig. 2.13 AP resection.

Stomas

Colostomy

Common locations	LIF or right hypochondrium
Features	May be permanent or planned for subsequent reversal; mucosa sutured directly to skin
Output	Soft/solid stool; intermittently passed
Indications	Colorectal cancer, diverticular disease, trauma, radiation enteritis, bowel ischaemia, obstruction, Crohn's disease

Ileostomy

Common locations	RIF
Features	May be permanent or planned for subsequent reversal; bowel mucosa sutured to form a 'spout' to avoid skin contact with bowel contents which are irritating (not flush with skin)
Output	Liquid stool (may be bile-stained); passed continuously
Indications	GI tract cancer, IBD, trauma, radiation enteritis, bowel ischaemia, obstruction

Urostomy

Sometimes referred to as a nephrostomy if originating in renal pelvis

Common locations	Left or right flank, lower anterior abdominal wall
Features	A ureteric catheter may be protruding from the skin into the stoma
Output	Clear urine passed continuously
Indications	Renal tract cancer, urinary tract obstruction, spinal column disorders, hydronephrosis, urinary fistulae

Common complications

- Electrolyte/fluid imbalance (see ⬚ p385–389)
- Ischaemia/necrosis shortly after formation
- Obstruction/prolapse/parastomal hernia
- Skin erosion/infection
- Psychosocial implications.

It is important to refer patients who are likely to need stomas to the stoma care nurse prior to the operation. Patients with stomas also need to alter their diet to avoid excess flatulence or overly watery stool, so should also be referred to the dietician. Troublesome 'high-output' stomas leading to fluid balance problems or excessive need for bag emptying require specialist gastroenterologist advice.

History and examination

Basic history

Taking a thorough history is an essential skill as a junior doctor and something you will become extremely practised at. These two pages show the basic features of a history, with details of how to perform a basic examination following after. The rest of the chapter shows how to adapt these basic approaches for specific situations.

Taking a history (OHCM9 📖 p20)
- Try to be in a setting that offers privacy and has a bed
- Establish the patient's name and check their date of birth
- Introduce yourself and begin with open-ended questions.

Presenting complaint Why has the patient come to hospital? Write their main problem(s) in their own words along with duration of symptoms and who referred them; if the referral letter has a different presenting complaint then document this too.

History of presenting complaint(s) Ask questions aimed at differentiating the causes of the presenting complaint and assessing its severity. Try to exclude potentially life-threatening causes first. Ask specifically about previous episodes and investigations/treatments. Use the SOCRATES questions for pain (site, onset, character, radiation, associations, timing, exacerbating/relieving factors, severity). Ask about the effect on their activities of daily living (ADLs). If there are multiple problems ask if they come on together or are related.

Risk factors Document recognised risk factors for important differentials.

Past medical history Ask about previous medical problems/operations and attempt to gauge the severity of each (eg hospital/ICU admissions, exercise tolerance (ET), treatment); use the drug history to prompt the patient's memory. Consider documenting specifically about asthma, DM, angina, ↑BP, MI, stroke, PE/DVT, epilepsy.

Drug history Document all drugs along with doses, times taken and any recent changes. Always document drug allergies along with the reaction precipitated. Alternatively if the patient has never had a drug allergy then document this.

Family history Ask about relevant illness in the family (eg heart problems, DM, cancer). Are other family members well at the moment?

Social history This is essential: **home** ask about who they live with, the kind of house (eg bungalow, residential home), any home help, own ADLs (cooking, dressing, washing); **mobility** walking aids (stick/frame), exercise tolerance (how far can they walk on level ground? can they climb stairs?); **lifestyle** occupation, alcohol (units/wk), smoking (cigarettes/d and pack years), recreational drugs:
- *Alcohol;* 1 unit = ½ pint of beer, glass of wine, measure of spirits; bottle of wine = 9units, 1l of strong cider = 8.5units
- *Smoking;* 20 cigarettes/d for 1yr = 1 pack year.

Systems' review Relevant systems' review will often be part of the HPC; a thorough systems' review is only necessary if you are unsure what is relevant or are struggling to explain the symptoms. See OHCM9 📖 p22.

CVS	Chest pain, palpitations, SOB, ankle swelling, orthopnoea
Resp	Cough (?blood), sputum, wheeze, SOB
Abdo	Abdo pain, nausea/vomiting, bowel habit (?blood), stool colour and consistency, distension, dysuria, frequency, urgency, haematuria
Neuro	Headache, photophobia, neck stiffness, weakness, change in sensation, balance, fits, falls, speech, changes in vision/hearing
Systemic	Appetite, weight loss/gain, fever/night sweats, malaise, stiff/swollen joints, fatigue, rashes/itch, sleep pattern

Summarising Ask if there are any other problems that have not been discussed and repeat back a summary of the history to the patient to check that they agree. It is a good idea to use the ICE questions (Ideas, Concerns, Expectations) at this point – ask the patient if they have any idea or suspicion of what might be wrong with them, if there's anything in particular that they're worried about (this may prompt them to admit specific concerns eg having cancer), and what they expect will happen to them whilst they are in hospital.

Most patients have no idea about tests and investigations and find being admitted to hospital a frightening event; they often value the opportunity to talk about possible options and ask questions.

Always finish your history by asking specifically if the patient has any further questions or any other issues they would like to discuss, as frequently they will be too embarrassed/shy/reticent to ask.

Should you take notes whilst clerking?

There is no simple answer to this. Taking notes while the patient talks may allow you to record important details accurately or even to write up your clerking as you go. This can be extremely useful during busy on-calls. Alternatively not taking notes allows you to give the patient your undivided attention and the opportunity to record the clerking having considered the whole picture. In the end it comes down to individual preference and workload.

After the history

By the end of taking the history you should have a reasonable idea of the differential diagnosis. Try to think of specific signs that would be present on examination to confirm or refute these differentials. A basic examination is described on the next page.

Basic examination

It is good practice to perform a brief CVS, RS, abdo and neuro exam on all patients but focus your examination according to their history. Check observations (temp, BP, HR, RR, O_2 sats):

- Ask a nurse to chaperone you if necessary
- Get consent before touching the patient, ask where it hurts
- First assess briefly whether the patient looks well or ill.

Hands (📖 p152)

- *Inspection* at the hands for signs of disease
- *Palpation* check the pulse for rate, rhythm and character (eg ?collapsing pulse).

Mouth

- *Inspection* central cyanosis, mucous membranes, stomatitis, beefy tongue (↓iron), candidiasis, ulcers, dental hygiene (risk factor for SBE).

Cardiovascular system (📖 p128)

- *Inspection* JVP (very useful if visible), swollen ankles
- *Palpation* temp of hands, capillary-refill, carotid pulse (volume and character), apex beat, heaves/thrills, hepatomegaly
- *Auscultation* heart sounds, added sounds/murmurs (timing, volume, radiation), carotid bruits, basal crackles.

Respiratory system (📖 p130)

- *Inspection* asterixis (flap), stridor, JVP, RR and effort (accessory muscles, recession), chest wall movement, peripheral oedema
- *Palpation* trachea, cervical lymphadenopathy, expansion
- *Percussion* does right equal left?, hyperresonant, dull, stony dull
- *Auscultation* air entry, crackles, wheeze, bronchial BS, rub.

Abdomen (📖 p131)

- *Inspection* jaundice, scars, distension, hernias, oedema
- *Palpation* start away from pain and watch patient's face: tenderness, peritonism (guarding, rebound, rigidity, percussion tenderness), masses, liver, spleen, kidneys and AAA (expansile mass), hernias, ±genitalia, PR (masses, stool, tenderness, prostate, blood/mucus/melaena)
- *Percussion* ascites (shifting dullness, fluid thrill), liver, spleen
- *Auscultation* bowel sounds (absent, reduced, increased, tinkling).

Peripheral nerves (📖 p134)

- *Inspection* posture, movement of limbs
- *Palpation* **tone**; **power** (5 normal, 4 weak, 3 against gravity only, 2 not even against gravity, 1 twitch, 0 none); **reflexes** tendons, plantars; **sensation**
- *Coordination* finger–nose, slide heel down opposite leg.

Cranial nerves (📖 p133)

- *Inspection* GCS, mental state (📖 p161), facial symmetry, scars, obvious gaze palsies, speech, posture
- *Eyes* (II, III, IV, VI) acuity, pupil reactivity, fields, movements, fundi
- *Face* (V, VII) sensation and power
- *Mouth* (IX, X, XII) tongue movements, palate position, cough
- *Other* (VIII) hearing, balance, gait (XI), shrug, head movements.

Recording your clerking

The initial clerking of a patient is one of the most important steps in their journey through the hospital. It will be reread by every team that looks after the patient and used as a benchmark for measuring the progress of the patient's condition. A good clerking gives the patient the best opportunity to receive the correct investigations and treatment.

Heading Your name, position, location, date, time; state clearly why the patient is being clerked (eg referred from ED with chest pain).

Format Follow a logical order setting out each section under the headings shown over these four pages. If a piece of information from a different section is really important then write it in the history of presenting complaint and/or under the social history.

Sources State where you got important information from (eg patient, relative (with name and relationship), notes, computer records). This makes it easy to check if the information is of critical importance.

Use the notes Don't rely on a patient's account of their previous medical history, especially for investigations and results. Try to find the official record of key investigations rather than relying on another doctor's comments.

Be thorough These pages represent a basic clerking; you should record all of the information described on these pages at the very least.

State the obvious What appears obvious now may not be to someone reading the notes or on the next shift, eg below-knee prosthetic leg, crying constantly.

Differential diagnosis What diseases are likely to explain the patient's symptoms? What serious diseases need to be excluded? Make a list of these after the examination. Consider recording the most critical evidence for and against each diagnosis.

Management plan This should be a detailed list of the steps you will take to diagnose and treat the differential diagnosis. It should be written in order of priority. Alongside investigations and treatment consider nursing measures, frequency of observations, what to do in the event of deterioration, referrals, best location (eg respiratory ward, HDU).

State what the patient was told This prevents confusion. If you are not telling the patient about a serious illness then state why.

See 🕮 p74 for other tips about writing in the notes.

Cardiovascular

History

Symptoms chest pain or heaviness, dyspnoea (exertional, orthopnoea, paroxysmal nocturnal) (see Table 3.1), ankle/limb swelling, palpitations, syncope or pre-syncope, limb pain (at rest or on exertion), fatigue, numbness, ulcers.

Past medical history IHD, MI, hypertension, palpitations, syncope, clotting problems, rheumatic fever, cardiac surgery, recent dental work, liver problems, renal problems, thyroid disease.

Table 3.1 *Functional status of established heart disease (NYHA)*

Class I	Disease present but no symptoms during ordinary activity
Class II	Angina or dyspnoea during ordinary activity (eg walking to shops)
Class III	Angina or dyspnoea during minimal activity (eg making cup of tea)
Class IV	Angina or dyspnoea at rest

Drug history cardiac medications (and compliance), allergies.

Social history tobacco, alcohol, and caffeine consumption, illicit drug use (?IV), occupation, exercise tolerance on flat and stairs.

Family history IHD, ↑lipids, cardiomyopathy, congenital heart disease.

Coronary artery disease risk factors previous IHD, smoking, ↑BP, ↑lipids, family history of IHD, DM, obesity and physical inactivity, male sex.

Palpation of central and peripheral pulses

Central
- **Carotid** two fingers, medial to the sternocleidomastoid muscle and lateral to the thyroid cartilage (do not palpate both sides together)
- **Abdominal aorta** both fingertips, halfway between umbilicus and xiphisternum.

Arms
- **Radial** two fingers pressed on the radial aspect of the inner wrist
- **Ulnar** two fingers pressed on the ulnar aspect of the inner wrist
- **Brachial** two fingers pressed into the antecubital fossa, just medial to the biceps tendon (ask patient to flex arm against resistance to find the tendon).

Legs
- **Femoral** two fingers pressed firmly into the middle of the crease in the groin, halfway between the symphysis pubis and the anterior superior iliac spine.
- **Popliteal** ask patient to flex their knee, put both your thumbs either side of the patella and press firmly with your fingertips into the popliteal fossa.
- **Posterior tibial** two fingers pressed 1cm posterior to the medial malleolus.
- **Dorsalis pedis** two fingers pressed between the 1st and 2nd metatarsals.

Examination (lying at 45°)

General inspection dyspnoea at rest, cyanosis, pallor, facial flushing, Marfan's, Turner's, Down's syndromes, rheumatological disorders, acromegaly.

Hands radial pulses (right and left, collapsing pulse), clubbing, splinter haemorrhages, Osler's nodes, peripheral cyanosis, xanthomata.

Face eyes (pallor, jaundice, xanthelasma), malar flush, mouth (cyanosis, high arched palate, dentition).

Neck JVP, carotids (pulse character).

Precordium inspection (scars, deformity, apex beat), palpate (apex beat, thrills, heave (Table 3.2)), auscultate (heart sounds (Table 3.3), murmurs – also auscultate with the patient in both left lateral and sitting forward positions).

Back scars, sacral oedema, pleural effusions, pulmonary oedema.

Abdomen palpate liver, spleen, aorta, ballot kidneys, percuss for ascites, femoral and renal artery bruits, radiofemoral delay.

Legs peripheral pulses, temperature, ulceration, oedema, calf tenderness, venous guttering, thin shiny skin, loss of hair, gangrene, varicose veins, eczema, haemosiderin pigmentation of the skin (particularly above the medial malleolus), lipodermatosclerosis ('inverted champagne bottle leg').

Blood pressure lying and standing, consider also left and right arms separately.

Other urine analysis, fundoscopy, temperature chart.

Table 3.2 *Characteristics of valve defects*

Mitral stenosis	Mid-diastolic rumbling murmur, loud 1st HS, opening snap, malar flush, AF, tapping apex, left parasternal heave
Mitral regurgitation	Pansystolic murmur radiating to the axilla, soft 1st HS, 3rd HS present, thrusting apex, left parasternal heave
Aortic stenosis	Ejection systolic murmur radiating to the neck, 4th HS, reversed HS splitting, slow rising pulse, systolic thrill
Aortic regurgitation	Early diastolic murmur (best heard in expiration), collapsing pulse, wide BP, pistol-shot femoral pulse, Corrigan's sign, Quincke's sign, de Musset's sign

Table 3.3 *Heart sounds*

1st (S_1)	Physiological; blocking of blood flow after closing of the mitral (M_1) and tricuspid (T_1) valves
2nd (S_2)	Physiological; blocking of blood flow after closing of the aortic (A_2) and pulmonary (P_2) valves; aortic precedes pulmonary and splitting can be heard during inspiration
3rd (S_3)	Sometimes pathological; caused by blood rushing into the ventricles after S_2; suggests increased volume of blood in athletes, pregnancy or heart failure
4th (S_4)	Pathological; blood pushing open a stiff ventricle before S_1; suggests LVF, aortic stenosis, cardiomyopathy

Respiratory

History

Symptoms cough, sputum, shortness of breath (see Table 3.4), wheeze, chest pain, fevers and sweats, weight loss, hoarseness, snoring, day sleepiness.

Past medical history chest infections/pneumonias (as child or adult), tuberculosis, HIV status and risk factors, allergy, rheumatoid disease.

Drug history respiratory drugs (inhalers, steroids, etc), vaccination history (especially BCG, Hib, pneumococcus), drugs known to cause respiratory problems (bleomycin, methotrexate, amiodarone, etc), allergies.

Social history tobacco use (expressed in pack years – ie 20 cigarettes a day for 1year = 1pack year) and social exposure to tobacco smoke if non-smoker, pets, exposure to other family members with respiratory problems (TB etc), illicit drug use (crack cocaine, cannabis).

Occupational history past and present jobs, asking specifically about dust exposure, asbestos, animal dander.

Family history asthma/atopy, cystic fibrosis, emphysema.

Table 3.4 *Functional status of breathlessness (NYHA)*

Class I	Disease present but no dyspnoea during ordinary activity
Class II	Dyspnoea during ordinary activities (eg walking to shops)
Class III	Dyspnoea during minimal activities (eg making cup of tea)
Class IV	Dyspnoea at rest

Examination (lying at 45°)

General inspection O_2 requirements, cough, audible wheeze or stridor, rate and depth of respiration, use of accessory muscles, body habitus.

Hands clubbing, peripheral cyanosis, tar staining, wasting/weakness of intrinsic muscles, HR, fine tremor of β-agonists, flapping tremor of CO_2 retention.

Face eyes (Horner's syndrome, anaemia), mouth (central cyanosis), voice.

Neck trachea position (±scars), JVP.

Chest anteriorly inspect (shape, scars, radiotherapy marks), palpate (supraclavicular nodes, axillary nodes, expansion, vocal fremitus, apex beat, parasternal heave), percuss, auscultate.

Chest posteriorly inspect, palpate (including cervical nodes), percuss, auscultate.

Other peripheral oedema, calf erythema/tenderness, temperature chart, breast examination (if suspect malignancy), abdominal examination, PEFR, sputum pot.

Recording PEFR

Ensure the meter is set to zero and fit a new disposable mouthpiece. Stand the patient up (or sit up if unable to stand) and give them clear instructions. They should take as deep a breath as possible, before placing the meter in their mouth and closing their lips around the mouthpiece. Encourage them to blow out as hard and as fast as possible. Record the reading obtained, then document the best of 3 efforts.

Gastrointestinal

History

Symptoms abdo pain, association with eating, vomiting or opening bowels, weight loss, appetite, bruising, bleeding, nausea, vomiting (appearance), dysphagia, dysuria, urinary frequency and urgency, possibility of pregnancy; **stool** change in bowel habit, frequency, consistency, colour, pain on passing, recurrent urge, blood (bowl or paper), offensive smell, mucus.

Past medical history GI bleeds, GORD, varices, gallstones, liver problems, jaundice, IBD, haemorrhoids, polyps.

Drug history NSAIDs, anticoagulants, hepatotoxic drugs (📖 p172), opioids, laxatives.

Social history foreign travel, illicit drug use (?IV).

Alcohol intake per day (in units, 📖 p124), CAGE questions (📖 p104).

Family history IBD, liver disease, cancer.

Examination (lying flat on back)

General inspection oedema, wasting, jaundice, anaemia, lymphadenopathy, breath odour, mouth ulcers, gynaecomastia, spider naevi, bruises.

Hands clubbing, nail colour, palm colour, flap, Dupuytren's.

Abdomen distension (fat, faeces, flatus, fluid, foetus), prominent veins, tenderness (guarding, rebound), masses, organomegaly (see Tables 3.5 and 3.6), ascites, hernial orifices (inguinal, femoral, incisional), bowel sounds.

PR visible haemorrhoids, fissures and skin tags, anal tone, prostate, rectal masses, appearance of faeces ±blood.

Table 3.5 *Common abdominal masses – if in doubt check with USS*

Liver	RUQ, extends to RLQ, unable to get above, dull to percussion
Spleen	LUQ extends to RLQ, unable to get above, notch
Kidney	RUQ and/or LUQ, ballotable, able to get above it, smooth outline
Faeces	Indentable mass away from umbilicus

Table 3.6 *Common causes of enlarged liver and spleen*

Hepatomegaly alcohol, hepatitis, EBV, CMV, thin patient, autoimmune hepatitis, toxins, liver metastases, lymphoma, leukaemia, haemochromatosis, amyloidosis, hyperexpanded chest eg COPD, heart failure

Splenomegaly chronic liver disease, autoimmune disease, thrombocytopenia, EBV, CMV, hepatitis, HIV, haemolytic anaemia, leukaemia, lymphoma, endocarditis, thalassaemia, sickle cell, myelofibrosis, sarcoid, amyloidosis, malaria, leishmaniasis

Hepatosplenomegaly hepatitis, EBV, CMV, chronic liver disease, leukaemia, lymphoma, myelofibrosis, amyloidosis

Neurological

History

Presenting complaint onset, duration, course (improving, worsening, relapsing–remitting), aggravating or alleviating factors, change with time of day, trauma.

Symptoms headache, pain, numbness, tingling, weakness, tremor, twitching, abnormal movements, loss of consciousness, seizures, abnormal smells, vision (loss, diplopia, flashing lights), hearing, swallowing, speech, balance, vertigo, nausea, vomiting, coordination, urinary incontinence or retention, impotence, faecal incontinence, constipation, personality, memory, language, visuospatial skills, change in intellect.

Corroborating history in many neurological conditions the patient may not be able to describe all the symptoms, eg seizure; try to get a history from a witness or family member.

Past medical history similar episodes, meningitis, migraines, strokes, seizures, heart problems, hypertension, DM, psychiatric problems.

Drug history neurological drugs (eg antiepileptics, Parkinson's medications), psychiatric drugs (eg antipsychotics, antidepressants), all others (especially cardiac and hypoglycaemic drugs).

Family history draw a family tree with all four grandparents and all their children and grandchildren, ask specifically about learning difficulties, disability, epilepsy, dementia, CVAs, psychiatric problems.

Social history alcohol, smoking, illicit drugs, occupation, travel abroad, dominant hand.

Examination

Obs GCS, BP (lying and standing), HR, RR, glucose.

General appearance posture, neglect, nutrition, mobility aids.

Cognition tested using the Mini-Mental State Exam (📖 p343) or 10-point Abbreviated Mental State Exam (📖 p341).

Meningism photophobia, neck stiffness, Brudzinski's sign (flexion of both knees on testing neck stiffness), Kernig's sign (hamstring spasm on attempting to straighten the knee with hip and knee flexed), straight leg raise (hamstring spasm on passively flexing the hip).

Skin birthmarks, vitiligo, café-au-lait spots, ash leaf macules, lumps, tufts of hair/dimples at the base of the spine.

See Table 3.7 for cranial nerve examination.

Table 3.7 *Cranial nerve examination*

Nerve		Function	Tests
Olfactory	I	Smell	Rarely tested
Optic (Fig. 3.1)	II	Vision	Visual acuity, visual fields, pupil reflexes, fundoscopy
Oculomotor	III	Eye movements, lift the eyelid, pupil constriction	Eye movements, pupil reflexes
Trochlear	IV	Superior oblique	Move eye down and out
Trigeminal	V	Sensation to face, movement of jaw muscles	Facial sensation, jaw power, corneal reflex
Abducens	VI	Lateral rectus muscle	Move eye laterally
Facial	VII	Facial muscle movement, taste (anterior 2/3rd), salivary and lacrimal glands, stapedius muscle	Facial power
Vestibulo-cochlear	VIII	Hearing and balance	Whispering numbers, Weber's (forehead), Rinne's (behind ear)
Glosso-pharyngeal	IX	Taste (posterior 1/3rd), parotid gland, sensation of pharynx, nasopharynx, middle ear	Saying 'Ahh', swallow, gag reflex
Vagus	X	Sensation of pharynx and larynx, movement of palate, pharynx, larynx	Saying 'Ahh' (deviates away from defect), cough, swallow, speech, gag reflex
Accessory	XI	Movement of sternomastoid and trapezius	Shrug shoulders, turn head
Hypoglossal	XII	Movement of tongue	Stick tongue out (deviates towards defect), speech

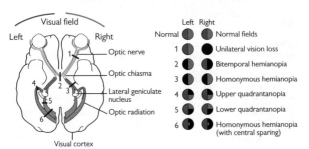

Fig. 3.1 Optic pathways and effect of a lesion on the visual fields at various locations.

Peripheral nerve examination

Appearance posture, tremor, muscle wasting, fasciculation, abnormal movements, facial expression and symmetry, neglect.

Hold out hands with palms up and eyes closed; look for drift (pyramidal defect), tremor or involuntary finger movement (loss of position sense).

Tone tone at wrist, elbow, knee and ankle (increased, decreased, clasp knife, cog-wheeling), clonus at the ankle (≥5 beats is abnormal).

Power isolate each joint with one hand so that only the muscle group you are testing can be used for the movement; compare each side (Table 3.8).

Table 3.8 *Medical Research Council (MRC) grading of muscle power*

Grade 0	No movement
Grade 1	Flicker of movement
Grade 2	Movement but not against gravity
Grade 3	Weakness but movement against gravity
Grade 4	Weakness but movement against resistance
Grade 5	Normal power

Table 3.9 *Root levels of main limb movements*

Joint	Movement	Root	Joint	Movement	Root
Shoulder	Abduction	C5	Hip	Flexion	L1–2
	Adduction	C5–7		Adduction	L2–3
Elbow	Flexion	C5–6		Extension	L5–S1
	Extension	C7	Knee	Flexion	L5–S1
Wrist	Flexion	C7–8		Extension	L3–4
	Extension	C7	Ankle	Dorsiflexion	L4
Fingers	Flexion	C8		Plantarflexion	S1–2
	Extension	C7	Big toe	Extension	L5
	Abduction	T1			

Reflexes deep tendon reflexes comparing each side (Table 3.10), if absent ask the patient to clench their teeth (reinforcement); plantar reflexes.

Table 3.10 *Tendon reflexes*

Grading of tendon reflexes		Root levels of tendon reflexes			
0	Absent	**Reflex**	**Root**	**Reflex**	**Root**
±	Present with reinforcement	Bicep	C5–6	Knee	L3–4
+	Reduced	Supinator	C5–6	Ankle	S1–2
++	Normal	Tricep	C7–8		
+++	Increased				
++++	Increased with clonus				

Coordination finger–nose, dysdiadochokinesia, tapping, heel–shin.

Romberg's tested with patient standing with eyes open then closed, positive if more unbalanced with eyes closed; suggests sensory ataxia.

Sensation pinprick, light touch, vibration, joint position; the spinal dermatomes of the front and back are shown in Fig. 3.2 and spinal tracts on 📖 p136.

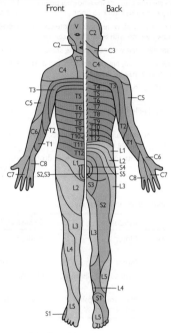

Fig. 3.2 Dermatomes of the front (L) and back (R).

Nerves of the hand
See Table 3.11 and Fig. 3.3.

Table 3.11 *Innervation of hand movements*

Movement	Nerve
Finger abduction and adduction	Ulnar
Thumb opposition and abduction	Median
Finger extension	Radial

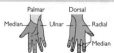

Fig. 3.3 Sensation of the hand.

Table 3.12 *Gait examination*

Gait	Description	Cause
Antalgic	Painful gait, limping, short weight-bearing on painful side	Mechanical injury, sciatica
Apraxic	Unable to lift legs despite normal power, magnetic steps/stuck to floor	Hydrocephalus, frontal lesions
Ataxic	Uncoordinated, wide-based, unsteady (as if drunk), worse with eyes shut if sensory	Cerebellar, sensory
Festinating	A shuffling gait with accelerating steps	Parkinson's
Hemiparetic	Knee extended, hip circumducts and drags leg; elbow may be flexed up	Hemiplegia, eg CVA
Myopathic	Waddling, leaning back, abdomen sticking out	Proximal myopathy
Shuffling	Short, shuffled steps, stooped, no arm swing	Parkinson's
Spastic	Restricted knee and hip movements, slow, shuffling, 'wading through water'	Pyramidal tract lesion eg MS
Steppage	High steps with foot slapping, 'foot drop'	Peripheral neuropathy

Table 3.13 *Spinal tracts and anatomy*

Tract	Modality	Crosses (decussates) at
Lateral corticospinal (pyramidal)	Motor	Medulla
Anterior corticospinal	Motor	Level of exit of the cord
Posterior columns (dorsal)	Light touch, vibration, position	Medulla
Spinothalamic	Hard touch, pain, temperature	Level of entry to the cord

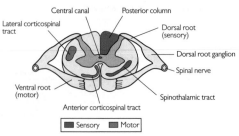

Fig. 3.4 Cross-section of the spinal cord showing spinal tracts.

Endocrine

History

Symptoms weight loss, weight gain, appetite, sweating, heat/cold intolerance, tremor, weakness, tiredness, dizziness, hirsuitism, joint pain/swelling, change in appearance (skin, hair, nails, face, eyes), change in clothes/shoe/hat size, altered sensation, ulcers, visual problems.

Cardiorespiratory features chest pain, breathlessness, palpitations, sleep apnoea.

GI/urinary features diarrhoea, constipation, nausea, vomiting, abdominal pain, thirst, polyuria.

Reproductive features menstrual irregularities, infertility, gynaecomastia, galactorrhoea, impotence.

Psychiatric features anxiety, mood changes, memory problems.

Eye features blurred vision, visual field defects, bulging eyes.

Past medical history thyroid surgery, stroke, heart failure, liver failure, renal artery stenosis, renal failure, adrenal surgery, brain surgery.

Drug history steroids, diuretics, OCP, HRT, levothyroxine, insulin.

Family history DM, thyroid disease, pituitary tumours.

Examination (lying at 45°)

General inspection body habitus, 'buffalo hump', facial appearance ('moon face'), striae, bruising, muscle wasting, hyperpigmentation, coarse skin, prominent jaw and brow ridge, goitre, gynaecomastia, hirsuitism, acanthosis nigricans, vitiligo, acne, necrobiosis lipoidica, pretibial myxoedema.

Hands temperature, sweating, size, tremor.

Eyes lid lag, proptosis, exophthalmos, bitemporal hemianopia, cranial nerve III, IV, or VI palsy, fundoscopy.

Neck goitre, thyroid lumps.

Cardiorespiratory ↑↓HR, ↑↓BP, postural hypotension, irregular pulse, peripheral oedema, bibasal crackles (LVF).

Neurological cranial nerve III/IV/VI palsy, peripheral neuropathy, slow relaxing reflexes, weakness (myopathy).

Other joints, skin, genitalia, fundoscopy, urine analysis, U+E, early morning cortisol, TFTs, short Synacthen® test (□ p571), GTT – more specialist tests on advice from an endocrinologist.

Skin

History

Presenting skin complaint **timing** how long present for, sudden or gradual onset, getting better or worse; *location* original site and subsequent sites affected; **symptoms** itch (localised or generalised), pain, burning, bleeding, weeping; **exacerbating factors** dietary components, drugs, sunlight (seasonal variability), pet dander, night-time, water; **relieving factors** emollient cream, topical/systemic steroids.

Current health anorexia, diarrhoea, fever, headache, fatigue, weight loss, depression, sore throat, joint pain.

Past medical history previous skin disease, DM, BD, asthma/atopy, varicose veins, peripheral arterial disease, cardiac problems, endocrine disease, neurological problems, ulcers, trauma, sarcoid, porphyria, SLE, malignancy, sensitivity of skin to sun exposure, lifelong history of sun exposure or use of sun beds.

Drug history dermatological agents being used at present and their effects, previous drugs used and their effects, oral and topical steroids, other drugs being taken, drug allergies.

Allergy hayfever, pet dander, dust mite etc.

Occupational history current and previous jobs and effect of work upon skin, exposure to chemicals; hobbies and recreational activities.

Family history anyone else in the family affected; need to differentiate inherited pathology versus infectious pathology.

Travel history recent foreign travel and relationship of any travel to skin disease – vaccinations/prophylaxis taken for foreign travel.

Function restricted actions, effect on life, mobility, occupation, dominant hand, hobbies/sports, smoking, social support.

Examination

The whole body should be examined in good natural light; patients complaining of a rash on their arm may well have other tell-tale signs elsewhere on the body. Don't be afraid to ask patients to strip, but remember to have a chaperone present and to explain why you are looking.

Distribution solitary lesion, flexor aspects of limbs/trunk, extensor aspects of limbs/trunk, scalp/eyebrows/gutters of nose, sun-exposed sites, tip of nose, helix of ear, in webspaces of hands or feet, periumbilical.

Morphology noting or describing the appearance of the rash using the terms on p139 (Tables 3.14–3.17) refines the list of differential diagnoses.

Hair alopecia (hair loss) may be generalised or localised, hirsuitism (hair in the typical male distribution), hypertrichosis (excessive hair growth).

Nails clubbing, pitting, ridging, onycholysis, nail loss, thinning of nail plate, discolouration.

Table 3.14 *Non-palpable skin lesions*

Ecchymosis	Bruising; discolouration from blood leaking into the skin
Macule	Flat well-defined area of altered skin pigmentation
Petechia	Non-blanching pinpoint-sized purple macule
Purpura	Purple lesion resulting from free red blood cells in the skin non-blanching
Telangiectasia	Abnormal visible dilatation of blood vessels (spider naevi)

Table 3.15 *Palpable skin lesions*

Nodule	Solid, mostly subcutaneous lesion (>0.5cm diameter)
Papule	Raised well-defined lesion (<0.5cm diameter)
Plaque	Raised flat-topped lesion, usually >2cm diameter
Weal	Transient raised lesion with pink margin
Urticaria	Weals with pale centres and well-defined pink margins

Table 3.16 *Blisters*

Abscess	Fluctuant swelling containing pus beneath the epidermis
Bulla	Fluid-filled blister larger than a vesicle (>0.5cm diameter)
Pustule	Well-defined pus-filled lesion
Vesicle	Fluid-filled blister (<0.5cm diameter)

Table 3.17 *Skin defects*

Excoriation	Linear break in the skin surface (a scratch)
Atrophy	Thinning and loss of skin substance
Crust	Dried brownish/yellow exudates
Erosion	Superficial break in the continuity of the epidermis
Abrasion	Scraping off superficial layers of the skin (a graze)
Fissure	Crack, often through keratin
Incisional wound	Break to the skin by sharp object
Laceration	Break to the skin caused by blunt trauma/tearing injury
Lichenification	Skin thickening with exaggerated skin markings
Scale	Fragment of dry skin
Ulcer	Loss of epidermis and dermis resulting in scar

Oncological/haematological

History

Symptoms weight loss, anorexia, weakness, lethargy, fatigue, cough, haemoptysis, shortness of breath, postural dizziness, nausea, vomiting, diarrhoea, constipation, PR bleeding, lumps, swelling, pain, fractures, bone pain, polyuria, prostatism, bruising, recurrent epistaxis, haemarthrosis, heavy menstrual loss, recurrent miscarriage, fevers, infections, focal neurology.

Past medical history DM, asthma, ↑BP, IHD, liver disease, jaundice, thyroid problems, anaemia, malignancy (and radiotherapy), epilepsy, gastric or small bowel surgery, malabsorption, chronic disease (eg RA), blood transfusions, splenectomy.

Drug history chemotherapy (regimen, date of last dose, response, side effects), iron, B_{12}/folate, aspirin, anticoagulants, vaccinations post-sple-nectomy, long-term antibiotics, OCP, allergies.

Social history smoking, alcohol, family support, living circumstances, home help, occupation, previous exposure to dyes/asbestos/coal tar, racial origin, diet (vegan, vegetarian), recreational drug use.

Family history malignancy, thalassaemia, sickle-cell anaemia, haemophilia, von Willebrand's disease, pernicious anaemia, spherocytosis, thrombophilia.

Examination

General inspection bruising, pigmentation, rashes and nodules, ulceration, cyanosis, plethora, jaundice, excoriations, racial origin (haemoglobinopa-thies and thalassaemias).

Hands nails (koilonychias, pallor, clubbing), palmar crease pallor, arthropathy.

Face eyes (jaundice, pallor), mouth (gum hypertrophy or bleeding, ulceration, candida, atrophic glossitis, angular stomatitis, gingivitis).

Lymph nodes cervical, axillary, epitrochlear (elbow), inguinal.

Bones bony pain in sternum, spine, clavicles, scapulae.

Abdomen hepatomegaly, splenomegaly, para-aortic nodes, ascites.

Legs vasculitis, bruising, pigmentation, ulceration, neurological signs.

Other fundi (haemorrhages, engorged veins, papilloedema), temperature chart, urinalysis.

Breast

History

Lump size, duration, mobility, pain, nipple discharge/bleeding/inversion, skin changes, previous breast lumps.

Past obs/gynae history number of pregnancies, age of first pregnancy, breastfeeding, menarche, menopause.

Past medical history DM, asthma, ↑BP, IHD, clotting problems, liver disease, anaemia, previous malignancy, epilepsy.

FH breast cancer, gynae cancer.

DH HRT, COC use.

Examination (lying at 45°)

Examine both breasts (normal side first):

Inspection asymmetry, scars, skin changes, nipple discharge/inversion, skin tethering, erythema, oedema.

Palpation ask the patient to show you where the lump is, palpate all four quadrants (see Fig. 3.5) and axillary tail, assess any palpable masses.

Lymphadenopathy axilla, cervical, supraclavicular.

Other liver, spine.

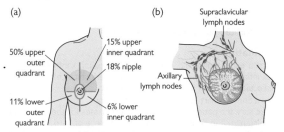

Fig. 3.5 Anatomy of the breast. (a) Quadrants of the breast showing proportion of breast cancer by location. (b) Glands and lymphatics of the right breast.

Eyes

History
Symptoms reduced/impaired vision or visual loss, red eye, discomfort (gritty or FB sensation), pain of the eye or soft tissues around the eye, dry eyes or excessive watering, itch, swelling, photophobia or haloes around lights, floaters or flashing lights, diplopia, discharge.

Past ophthalmic history glaucoma, myopia, cataracts, previous surgery, glasses/contact lens prescription and last optometry check-up.

Past medical history numerous systemic diseases can affect the eye, including DM, ↑BP, vascular disease, RA, SLE, thyroid disease, MS.

Drug history ophthalmic medications, steroids, medications for coexisting disease; allergies.

Family history glaucoma, retinoblastoma.

Social history ability to self-care, impact eye disease has upon ADLs and home support received/needed.

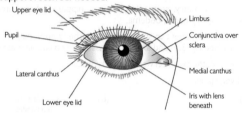

Fig. 3.6 Surface anatomy of the right eye.

Examination
Inspection exophthalmos, proptosis, jaundice, pallor, xanthelasma, eyelids (cysts, inflammation), red eye, corneal arcus, periorbital cellulitis (Fig. 3.6).

Visual acuity this **must** be tested in **all** patients:
- Use a Snellen chart at 6m to test visual acuity
- Make sure the patient is using the correct glasses for the test (reading vs. distance) if in doubt use a pin-hole in a piece of card
- If visual acuity is very bad assess ability to **count fingers, awareness of movement** (waving hand) or **perception of light** (pen torch).

Pupillary response and reflexes check the pupils are equal, reacting to light and accommodation (PERLA) and for a relative afferent papillary defect. Look for the red reflex (absent in dense cataracts).

Visual fields confrontation testing to identify any visual field loss and to establish if the defect is unilateral or bilateral (📖 p133).

Ocular movements look for loss of conjugate gaze or nystagmus.

Ophthalmoscopy
- With the ophthalmoscope set on +10 the cornea and anterior chambers can be examined. 1 or 2 drops of fluorescein highlights corneal ulcers, abrasions and foreign bodies, especially under the blue light
- With the ophthalmoscope set on 0 the user can visualise the retina. It is important to dilate the pupil with 1 or 2 drops of a weak mydriatic (eg 0.5% or 1% tropicamide) to allow full visualisation of the retina. The risk of causing acute glaucoma with mydriatics is small.

Table 3.18 Descriptive terms in ophthalmology

Accommodation	Alteration in lens and pupil to focus on near/far objects
Acuity	Ability of the eye to discriminate fine detail
Anterior chamber	Chamber anterior to the lens, containing aqueous
Aqueous	Fluid-like jelly in the anterior chamber of the eye
Blepharitis	Inflammation/infection of eyelids
Canthus	Medial or lateral junction of the upper and lower eyelids
Chemosis	Conjunctival oedema
Choroid	Layer sandwiched between retina and sclera
Conjunctiva	Mucous membrane covering sclera and cornea anteriorly
Cycloplegia	Ciliary muscle paralysis preventing accommodation
Dacryocystitis	Inflammation of the lacrimal sac
Ectropion	Eyelids evert outwards (away from the cornea)
Entropion	Eyelids invert towards the cornea (lashes irritate cornea)
Fovea	Highly cone-rich area of the macula (yellow-spot)
Fundus	Area of the retina visible with the ophthalmoscope
Hyphaema	Blood in the anterior chamber seen as a red fluid level
Hypopyon	Pus in the anterior chamber seen as a white fluid level
Limbus	Border between cornea and sclera
Macula	Rim around the fovea, rich in cone cells
Miotic	Agent resulting in pupillary constriction (eg pilocarpine)
Mydriatic	Agents resulting in pupillary dilatation (eg tropicamide)
Optic cup	Depression in the centre of the optic disc
Optic disc	Optic nerve head seen as white opacity on fundoscopy
Posterior chamber	Chamber between the iris and ciliary body
Presbyopia	Age-related reduction in near acuity (long-sightedness)
Ptosis	Drooping eyelid(s)
Sclera	The visible white fibrous layer of the eye
Scotoma	Defect resulting in loss of a specific area of vision
Strabismus	Squint, loss of conjugate gaze
Tonometer	Apparatus for indirectly measuring intraocular pressure
Vitreous	Jelly-like matter which occupies the globe behind the lens

Head and neck

History

As well as a good general history, specific symptoms to note include:

- *Ears* pain, blocked ears, wax, discharge, tinnitus, deafness, unilateral/ bilateral features, vertigo, trauma, itching, foreign bodies (FB), noise exposure, occupation
- *Nose* blocked nose, watery discharge, sneezing, itching, coughing, change in voice, altered sensation of smell/taste, external deformity/ recent trauma, epistaxis, sinusitis; ask about daytime variation in symptom severity, pattern of obstruction, effects on speech and sleep
- *Throat* dysphagia, pain on swallowing, hoarseness, difficulty opening jaw (trismus), stridor, sleep apnoea/snoring; ask about neck lumps, vomiting, heartburn, waterbrash (acid regurgitation or filling of mouth with saliva).

Examination

- *Ears* **inspect** the pinna, auditory meatus, tenderness over pinna or mastoid; **otoscopy** examine all four quadrants of the eardrum (see Fig. 3.7) (colour, bulging/retraction, perforation, exudate); **test hearing** (see 'Hearing tests')
- *Nose* **look** for obvious scars, deviations/deformities, tilt the head back and look down each nostril (Fig. 3.8); **rhinoscopy** (administer lidocaine spray first), look for polyps, inflamed turbinates, pus
- *Throat* **inspect** the lips, around and inside the mouth; **examine** the tongue and tonsils using a torch and tongue depressor, check palate movements by asking the patient to say 'ah' (Fig. 3.9)
- *Neck* **look** for swellings, asymmetry, scars; **ask** the patient to swallow, protrude the tongue; **palpate** the neck from behind and ask the patient to take a sip of water; **feel** for tracheal deviation, lymphadenopathy, tenderness; **auscultate** for a bruit; **examine** any lumps (see 📖 p458).

Hearing tests (OHCS8 📖 p540)

- *Whisper* a different number into each ear, standing 30cm away whilst blocking the other ear. Ask the patient to repeat it in turn.
- **Tuning fork tests**:
  - *Rinne's test* place the tuning fork on the patient's mastoid bone until it is no longer heard; then place the fork near the external auditory meatus where it is still heard in a normal ear, but not in an ear with conductive deafness
  - *Weber's test* place the tuning fork in the middle of the forehead and ask which side the sound is loudest; in nerve deafness the sound is loudest in the normal ear, in conductive deafness the sound is loudest in the abnormal ear.

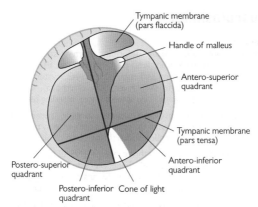

Tympanic membrane (pars flaccida)

Handle of malleus

Antero-superior quadrant

Tympanic membrane (pars tensa)

Antero-inferior quadrant

Cone of light

Postero-inferior quadrant

Postero-superior quadrant

Fig. 3.7 Structures and quadrants of the right tympanic membrane (eardrum) as seen on otoscopy.

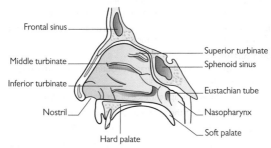

Frontal sinus

Middle turbinate

Inferior turbinate

Nostril

Hard palate

Superior turbinate

Sphenoid sinus

Eustachian tube

Nasopharynx

Soft palate

Fig. 3.8 Anatomy of the nose.

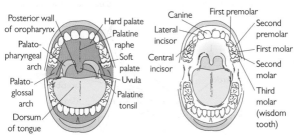

Posterior wall of oropharynx

Palato-pharyngeal arch

Palato-glossal arch

Dorsum of tongue

Hard palate

Palatine raphe

Soft palate

Uvula

Palatine tonsil

Canine

Lateral incisor

Central incisor

First premolar

Second premolar

First molar

Second molar

Third molar (wisdom tooth)

Fig. 3.9 Anatomy of the mouth and oropharynx.

Musculoskeletal

History

Symptoms joint pain, swelling, deformity, morning stiffness, instability, sensory changes, back pain, limb pain, muscle/soft tissue aches, cold fingers and toes, dry eyes and mouth, red eyes, systemic symptoms (fatigue, weight loss, tight skin, fever, rash, diarrhoea), injury/trauma (mechanism, timing, change in symptoms since), bleeding tendency.

Past medical history previous trauma/surgery, recent infections (streptococcal, gonorrhoeal, tuberculosis etc), insect/tick bites, IBD, skin disease (psoriasis), childhood arthritis, haemophilia.

Drug history previous anti-arthritic agents (NSAIDs, steroids (oral/intra-articular), DMARDs) with beneficial/side effects, long-standing steroids, Ca^{2+} supplements, vitamin D analogues, bisphosphonates, other concurrent medications (antihypertensives etc), allergies.

Activities of daily living ability to: bathe, dress (and undress), eat, transfer from bed to chair and back, use of the toilet; ?change with symptoms.

Social history domestic arrangements (who else is at home, location of bathroom in relation to bed), smoking history, drug and alcohol use.

Family history rheumatoid, gout, osteoarthritis, haemochromatosis, inflammatory bowel disease, haemophilia.

Examination

Each joint has a specific examination routine, though the underlying principles for each are very similar:

General inspection overall appearance of the patient and their gait.

Look close inspection of the joint, comparing left to right if possible.

Feel assessment of warmth, tenderness, crepitus, effusions etc.

Move active (patient moving the joint) and passive (examiner moving joint) movements; stressing joint where appropriate.

Measure range of movements (in degrees) and degree of joint laxity.

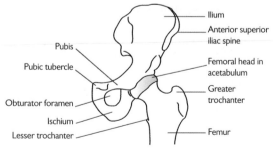

Fig. 3.10 Anatomy of the left hip joint.

Hip (OHCS8 📖 p680) (Fig. 3.10)

Inspection leg shortening, internal rotation (hip dislocation), external rotation (fractured neck of femur), scars, sinuses, cellulitis, bruising.

Palpation check bony landmarks (greater trochanter, anterior superior iliac crest) are symmetrical, warmth, crepitus and clicks on movement.

Supine active and passive range of movement; flexion (straight leg flexion 0–90°, flexion with knee bent 0–135°), abduction (0–50°), adduction, internal (0–45°) and external (0–45°) rotation, fixed flexion deformity (with hand in lumbar lordosis, check the popliteal fossa can touch the couch).

Prone active and passive range of movement; extension (0–20°).

Stressing is not generally undertaken for the hip.

Gait Trendelenburg gait (📖 p136), walking aids.

Other joints knee (Fig. 3.11) and lower spine/sacroiliac (📖 p149).

Knee (OHCS8 📖 p686)

Inspection swelling, erythema, resting position, varus (bow-legs) or valgus (knock-knees) deformity, scars, sinuses, cellulitis, muscle wasting of thigh muscles compared to the other side (especially vastus medialis).

Palpation temperature, bony landmarks (head of fibula, medial and lateral joint lines, patella), effusion (if large infra-patella sulci will be bulging outwards with a positive patella tap, if small try milking fluid down from thigh and stroking fluid from one side to the other), crepitus, clunks or clicks on movement, patella position, tenderness and mobility.

Supine active and passive movement; flexion (0–135°), extension (0°).

Prone popliteal fossa cysts or aneurysms.

Stressing cruciates flex knee to 90°, immobilise the patient's foot by sitting on it and check the integrity of the anterior and posterior cruciate ligaments by pulling and pushing the lower leg, respectively **collaterals** flex knee to 30°, fix the thigh with your left hand and test medial collateral (pull lower leg laterally) and then lateral collateral (push lower leg medially).

Gait limp, walking aids.

Other joints hip (see previous section) and ankle (📖 p148).

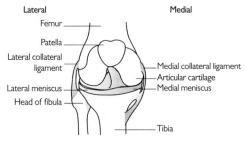

Lateral   Medial

- Femur
- Patella
- Lateral collateral ligament
- Lateral meniscus
- Head of fibula
- Medial collateral ligament
- Articular cartilage
- Medial meniscus
- Tibia

Fig. 3.11 Anatomy of the right knee joint.

Ankle (OHCS8 📖 p692) (Fig. 3.12)
Inspection swelling, erythema, resting position (consider fracture–dislocation and get immediate senior help if there is marked deviation of the foot following trauma (📖 p434).
Palpation temperature, bony landmarks (medial and lateral malleolus, tibiotalar joint), crepitus, pain, swelling, effusion, crepitus, clicks **trauma** palpate proximal fibula head to exclude its fracture, foot pulses (📖 p128), distal sensation and cap-refill.
Movement active and passive movement; plantarflexion (0–50°), dorsiflexion (0–15°), inversion (0–30°), eversion (0–15°).
Stressing is not generally undertaken for the ankle.
Gait limp, walking aids, ability to walk two paces unaided.
Other joints knee (📖 p147) and foot (📖 p148).

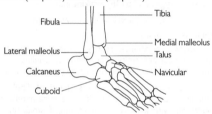

Fig. 3.12 Anatomy of the right ankle joint.

Foot (Fig. 3.13)
Inspection swelling, erythema, resting position, high-arch, bunions.
Palpation temperature, pain or crepitus along each metatarsal and phalanx, forefoot bones (navicular, cuboid and medial, intermediate and lateral cuneiform), foot pulses (📖 p128), distal sensation and cap-refill.
Movement as for ankle examination but also adduction and abduction across the talonavicular and calcaneocuboid joints.
Stressing is not generally undertaken for the foot.
Gait limp, walking aids, ability to walk two paces unaided.
Other joints ankle (📖 p148).

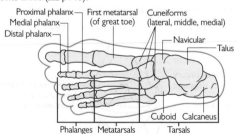

Fig. 3.13 Anatomy of the left foot.

Back (OHCS8 📖 p670) (Fig. 3.14)

Inspection deformity, loss or exaggeration of thoracic kyphosis or lumbar lordosis, lateral deviation from the midline (scoliosis).

Palpation with patient standing palpate each vertebra for pain; with patient prone palpate each side of pelvis for sacroiliac tenderness.

Movement **active** flexion (touch toes with knees together and legs straight; most people can touch their shins), extension (leaning backwards), lateral bending (lateral flexion) and rotation (best assessed with patient seated so pelvis is fixed) **passive** with patient supine, perform straight leg raise by elevating each leg in turn (0–85°).

Measure Schober's test for lumbar flexion (mark the level of the posterior iliac spine in the midline; make a further two marks, one 5cm below this and one 10cm above this; the distance between these two new marks measured when the patient is standing and then in full flexion – an increase of <5cm suggests limited lumbar flexion).

Other joints hip (📖 p147) and knee (📖 p147).

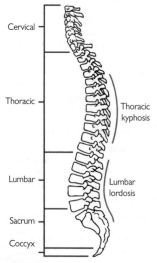

Cervical

Thoracic

Thoracic kyphosis

Lumbar

Lumbar lordosis

Sacrum

Coccyx

Fig. 3.14 Anatomy of the spine.

Pelvis

The joints in the pelvis are fixed, however the sacroiliac joint can be palpated for tenderness from behind; in a trauma emergency a senior member of the trauma team may test the pelvis for instability. See Fig. 3.15.

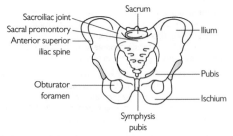

Fig. 3.15 Anatomy of the pelvis.

Shoulder (OHCS8 📖 p662) (Fig. 3.16)

Inspection swelling, erythema, deformity, resting position, (check from the front, side and back), scars, sinuses, cellulitis, swelling, muscle wasting (deltoid, supraspinatus, infraspinatus).

Palpation temperature, bony landmarks (acromion, clavicle, spine of scapula, cervical and upper thoracic vertebrae), crepitus, clicks.

Movement active and passive movement; abduction (0–90° with elbow flexed, 0–180° with elbow extended), adduction, internal (0–90°) and external (0–65°) rotation, flexion (0–180°) and extension (0–65°), passive abduction should be undertaken carefully if painful.

Stressing **Impingement test** arm held at 90° abduction and internally rotated, if pain detected it is a positive test **Scarf test** patient's left hand placed over their right shoulder and vice versa, if pain detected it is a positive test (acromioclavicular joint pathology).

Other joints elbow (📖 p151) and back (📖 p149).

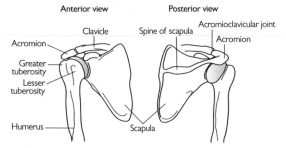

Fig. 3.16 Anatomy of the right shoulder joint.

Elbow (OHCS8 📖 p666) (Fig. 3.17)

Inspection swelling, erythema, inflamed bursae, rheumatoid nodules or psoriatic plaques over the olecranon, scars.

Palpation temperature, bony landmarks (medial and lateral epicondyles, olecranon), crepitus, clicks, instability.

Movement active and passive movement; flexion (0–150°) and extension (0°); pronation, supination.

Stressing is not generally undertaken for the elbow.

Other joints shoulder (Fig. 3.16 📖 p150) and wrist (Fig. 3.18).

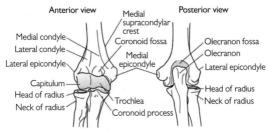

Fig. 3.17 Anatomy of the right elbow.

Wrist (OHCS8 📖 p668) (Fig. 3.18)

Inspection swelling, erythema, deformity (eg Colles' fracture), features of rheumatoid disease (📖 p454), scars.

Palpation temperature, bony landmarks (styloid process of radius, head and styloid process of ulna), scaphoid (base of the anatomical snuff-box).

Movement active and passive movement; flexion (0–75°), extension (0–75°), radial (0–20°), ulnar deviation (0–20°), pronation, supination.

Stressing is not generally undertaken for the wrist.

Other joints elbow (📖 p151) and hand (📖 p152).

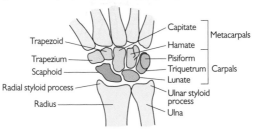

Fig. 3.18 Anatomy of the wrist and hand.

Hand (OHCS8 📖 p668) (Fig. 3.19)

Inspection erythema, swelling, breaks to the skin, features of rheumatoid disease (📖 p454) or osteoarthritis (📖 p454), deformity, dislocation, muscle wasting, nail pitting.

Palpation temperature, palpate each metacarpal and phalanx for pain or crepitus, distal cap-refill and sensation.

Movement active and passive movement; flexion and extension of every MTPJ, PIPJ and DIPJ, abduction and adduction of every MTPJ, opposition and circumduction of the thumb MTPJ; ask the patient to: hold a pencil and write, pick up a mug, undo a button, oppose their thumb and little finger (check strength of this against your own); check strength of extension and flexion following penetrating or lacerating trauma to identify tendon injury.

Stressing collateral ligaments of the digits following trauma or dislocation by attempting to deviate the phalanges medially or laterally.

Other joints wrist (📖 p151) and inspect the elbow.

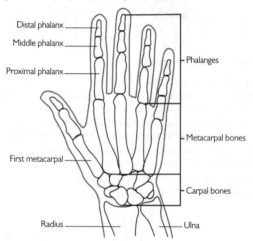

Fig. 3.19 Anatomy of the hand, thumb and fingers.

Urological

History

Symptoms polyuria, anuria, prostatism (urgency, hesitancy, poor stream, terminal dribble, nocturia), haematuria, dysuria, oedema, renal colic, incontinence, malaise, lethargy, N+V, anorexia, weight loss, itching, passing stones in the urine, incontinence, impotence, infertility, bone pain, genital discharge, genital/perineal lesion, scrotal pain, dyspareunia (pain on intercourse), foreign body (vaginal, urethral, anal), anal/peri-anal problems.

Past medical history DM, ↑BP, recurrent UTIs, renal/ureteric stones, myeloma, known renal impairment/failure, previous vesicoureteric reflux, gout, immunosuppression (steroids, HIV), neurological disease, long-term urinary catheter, STIs, spinal cord pathology; *male* tight foreskin, recurrent balanitis, testicular pain/swelling; *female* number of children, mode of delivery and any complications, last cervical smear and result.

Drug history nephrotoxics (including NSAIDs, ACEi, aminoglycosides), bladder neck relaxants, infertility or impotence drugs, antiandrogens; allergies.

Social history foreign travel, ability to cope with ADLs, sex abroad, illicit drug use (smoke, oral, IV).

Sexual history
- Last sexual intercourse (LSI) – gender of partner, type of intercourse (vaginal, anal, oral), barrier contraception used, relationship of partner (casual, long-term), problems or symptoms in partner, date of LSI
- Repeat the above for all partners in the last 3mth
- All men should also be asked if they have ever had sex with another man in the past as this affects risk and types of STI to consider.

Occupational history past and present jobs, exposure to dyes.

Family history polycystic kidney disease, DM, ↑BP.

Examination (lying flat, supine) (Fig. 3.20)

General inspection mental state, RR (?Kussmaul breathing), hiccups, pallor, hydration (*dehydrated*: sunken eyes, dry lips/tongue; *fluid-overload*: peripheral oedema, pulmonary oedema).

Hands leuconychia, brown nails, pale nail beds.

Arms bruising (purpura), pigmentation, scratch marks, fistula, BP (lying and standing).

Face eyes (anaemia, jaundice), mouth (dehydration, ulcers, fetor), rash.

Neck JVP.

Abdomen inspect (distended bladder, scars, transplanted kidney, dialysis port), palpate (ballot kidneys, bladder, liver, spleen, lymph nodes), percuss (enlarged bladder, ascites), auscultate (renal artery bruits), PR for prostate.

Rectum size, surface, consistency and symmetry of prostate in men, faecal impaction (will worsen urinary retention).

Back oedema, loin tenderness on percussion.

Chest CVS and RS examination (pericarditis, heart failure, fluid overload).

Legs oedema, bruising, pigmentation, scratch marks, neuropathy, proximal weakness (myopathy), altered reflexes, muscle wasting.

Urinalysis glucose, blood, protein, nitrites, leucocytes.

Other fundoscopy (DM and ↑BP changes), blood glucose, weight.

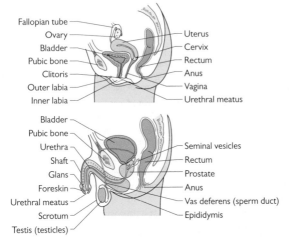

Fig. 3.20 Anatomy of the female (L) and male (R) urogenital systems.

Examination of male genitalia

Inspection look for any ulceration (including retracting foreskin and checking the glans), warts, scars, or sinuses, urethral discharge, tight foreskin (phimosis) or retracted foreskin which is stuck leaving the glans exposed (paraphimosis). Observe the scrotum for skin changes or oedema and, whilst the patient is standing, the lie of the testes (the left testis usually hangs lower than the right and both testes lie longitudinally – a high testis with a transverse lie may indicate torsion, though a torted testis may also appear normal).

Palpate each testis in turn between the fingers and the thumb feeling for texture, tenderness, nodules, and to compare left to right. An absent testis may be maldescended and trapped in the inguinal canal. Examine epididymis and follow it up superiorly to the spermatic cord and up into the inguinal ring. Palpate inguinal lymph nodes or maldescended testis.

Examination of female genitalia
See 📖 p156.

Female reproductive system

History

Menstrual history date of last period, length of menstrual cycle (regular or irregular), length of period, associated pain/symptoms (Table 3.19), age when periods started/stopped; bleeding/discharge severity of periods (number of pads/tampons, clots, flooding), bleeding between periods, after intercourse (vaginal, anal, oral), or after menopause, rectal/urinary bleeding, effect on lifestyle, other vaginal discharge (colour, consistency and smell).

Sexual history pain on superficial or deep penetration (dyspareunia), type of intercourse (vaginal, anal, oral), use of contraception, intercourse in foreign countries, previous sexually transmitted infections; **contraception** current and previous types, problems/benefits.

Cervical smear date of last test and result, previous results and any treatment (repeat smears, colposcopy clinic, laser ablation).

Past gynae history previous problems and/or operations (where and name of surgeon), breast or thyroid problems, use of HRT, prolapse.

Past obstetric history number of pregnancies, number of births, type of delivery, complications, subfertility (see 🕮 p158 for obstetric history).

Past medical history clotting problems, thyroid problems, anaemia, malignancy.

Urinary problems incontinence (on laughing/coughing/exercising or spontaneous), dysuria, urgency, frequency, haematuria, if symptomatic ask about fluid intake, leg weakness, faecal incontinence, back pain and previous spinal problems/surgery, effect on lifestyle.

Other vaginal lumps, weight loss, other concerns.

Examination

Always have a chaperone who can also guard the door. Ask friends and family members to leave, unless the patient wants them to stay (this also provides an opportunity to ask questions which the patient may not have answered fully with others present). As with any examination it is essential to keep the patient informed about what you are going to do. Start with the patient lying flat on their back with arms by their sides. See Fig. 3.21.

Abdominal Assess for scars, striae, hernias, body hair distribution, everted umbilicus, distension, tenderness including loins (±guarding, rebound), masses, organomegaly, percuss (masses, shifting dullness).

Ask the patient to move her feet apart, bend her knees and let her legs flop outwards. Have a strong light source directed at the vulva and gloves on both hands.

Vulval Look for rashes, ulcers, warts, lumps or other lesions; spread the labia majora using your non-dominant thumb and index finger and look for lesions, lumps, discharge (urethral/vaginal), bleeding; ask the patient to push down (look for prolapse) and cough.

Vaginal Insert a well-lubricated index and middle finger (dominant hand) into the vagina and feel for the cervix, noting the size, shape, consistency and whether it is mobile or tender. Feel above, below and to the sides (adnexae) for masses or tenderness. Finally palpate the uterus by placing your other hand above the pubic symphysis and press down with the fingers at the cervix; pressing up feel for uterine position (anteverted/retroverted), size, shape, consistency, mobility and tenderness. Inspect the finger afterwards for blood or discharge.

Cusco's speculum Whilst the patient is in the same position insert a well lubricated and warmed speculum into the vagina. Look at the cervix for ulceration, bleeding, cysts or other lesions and the cervical os. If required take swabs and/or a cervical smear.

Consider Sims' speculum (for examining prolapses), rectal examination.

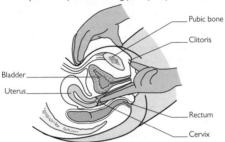

Fig. 3.21 Examination of the female reproductive system.

Table 3.19 *Descriptive terms in gynaecology*
Anatomy
Introitus the entrance to the vagina
Adnexae the areas lateral to the cervix where the ovaries are located
Abnormal bleeding
Climacteric phase of irregular periods and associated symptoms prior to menopause
Intermenstrual bleeding between periods
Oligomenorrhoea infrequent menstruation, >42d menstrual cycle
Menopause the end of menstruation
Menorrhagia excessive blood loss during menstruation (>80ml/cycle)
Postcoital bleeding after sexual intercourse
Postmenopausal bleeding >6mth after the menopause
Primary amenorrhoea failure to start menstruating by 16yr
Secondary amenorrhoea absence of menstruation for >6mth after menstruation has started and not due to pregnancy
Pain
Dysmenorrhoea pain associated with menstruation
Dyspareunia pain associated with sexual intercourse, can be superficial (eg vulval or entrance to vagina) or deep (only on deep penetration)

Obstetric

History

Current pregnancy estimated due date (EDD), gestation, last menstrual period (LMP), method of conception, scan results, site of placenta, rhesus status, concerns, attitude to pregnancy; **current symptoms** bleeding, other vaginal discharge, headache, visual disturbance, dysuria, urinary frequency or urgency, constipation, vomiting, GORD.

Previous pregnancies number of pregnancies (gravidity), number of deliveries ≥24/40wks (parity), miscarriages, terminations (reason, gestation, method), stillbirths, complications: vomiting, anaemia, bleeding, group B strep, BP, proteinuria, gestational DM, poor foetal growth, admission.

Delivery history method of delivery and reason (vaginal, ventouse, forceps, elective/emergency Caesarean), gestation, birthweight, sex, complications (fever, prolonged rupture of membranes, CTG trace), postnatal baby problems (feeding, infection, jaundice), admission to SCBU/NNU, outcome (how is the child now), postnatal maternal problems (pain, fever, bleeding, depression).

Past gynae history previous problems, operations, STIs.

Past medical history DVT, PE, DM, admissions, psychiatric problems.

Family history DM, ↑BP, pre-eclampsia, congenital abnormalities, DVT, PE, multiple pregnancies.

Social history support from family/partner, type of housing, employment, financial problems, smoking, alcohol, substance abuse.

Table 3.20 *Antenatal care*

Gestation (wk)	Standard antenatal care: purpose of each visit
Booking	FBC, G+S, red cell antibodies, rubella, syphilis, hepatitis B, HIV serology, sickle-cell disease, BMI, BP, urine dipstick and culture
11–14	USS for gestational assessment and nuchal screening
16	Urine, BP, serum screening (for Down's and neural tube defects)
20	USS for foetal anomalies and growth and placental position
28	Fundal height, BP, urine, FBC, red cell antibodies, anti-D if rhesus −ve
25*, 31*	Fundal height, BP, urine
34	Fundal height, BP, urine, anti-D if rhesus −ve
36, 38, 40*	Foetal position, fundal height, BP, urine
41	Discuss induction, foetal position, fundal height, BP, urine

* For the first pregnancy only.

Examination

Foetal heart Audible from 12wk using a Doppler ultrasound and 24wk using a Pinard stethoscope; it is faster than the mother's (110–160bpm).

Weight Plot mother's weight and BMI (📖 p604) at the booking visit.

Inspection Striae, linea nigra (line of pigmentation from the pubic symphysis to the navel that darkens during the 1st trimester), venous distension, scars, oedema.

Fundal height The fundus (top of the uterus) is palpable from about 12wk gestation; it should be measured from the top of the pubic symphysis to the top of the fundus with a tape measure. Between 16 and 36wk the fundal height in centimetres should be the same as the gestation ±2cm, eg 23–27cm at 25wk. Fundal height is unreliable after 36wk. See Fig. 3.22.

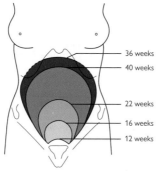

Fig. 3.22 Location of the fundus as pregnancy progresses.

Foetal lie After 32wk it is possible to assess the position of the foetus by palpating across the abdomen for the foetal head:
- **Longitudinal** head palpable in midline
- **Oblique** head palpable in iliac fossa
- **Transverse** head palpable in lateral abdomen.

Presentation Palpation after 32wk can also assess the presentation though this is liable to change until about 36wk. By palpating both ends of the foetus the position of the head can be determined:
- **Cephalic** head is at the bottom
- **Breech** head is at the top.

Engagement This is assessed by palpating the base of the uterus above the pubic symphysis between two hands to assess how much of the presenting part is palpable. If only the top 1/5th of the presenting part is palpable the foetus has 'engaged'.

Blood pressure must be monitored regularly to assess for pregnancy induced ↑BP; consider urine dipstick and fundoscopy too.

Urine dipstick for protein (pre-eclampsia) and glucose (DM).

USS Lie, presentation and engagement can be confirmed on USS.

Psychiatric

History

Are you safe? sit so the patient is not between you and the door, remove all potential weapons, be familiar with the panic alarm, check notes/ask staff about previous violence, low threshold for a chaperone.

Set the scene make sure you are both comfortable, ensure privacy and that you will not be disturbed, eg give the bleep to someone else, have tissues available, emphasise confidentiality.

Basics full name, age, marital status, occupation, who were they referred by, current status under Mental Health Act.

Past psychiatric history previous psychiatric diagnoses, in-patient/day patient/out-patient care, do they have a community psychiatric nurse (CPN), previous deliberate self-harm (DSH), previous treatments and effects, ever been admitted under the Mental Health Act.

Medication history current and previous medications, effects, did they/do they take it, allergies/reactions, alternative/herbal remedies.

Personal history
- *Childhood* pregnancy, birth, development (📖 p164), associated memories, names of schools attended, reason if changed schools, types of school (mainstream/specialist), age of leaving school, qualifications.
- *Employment* loss of jobs, which did they enjoy, why did they change, ask about unemployment and why.
- *Relationships* current relationship(s) and sexual orientation, list of major relationships and reasons for ending, any children and who they live with and relationship to patient.

Forensic contact with police, convictions or charges, sentences, outstanding charges.

Personality how would they describe their personality now and before the illness? How would others describe it?

Social history occupation and duration of employment/unemployment, where they live, concerns over money, friends and relationships, hobbies.

Drug and alcohol smoking, alcohol, illicit drugs.

Family history family tree with parents and siblings, ages, occupations, relationships, illnesses.

Examination

Psychiatrists examine the mind through talking to the patient. Much of the information is gleaned whilst taking the history and should be organised under the following headings:

Appearance racial origin, age, dress, make-up, hairstyle, jewellery, tattoos, cleanliness, neglect, physical condition.

Behaviour appropriateness, posture, movement (excessive, slow, exaggerated), gestures, tics, facial expression, eye contact, anxiety, suspiciousness, rapport, abnormal movements, aggression, distraction, concentration.

Mood the patient's subjective assessment of their mood.

Affect interviewer's objective assessment of mood and appropriateness of patient's response, eg flat, reactive, blunted.

Speech form accent, volume, rate, tone, quantity, hesitations, stuttering; **content** associations (derailment, changing between subjects), puns.

Thought form rate, flow (eg blocked), connection (eg flight of ideas, derailment); **content** beliefs about self, beliefs about others, thought insertion/withdrawal/control/broadcast, beliefs about the world/future, delusions, overvalued ideas, obsessions, compulsions, ruminations, rituals, phobias.

Perception illusions, hallucinations (visual, auditory, tactile, olfactory), unusual experiences, depersonalisation, derealisation.

Cognition this can be tested formally using the Mini-Mental State Examination (MMSE) on 📖 p343, often the Abbreviated Mental Test Score (AMTS) is used instead (📖 p341).

Risk thoughts of deliberate self-harm, suicide, harming others, plans, acquiring equipment, writing notes, previous suicide attempts.

Insight awareness of illness and need for treatment.

Defining 'mental illness'

What constitutes abnormal behaviour to the extent of constituting a mental illness can be a controversial and difficult area, subject to allegations of cultural and political bias and even suggestions of undue influence from the pharmaceutical industry. Two main classification systems are accepted:

- The *Diagnostic and Statistical Manual of Mental Disorders*, produced by the American Psychiatric Association; the 5th edition (2013) is currently in use: DSM-5
- The *International Classification of Diseases*, published by the World Health Organization (covers all of medicine); 10th edition (1992) is currently in use: ICD-10.

Each classification carries a slightly different emphasis and diagnostic criteria; in rare instances, this results in an abnormal condition recognised in one, but not the other.

Common terms in psychiatry

Affect pattern of observable behaviours which reflects **emotions** experienced

Anxiety feeling of apprehension caused by anticipation of perceived danger

Approved clinician a doctor entitled to recommend compulsory admission for treatment under the 2007 Mental Health Act

Cognition the process of thinking, reasoning and remembering

Compulsion repetitive behaviours in response to obsessions; often to relieve the distress caused by them, eg washing hands

Delirium acute onset of disordered cognition with attentional deficits; typically involves changes in arousal and may be associated with hallucinations

Delusion a fixed, false belief that goes against available evidence and is not explained by the person's religious or cultural background

Dementia global organic deterioration of cognition with preserved consciousness

Depersonalisation altered sense of self as if detached or outside the body

Derealisation altered sense of reality as if detached from surroundings

Emotion a complex state of feeling that results in physical and psychological changes that influence thought and behaviour

Euphoria pathologically exaggerated feeling of wellbeing

Flight of ideas rapid switching of topics where the thread of connection can be determined (eg sound, content)

Formal admission admission under a section of the Mental Health Act

Hallucination a false sensory perception in absence of a real stimulus, eg hearing voices; feature of psychosis if the subject lacks recognition of the false nature

Illusion false interpretation of a real external stimulus, eg seeing a shadow and thinking it is a person

Informal admission voluntary admission as a psychiatric in-patient

Insight the ability of a person to recognise their mental illness

Mania abnormal elevation of mood with grandiose ideas, increased energy and agitation, pressure of speech, distractibility, and pleasure seeking

Mood emotional state that colours the person's perception of the world

Obsession recurrent unwanted thoughts or images, eg my hands are dirty

Passivity delusional belief in external control of a person's actions or thoughts

Personality disorder enduring and inflexible behavioural patterns that markedly differ to societal norms

Phobia persistent, irrational fear of an activity, object or situation, leading to the desire to avoid the feared stimulus; beyond voluntary control

Psychosis disordered thinking and perception without **insight**, often accompanied by delusions or hallucinations

Ruminations a compulsion to consider an idea or phrase

Stereotype repeated pattern of movement or speech without any goal

Thought insertion delusional belief by a person that an external agency is putting thoughts into his/her mind (a **passivity** phenomenon)

Neonatal examination

The baby check is a key component of life in paediatrics. All neonates should be examined within 72h of birth with the aim of:
- Identifying unwell babies (tone and respiratory rate are very important)
- Identifying abnormalities (especially reversible ones).

Preparation prior to the examination you should check the maternal notes for: significant maternal illness, gestation at birth, birthweight, type of delivery, problems at delivery (meconium, premature rupture of membranes (PROM), group B strep, low Apgar scores).

Introduction introduce yourself to the mother/parents, offer congratulations and explain that you've come to examine their baby. Ask if the baby has passed **faeces** and **urine**, is **feeding** well and if there are any concerns; ask them to undress the baby to the nappy while you wash your hands.

> *Settled baby* consider doing the following first as they are difficult if the baby is crying: listening to the heart and feeling the apex beat, counting the respiratory rate, feeling the femoral pulse and looking in the eyes.
>
> *Crying baby* try getting the baby to suck (pacifier, breast, bottle, parent's little finger, your little finger), if this fails swaddle the baby and ask the parents to give the baby a feed then return in 30min.

Overall take a few moments just to look, ask yourself is the baby: jaundiced, blue, dysmorphic, moving normally, breathing normally?

Neuro **tone** (degree of head support, spontaneous symmetrical limb movements), Moro reflex is not routinely performed.

Head anterior and posterior **fontanelle** (bulging, sunken), **head circumference**, eyes **red reflex** (paler in pigmented babies), **face** (dysmorphic?), **ear** shape and position (tags, pits, top of insertion of pinna should be at the level of the eyes), **palate** (with your little finger), **suck reflex**.

Hands/arms **fingers** (number, shape, colour), **palms** (single crease in 60% of Down's and 1% of non-Down's), symmetrical arm movement.

Chest **respiratory rate** (RR >60 is abnormal), listen to the **heart**, apex beat, gently feel the clavicles for fractures.

Abdo **palpate** (to exclude hepatomegaly, splenomegaly, masses), descended **testes**, patent **anus**, enlarged clitoris, **femoral pulses**.

Hips/feet anterior hip creases (symmetrical?), **Barlow** test (flex hip to 90°, press posteriorly, feel for a click/clunk if the hip dislocates), **Ortolani** test (after Barlow's abduct the hips one at a time whilst pressing on the greater trochanter with your middle finger, feel for a click/clunk as the hip relocates), note repetition of these tests can cause hip instability, **ankles** (talipes, correctable or not), **toes** (number, shape, colour).

Turn baby over **spine** (straight), **sacrum** (lumps, dimples, hair tufts, skin defects), **buttocks** (blue spots – make a note), posterior hip creases.

Plot in the red book: weight, head circumference, examination.

Paediatric

History

Basics age in days (until 1mth), weeks (until 2mth), months (until 2yr) or years, gender, who gave the history, who was present.

Current state feeding and drinking, weight gain, wetting nappies/passing urine, fever, bowels, crying, runny nose (coryza), cough, breathing problems, pulling ears, drawing up legs, rash.

Birth pregnancy problems and medications, gestation at birth (37–42/40 is normal), type of delivery (NVD, induced, ventouse, forceps, if LSCS ask why), resuscitation, special care, birthweight, premature rupture of membranes (PROM), group B strep (GBS), meconium, maternal pyrexia during labour, vitamin K (IM or oral), feeding (breast, bottle, type of milk).

Immunisations check the child is up to date with vaccinations (Table 3.21); jabs will be postponed if the child is unwell or febrile beforehand and children often get a slight fever for <24h afterwards.

Table 3.21 *UK vaccination schedule*

Birth	May get tuberculosis (BCG) and/or hepatitis B if at risk
2mth	Diphtheria, tetanus, pertussis, polio and *Haemophilus influenzae* type b (DTaP/IPV/Hib), pneumococcal disease (PCV) and rotavirus
3mth	Diphtheria, tetanus, pertussis, polio and *Haemophilus influenzae* type b (DTaP/IPV/Hib), meningococcal group C disease (MenC) and rotavirus
4mth	Diphtheria, tetanus, pertussis, polio and *Haemophilus influenzae* type b (DTaP/IPV/Hib) and pneumococcal disease (PCV)
12–13mth	Measles, mumps, rubella (MMR), *Haemophilus influenzae* type B (Hib), pneumococcal (PCV), meningococcal group C disease (MenC)
2yr and 3yr	Influenza
3yr4mth–5yr	Diphtheria, tetanus, pertussis and polio (DTaP/IPV), MMR
12–13yr	Human papilloma virus (girls only)
14yr	Tetanus, diphtheria and polio (Td/IPV) and meningococcal group C disease (MenC)

Development see Table 3.22 and ask about school performance.

Social history who the child lives with, who has parental responsibility, parental jobs, smoking, nursery/school attendance, type of school (mainstream, special needs), academic ability, sporting ability, friends at school, enjoyment of school, foreign travel.

Family history family tree with parents and siblings, ask diplomatically about consanguinity if relevant, any illnesses in the family, how are their parents and siblings at the moment, asthma, eczema, hayfever, DM, epilepsy, other diseases specific to presenting complaint.

Examination

Much of the examination can be performed by simply observing the child; this usually has the advantage of limiting tears. Approach younger children gently whilst they are sitting on a parent's knee and feeling secure. Examination is much the same as for adult patients, but include the following:

If unwell ABC and resuscitate, see 📖 p234.

Chaperone ask a nurse to accompany you if a child of either sex is over 10yr, there is a child protection issue or whenever you feel it is necessary.

Hydration fontanelle, capillary-refill (≤2s), warm peripheries, mucous membranes, tears if crying, skin turgor, sunken eyes, tachycardia, lethargy.

Respiratory grunting, head bobbing, nasal flaring, tracheal tug, cervical lymphadenopathy, recession (sternal, subcostal, intercostal).

Cardiovascular cyanosis (check mouth), clubbing, mottled skin, murmurs may radiate to the back, femoral pulses (coarctation), radiofemoral delay, dextrocardia, hepatomegaly (heart failure).

Abdominal check the external genitalia if young, relevant or boys with abdominal pain (torsion), never do a PR (though seniors might).

Neurological AVPU (**A**lert, responds to **V**oice, responds to **P**ain, **U**nresponsive), fontanelles, tone, reflexes (including Moro and grasp reflex if young), head circumference (growth chart), development (Table 3.22).

Table 3.22 *Key stages in childhood development*

Age	Gross motor	Fine motor	Speech	Social
6wk	Holds head in line	Eyes follow 90°	Startles to sound	Smiles
3mth	Lifts head up	Eyes follow 180°	Coos	Laughs
6mth	Sits unsupported	Transfers objects	Babbles	Objects to mouth
9mth	Pulls to stand	Finger–thumb grip	'Mama, dada'	Waves goodbye
12mth	Walks unsupported	Points	First words	Finger foods
18mth	Running	Scribbles	Asks for 'wants'	Feeds alone
2yr	Jumps	Copies line	2–3-word sentences	Uses fork
3yr	Uses tricycle	Copies circle	Name and age	Dry by day
4yr	Hops	Copies cross	Counts to 10	Dry by night

ENT always check the ears and throat if there is a suspicion of infection; describe the colour, appearance and if an effusion or pus is present.

Weight, height should be plotted on a sex-specific growth chart.

Head circumference this is especially important in infants and those with neurological disease; the measurement should be plotted on a sex-specific chart.

Prescribing

Prescribing – general considerations

Prescribing medicines is rarely taught well in medical school, yet it is one of the first tasks you'll be asked to do on day one. Even the most experienced of doctors will only know by heart the dose and frequency of a maximum of 30–40 drugs, so do not worry if you cannot even remember the dose of paracetamol; for adults it's 1g/4–6h PO max 4g/24h in divided doses (p211).

Many medical errors in hospital involve drugs so it is important to consider a few things every time you want to prescribe a drug, rather than just writing a prescription as a knee-jerk reaction.

Indication Is there a valid indication for the drug? Is there an alternative method to solve the problem in question (such as move to a quiet area of the ward rather than prescribe night-time sedation)?

Contraindications Are there contraindications to the drug you are about to prescribe? Does the patient have asthma or suffer with Raynaud's syndrome, in which case β-blockers may create more problems than they solve.

Route of administration If a patient is nil by mouth, then it is pointless prescribing oral medications; use the *BNF* or ask the pharmacist to help you use alternative routes of administration. Remember IM and SC injections are painful, so avoid these if possible.

Drug interactions Some drugs are incompatible when physically mixed together (eg IV furosemide and IV metoclopramide), and other drug combinations should ring alarm bells (eg ACEi with K^+-sparing diuretics). Look through the patient's drug chart to spot potential drug interactions (p171).

Adverse effects All drugs have side effects. Ensure the benefits of treatment outweigh the risk of side effects and remember some patients are more prone to some side effects than others (eg Reye's syndrome in children with aspirin, or oculogyric crises in young females with metoclopramide). Some side effects should prompt urgent action (such as stopping statin drugs in patients who complain of muscle pains, or patients who get wheezy with β-blockers), but others can be advantageous if they are not exposing the patient to unnecessary risks (such as slight sedation with some antihistamines).

Administering drugs Sometimes it's necessary for doctors to prescribe and administer a drug to the patient. Always double check the drug prescription and the drug with another member of staff (qualified nurse or doctor). This is not a sign of uncertainty, this is a sign that you are meticulous and will greatly limit the chance of a drug error occurring, which would make you look careless.

> **If in doubt** Never prescribe or administer a drug you are unsure about; even if it is a dire emergency seek senior help or consult the *BNF* or a pharmacist.

How to prescribe – best practice

Knowing how drugs work and their common side effects is very useful, but you must also be able to safely prescribe them. There are a few basic rules about prescribing, and even if you are slightly unsure ask the ward or hospital pharmacist or consult the *BNF*; it's not a sign of failure.

The basics There are usually at least four drug sections on the drug card (Figs 4.1–4.3); once-only, regular medications, PRN ('as required') medications, and infusions (fluids) (□ p380). Other sections might include O_2, anticoagulants, insulin, medications prior to admission, and nurse prescriptions.

Labelling the drug card As with the patient's notes, the drug card should have at least three identifying features: name, DoB, and NHS number (the NPSA advice is that the NHS number should be used whenever possible to help avoid errors). There are usually spaces to document the ward, consultant, date of admission and number of drug cards in use (1 of 2, 2 of 2, etc).

The allergy box Ask the patient about allergies; check old drug cards if available. Document any allergies in this box and the reaction precipitated; eg penicillin → rash. If there are no known drug allergies then record this too. Nurses are unable to give any drugs unless the allergy box is complete.

Writing a prescription Use black pen and write clearly, ideally in capitals. Use the generic drug name (eg diclofenac, not Voltarol®) and clearly indicate the dose, route, frequency of administration, date started, and circle the times the drug should be given (Figs 4.2 and 4.3). Record any specific instructions (such as 'with food') and sign the entry, writing your name and bleep number clearly on the first prescription.

Common abbreviations

IV – intravenous	od – once a day/24h
PO – by mouth	om – every morning
IM – intramuscular	on – every night
SC – subcutaneous	bd – twice a day/12h
PR – by rectum	tds – three times a day/8h
INH – inhaled	qds – four times a day/6h
NEB – nebulised	units – avoid 'IU' or 'U'
STAT – immediately	PRN – as required
g – gram	mg – milligram
microgram avoid mcg or µg	ml – millilitre
T̄, T̄T̄ one tablet, two tablets	

Controlled drugs See □ p173.

Changes to prescriptions If a prescription is to change do not amend the original; cross it out clearly and write a new prescription (Fig. 4.1) (see □ p170). Initial and date any cancelled prescriptions and record a reason if appropriate (eg β-blocker stopped in wheezy asthmatic patient).

Rewriting drug cards When rewriting drug cards ensure the correct drugs, doses and original start dates are carried over and that the old drug card(s) are crossed through and filed in the notes.

Drug			Date/Time	--/--/--	--/--/--
PARACETAMOL			0600		
Route	Dose	Start	0800		
PO	1g	05.08.14	1000		
Additional instructions			1200		
			1400		
Signature	Pharmacy		1800		
Dr C J Flint			2200		
			0000		

Fig. 4.1 Example of cancelled drug prescription for a regular medication.

Drug			Date	05.08.14	
IBUPROFEN					
Route	Dose	Start	Time	12:35	
PO	400mg	05.08.14			
Max frequency		Max dose/24h	Dose	400mg	
6 hourly		1.2g			
Indications for use			Route	PO	
Analgesia/fever					
Signature	Pharmacy		Given by	SN Jones	
Dr C J Flint					

Fig. 4.2 Example of drug prescription for a PRN medication.

Date	Drug	Dose	Route	Time	Prescribed	Given by	Time
03.08.14	ASPIRIN	300mg	PO	STAT	C J Flint	SN Jones	15:35

Fig. 4.3 Example of a once-only (STAT) medication.

Verbal prescriptions

Verbal prescriptions are only generally acceptable for emergency situations, and the drug(s) should be written up at the first opportunity. If a verbal prescription is to be used, say the prescription to two nurses to minimise the risk of the wrong drug or dose being given. Check your local prescribing policy first.

Self-prescribing

F1s can only prescribe on in-patient drug cards and TTOs. The GMC's Good Medical Practice (2013) guidance states you should 'avoid providing medical care to yourself or anyone with whom you have a close personal relationship'.

Drug interactions

A list of specific drug interactions are shown in **Appendix 1** of the *BNF*.

Pharmacokinetic interactions occur when one drugs alters the *absorption, distribution, metabolism,* or *excretion* of another drug which alters the fraction of active drug, causing an aberrant response to a standardised dose. See the following examples:

- *Absorption* metal ions (Ca^{2+}, Fe^{3+}) form complexes with tetracyclines and decrease their absorption and therefore bioavailability
- *Distribution* warfarin is highly bound to albumin, so drugs such as the sulfonamides which compete for binding sites cause displacement of warfarin, increasing both its free fraction and anticoagulant effect
- *Metabolism* rifampicin is a potent enzyme inducer (📖 p174) and increases metabolism of the OCP, reducing its clinical effectiveness; other forms of contraception should be used in such circumstances
- *Excretion* quinidine reduces the renal clearance of digoxin, resulting in higher than anticipated levels of serum digoxin and increasing the risk of digoxin side effects and/or toxicity.

Pharmacodynamic interactions occur when two or more agents have affinity for the same site of drug action, such as:

- Salbutamol and propranolol (a non-specific β-blocker) have opposing effects at the β-adrenergic receptor; clinical effect is determined by the relative concentrations of the two agents and their receptor affinity.

Drugs which commonly have interactions include digoxin, warfarin, antiepileptics, many antibiotics, antidepressants, antipsychotics, theophylline and amiodarone. If in doubt, look in the *BNF*.

Reporting adverse drug reactions

The Yellow Card Scheme has been running for over 40 years, and is coordinated by the Medicines and Healthcare products Regulatory Agency (MHRA). During drug development, side effects with a frequency of 1:1000 or greater (more common) are likely to be identified, so the Yellow Card Scheme is important in detecting rarer side effects once a drug is in general use and all doctors have a duty to contribute to this. Yellow tear-out slips in the back of the *BNF* are completed and sent off and used to monitor adverse drug reactions. The forms can be completed by any healthcare worker and even by patients.

Common drug reactions such as constipation from opioids, indigestion from NSAIDs, and dry mouth with anticholinergics are well recognised and considered minor effects and do not need reporting.

Sinister drug effects such as anaphylaxis, haemorrhage, severe skin reactions etc must be reported via the Yellow Card Scheme, irrespective of how well documented they already are. Any suspected reaction from a new drug (drugs marked with an inverted triangle (▼) in the *BNF*) must also be reported by this scheme.

Special considerations

Every prescription should be carefully considered with specific reflection of the patient in question. If in doubt, consult the *BNF* or speak to the pharmacist or a senior. There are some groups of patients for whom prescriptions must be even more carefully considered.

Patients with liver disease The liver has tremendous capacity and reserve so liver disease is often severe by the time the handling of most drugs is altered. The liver clears some drugs directly into bile (such as rifampicin) so these should be used cautiously if at all. The liver also manufactures plasma proteins and hypoproteinaemia can result in increased free fractions of some agents (phenytoin, warfarin, prednisolone) and result in exaggerated pharmacodynamic responses. Hepatic encephalopathy can be made worse by sedative drugs (night sedation, opioids etc), and fluid overload by NSAIDs and corticosteroids is well documented in liver failure. Hepatotoxic drugs (such as methotrexate and isotretinoin) should only be used by experts as they may precipitate fulminant hepatic failure and death. Patients with established liver failure have an increased bleeding tendency so avoid IM injections and employ caution if using any anticoagulant drugs. Paracetamol can be used in liver disease, but consider a reduced dose; consult *BNF*/pharmacist. *Special considerations for patients with liver disease are listed under each drug monograph in the BNF.*

Patients with renal disease Patients with *impaired* renal function should only be given nephrotoxic drugs with extreme caution as these may precipitate fulminant renal failure; these include NSAIDs, gentamicin, lithium, ACEi, and IV contrast. Any patient with renal disease (impairment or end-stage renal failure) will have altered drug handling (metabolism, clearance, volume of distribution etc) and more careful thought must be given when prescribing for the patients with GFR <60ml/min, and senior input sought when GFR <30ml/min (*BNF*, pharmacist or senior); the amount, dosing frequency, and choice of drug needs careful thought. Remember that a creatinine in the 'normal' range does not mean normal renal function, see 📖 p373. *Special considerations for patients with renal disease are listed under each drug monograph in the BNF.*

Pregnant patients Many drugs can cross the placenta and have effects upon the foetus. In the first trimester (weeks 1–12) this usually results in congenital malformations, and in the second (weeks 13–26) and third trimesters (weeks 27–42) usually results in growth retardation or has direct toxic effects upon foetal tissues. There are no totally 'safe' drugs to use in pregnancy, but there are drugs known to be particularly troublesome. The minimum dose and the shortest duration possible should be used when prescribing in pregnancy and all drugs avoided if possible in the first trimester.

- *Drugs considered acceptable* penicillins, cephalosporins, heparin, ranitidine, paracetamol, codeine
- *Drugs to avoid* tetracyclines, streptomycin, quinolones, warfarin, thiazides, ACEi, lithium, NSAIDs, alcohol, retinoids, barbiturates, opioids, cytotoxic drugs and phenytoin.

Special considerations for pregnant patients are listed under each drug monograph in the BNF.

Breastfeeding patient As with pregnant patients, drugs given to the mother can get into breast milk and passed on to the feeding baby. Some drugs become more concentrated in breast milk than maternal plasma (such as iodides) and can be toxic to the child. Other drugs can stunt the child's suckling reflex (eg barbiturates), or act to stop breast milk production altogether (eg bromocriptine). Speak to a pharmacist before prescribing any drug to a mother who is feeding a child breast milk. *Special considerations for patients who are breastfeeding are listed under each drug monograph in the BNF.*

Children see the ***British National Formulary for Children***. Neonates are more unpredictable in terms of pharmacokinetics and pharmacodynamics than older children; prescriptions for this age group should be undertaken by experienced neonatal staff and drugs double-checked prior to administration. After the first month or two the gut, renal system and metabolic pathways become more predictable. Almost all drug doses still need to be calculated by weight (eg mg/kg) or by body-surface area (BSA). There are a few drugs which should never be prescribed in children by a non-specialist, including tetracycline (causes irreversible staining of bones and teeth), aspirin (predisposes to Reye's syndrome); others should be used with caution such as prochlorperazine and isotretinoin. *Always consult the BNF for children when prescribing for paediatric patients.*

Controlled drugs

Controlled drugs (CDs) are those drugs which are addictive and most often abused or stolen, and are subject to the prescription and storage requirements of the Misuse of Drugs Regulations 2001; they include the strong opioids (morphine, diamorphine, pethidine, fentanyl, alfentanil, remifentanil, methadone), amphetamine-like agents (methyl-phenidate (Ritalin®), and cocaine (a local anaesthetic). These agents are stored in a locked cabinet and a record of their use on a named patient basis is required to be kept by law. Some other drugs may be kept in the CD cupboard such as concentrated KCl, ketamine, benzodiazepines and anabolic steroids, but this is not a legal requirement and will depend upon local policy. The weaker opioids (codeine, tramadol) are not treated as controlled drugs though they are still often misused.

Prescribing controlled drugs for in-patients is just like prescribing any other drug and the benefits should be balanced against potential side effects for each individual patient. Morphine, diamorphine and pethidine are the most commonly prescribed CDs on the ward. As with all prescrip-tions, write the details clearly and make sure a maximum dose and a minimal interval between doses is documented (see 📖 p86 for management of pain).

Controlled drugs for TTOs see 📖 p78.

Enzyme inducers and inhibitors

The term *enzyme inducers* is used to describe agents (usually drugs, but not always) which alter the activity of hepatic enzymes, namely the cytochrome P450 enzymes which are involved in phase 1 metabolism (typically oxidation, reduction and hydrolysis reactions). Agents which *induce* cytochrome P450 activity result in increased metabolism of affected drugs and reduced activity of affected drugs; *inhibitors* of cytochrome P450 have the reverse effect and result in exaggerated drug responses as more of the affected drug remains available to exert its effect. Common inducers and inhibitors are listed here.

Inducers

Table 4.1 shows drugs that induce metabolic enzymes. Each of the drugs on the left can induce the enzymes so that all of the drugs on the right (and any of the other drugs on the left) will have reduced plasma levels:

Table 4.1 *Enzyme inducers*

Enzyme inducers	Plasma levels reduced
Phenobarbital/barbiturates	Warfarin
Rifampicin	Oral contraceptives
Phenytoin	Corticosteroids
Ethanol (chronic use)	Ciclosporin
Carbamazepine	(all drugs on left)

Inhibitors

Table 4.2 shows some drugs which inhibit enzymes. Each of the drugs on the left can influence the metabolic enzymes responsible for breaking down the drug on the right; this has the effect of increasing the plasma level of this latter drug, exaggerating its biological effect:

Table 4.2 *Enzyme inhibitors*

Enzyme inhibitors	Plasma levels increased
Disulfiram	Warfarin
Chloramphenicol	Phenytoin
Corticosteroids	Tricyclic antidepressants
Cimetidine	Amiodarone, phenytoin, pethidine
MAO inhibitors	Pethidine
Erythromycin	Theophylline
Ciprofloxacin	Theophylline

Endocarditis prophylaxis[1]

Adults and children with structural cardiac conditions

Regard people with the following cardiac conditions as being at risk of developing infective endocarditis:
- Acquired valvular heart disease with stenosis or regurgitation
- Valve replacement
- Structural congenital heart disease, including surgically corrected or palliated structural conditions, but excluding isolated atrial septal defect, fully repaired ventricular septal defect or fully repaired patent ductus arteriosus, and closure devices that are judged to be endothelialised
- Hypertrophic cardiomyopathy
- Previous infective endocarditis.

Advice

Offer people at risk of infective endocarditis clear and consistent information about prevention, including:
- The benefits and risks of antibiotic prophylaxis, and an explanation of why antibiotic prophylaxis is no longer routinely recommended
- The importance of maintaining good oral health
- Symptoms that may indicate infective endocarditis and when to seek expert advice
- The risks of undergoing invasive procedures, including non-medical procedures such as body piercing or tattooing.

When to offer prophylaxis

Do not offer antibiotic prophylaxis against infective endocarditis:
- To people undergoing dental procedures
- To people undergoing non-dental procedures at the following sites:
  - upper and lower gastrointestinal tract
  - genitourinary tract; this includes urological, gynaecological, and obstetric procedures, and childbirth
  - upper and lower respiratory tract; this includes ear, nose, and throat procedures and bronchoscopy.

Do not offer chlorhexidine mouthwash as prophylaxis against infective endocarditis to people at risk undergoing dental procedures.

Managing infection

- **Investigate and treat promptly** any episodes of infection in people at risk of infective endocarditis to reduce the risk of endocarditis developing.
- **Offer** an antibiotic that covers organisms that cause infective endocarditis if a person at risk of infective endocarditis is receiving antimicrobial therapy because they are undergoing a gastrointestinal or genitourinary procedure at a site where there is a suspected infection.

[1] NICE clinical guidelines available at ⌂guidance.nice.org.uk/CG64

Night sedation

Patients develop tolerance and dependence to hypnotics (sedating drugs) if they are taken long term. They are only licensed for short-term use and should be avoided if possible.

> **Causes of insomnia** Anxiety, stress, depression, mania, alcohol, pain, coughing, nocturia (diuretics, urge incontinence), restless leg syndrome, steroids, aminophylline, SSRIs, benzodiazepine/opioid withdrawal, sleep apnoea, poor sleep hygiene, levothyroxine.

Try to dose regular medications so that stimulants (steroids, SSRIs, aminophylline) are given early in the day, whilst sedatives (tricyclics, antihistamines) are at night. Encourage sleep hygiene (below), ear plugs, eye shades and treat any causes of insomnia.

> **Sleep hygiene** *Avoid* caffeine in evening (tea, coffee, chocolate), alcohol, nicotine, daytime naps, cerebral activity before sleep; *encourage* exercise, light snack 1–2h before bed, comfortable and quiet location (ear plugs and eye shades), routine.

If the patient is still unable to sleep and there is a temporary cause (eg post-op pain, noisy ward) then it is appropriate to prescribe a one-off or short course (≤ 5d) of hypnotics (Table 4.3). Some patients may be on long-term hypnotics; these are usually continued in hospital. If long-term hypnotics are stopped the dose should be weaned to minimise withdrawal.

Table 4.3 *Common oral hypnotics*

Diazepam	5–15mg/24h	Significant hangover effect, useful for anxious patients
Temazepam	10–20mg/24h	Shorter action than diazepam, less hangover
Zopiclone	3.75–7.5mg/24h	Less dependence and risk of withdrawal than diazepam and less hangover effect

Contraindications Respiratory failure and sleep apnoea.

Side effects Include hangover (morning drowsiness), confusion, ataxia, falls, aggression and a withdrawal syndrome similar to alcohol withdrawal if long-term hypnotics are stopped suddenly.

Discharge If a patient is not on hypnotics when they enter hospital they should not be on hypnotics when they leave. It is bad practice to discharge patients with supplies of addictive and unnecessary medications.

Violent/aggressive patients See 🕮 p105 for emergency sedation.

Pre-op sedation Diazepam and temazepam can be used for sedation before a procedure or anaesthetic; this is usually prescribed by the anaesthetist 1–2h beforehand. Midazolam is a rapidly acting IV sedative; it should only be used by experienced doctors under monitored conditions (sats, RR, BP, and cardiac monitor) with a crash trolley available. Give 1–2mg boluses then wait 5min for the full response before repeating; >5mg is rarely needed.

Steroid therapy

Steroids given for >3wk should never be abruptly discontinued as this can precipitate an Addisonian crisis (📖 p332). Patients can need >60mg prednisolone per day for severe inflammatory disease and this must be converted to an appropriate IV corticosteroid dose if they are unable to take regular PO doses (Table 4.4). Long-term steroid use should prompt consideration of osteoporosis prophylaxis (📖 p437).

Table 4.4 *Conversion of oral prednisolone to IV hydrocortisone*

Normal prednisolone dose	Suggested hydrocortisone dose[1]
≥60mg/24h PO	100mg/6h IV
20–50mg/24h PO	50mg/6h IV
≤20mg/24h PO	25mg/6h IV

Steroid conversion (see *BNF* 6.3.2)

These are equivalent corticosteroid doses compared to 5mg predni-solone, but do not take into account dosing frequencies or mineralo-corticoid effects:

- Hydrocortisone 20mg; usually given IV 6–8h
- Methylprednisolone 4mg; usually given once daily
- Dexamethasone 750micrograms; usually given once daily.

Withdrawing steroid therapy It is an art and must be performed gradually if steroids have been used for >3wks. Large doses (>20mg prednisolone or equivalent) can be reduced by 5–10mg/wk until dose is 7.5mg prednisolone/d. Thereafter the doses must be reduced more slowly, eg by 2.5mg/wk until the dose is 2.5mg/d. Thereafter reduce the dose by eg 1mg/wk down to zero. Aim to taper dose to zero over 6–8wk.

Steroid side effects and treatment and monitoring options

GI ulceration	Consider PPI or H$_2$-receptor antagonist
Infections and reactivation of TB	Low threshold for culturing samples or CXR
Skin thinning/poor wound healing	Pressure care and wound care
Na$^+$ and fluid retention	Twice-daily BPs
Hyperglycaemia	Twice-daily BMs if taking high-dose steroids
Osteoporosis (📖 p437)	Bone protection (Ca^{2+} + bisphosphonate)
Hypertension	Twice-daily BPs

[1] If patients with known adrenal insufficiency, or those who have been on any dose of oral corticosteroids for >3wks present unwell, consider an initial dose of 100mg hydrocortisone IV STAT, then d/w senior as to regular steroid dose. If unable to tolerate PO administration, ensure equivalent IV steroids given, as per steroid conversion box.

Topical corticosteroids

Topical steroids are used in the treatment of many inflammatory skin diseases. As with corticosteroids given orally or intravenously, the mechanism of action is complex. Corticosteroids offer symptomatic relief but are seldom curative. The least potent preparation (see Table 5.20 📖 p219) should be used to control symptoms. Withdrawal of topical steroids often causes a rebound worsening of symptoms and the patient should be warned about this. The amount of steroid needed to cover various body parts is shown in Fig. 4.4. Always wash hands after applying topical steroids.

Side effects local thinning of the skin, worsening local infection, striae and telangiectasia, acne, depigmentation, hypertrichosis; systemic rarely adrenal suppression, Cushing's syndrome (subsequent withdrawal of topical steroids can precipitate an Addisonian crisis).

Potency see 📖 p219 for a list of the common topical steroids used arranged by potency.

ONE adult fingertip unit (FTU)*

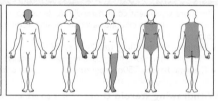

Age	Number of fingertip units (FTUs)				
	Face & neck	Arm & hand	Leg & foot	Trunk (front)	Trunk (back) inc. buttocks
Adult	2½	4	8	7	7
Children:					
3–6 months	1	1	1½	1	1½
1–2 years	1½	1½	2	2	3
3–5 years	1½	2	3	3	3½
6–10 years	2	2½	4½	3½	5

Fig. 4.4 Amount of topical steroid required to treat various body parts. * One adult fingertip unit (FTU) is the amount of ointment or cream expressed from a tube with a standard 5mm diameter nozzle, applied from the distal crease on the tip of the index finger.
Reproduced with permission from Long, C.C. and Finlay, A.Y. (1991) *Clinical and Experimental Dermatology*, **16**: 444–7. Blackwell Publishing.

Empirical antibiotic treatment

Choice of suitable antibiotic depends upon likely pathogen and its usual antimicrobial sensitivity, patient factors (age and coexisting disease), drug availability, and local guidelines. Some common infections and suggested antibiotic regimens are listed below (suitable for an otherwise healthy 70kg adult); more detailed options, including choices for patients with penicillin allergies are listed on 📖 p649.

Local antibiotic guidelines are written to ensure the most appropriate antibiotics are used prior to knowing the pathogen and its antimicrobial sensitivities.

Taking cultures prior to commencing antibiotic therapy is important as it allows subsequent therapy to be more specifically tailored. However, cultures should not delay treatment in the septic patient.

Urinary tract	Co-amoxiclav 625mg/8h PO
Cellulitis	Flucloxacillin 1g/6h PO/IV
Wound infection	As for cellulitis if after 'clean' surgery; for 'dirty' surgery or trauma, use co-amoxiclav 1.2g/8h IV
Meningitis	Ceftriaxone 4g IV STAT then 2g/12h IV for 5-10d. Consider addition of amoxicillin 2g/4h IV if patient >50yr, pregnant or immunocompromised and/or vancomycin 1g/12h IV if pneumococcal meningitis suspected
Encephalitis	As for meningitis + aciclovir 10mg/kg/8h IV
Endocarditis	<u>Acute presentation</u>: flucloxacillin 2g/6h IV + gentamicin 5mg/kg/24h IV <u>Indolent presentation</u>: benzylpenicillin 1.2g/4h IV + gentamicin 5mg/kg/24h IV
Septic arthritis	Co-amoxiclav 1.2g/8h IV

Pneumonia 📖 pp 276–7

Community-acquired (CAP), CURB65=0-1	Amoxicillin 500mg–1g/8h PO
CAP, CURB65=2	Amoxicillin 1g/8h PO/IV + clarithromycin 500mg/12h PO/IV
CAP, CURB65≥3	Co-amoxiclav 1.2g/8h IV + clarithromycin 500mg/12h IV
Hospital-acquired	Co-amoxiclav 1.2g/8h IV (if severe: Tazocin® 4.5g/8h IV)
Aspiration pneumonia	Co-amoxiclav 1.2g/8h IV + metronidazole 400mg/8h PO or 500mg/8h IV

Septicaemia

Urinary tract sepsis	Co-amoxiclav 1.2g/8h IV + gentamicin 5mg/kg IV STAT
Intra-abdominal sepsis	Tazocin® 4.5g/8h IV
Meningococcal sepsis	Ceftriaxone 4g IV STAT then 2g/24h IV
Neutropenic sepsis	Tazocin® 4.5g/8h IV + gentamicin 5mg/kg/24h IV
Skin/bone source	Flucloxacillin 2g/6h IV
Severe sepsis/septic shock, no clear focus	Tazocin® 4.5g/8h IV + gentamicin 5mg/kg STAT

Clostridium difficile (C. diff)

Bacteriology C. difficile is a Gram-positive spore-forming anaerobic bacillus, which colonises the intestines of some individuals (often those in long-term care). The use of antibiotics alters the balance of the gut flora, and can allow the overgrowth of C. difficile.

Transmission via the faeco-oral route. The spores are heat-resistant and can lay dormant in the environment for long periods. They are resistant to stomach acid and germinate once in the colon.

Symptoms diarrhoea and abdominal pains are the commonest features of C. difficile overgrowth; when severe this can evolve into pseudomembranous colitis. In the elderly and frail this can result in dehydration and even death.

Detection is through urgent testing of stool as soon as suspicion of C. difficile arises.[1] Currently this involves a 2-stage process, with a rapid, screening test for a C. difficile protein (or PCR for the C. difficile toxin gene), followed by a more specific immunoassay for the C. difficile toxin. Speak to the laboratory if there is any doubt. Consider an urgent AXR to rule out toxic megacolon.

Treatment is with metronidazole 400mg/8h PO or vancomycin 125mg/6h PO initially. More intensive regimens including higher doses of oral vancomycin, metronidazole IV or vancomycin PR may be required in patients who fail to respond or who relapse after initial treatment. Faecal transplantation (introduction of a suspension prepared from the fresh faeces of a screened donor either directly into the colon via enema or colonoscope, or through the upper GI tract after NJ delivery) is emerging as a highly effective, if cosmetically unappealing, method of treatment for refractory cases.[2] Barrier nursing and thorough hand hygiene are important to prevent transmission to other patients (the spores are resistant to alcohol hand gels so thorough hand washing with soap is essential).[3]

Surveillance as C. difficile is now regarded as a major cause of hospital-acquired infections (HAI); local infection control teams should be made aware if a case is identified or even suspected; they will often advise ward and medical staff on how the patient should be managed.

Ecology, Clostridium difficile and antibiotics

Intestinal carriage of Clostridium difficile does not equate with disease – what matters is when C. difficile is able to outgrow other commensal bacteria in the colon to the detriment of normal colonic ecology. Hence controlling the transmission of C. difficile is not sufficient. Instead, we need to avoid perturbations in the colonic flora through the indiscriminate use of broad-spectrum antibiotics. As part of this approach, most trusts are limiting the use of cephalosporins, quinolones, and clindamycin, as well as drawing up helpful guidelines regarding antibiotic selection. Always check local antibiotic guidelines and consider risk and benefit before prescribing any antibiotics.

[1] Bristol Stool Chart types 5-7 stool not attributable to an underlying condition (eg overflow) or therapy (eg laxatives) from hospital patients aged >2 years, all community patients aged >65 years, and from community patients aged <65 years, wherever clinically indicated. See DH guidance at www.gov.uk/government/uploads/system/uploads/attachment_data/file/215135/dh_133016.pdf
[2] See Rohlke and Stollman, *Therap Adv Gastroenterol* 2012 **5**:403 for a good review of trial data, available free at www.ncbi.nlm.nih.gov/pmc/articles/PMC3491681
[3] Much emphasis is rightly placed on the prevention of in-hospital C. difficile transmission, with all sorts of policies introduced in the name of infection control. However, community transmission appears to be at least as important, if not more so; see, for example, Eyre, D.W. et al. *NEJM* 2013 **369**:1195 available free at www.nejm.org/doi/full/10.1056/NEJMoa1216064

Pharmacopoeia

Pharmacopoeia

Users are advised to always check local prescribing guidelines and formularies and to consult the *BNF* when prescribing drugs.

ACEi angiotensin-converting enzyme inhibitor *Dose* see Table 5.1, and see Table 5.2 on how to commence a patient on an ACEi ***Indications*** heart failure, hypertension, diabetic nephropathy, prophylaxis of cardiovascular events ***Caution*** pregnancy and breastfeeding, patients already taking diuretics, renal artery stenosis/renal impairment, aortic stenosis, hyperkalaemia, known allergy to ACEi. May not be effective in African-Caribbean patients ***SE*** postural hypotension, renal impairment and hyperkalaemia, dry cough, taste disturbance, urticaria and angioedema. If cough is problematic for the patient, consider AT II receptor antagonist, or other antihypertensive agent ***BNF*** 2.5.5.1.

Table 5.1 *ACEi **BNF** 2.5.5.1*

Enalapril	***Dose*** initially 5mg/24h PO up to max 40mg/24h PO
Fosinopril	***Dose*** initially 10mg/24h PO up to max 40mg/24h PO
Lisinopril	***Dose*** initially 5–10mg/24h PO up to max 80mg/24h PO
Perindopril erbumine	***Dose*** initially 4mg/24h PO up to max 8mg/24h PO
Perindopril arginine	***Dose*** initially 5mg/24h PO up to max 10mg/24h PO
Ramipril	***Dose*** initially 1.25–2.5mg/24h PO up to max 10mg/24h PO

Table 5.2 *Starting an ACE inhibitor*

Patients with significant comorbidity and/or taking other antihypertensive medications, as well as the frail and elderly, may need more cautious management when starting an ACEi and when increasing the dose	
Before starting	Check U+E, document starting BP, identify target BP
First dose	Start with lowest dose and consider giving at bedtime to limit any problems with first-dose hypotension
In hospital	Increase dose daily/alternate days as BP allows, monitor U+E daily/alternate days
In community	Check U+E and BP at 7–10d after starting therapy or increasing dose. Increase dose every 14d until target BP reached

Acetylcysteine (Parvolex®) amino acid derivative *Dose* 150mg/kg (max 16.5g) in 200ml 5% glucose IVI over 15min; then 50mg/kg (max 5.5g) in 500ml 5% glucose IVI over 4h; then 100mg/kg (max 11g) in 1l 5% glucose IVI over 16h ***Indication*** mainly used in known or suspected paracetamol overdose ***Caution*** asthma ***SE*** allergic-like reactions, rash, bronchospasm, anaphylaxis ***BNF*** emergency treatment of poisoning.

Actrapid® insulin see insulins.

Adenosine nucleoside (antiarrhythmic) Dose 6mg rapid IV bolus; if needs repeated dose 12mg rapid IV bolus, then 12mg rapid IV bolus **Indication** supraventricular tachycardia **CI** 2nd/3rd degree heart block, sick sinus syndrome (unless pacemaker fitted), long QT syndrome, COPD/asthma **Caution** pregnancy, recent MI, pericarditis, heart block, bundle branch block, accessory pathway, hypovolaemia, valvular lesions **SE** nausea, sinus pause, bradycardia/asystole, flushing, angina, dizziness **BNF** 2.3.2.

Adrenaline (epinephrine); anaphylaxis catecholamine Dose 0.5mg/STAT IM (0.5ml of 1:1000); repeat after 5min if inadequate response **Indication** suspected anaphylaxis; if in doubt <u>give it</u> **Caution** cerebro- and cardiovascular disease **SE** ↑HR, ↑BP, anxiety, sweats, tremor, arrhythmias **BNF** 3.4.3.

Adrenaline (epinephrine); cardiac arrest catecholamine Dose 1mg/STAT IV (10ml of 1:10,000); repeat as per ALS algorithm **Indication** cardiac arrest **Caution** as above **SE** as above **BNF** 2.7.3.

Aggrastat® glycoprotein IIb/IIIa inhibitor see tirofiban.

Alteplase plaminogen activator see fibrinolytics.

Amiloride potassium-sparing diuretic Dose 5-10mg/24h PO (max 20mg/24h PO) **Indication** oedema, potassium conservation when used as an adjunct to thiazide or loop diuretics for hypertension, congestive cardiac failure, hepatic cirrhosis with ascites **CI** hyperkalaemia, anuria, Addison's disease **Caution** renal impairment, DM, pregnancy and breastfeeding **SE** abdominal pain, GI disturbances including bleeding **BNF** 2.2.3.

Aminophylline; IV theophylline/methylxanthine Dose <u>Loading</u>: 5mg/kg (based on ideal body weight) in 100ml 0.9% saline IVI over 20min. <u>Maintenance</u>: 0.5mg/kg/h, make up 500mg in 500ml 0.9% saline (concentration = 1mg/ml) IVI **Indication** reversible airways disease, severe acute asthma **Caution** avoid loading dose if patient taking oral theophylline; cardiac disease, hypertension, epilepsy **SE** tachycardia, palpitations, arrhythmia, convulsions **Info** theophylline is only available as an oral preparation; aminophylline consists of theophylline and ethylenediamine which simply improves the drug's solubility **BNF** 3.1.3.

Monitoring aminophylline (theophylline)	Stop infusion 15min prior to sampling, take sample *4–6h after commencing an infusion* 10–20mg/l (55–110micromol/l); *toxic* >20mg/l (>110micromol/l); *signs of toxicity* arrhythmia, anxiety, tremor, convulsions (OHAM3 🕮 p731)

Amiodarone; cardiac arrest class III antiarrhythmic *Dose* 300mg IV/STAT after third shock if patient remains in VF/pulseless VT *Indication* VF/pulseless VT *BNF* 2.7.3.

Amiodarone; arrhythmias class III antiarrhythmic *Dose* <u>oral loading</u>: 200mg/8h PO for 1wk, then 200mg/12h PO for 1 wk, then 200mg/24h PO as maintenance dose, <u>IV loading</u>: initially 5mg/kg over 20–120min IVI (with ECG monitoring) then further infusion if necessary of up to 1.2g over 24h IVI *Indication* SVT, nodal and ventricular tachycardias, atrial fibrillation and flutter, ventricular fibrillation (see above) *CI* bradycardia, sino-atrial heart block, thyroid dysfunction, iodine sensitivity *Caution* pregnancy, breastfeeding, thyroid disease, hypokalaemia, heart failure, elderly, bradycardia *SE* N+V, taste disturbance, raised transaminases, jaundice, bradycardia, hypotension, pulmonary toxicity, corneal deposits, skin discolouration *Info* monitor LFTs and TFTs every 6mth *BNF* 2.3.2.

Amlodipine see calcium-channel blockers.

Amoxicillin beta-lactam *Dose* 500mg–1g PO/IV 8h *Indication* infection *CI* penicillin allergy *Caution* glandular fever, CMV infection, ALL/CLL *SE* N+V, diarrhoea, rash *BNF* 5.1.1.3.

Ampicillin beta-lactam *Dose* 500mg–1g PO/IV 6h *Indication* infection *CI* penicillin allergy *Caution* glandular fever, CMV infection, ALL/CLL *SE* N+V, diarrhoea, rash *BNF* 5.1.1.3.

Antacids/Alginates *Dose* see Table 5.3 *Indications* acid reflux disease *Caution* hepatic and renal impairment; if symptoms are severe or persist seek expert opinion *SE* depends upon preparation used, see Table 5.3 *Info* the sodium load in these preparations can be significant and they should be used with caution in patients with hepatic impairment. The alginates increase the viscosity of the stomach contents and can protect the oesophageal mucosa from acid attack; the raft-forming alginates float on the surface of the stomach contents and may further reduce the symptoms of reflux *BNF* 1.1.1/1.1.2.

Table 5.3 *Antacids BNF 1.1.1; alginates BNF 1.1.2*

Classification	
Aluminium hydroxide	eg Alu-Cap® **Dose** 1 capsule 4 times daily and at bedtime **CI** hypophosphataemia, neonates **SE** constipation
Magnesium carbonate	**Dose** 10ml 3 times daily in water **CI** hypophosphataemia **SE** diarrhoea, belching (due to CO_2 liberation)
Magnesium trisilicate	**Dose** depends upon preparation, see **BNF** 1.1.1 **CI** and **SE** see magnesium carbonate
Alginate raft-forming suspensions	eg Peptac® **Dose** 10–20ml after meals and at bedtime **SE** usually none
Other alginate preparations	eg Gastrocote® **Dose** 5–15ml 4 times daily (after meals and at bedtime) **SE** usually none

Antiemetics Dose see Table 5.5 **Indications** N+V see Table 5.4; not all antiemetics are effective for all causes of N+V **Caution** and **SE** see Table 5.5 **Info** it is important to establish the cause of N+V **BNF** 4.6.

Table 5.4 *Causes of N+V and suggested antiemetic* **BNF** 4.6

Likely cause	Suggested antiemetics
Pregnancy	Promethazine, prochlorperazine, metoclopramide
Post-operative	In no particular order: 5HT₃ antagonists, antihistamines (eg cyclizine), dexamethasone, phenothiazines (eg prochlorperazine), metoclopramide.
Bowel obstruction	Treat the cause. Avoid metoclopramide
Motion sickness	Hyoscine hydrobromide, promethazine, cyclizine
Vestibular disorders	Betahistine (see BNF 4.6), antihistamine (eg cinnarizine, see BNF 4.6), phenothiazine (eg prochlorperazine)
Cytotoxic chemotherapy	Pre- and post-treatment with domperidone or metoclopramide; add in dexamethasone, 5HT₃ antagonists. See BNF 8.1
Palliative care	Depends upon cause. See 🕮 p91

Table 5.5 *Antiemetic classification* **BNF** 4.6

Antihistamines	Cinnarizine, cyclizine, promethazine
Cyclizine	**Dose** 50mg/8h PO/IV/IM **CI** heart failure **SE** drowsiness, pain on injection, urinary retention, dry mouth, blurred vision
Phenothiazines	Chlorpromazine, droperidol, perphenazine, prochlorperazine, trifluoperazine
Prochlorperazine	**Dose** consult *BNF*; 10mg/8h PO, 12.5mg/24h IM, 3–6mg/12h BUCCAL **CI** Parkinson's, epilepsy **SE** extrapyramidal effects, hypotension, drowsiness, agitation
Dopamine antagonists	Domperidone, metoclopramide
Metoclopramide	**Dose** 10mg/8h PO/IV/IM **CI** avoid in patients <21y (especially ♀) and in bowel obstruction **SE** extrapyramidal effects
5HT₃ antagonists	Granisetron, ondansetron, palonosetron
Ondansetron	**Dose** 4–8mg/8h PO/IV/IM **CI** QT prolongation **SE** constipation, headache, flushing, bradycardia, hypotension
Miscellaneous	Dexamethasone, benzodiazepines, hyoscine hydrobromide, nabilone, neurokinin receptor antagonists

Antihistamines H₁ receptor antagonists *Dose* see Table 5.6 *Indications* symptomatic relief of allergy (eg hayfever, allergic rhinitis, urticaria) *Caution* avoid if possible in pregnancy and breastfeeding; consult *BNF* if renal or hepatic impairment; all antihistamines have the potential to cause sedation, some more so than others (see Table 5.6); the sedating antihistamines also possess significant antimuscarinic activity and should be used with caution in prostatic hypertrophy, urinary retention, and in patients with angle-closure glaucoma *SE* drowsiness, headache, antimuscarinic effects *Info* the drugs in this section are all antagonists at H₁ receptor; cimetidine and ranitidine antagonists at the H₂ receptor and are useful for gastric acid suppression (see ranitidine) *BNF* 3.4.1.

Table 5.6 *Antihistamines* **BNF** *3.4.1*

Non-sedating antihistamines; acrivastine, cetirizine, desloratadine, fexofenadine, levocetirizine, loratadine, mizolastine, rupatadine	
Cetirizine	**Dose** 10mg/24h PO **Caution** halve dose if eGFR <30ml/min
Desloratadine	**Dose** 5mg/24h PO
Loratadine	**Dose** 10mg/24h PO
Sedating antihistamines; alimemazine, chlorphenamine, clemastine, cyproheptadine, hydroxyzine, ketotifen, promethazine	
Chlorphenamine (chlorpheniramine)	**Dose** 4mg/4–6h PO (max 24mg/24h); 10mg/8h IV/IM (over 1min if given IV)

Arthrotec® NSAID see diclofenac.

Asacol® aminosalicylate see mesalazine.

Aspirin; antiplatelet NSAID *Dose* <u>anti-platelet</u> 75mg/24h PO; <u>ACS/MI</u> 300mg/STAT PO; <u>non-haemorrhagic stroke</u> 300mg/24h PO for 14d then 75mg/24h PO *Indication* secondary prevention of thrombotic cerebrovascular and cardiovascular events *CI* active bleeding, children under 16 (Reye's syndrome) *Caution* pregnancy, breastfeeding, asthma, peptic ulceration, concomitant use of other anticoagulants *SE* bronchospasm, GI irritation/haemorrhage *BNF* 2.9.

Aspirin; analgesic/antipyretic NSAID *Dose* 300–900mg/4–6h PO; max 4g/24h *Indication* pain, pyrexia *CI* as above *Caution* as above *SE* as above *BNF* 4.7.1.

AT II receptor antagonists *Dose* see Table 5.7; commence therapy in the same way as starting an ACEi (see 📖 p182) *Indications* patients intolerant of ACEi; heart failure, hypertension, diabetic nephropathy, prophylaxis of cardiovascular events *Caution* pregnancy and breast-feeding, renal artery stenosis/renal impairment, aortic stenosis, hyperkalaemia, known allergy to ACEi. May not be effective in African-Caribbean patients *SE* postural hypotension, renal impairment and hyperkalaemia, taste disturbance, urticaria and angioneurotic oedema; cough can occur but is less common than with ACEi *BNF* 2.5.5.2.

Table 5.7 *AT II receptor antagonists* **BNF** 2.5.5.2

Candesartan	*Dose* initially 4-8mg/24h PO up to max 32mg/24h PO
Irbesartan	*Dose* initially 75–150mg/24h PO up to max 300mg/24h PO
Losartan	*Dose* initially 25–50mg/24h PO up to max 100mg/24h PO
Valsartan	*Dose* initially 80mg/24h PO up to max 320mg/24h PO

Atenolol see beta-blockers.

Atorvastatin HMG CoA reductase inhibitor see statins.

Atropine; bradycardia anticholinergic *Dose* 500micrograms/STAT IV every 3–5min; max 3mg/24h *Indication* bradycardia *CI* glaucoma, myasthenia gravis, pyloric stenosis, prostatic enlargement *Caution* Down's syndrome, GORD *SE* transient bradycardia, antimuscarinic effects (constipation, urinary urgency and retention, pupil dilatation/loss of accommodation, dry mouth) *BNF* 15.1.3.

Atropine; cardiac arrest anticholinergic *Dose* 3mg/STAT IV *Indication* non-shockable cardiopulmonary arrest *Caution* none in the arrest situation *SE* as above *Info* atropine is no longer recommended for routine use in non-shockable cardiopulmonary arrest (see 2010 Resuscitation Guidelines) *BNF* 2.7.3.

Bactroban® antibacterial see mupirocin.

Beclometasone corticosteroid *Dose* 200–400micrograms/12h INH *Indication* chronic asthma (step 2 BTS guidelines) *Caution* TB *SE* oral candidiasis, hoarse voice, paradoxical bronchospasm (rare) *Info* different preparations/devices are not interchangeable and should be prescribed by brand name *BNF* 3.2.

Bendroflumethiazide thiazide diuretic *Dose* <u>Oedema</u>; 5–10mg/alternate days PO <u>Hypertension</u>; 2.5mg/24h PO *Indication* oedema, hypertension *Caution* DM, gout, SLE *SE* dehydration, hypotension, electrolyte imbalance (especially ↓K⁺) *Interaction* ↑lithium levels and NSAIDs decrease effect *BNF* 2.2.1.

Benzylpenicillin (penicillin G) beta-lactam Dose 0.6–1.2g/6h IV (max 4.8g/24h in divided doses) **Indication** infection; skin, throat, endocarditis **CI** penicillin allergy **Caution** history of allergy **SE** diarrhoea **Interaction** decrease effects of oral contraceptive pill, allopurinol increases risk of rash **BNF** 5.1.1.1.

Beta-blockers Dose see Table 5.8 **Indications** generic indications include: hypertension, angina, myocardial infarction, arrhythmias, heart failure, thyrotoxicosis, anxiety, migraine prophylaxis, benign essential tremor; topically for glaucoma **Caution** pregnancy, breastfeeding, avoid abrupt withdrawal especially in patients with IHD (risk of rebound ↑HR/↑BP), 1st-degree AV block, DM (may mask symptoms ↓glucose), COPD **CI** asthma, uncontrolled heart failure, marked bradycardia, ↓BP, 2nd/3rd-degree AV block, severe peripheral arterial disease **SE** bradycardia, hypotension (especially postural), heart failure, bronchospasm, conduction disorders, peripheral vasoconstriction, headache, fatigue, sleep disturbance (often nightmares, insomnia), impotence **Info** the cardioselective β-blockers (below) have less effect on $β_2$ receptors but are not cardiospecific and bronchoconstriction can still occur in susceptible patients. Water-soluble β-blockers (atenolol, nadolol, sotalol) are excreted by the kidneys and a dose reduction is often necessary in renal impairment; these also are less likely to cause sleep disturbance and nightmares.

Table 5.8 β-blockers **BNF** 2.4 Doses below show initial dose range for treatment of hypertension, doses vary with indication; consult **BNF**

Cardioselective	
Atenolol	**Dose** 25–50mg/24h PO (100mg/24h max); also available IV
Bisoprolol	**Dose** 5–10mg/24h PO (20mg/24h max)
Metoprolol	**Dose** 50–100mg/24h PO (400mg/24h max); also available IV
Non-cardioselective	
Carvedilol	**Dose** 12.5mg/24h PO (max 50mg/24h in divided doses)
Labetalol	**Dose** 100mg/12h PO (max 2.4g/24h in divided doses); also available IV
Propranolol	**Dose** 40–80mg/12h PO, increase weekly (max 320mg/24h in divided doses)
Sotalol	Used only to treat arrhythmias. Only commence after seeking expert advice **Dose** 40mg/12h PO (usual maintenance dose 80–160mg/12h PO); also available IV
Timolol	Used predominantly as eye drops for the treatment of glaucoma; case reports exist of this resulting in systemic effects

Betamethasone cream see topical corticosteroid.

Bezafibrate fibrate Dose 200mg/8h PO; modified release preparations available, check BNF **Indication** hyperlipidaemias unresponsive to diet and other measures **CI** hypoalbuminaemia, primary biliary cirrhosis, gall bladder disease, nephrotic syndrome, pregnancy and breastfeeding **Caution** renal impairment (see **BNF** for reduced dosing), hepatic impairment, hypothyroidism **SE** GI disturbance, anorexia, cholestasis **BNF** 2.12.

Bisoprolol see beta-blockers.

Bowel cleansing preparations laxative Dose consult **BNF** 1.6.5 or local guideline **Indications** prior to surgery, colonoscopy or radiological examination **CI** bowel obstruction, toxic megacolon **Caution** elderly, children, dehydration **SE** N+V, abdominal pain and distension, dehydration, electrolyte disturbance **Info** these agents should not be used in the treatment of constipation (see also laxatives) **BNF** 1.6.5.

Bricanyl® β_2 **agonist** see terbutaline.

Buccastem® see antiemetics (phenothiazine).

Budesonide corticosteroid Dose 100–800micrograms/12h INH; 1–2mg/12h NEB **Indication** chronic asthma (step 2 BTS guidelines) **Caution** TB **SE** oral candidiasis, hoarse voice, paradoxical bronchospasm (rare) **BNF** 3.2.

Bupropion (Zyban®) treatment of nicotine dependence Dose commence 1–2 wk before target smoking cessation date, initially 150mg/24h PO for 6d, then 150mg/12h PO (max single dose 150mg; max total daily dose 300mg) **Indication** smoking cessation **CI** acute alcohol or benzodiazepine withdrawal, severe hepatic cirrhosis, CNS tumour, history of seizures **Caution** hepatic impairment, renal impairment, pregnancy and breastfeeding **SE** dry mouth, GI disturbances, taste disturbance, agitation, anxiety **BNF** 4.10.2.

Buscopan® antimuscarinic see hyoscine butylbromide.

Calcichew®/Calcichew® D₃ calcium salt see calcium carbonate.

Calcium carbonate calcium salt Dose see BNF **Indication** osteoporosis, ↓Ca²⁺ **CI** ↑Ca²⁺ (urine/serum) eg malignancy **Caution** history of renal stones, sarcoid, renal impairment **SE** GI disturbance, ↓HR, arrhythmias **BNF** 9.5.1.

Calcium-channel blockers dihydropyridines *Dose* see Table 5.9 *Indications* ↑BP, prophylaxis of angina *CI* unstable angina, cardiogenic shock, significant aortic stenosis, acute porphyria *Caution* pregnancy, breastfeeding, heart failure *SE* abdominal pain, N+V, flushing, palpitations, ↓BP, oedema, headache, sleep disturbance, fatigue *Info* the dihydropyridines relax smooth muscle and dilate both coronary and peripheral arteries. Nimodipine preferentially acts upon cerebral vascular smooth muscle and is used in the prevention and treatment of ischaemic neurological deficits following aneurysmal subarachnoid haemorrhage *BNF* 2.6.2.

Table 5.9 *Calcium-channel blockers (dihydropyridines)* **BNF** 2.6.2

Amlodipine	**Dose** initially 5mg/24h PO up to max 10mg/24h PO.
Felodipine	**Dose** initially 5mg/24h PO up to max 10–20mg/24h PO
Nifedipine	**Dose** depends upon preparation. Always specify specific brand for modified release (MR) preparations; consult **BNF** 2.6.2
Nimodipine	**Dose** 60mg/4h PO starting within 4d of subarachnoid haemorrhage and continue for 21d; IV preparation available, consult **BNF** 2.6.2

Calcium-channel blockers verapamil, diltiazem *Dose* see Table 5.10 *Indications* ↑BP, prophylaxis of angina; verapamil is also used in the management of tachyarrhythmias *CI* left ventricular failure, bradycardia, 2nd- or 3rd-degree AV dissociation, sick sinus syndrome *Caution* pregnancy, patients taking β-blockers or other negatively chronotropic drugs, 1st-degree AV dissociation, acute phase of MI *SE* bradycardia, ↓BP, heart block, dizziness, flushing, headache, oedema, GI disturbance *Interactions* unlike the dihydropyridines diltiazem and verapamil are negatively chronotropic and inotropic and should not generally be used in conjunction with β-blockers or other negatively chronotropic drugs *BNF* 2.6.2.

Table 5.10 *Calcium-channel blockers (verapamil, diltiazem)* **BNF** 2.6.2

Diltiazem	**Dose** depends upon preparation; consult. Always specify specific brand for modified release (MR) preparations; consult BNF 2.6.2
Verapamil	**Dose** typically 40–120mg/8h PO for SVT; 80–120mg/8h PO for angina prophylaxis; 80–160mg/8h PO for ↑BP; 5–10mg over 5min IV with ECG monitoring for treatment of acute SVT (seek senior help before giving IV inotropes/chronotropes)

Calcium chloride calcium salt *Dose* 10ml of 10%; give 1ml/min IV *Indication* Emergency management of ↓Ca^{2+} *CI* ↑Ca^{2+} *Caution* history of renal stones, sarcoid, renal impairment *SE* peripheral vasodilatation, ↓BP, injection-site reactions; more irritant than calcium gluconate *BNF* 9.5.1.

Calcium gluconate calcium salt *Dose* 10ml of 10%; give over 3min IV *Indication* Emergency management of ↓Ca^{2+}, ↑K$^+$ *CI* ↑Ca^{2+} *Caution* history of renal stones, sarcoid, renal impairment *SE* peripheral vasodilatation, ↓BP, injection-site reactions *BNF* 9.5.1.

Calcium Resonium® **calcium salt** **Dose** 15g/6-8h PO; PR preparations also available (see *BNF*) **Indication** ↑K+ (mild to moderate) **Caution** pregnancy, breastfeeding **SE** GI disturbance **Info** monitor K+ **BNF** 9.2.1.1.

Calpol® **simple analgesic** see paracetamol.

Candesartan see AT II antagonists.

Canesten® **imidazole anti-fungal** see clotrimazole.

Captopril see ACEi.

Carbamazepine **antiepileptic** **Dose** <u>Initially</u>: 100mg/12h PO; <u>Increase</u> to max 2g/24h in divided doses; PR preparations available (see *BNF*) **Indication** anti-epileptic; generalised tonic-clonic, chronic pain, eg trigeminal neuralgia (see *BNF* for dosing) **CI** AV conduction abnormalities, history of bone marrow depression, acute porphyria **Caution** pregnancy, breastfeeding, cardiac disease, Hong Kong Chinese/Thai origin, history of skin conditions **SE** N+V, dizziness, drowsiness, headache, ataxia, visual disturbance, cytopenias, hepatic dysfunction, skin disorders **Interaction** enzyme inducer **BNF** 4.8.1.

Monitoring **carbamazepine**	*random sample* 20–50micromol/l (4–12mg/l); *toxic* >50micromol/l (>12mg/l)

Carbimazole **antithyroid** **Dose** <u>Initially</u>: 15–40mg/24h PO; <u>Once euthyroid</u>: 5–15mg/24h PO as maintenance dose usually given for 12–18mth **Indication** hyperthyroidism **CI** severe blood disorders **Caution** pregnancy, breastfeeding, hepatic impairment **SE** N+V, pruritus, rash, agranulocytosis **BNF** 6.2.2.

Carvedilol see beta-blockers.

Cefaclor see cephalosporin.

Cefalexin see cephalosporin.

Cefotaxime see cephalosporin.

Cefradine see cephalosporin.

Ceftazidime see cephalosporin.

Ceftriaxone see cephalosporin.

Cefuroxime see cephalosporin.

Celecoxib (Celebrex®) **NSAID/COX2 inhibitor** **Dose** 100–200mg/12h PO (max 400mg/24h in divided doses) **Indication** pain and inflammation; osteoarthritis, rheumatoid arthritis and ankylosing spondylitis **CI** IHD, CVD, HF, allergy to any NSAID **Caution** pregnancy, breastfeeding, hepatic impairment, renal impairment **SE** GI disturbance/bleeding, headache, dizziness **Interaction** decreases effects of antihypertensives, increases toxicity of methotrexate, increased risk of renal impairment with ACEi, AT II antagonists or ciclosporin **BNF** 10.1.1.

Cephalosporin Dose see Table 5.11 **Indications** infections [with known or suspected antimicrobial sensitivity (consult local guidelines)], surgical prophylaxis, other prophylaxis **Caution** not known to be harmful in pregnancy, present in breast-milk in low concentration; 0.5–6.5% of patients who are penicillin-allergic will display allergy to cephalosporins as cephalosporins contain a beta-lactam ring as do the penicillins and carbapenems **SE** diarrhoea (rarely antibiotic-associated colitis), N+V, abdominal discomfort, headache, allergic reactions **Info** cephalosporins are amongst the antibiotics which are most likely to result in *Clostridium difficile* diarrhoea, the others being quinolones and clindamycin. As with all antibiotics, it is important to consult local guidelines as infectious agents have differing susceptibility depending upon geographical location **BNF** 5.1.2.1.

Table 5.11 *Cephalosporins* **BNF** 5.1.2.1 (consult local guidelines)		
First generation		
Cefalexin	**Dose 500mg** (250–500mg) 8h PO **Indications** UTIs, respiratory tract infections, otitis media, sinusitis, skin and soft tissue infections	
Cefradine	**Dose**; **500mg** (250–500mg) 6h PO **Indications** surgical prophylaxis but generally not used widely now	
Second generation		
Cefuroxime	**Dose 750mg** (750–1500mg) 8h IV, **500mg** (250–500mg) 12h PO; **Indications** Gram-positive and Gram-negative bacteria; surgical prophylaxis	
Third generation		
Cefotaxime	**Dose 1g** (1–2g) 12h IV **Indications** better Gram-negative activity, but poorer coverage against Gram-positive bacteria than cefuroxime; penetrates the CSF	
Ceftriaxone	**Dose 1g** (1–4g) 24h IV **Indications** better Gram-negative activity, but poorer coverage against Gram-positive bacteria than cefuroxime; penetrates the CSF	
Ceftazidime	**Dose 1g** (1-2g) 8h IV or 2g/12h IV; **Indications** better Gram-negative activity, but poorer coverage against Gram-positive bacteria than cefuroxime; good activity against *Pseudomonas*	

Cetirizine H1-antagonist see antihistamine.

Chloramphenicol; eye drops antibiotic Dose 1 drop 0.5%/2h TOP; reduce frequency as infection is controlled. Continue for 48h after symptoms resolve **Indication** conjunctivitis, corneal abrasions, post eye surgery **SE** transient stinging **BNF** 11.3.1.

Chlordiazepoxide benzodiazepine *Dose* see Table 5.12 *Indications* acute alcohol withdrawal treatment/prophylaxis *Caution* pregnancy, breastfeeding, liver disease, renal impairment, respiratory disease (sleep apnoea, respiratory failure), reduce dose in the elderly, avoid abrupt withdrawal *SE* respiratory depression, drowsiness, confusion, ataxia, amnesia, dependence *Info* symptoms of acute alcohol withdrawal tend to occur 12–48h after the last alcoholic drink and usually subside 5–7d after the last drink. A reducing dose of chlordiazepoxide acts as a surrogate CNS depressant (which is the effect alcohol has upon the CNS) and it is uncommon for physical symptoms of withdrawal to present if patients are treated with this sort of regimen; always consider vitamin supplementation in these patients (📖 p103); consult local guidelines *BNF* 4.1.2.

Table 5.12 *Chlordiazepoxide regimen for alcohol withdrawal*

Day 1	20mg/6h PO	Day 5	5mg/6h PO
Day 2	20mg/8h PO	Day 6	5mg/8h PO
Day 3	10mg/6h PO	Day 7	5mg/12h PO
Day 4	10mg/8h PO	Day 8	STOP

Local guidelines may differ from this suggested regimen

Chlorhexidine antiseptic *Indication* skin preparation prior to surgery or other invasive procedures (eg vascular access, spinal/epidural anaesthesia), surgical hand scrub, oral hygiene, antiseptic lubricant (eg Hibitane®) *CI* avoid contact with eyes, brain, meninges, middle ear and other body cavities *SE* sensitivity, mucosal irritation *BNF* 13.11.2/12.3.3.

Chlorphenamine (H$_1$-antagonist) see antihistamine.

Cimetidine antihistamine (H$_2$-antagonist) see ranitidine.

Ciprofloxacin quinolone *Dose* 500–750mg/12h PO; 400mg/12h IV *Indication* infections: GI, respiratory, urinary *CI* pregnancy, breastfeeding, allergy to quinolones *Caution* myasthenia gravis, seizures (reduced seizure threshold), adolescents/children, renal impairment *SE* N+V, diarrhoea, tendonitis (including tendon rupture) *Interaction* NSAIDs increase risk of seizure, increase levels of theophyllines, increase nephrotoxicity of ciclosporin, increase effect of warfarin *BNF* 5.1.12.

Citalopram selective serotonin re-uptake inhibitor *Dose* 20mg/24h PO (max 40mg/24h) *Indication* depression, panic disorder *CI* active mania, QT interval prolongation *Caution* pregnancy, epilepsy, cardiac disease, DM *SE* GI disturbance, anorexia, weight loss, ↓Na$^+$, agitation *Interaction* MAOI within 2wk *BNF* 4.3.3.

Clarithromycin macrolide antibiotic *Dose* 250–500mg/12h PO/IV *Indication* atypical pneumonias, *H. pylori* *CI* allergy *Caution* pregnancy, breastfeeding, hepatic or renal impairment, concomitant use with statins *SE* GI upset, irritant to veins *BNF* 5.1.5.

Clindamycin antibiotic *Dose* 150–450mg/6h PO; up to 4.8g/24h IV in 2–4 doses for life-threatening infections (consult *BNF*) *Indication* Gram-positive cocci and anaerobes; osteomyelitis, intra-abdominal infections, MRSA *CI* diarrhoea *Caution* breastfeeding, acute porphyria *SE* GI disturbance, antibiotic-associated colitis (namely *C. diff*), hepatotoxicity, arthralgia; discontinue drug if patient develops new onset diarrhoea *Interaction* increases neuromuscular blockade *BNF* 5.1.6.

Clobetasol propionate cream see topical corticosteroids.

Clopidogrel antiplatelet *Dose* Loading: 300mg/STAT PO. Maintenance: 75mg/24h PO *Indication* prevention of atherothrombotic events following MI/ACS/CVA *CI* pregnancy, breastfeeding, active bleeding *Caution* hepatic impairment, increased risk of bleeding, recent trauma/surgery *SE* GI disturbance, bleeding disorders *Interaction* increased risk of bleeding with NSAIDs and anticoagulants; proton pump inhibitors may reduce effectiveness of clopidogrel *BNF* 2.9.

Clotrimazole imidazole anti-fungal *Dose* 1% cream 2–3 applications/24h *Indication* fungal skin infections, vaginal candidiasis *Caution* avoid contact with eyes and mucous membranes, can damage condoms and diaphragms *SE* local irritation *BNF* 13.10.2.

Co-amoxiclav beta-lactam with clavulanic acid *Dose* 375–625mg/8h PO; 1.2g/8h IV *Indication* infection; where amoxicillin alone is not appropriate *CI* penicillin allergy *Caution* renal impairment, glandular fever, CMV infection, ALL/CLL *SE* N+V, diarrhoea, rash *BNF* 5.1.1.3.

Co-beneldopa levodopa and dopa-decarboxylase inhibitor (benserazide) *Dose* initially 50mg/6-8h PO, increased to 100mg/24h or 100mg/twice a week according to response; usual maintenance dose 400-800mg/day in divided doses *Indication* Parkinson's disease *Caution* severe pulmonary or cardiovascular disease, psychiatric illness, endocrine disorders, pregnancy and breastfeeding *SE* GI disturbances, taste disturbances, dry mouth, anorexia, arrhythmias and palpitations, postural hypotension, drowsiness, dystonia, dyskinesia *BNF* 4.9.1.

Co-careldopa levodopa and dopa-decarboxylase inhibitor (carbidopa) *Dose* depends upon preparation, consult BNF *Indication* Parkinson's disease *Caution* severe pulmonary or cardiovascular disease, psychiatric illness, endocrine disorders, pregnancy and breastfeeding *SE* GI disturbances, taste disturbances, dry mouth, anorexia, arrhythmias and palpitations, postural hypotension, drowsiness, dystonia, dyskinesia *BNF* 4.9.1.

Co-codamol weak opioids with paracetamol *Dose* 8/500mg two tablets/4–6h PO (max eight tablets/24h in divided doses); 30/500mg two tablets/4–6h PO (max eight tablets/24h in divided doses) *Indication* pain *CI* acute respiratory depression, paralytic ileus; codeine containing medicines should not be used in children under 12yr, or in any patient under the age of 18yr who undergoes removal of tonsils or adenoids for the treatment of sleep apnoea *Caution* pregnancy (especially delivery), COPD, asthma, renal impairment, hepatic impairment *SE* N+V, constipation *Info* co-prescribe laxatives if using opioids for >24h *BNF* 4.7.1.

Codeine phosphate weak opioid *Dose* 30–60mg/4h PO/IM (max 240mg/24h in divided doses) *Indication* pain *CI* acute respiratory depression, paralytic ileus; codeine containing medicines should not be used in children under 12yr, or in any patient under the age of 18yr who undergoes removal of tonsils or adenoids for the treatment of sleep apnoea *Caution* pregnancy (especially delivery), COPD, asthma, renal impairment, hepatic impairment; never give codeine phosphate IV *SE* N+V, constipation *Info* co-prescribe laxatives if using opioids for >24h *BNF* 4.7.2.

Combivent® antimuscarinic with ß₂ agonist *Dose* 500micrograms ipratropium bromide with 2.5mg salbutamol/PRN NEB *Indication* asthma and other reversible airway obstruction, COPD *Caution* prostatic hyperplasia, glaucoma *SE* antimuscarinic effects (commonly dry mouth), fine tremor, tension headaches, arrhythmias *BNF* 3.1.4.

Corsodyl® antiseptic see chlorhexidine.

Cyclizine antihistamine (H₁ antagonist) see antiemetics.

Dalteparin low-molecular-weight heparin *Dose* consult *BNF* *Indication* DVT/PE treatment and prophylaxis, ACS *CI* bleeding disorders, thrombocytopenia, severe hypertension, recent trauma *Caution* hyperkalaemia, hepatic or renal impairment *SE* haemorrhage, thrombocytopenia, hyperkalaemia *Interaction* NSAIDs increase bleeding risk, effects increased by GTN *BNF* 2.8.1.

Desloratadine antihistamine (H₁ antagonist) see antihistamines.

Dexamethasone corticosteroid *Dose* see *BNF* *Indication* cerebral oedema (malignancy), suppression of inflammation/allergic disorders, diagnosis of Cushing's disease, chemotherapy induced N+V *CI* systemic infection *Caution* adrenal suppression, may precipitate tumour lysis syndrome in patients with some haematological malignancies *SE* Cushing's syndrome, DM, osteoporosis, psychiatric reactions, raised WCC (specifically neutrophilia) *BNF* 6.3.2.

Diamorphine opioid *Dose* 2.5–5mg/4h SC/IM/IV *Indication* severe pain, ACS/acute MI, acute pulmonary oedema, palliative care *CI* respiratory depression, paralytic ileus, raised ICP/head trauma, comatose patients, phaeochromocytoma *Caution* pregnancy (especially delivery), COPD, asthma, renal impairment, hepatic impairment *SE* N+V, constipation, respiratory depression, dry mouth *Interaction* MAOI *Info* co-prescribe laxatives if using opioids for >24h *BNF* 4.7.2.

Diazepam benzodiazepine *Dose* status epilepticus: 5–10mg over 10min IV (max 20mg) or 10–40mg PR; other short-term usage: 2mg/8h PO (max 30mg/24h in divided doses) *Indication* seizures, status epilepticus; short term: anxiety, alcohol withdrawal, muscle spasms *CI* respiratory depression, sleep apnoea, unstable myasthenia gravis, hepatic impairment *Caution* pregnancy, breastfeeding, history of drug abuse, respiratory disease, muscle weakness, renal impairment *SE* drowsiness, confusion, muscle weakness *BNF* 4.1.2/4.8.2.

Diclofenac NSAID *Dose* 50mg/8h PO/PR (max 150mg/24h in divided doses) *Indication* pain, inflammation *CI* pregnancy, peptic ulcer disease, hepatic impairment, congestive heart failure, ischaemic heart disease, peripheral arterial disease, cerebrovascular disease *Caution* breastfeeding, renal impairment, asthma, GI disease, patients with significant risk factors for cardiovascular events (eg ↑BP, ↑lipids, DM, smoking) *SE* GI disturbance/bleeding, headache, dizziness *Info* Arthrotec® is a preparation of diclofenac with misoprostol and may reduce GI side effects *BNF* 10.1.1.

Digoxin cardiac glycoside *Emergency IV loading dose* 0.75–1mg over at least 2h IV *Rapid oral loading dose* 0.75–1.5mg over 24h in 3 divided doses PO (typically 500micrograms PO initially, followed by 250micrograms PO 6h later, and further 250micrograms PO 12h later if still tachycardic *Maintenance dose* 62.5–125micrograms/24h PO *Indications* often 2nd-line agent in supraventricular tachyarrhythmias (commonly AF and atrial flutter), heart failure *CI* 2nd- or 3rd-degree AV dissociation, accessory conducting pathways (eg WPW) *Caution* pregnancy, recent MI, sick sinus syndrome, renal impairment, elderly patients, ↓K+, ↓Mg^{2+} or ↑Ca^{2+} *SE* N+V, diarrhoea, bradyarrhythmias, tachyarrhythmias, dizziness, blurred or yellow vision *Therapeutic monitoring* (see Table 5.13) should be undertaken if toxicity is considered (usually presents with N+V) or if rate control is poor *Info* digoxin is now rarely used for rapid rate control, with other agents often being used in preference (📖 p250) or DC cardioversion (📖 p532). Digoxin is most often used in the chronic rate control of supraventricular tachyarrhythmias and in heart failure. Digoxin does not restore sinus rhythm, it merely slows conduction at the atrio-ventricular node, limiting the number of impulses passing from the atria through to the ventricles thus controlling ventricular rate. It also acts as a positive inotrope, increasing the force of ventricular contraction *If rate not adequately controlled* after loading with digoxin, discuss with senior or cardiologist *BNF* 2.1.1.

Monitoring digoxin	Optimum sampling time *6–12h post oral dose* 1–2.6nmol/l (0.8–2microg/l); typically takes 7d to get to steady state *toxic* >2.6nmol/l (>2microg/l). Toxicity can occur at levels <1.3nmol/l if patient has ↓K+ *signs of toxicity* (see Table 5.13 and OHAM3 📖 p708)

Table 5.13 *Digoxin toxicity*

Symptoms	N+V, confusion, diarrhoea, yellow and blurred vision
Bloods	Toxicity precipitated by renal failure, ↓K+, ↓Mg^{2+} and ↓T$_4$ Check digoxin level (📖 see box); toxic if >2.6nmol/l (>2microg/l)
ECG	Tachy- and bradyarrhythmias. ST depression/T-wave inversion
Complications	↑K+, cardiac dysrhythmias (tachy- and bradyarrhythmias)
Management	Airway, breathing, and circulation Continuous ECG monitoring Treat arrhythmias Consider *digoxin-binding antibody fragments* (DigiFab®, **BNF** 2.1.1) if known or suspected digoxin overdose

Dihydrocodeine weak opioid *Dose* 30mg/4–6h PO (max 240mg/24h in divided doses); 50mg/4–6h IM *Indication* pain *CI* acute respiratory depression, paralytic ileus *Caution* pregnancy (especially delivery), COPD, asthma, renal impairment, hepatic impairment; never give dihydrocodeine IV *SE* N+V, constipation *Info* co-prescribe laxatives if using opioids for >24h *BNF* 4.7.2.

Diltiazem see calcium-channel blockers.

Dipyridamole antiplatelet *Dose* 200mg modified release/12h PO (max 600mg/24h in divided doses), non-modified release preparations also available (see *BNF*) *Indication* secondary prevention of ischaemic stroke and TIA, adjunct to oral anticoagulation for prophylaxis of thromboembolism associated with prosthetic heart valves *Caution* breastfeeding, aortic stenosis, unstable angina, recent MI *SE* GI disturbance, dizziness, headache, myalgia *Interaction* increases effect of warfarin, decreases effect of cholinesterase inhibitors *BNF* 2.9.

Docusate sodium see laxatives.

Doxazosin α_1 **antagonist** *Dose* 1mg/24h PO; increase gradually to 2–4mg/24h (max 16mg/24h) *Indication* benign prostatic hyperplasia, hypertension *CI* breastfeeding, hypotension *Caution* pregnancy, hepatic impairment *SE* postural hypotension, headache, dizziness, urinary incontinence *Interaction* increases effects of antihypertensives *BNF* 2.5.4.

Doxycycline tetracycline *Dose* 100–200mg 12–24h PO (consult *BNF*) *Indication* respiratory tract infections, GU infections, anthrax, malaria prophylaxis *CI* pregnancy, breastfeeding, renal impairment, age <12yr (stains growing teeth and bones) *Caution* myasthenia gravis may worsen, exacerbates SLE *SE* GI disturbance including, dysphagia/oesophageal irritation, photosensitivity *Interaction* decreased absorption with milk, decreases effects of oral contraceptive pill, mildly increases effects of warfarin *BNF* 5.1.3.

Enalapril see ACEi.

Enoxaparin low-molecular-weight heparin *Dose* <u>DVT/PE prophylaxis:</u> 20–40mg/24h SC (see 📖 p407); <u>DVT/PE treatment:</u> 1.5mg/kg/24h SC; <u>ACS treatment:</u> 1mg/kg/12h *Indication* DVT/PE treatment and prophylaxis, ACS *CI* bleeding disorders, thrombocytopenia, severe hypertension, recent trauma *Caution* hyperkalaemia, hepatic or renal impairment *SE* haemorrhage, thrombocytopenia, hyperkalaemia *Interaction* NSAIDs increase bleeding risk, effects increased by GTN *BNF* 2.8.1.

Epilim® **antiepileptic** see valproate.

Erythromycin macrolide antibiotic *Dose* 500–1000mg/6h PO; 50mg/kg/24h IV in divided dose (typically 500–1000mg/6h IV) *Indication* infection; atypical pneumonias. Commonly used in patients allergic to penicillins *CI* allergy *Caution* pregnancy, breastfeeding, hepatic or renal impairment, concomitant use with statins *SE* GI upset, irritant to veins *BNF* 5.1.5.

Esomeprazole proton pump inhibitor Dose 20–40mg/24h PO **Indication** PUD, GORD, *H. pylori* eradication **CI** breastfeeding **Caution** pregnancy, hepatic impairment, gastric cancer **SE** GI disturbance, headache **Interaction** proton pump inhibitors may reduce effectiveness of clopidogrel **BNF** 1.3.5.

Felodipine see calcium-channel blockers.

Ferrous fumarate iron supplement Dose consult *BNF* as depends upon formulation **Indication** iron deficiency anaemia **SE** GI disturbance, dark stools **BNF** 9.1.1.1.

Ferrous gluconate iron supplement Dose 600mg/8h PO (see *BNF*) **Indication** iron deficiency anaemia **SE** GI disturbance, dark stools **BNF** 9.1.1.1.

Ferrous sulfate iron supplement Dose 200mg/8h PO **Indication** iron deficiency anaemia **SE** GI disturbance, dark stools **BNF** 9.1.1.1.

Fibrinolytic drugs plasminogen activator Dose & Indications depends upon specific agent, see Table 5.14 (see also 🔲 p536) **CI** recent haemorrhage, trauma or surgery, coagulopathies, aortic dissection, aneurysm, coma, history of cerebrovasalar disease, peptic ulceration, menorrhagia, hepatic impairment; streptokinase should not be used again beyond 4d of first administration due to antibody formation and risk of allergic reactions **Caution** pregnancy, following external chest compression, old age, hypertension **SE** N+V, bleeding, hypotension **BNF** 2.10.2.

Table 5.14 *Fibrinolytic drugs* **BNF** 2.10.2
In acute STEMI, fibrinolytic drugs should be used where primary cutaneous intervention (PCI) is not immediately available

Alteplase	**Indications** acute MI, massive PE, acute ischaemic stroke **Dose** consult *BNF*; given as an IV bolus followed by an IV infusion, followed by heparin infusion
Reteplase	**Indications** acute MI **Dose** consult *BNF*; given as two IV boluses 30min apart, followed by heparin infusion
Streptokinase	**Indications** acute MI, DVT, PE, acute arterial thromboembolism, central retinal venous or arterial thrombosis **Dose** consult *BNF*; typically 1.5million units in 100ml 0.9% saline over 1h IV. Do not repeat administration after 4d of initial dose due to risk of allergic reaction
Tenecteplase	**Indications** acute MI **Dose** consult *BNF*; given as an IV bolus, followed by heparin infusion
Urokinase	**Indications** thromboembolic occlusive vascular disease; DVT, PE and peripheral vascular occlusion; occluded intravenous catheters and cannulae blocked by fibrin clot **Dose** consult *BNF*

Finasteride antiandrogen *Dose* <u>BPH:</u> 5mg/24h PO; <u>male-pattern baldness:</u> 1mg/24h PO *Indication* BPH, male-pattern baldness *CI* females and adolescents *Caution* prostate cancer, urinary tract obstruction *SE* gynaecomastia, testicular pain, sexual dysfunction *BNF* 6.4.2/13.9.

Flagyl® antibiotic see metronidazole.

Flecainide class Ic antiarrhythmic *Dose* <u>initially:</u> 100mg/12h PO; <u>reduce to</u> lowest effective dose over 3–5d; 2mg/kg over 10–30min slow IV (max 150mg) *Indication* VT, SVT *CI* HF, history of MI, heart block, bundle branch block *Caution* patients with pacemakers, AF *SE* GI disturbance, dizziness, oedema, fatigue *Interaction* duration of action increased by amiodarone, fluoxetine, quinine; myocardial depression with β-blockers/verapamil *BNF* 2.3.2.

Flixotide® corticosteroid see fluticasone.

Flucloxacillin beta-lactam *Dose* 250–500mg/6h PO; 250–2000mg/6h IV *Indication* penicillin sensitive infections, endocarditis, osteomyelitis *CI* history of flucloxacillin-related jaundice, penicillin allergy *SE* diarrhoea, abdominal pain *Caution* renal impairment *Interaction* decrease effects of oral contraceptive pill, allopurinol increases risk of rash *BNF* 5.1.1.2.

Fluconazole triazole antifungal *Dose* 50–400mg/24h PO/IV dependent on indication *Indication* fungal meningitis, candidiasis, fungal prophylaxis *CI* pregnancy, acute porphyria *Caution* breastfeeding, hepatic or renal impairment *SE* GI disturbance *BNF* 5.2.

Fludrocortisone mineralocorticoid *Dose* 50–300micrograms/24h PO *Indication* Addison's disease, other adrenal insufficiency, postural hypotension *CI* systemic infection without antibiotic cover *Caution* adrenal suppression *SE* sodium and water retention, hypertension *BNF* 6.3.1.

Flumazenil benzodiazepine antagonist *Dose* 200micrograms/STAT IV, followed by 100micrograms/1min if required (max 1mg) *Indication* benzodiazepine OD/toxicity *CI* conditions dependent on benzodiazepines, eg status epilepticus *Caution* benzodiazepine dependence, mixed OD *SE* N+V, dizziness, arrhythmias *BNF* 15.1.7.

Fluoxetine selective serotonin re-uptake inhibitor *Dose* 20mg/24h PO (max 60mg/24h) *Indication* depression, bulimia nervosa and OCD *CI* active mania *Caution* pregnancy, epilepsy, cardiac disease, DM, bleeding disorders, glaucoma *SE* GI disturbance, anorexia, weight loss, ↓Na⁺, agitation *Interaction* MAOI within 2wk *BNF* 4.3.3.

Fluticasone corticosteroid *Dose* 100–500micrograms/12h INH (consult *BNF*) *Indication* chronic asthma (step 2 BTS guidelines) *Caution* TB *SE* oral candidiasis, hoarse voice, paradoxical bronchospasm (rare) *BNF* 3.2.

Folic acid vitamin B9 *Dose* 400micrograms/24h PO before conception and until week 12 of pregnancy; 5mg/wk for preventing methotrexate side effects *Indication* pregnancy, folate deficient megaloblastic anaemia, long-term methotrexate *CI* malignancy *Caution* never give alone for pernicious anaemia; can cause degeneration of spinal cord, undiagnosed megaloblastic anaemia *SE* GI disturbance *BNF* 9.1.2.

Fondaparinux factor Xa inhibitor *Dose* 2.5mg/24h SC (2.5mg loading dose 6h post-op) *Indication* VTE prophylaxis and treatment, ACS *CI* active bleeding, bacterial endocarditis *Caution* pregnancy, breastfeeding, bleeding disorders, active PUD, recent surgery, epidural/spinal anaesthesia, hepatic or renal impairment *SE* bleeding, purpura, anaemia, thrombocytopenia *BNF* 2.8.1.

Frusemide loop diuretic see furosemide.

Furosemide loop diuretic *Dose* typically 20–80mg/24h PO/IV *Indication* oedema (LVF, pulmonary oedema), resistant hypertension *CI* severe ↓K⁺ and ↓Na⁺, hypovolaemia, renal impairment *Caution* hypotension *SE* GI disturbance, hypotension, electrolyte disturbances (↓K⁺, ↓Na⁺, ↓Mg²⁺) *Interaction* increases toxicity of gentamicin, digoxin, NSAIDs *Info* IV doses >80mg should be infused at <4mg/min (risk of deafness) *BNF* 2.2.2.

Fusidic acid antibiotic *Dose* 2% topical cream 3–4 applications/24h; oral and IV preparations available (see *BNF*) *Indication* staphylococcal skin infections; <u>IV treatment</u> osteomyelitis, penicillin-resistant staphylococcal infections *Caution* pregnancy, breastfeeding, monitor LFTs *SE* GI disturbance, reversible jaundice *BNF* 5.1.7/13.10.1.2.

Fybogel® see laxatives.

Gabapentin antiepileptic *Dose* <u>day 1:</u> 300mg/24h PO; <u>continued:</u> increase by 300mg/24h up to max 3.6g/24h in 3 divided doses *Indication* epilepsy, neuropathic pain *Caution* pregnancy, breastfeeding, renal impairment, DM, avoid abrupt withdrawal *SE* GI disturbance, headache, sleep disturbance *Interaction* effects decreased by antidepressants *BNF* 4.8.1.

Gentamicin aminoglycoside *Dose* <u>Once daily:</u> 5–7mg/kg/24h IV adjust to serum concentration; other dosing regimens may be used (consult local guidelines) *Indication* infection; sepsis, meningitis, endocarditis *CI* myasthenia gravis *Caution* pregnancy, breastfeeding, renal impairment *SE* ototoxic, nephrotoxic *Interaction* effects increased by loop diuretics, increases effects of warfarin *BNF* 5.1.4.

Monitoring gentamicin	*Peak 1h post IV dose* 9–18micromol/l (5–10mg/l); *trough* <4.2micromol/l (<2mg/l); *toxic* >12mg/l (22micromol/l); *signs of toxicity* tinnitus, deafness, nystagmus, vertigo, renal failure (OHCM9 🔲 p766). Will vary with once-daily regimen, check locally.

Glibenclamide see sulphonylureas.

Gliclazide see sulphonylureas.

Glipizide see sulphonylureas.

Glucagon peptide hormone *Dose* 1mg/PRN IM/SC/slow IV *Indication* hypoglycaemia, in treatment of β-blocker overdose *CI* phaeochromocytoma *Caution* insulinoma, glucagonoma, chronic hypoglycaemia *SE* GI disturbance, ↓K⁺, hypotension *BNF* 6.1.4.

Glycerin suppositories see laxatives.

Glyceryl trinitrate nitrate see GTN.

GTN sublingual/transdermal nitrate Dose 1–2 sprays/PRN SL; 0.3–1mg/PRN SL **Indication** prophylaxis and treatment of angina, left ventricular failure **CI** hypotensive conditions, hypovolaemia, aortic stenosis **Caution** pregnancy, breastfeeding, hypothyroidism, recent MI, head trauma **SE** postural hypotension, tachycardia, headache **Info** transdermal patches are available, see *BNF* – patients may develop tolerance (tachyphylaxis) to nitrates and as such it is suggested to ensure patients have a nitrate-free period for 4–8h to prevent this; it is usual to have this period overnight when the effects of nitrates are least likely to be needed **BNF** 2.6.1.

GTN IV infusion nitrate Dose 10–200micrograms/min IVI GTN eg typical prescription: "50mg in 50ml 0.9% saline, start at 2ml/h and titrate up by 2ml/hr every 10min according to pain and BP; keep systolic BP >90mmHg" **Indication** left ventricular failure, ongoing ischaemic chest pain refractory to SL nitrates **CI** hypotensive conditions, hypovolaemia, aortic stenosis **Caution** pregnancy, breastfeeding, hypothyroidism, recent MI, head trauma **SE** postural hypotension, tachycardia, headache **Info** patients may develop tolerance (tachyphylaxis) to nitrates and as such it is suggested to ensure patients have a nitrate-free period for 4–8h to prevent this; it is usual to have this period overnight when the effects of nitrates are least likely to be needed **BNF** 2.6.1.

Haloperidol antipsychotic (butyrophenone) Dose <u>antiemetic</u>: 0.5–3mg/8h PO/IV; <u>other</u>: 0.5–10mg/8h PO/IM/IV **Indication** schizophrenia, agitation, N+V, motor tics, intractable hiccups **CI** comatose/ CNS depression **Caution** pregnancy, breastfeeding, hepatic or renal impairment, cardiovascular disease, Parkinson's, epilepsy **SE** extrapyramidal symptoms, cardiac arrhythmias (QTc prolongation) **BNF** 4.2.1/4.9.3.

Heparin glycosaminoglycan (potentiates antithrombin III) Dose <u>Loading dose</u>: 5000units or 75units/kg IV; <u>maintenance</u>: 18units/ kg/h IVI (titrate dose to keep APTT within therapeutic range); <u>prophylactic dose</u>: 5000units/12h SC (seldom used as LMWH have similar benefits and fewer side effects) **Indication** rapid anticoagulation, treatment and prophylaxis of DVT/PE, ACS **CI** bleeding disorders, thrombocytopenia, severe hypertension, recent trauma, history of heparin-induced thrombocytopenia (HIT, see 📖 p406) **Caution** ↑K⁺, hepatic or renal impairment **SE** haemorrhage, thrombocytopenia, ↑K⁺ **Interaction** NSAIDs increase bleeding risk, effects increased by GTN **BNF** 2.8.1.

Humalog® see insulin.

Humalin® see insulin.

Hydralazine vasodilator (arterial>>venous) *Dose* <u>hypertension:</u> 25–50mg/12h PO; 5–10mg slow IV titrated to effect (can repeat after 30min); <u>heart failure:</u> 25–75mg/6h PO *Indication* hypertension, heart failure *CI* SLE, severe tachycardia, myocardial insufficiency *Caution* pregnancy, breastfeeding, hepatic or renal impairment, ischaemic heart disease, cerebrovascular disease *SE* tachycardia, palpitation, hypotension, SLE-like syndrome after long-term, rebound hypertension on stopping therapy, fluid retention *BNF* 2.5.1.

Hydrocortisone cream see topical corticosteroids.

Hydrocortisone IV/PO corticosteroid *Dose* <u>acute</u>: 100–500mg/6h IV; <u>chronic</u>: 20–30mg/24h PO in divided doses *Indication* adrenocortical insufficiency, acute allergic/inflammatory reactions *CI* Systemic infection *Caution* adrenal suppression *SE* Cushing's syndrome, DM, osteoporosis, dyspepsia *BNF* 6.3.2.

Hydroxocobalamin vitamin B$_{12}$ *Dose* <u>macrocytic anaemia</u> **without** <u>neurological involvement</u>: initially 1mg three times a week IM, after 2 wk 1mg/3mth IM; <u>macrocytic anaemia</u> **with** <u>neurological involvement</u>: initially 1mg on alternate days IM until no further improvement, then 1mg/2mth IM *Indication* pernicious anaemia, other macrocytic anaemias with neurological involvement *Caution* do not give before diagnosis fully established *SE* N+V, headache, dizziness *BNF* 9.1.2.

Hyoscine butylbromide anticholinergic *Dose* 20mg/6h PO (max 80mg/24h in divided doses); 20mg/STAT IV/IM repeated after 30min (max 100mg/24h in divided doses) *Indication* GI/GU smooth muscle spasm *CI* myasthenia gravis *Caution* pregnancy, glaucoma, GI obstruction, prostatic hyperplasia, urinary retention *SE* antimuscarinic effects, drowsiness *BNF* 1.2.

Hyoscine hydrobromide anticholinergic *Dose* <u>antiemetic</u>: 300micrograms/6h PO (max 900micrograms/24h in divided doses) <u>excessive respiratory secretions</u>: 200–600micrograms/4–8h SC *Indication* motion sickness, excessive respiratory secretions *CI* glaucoma *Caution* pregnancy, GI obstruction, prostatic hyperplasia, urinary retention *SE* antimuscarinic effects, sedative *Interaction* decreases effects of sublingual GTN *BNF* 4.6/15.1.3.

Ibuprofen NSAID *Dose* 200–400mg/6h PO (max 2.4g/24h in divided doses) *Indication* pain, inflammation *CI* pregnancy, peptic ulcer disease *Caution* breastfeeding, hepatic or renal impairment, asthma, GI disease *SE* GI disturbance/bleeding, headache *Interaction* decreases effects of antihypertensives, increases toxicity of methotrexate *BNF* 10.1.1.

Insulatard® see insulin.

Insulin *Dose* when starting or changing SC doses liaise with diabetes team (eg diabetes nurse specialist); infusion see Table 5.16 *Indications* DM, diabetic ketoacidosis, hyperkalaemia, maintenance of euglycaemia in critical care and post MI *CI* hypoglycaemia *Caution* may need dose adjustments in pregnancy, breastfeeding, renal and hepatic impairment, see *BNF* 6.1.1 *SE* hypoglycaemia, local reactions and fat hypertrophy at injection site, rarely allergic reactions *Info* Table 5.15 is not an exhaustive list of insulins. In addition to these single preparations of insulin, so called biphasic mixtures of two different insulins are also used and often consist of a rapid or short acting insulin and a longer acting insulin (in different proportions) *BNF* 6.1.1.

Table 5.15 *Properties of common subcutaneous insulins* **BNF** 6.1.1

Type of insulin	Example	Onset	Peak	Max Duration
Rapid-acting				
Aspart	Novorapid®	15–30min	0.5–1.25h	4–6h
Lispro	Humalog®	15–30min	0.5–1.25h	4–6h
Glulisine	Apidra®	15–30min	0.5–1.25h	4–6h
Short-acting				
Soluble	Actrapid®	30–60min	2–3h	6–8h
Intermediate and long-acting				
Isophane	Insulatard®	2–4h	6–10h	14–18h
Glargine	Lantus®	3–4h	8–16h	20–24h
Detemir	Levemir®	3–4h	6–8h	~20h

Table 5.16 *IV infusions of insulins*

Indication	
Hyperkalaemia (📖 p385)	50ml of 50% glucose with 10units soluble insulin (eg Actrapid®) IVI over 10min
Sliding scale (📖 p327)	50ml of 0.9% saline with 50units soluble insulin (eg Actrapid®), often infused at 0–7ml/h depending upon the patient's blood sugar

Ipratropium anticholinergic *Dose* <u>Chronic:</u> 20–40micrograms/6h INH (max 80micrograms/6h) <u>Acute:</u> 250–500micrograms/4–6h NEB *Indication* bronchospasm; chronic and acute *Caution* glaucoma, prostatic hyperplasia *SE* minimal antimuscarinic effects *BNF* 3.1.2.

Iron see ferrous preparations.

ISMN nitrate see isosorbide mononitrate.

ISMO nitrate see isosorbide mononitrate.

Isoket® **nitrate** see isosorbide dinitrate.

Isosorbide dinitrate IV infusion nitrate Dose 2–10mg/h IVI **Indication** left ventricular failure, ischaemic chest pain **CI** hypotensive conditions, hypovolaemia, aortic stenosis **Caution** pregnancy, breastfeeding, hypothyroidism, recent MI, head trauma **SE** postural hypotension, tachycardia, headache **Info** patients may develop tolerance (tachyphylaxis) to nitrates if infused for prolonged periods, though there are obvious risks about stopping a nitrate infusion; consult senior **BNF** 2.6.1.

Isosorbide mononitrate nitrate Dose <u>initially:</u> 20mg breakfast and lunchtime PO <u>then:</u> 40mg breakfast and lunchtime PO (max 120mg/24h in divided doses) **Indication** prophylaxis of angina, adjunct in congestive heart failure **Caution** as GTN **SE** postural hypotension, tachycardia, headache **Info** patients may develop tolerance (tachyphylaxis) to nitrates and as such it is suggested to ensure patients have a nitrate-free period for 4–8h to prevent this; it is usual to have this period overnight when the effects of nitrates are least likely to be needed, hence prescribing them to be given at breakfast and lunchtime rather than 8am and 8pm **BNF** 2.6.1.

Istin® see calcium-channel blockers.

Lactulose see laxative.

Lamotrigine antiepileptic Dose <u>initially:</u> 25mg/24h PO for 14d <u>then:</u> 50mg/24h PO for 14d, increase by max 50–100mg/24h every 7–14d until seizures controlled (max 500mg/24h) **Indication** epilepsy **Caution** requires close monitoring of serum levels, pregnancy, breastfeeding, hepatic or renal impairment, avoid rapid withdrawal **SE** rash/severe skin reactions, cerebellar symptoms, cytopenias **BNF** 4.8.1.

Lansoprazole proton pump inhibitor Dose 30mg/24h PO for 4–8wk, 15mg/24h PO maintenance **Indication** prophylaxis and treatment of peptic ulcers, GORD, *H. pylori* eradication, Zollinger–Ellison syndrome **CI** pregnancy **Caution** breastfeeding, hepatic impairment, gastric cancer **SE** GI disturbance, headache **Interaction** proton pump inhibitors may reduce effectiveness of clopidogrel **Info** also available as a FasTab® which dissolves in the mouth and is useful in patients who are NBM **BNF** 1.3.5.

Laxative *Dose* see Table 5.17 *Indications* treatment and prophylaxis of constipation (see 📖 p310) *Caution* confirm the patient is constipated and consider causes of constipation *SE* see Table 5.17 *Info* chronic use of laxatives can lead to electrolyte imbalances and gut dysmotility. Ensure adequate water intake and increase fibre intake where possible. Always consider faecal impaction and other causes of obstruction before commencing oral laxatives. Combinations of laxatives from different groups can be used in severe constipation (eg lactulose and senna) *BNF* 1.6.

Table 5.17 *Laxative* **BNF** 1.6

Classification	
Bulk-forming laxatives BNF 1.6.1	eg Fybogel®, Normacol® *CI* difficulty in swallowing, intestinal obstruction, colonic atony, faecal impaction *SE* diarrhoea, flatulence, abdominal distension, gastrointestinal obstruction
Fybogel®	1 sachet or two 5ml spoons in water/12h PO
Stimulant laxatives BNF 1.6.2	eg bisacodyl, docusate, glycerol, senna *CI* intestinal obstruction, acute surgical abdomens, active inflammatory bowel disease, dehydration *SE* diarrhoea, hypokalaemia, abdominal pain, N+V *Info* co-danthramer should only be used in the terminally ill as potentially carcinogenic
Bisacodyl	5–10mg/nocte PO or 10mg/mane PR
Co-danthramer	1–2 capsules/nocte PO
Docusate sodium	200mg/12h PO (max 500mg/24h PO in divided doses)
Glycerin supps	1 suppository/PRN PR, max 4 in 24h
Senna	2 tablets/nocte PO or 10ml/nocte PO
Faecal softeners BNF 1.6.3	eg arachis oil, liquid paraffin *Info* infrequently used *CI* peanut allergy
Osmotic laxatives BNF 1.6.4	eg lactulose, Movicol®, magnesium salts, rectal phosphates (eg Fleet® enema), rectal sodium citrate (eg Microlette®) *CI* intestinal obstruction, colonic atony *SE* diarrhoea, flatulence, abdominal distension and discomfort, nausea; local irritation with rectal preparations
Lactulose	10–15ml/12h PO
Movicol®	1–3 sachets/24h PO
Phosphate enemas	1/PRN PR, max 2 in 24h
Microlette®	1/PRN PR, max 2 in 24h

Levothyroxine thyroid hormone (T$_4$) *Dose* typically 50–200micrograms/24h PO at breakfast *Indication* hypothyroidism *CI* thyrotoxicosis *Caution* pregnancy, breastfeeding, panhypopituitarism, adrenal insufficiency, cardiovascular disorders, DM *SE* hyperthyroid-like symptoms; GI disturbance, tremors, restlessness, flushing *Interaction* increases effects of TCAs and warfarin, decreases effects of propranolol **BNF** 6.2.1.

Lidocaine local anaesthetic (amide) *Dose* local anaesthesia: 1/2/4% solution SC (max 3mg/kg [max total dose 200mg]) anti-arrhythmic: see *BNF* **Indication** local anaesthesia, ventricular arrhythmias (alternative to amiodarone) *CI* myocardial depression, atrioventricular block, sinoatrial node disorders **Caution** pregnancy, hepatic or renal impairment, epilepsy, severe hypoxia/hypovolaemia *SE* dizziness, drowsiness, confusion, tinnitus **Interaction** increased myocardial depression with β-blockers and other anti-arrhythmics, increased risk of arrhythmias with antipsychotics *BNF* 15.2.

Lignocaine local anaesthetic (amide) see lidocaine.

Lisinopril see ACEi.

Lithium lithium salt (mood stabiliser) *Dose* see *BNF* **Indication** mania, bipolar disorder *CI* pregnancy, breastfeeding, untreated hypothyroidism, Addison's disease **Caution** thyroid disease, myasthenia gravis *SE* GI upset, thirst, polyuria **Interaction** diuretics, NSAIDs **Info** lithium citrate and lithium carbonate doses are not simply interchangeable d/w senior/pharmacist; on stable regiments monitor level every 3mth. The NPSA have published guidance on the 'safer use of lithium' and this should be consulted before commencing lithium therapy[1] *BNF* 4.2.3.

Monitoring lithium	Optimum sampling time 4–7d after commencing treatment *12h post dose* 0.4–1mmol/l; *early signs of toxicity* (Li$^+$ >1.5mmol/l) tremor, agitation, twitching, thirst, polyuria, N+V; *late signs of toxicity* (Li$^+$ >2mmol/l) spasms, coma, fits, arrhythmias, renal failure (OHAM3 📖 p716)

Loperamide opioid (antimotility) *Dose* 4mg PO initially then 2mg PO following every loose stool (max 16mg/24h in divided doses) **Indication** diarrhoea, control of high output stoma *CI* pregnancy, IBD, any condition where peristalsis should not be stopped; constipation, ileus, megacolon **Caution** hepatic impairment, can promote fluid and electrolyte depletion in the young *SE* abdominal cramps, constipation, dizziness **Info** loperamide should not be used in infective diarrhoeas or diarrhoea associated with IBD *BNF* 1.4.2.

Loratadine H1-antagonist see antihistamine.

Lorazepam benzodiazepine *Dose* sedation/anxiety: 1–4mg/24h PO/IM/IV seizures: 4mg slow IV (repeated once after 10min if needed) **Indication** sedation, seizures, status epilepticus *CI* respiratory depression, sleep apnoea, unstable myasthenia gravis, severe hepatic impairment **Caution** pregnancy, breastfeeding, history of drug abuse, respiratory disease, muscle weakness, renal impairment *SE* drowsiness, confusion, muscle weakness *BNF* 4.1.2/4.8.2.

[1] 🖱www.nrls.npsa.nhs.uk/resources/type/alerts/?entryid45=65426

Losartan see AT II antagonists.

Magnesium sulfate magnesium salt *Dose* 2–4g IV over 5–15min often followed by an infusion (see *BNF*) *Indication* arrhythmias, MI, acute severe asthma, pre-eclampsia/eclampsia, ↓Mg^{2+} *Caution* pregnancy, monitor BP, RR, urinary output, hepatic or renal impairment *SE* N+V, hypotension, thirst, flushed skin *Interaction* risk of hypotension with calcium-channel blockers *Info* magnesium sulphate 1g equivalent to approximately 4mmol *BNF* 9.5.1.3.

Monitoring magnesium	Levels should be checked every 6h whilst on IV therapy or more urgently if indicated *therapeutic range* 1.7–3.5mmol/l
0.7–1.0mmol/l	Normal plasma range
1.7–3.5mmol/l	Therapeutic range
2.5–5.0mmol/l	ECG changes (QRS widens)
4.0–5.0mmol/l	Reduction in tendon reflexes
>5.0mmol/l	Loss of deep tendon reflexes
>7.5mmol/l	Heart block, respiratory paralysis, CNS depression
>12mmol/l	Cardiac arrest

Maxolon® **antiemetic (dopamine antagonist)** see metoclopramide.

Mannitol polyol (osmotic diuretic) *Dose* 0.25–2g/kg/4–8h over 30–60min IVI (max 3 doses) *Indication* cerebral oedema, glaucoma *CI* pulmonary oedema, cardiac failure *Caution* pregnancy, breastfeeding, renal impairment *SE* hypotension, fluid and electrolyte imbalance *BNF* 2.2.5.

Mebeverine antispasmodic (antimuscarinic) *Dose* 135–150mg/8h PO (20min before food) *Indication* GI smooth muscle cramps; IBS/diverticulitis *CI* paralytic ileus *Caution* pregnancy, acute porphyria *SE* very rarely rash, urticaria *BNF* 1.2.

Meropenem carbapenem antibiotic *Dose* 500–1000mg/8h IV (dose doubled in severe infections) *Indication* aerobic and anaerobic Gram-positive and Gram-negative infections *Caution* pregnancy, breastfeeding, hepatic or renal impairment, sensitivity to beta-lactams *SE* GI disturbance including antibiotic associated colitis, headache, deranged LFTs *BNF* 5.1.2.2.

Mesalazine aminosalicylate *Dose* depends upon formulation, consult *BNF*; PO and PR preparations available *Indication* mild/moderate active ulcerative colitis and maintenance of remission *CI* salicylate allergy, coagulopathies *Caution* pregnancy, breastfeeding, hepatic or renal impairment *SE* GI upset, bleeding disorders *BNF* 1.5.1.

Metformin biguanide *Dose* <u>initially:</u> 500mg/24h PO with breakfast; <u>after 1wk:</u> 500mg/12h PO; <u>after further 1wk:</u> 500mg/8h PO if required (max 2g/24 in divided doses) *Indication* type 2 DM, polycystic ovarian syndrome *CI* hepatic or renal impairment *Caution* ketoacidosis, potential increased risk of lactic acidosis, iodine-containing contrast, general anaesthesia *SE* GI disturbance, metallic taste *BNF* 6.1.2.2.

Methadone opioid *Dose* usual range 60–120mg/24h PO; should not be given more frequently than 12h if on prolonged use; establish the patient's dose from the usual dispensing pharmacy, the patient may not tell you accurate information *Indication* aid in withdrawal from opioid dependence, chronic pain *CI* acute respiratory depression, paralytic ileus, raised ICP/head trauma, comatose patients, phaeochromocytoma *Caution* pregnancy (especially delivery), arrhythmias, hepatic or renal impairment *SE* N+V, constipation, respiratory depression, dry mouth *Interaction* MAOI within 2wk *BNF* 4.10.3.

Methotrexate dihydrofolate reductase inhibitor *Dose* 2.5–10mg/wk PO (max 25mg/wk) *Indication* rheumatoid arthritis, Crohn's disease, psoriasis, ALL, non-Hodgkin's lymphoma *CI* pregnancy, breast-feeding, hepatic or renal impairment, active infection, immunodeficient syndromes *Caution* blood disorders, effusions (especially ascites), peptic ulcer, ulcerative colitis *SE* GI disturbance/mucositis, pulmonary fibrosis, pneumonitis, myelosuppression *Interaction* NSAIDs, co-trimoxazole, trimethoprim *Info* patients usually also prescribed folic acid during treatment with methotrexate *BNF* 1.5.3/10.1.3.

Methylprednisolone corticosteroid *Dose* 2–40mg/24h PO; 10–500mg/24h IV/IM (exceptionally, up to 1g/24h for up to 3d) *Indication* acute inflammatory disease, cerebral oedema (associated with malignancy), graft rejection *CI* systemic infection *Caution* adrenal suppression *SE* Cushing's syndrome, DM, osteoporosis *Interaction* duration decreased by rifampicin, carbamazepine, phenytoin; duration of action increased by erythromycin, ketoconazole, ciclosporin *BNF* 6.3.2.

Metoclopramide dopamine antagonist see antiemetic.

Metoprolol see beta-blockers.

Metronidazole antibiotic *Dose* 400mg/8h PO; 500mg/8h IV *Indication* anaerobic and protozoal infections, abdominal sepsis, *Clostridium difficile* diarrhoea *Caution* pregnancy, breastfeeding, hepatic impairment, alcohol use *SE* GI disturbance, metallic taste, oral mucositis *Interaction* can increase lithium and phenytoin levels, increases effects of warfarin *BNF* 5.1.11.

Midazolam benzodiazepine *Dose* 1–10mg IV titrated to effect *Indication* conscious sedation, sedation in anaesthesia *CI* breastfeeding, respiratory depression, sleep apnoea, unstable myasthenia gravis *Caution* pregnancy, hepatic or renal impairment, history of drug abuse, respiratory disease, muscle weakness *SE* drowsiness, confusion, muscle weakness *BNF* 15.1.4.1.

Misoprostol prostaglandin E_1 analogue *Dose* treatment: 800micrograms/24h PO in divided dose; prophylaxis: 200micrograms/6–12h PO *Indication* prophylaxis and treatment of peptic ulcers *CI* pregnancy, breastfeeding *Caution* cardiovascular/cerebrovascular disease *SE* diarrhoea *BNF* 1.3.4.

Mixtard® see insulin.

Montelukast leukotriene receptor antagonist *Dose* 10mg/24h PO in evening *Indication* chronic asthma (BTS guidelines), allergic rhinitis *Caution* pregnancy, breastfeeding *SE* abdominal pain, headache, rarely Churg–Strauss syndrome *BNF* 3.3.2.

Morphine opioid *Dose* 2.5–10mg/4h IV titrated to effect; 5–10mg/4h IM/SC *Indication* acute severe pain, chronic pain, acute MI, acute LVF *CI* acute respiratory depression, paralytic ileus, raised ICP/head trauma, comatose patients *Caution* pregnancy (especially delivery), COPD, asthma, arrhythmias, renal impairment, hepatic impairment *SE* N+V, constipation, respiratory depression, dry mouth *Info* co-prescribe laxatives if using opioids for >24h *BNF* 4.7.2.

MST Continus® opioid see oral morphine.

Mupirocin antibacterial *Dose* apply to skin up to 3 times/24h *Indication* bacterial skin infections *Caution* pregnancy, breastfeeding, renal impairment *SE* local reactions; urticarial, pruritus, burning sensation, rash *BNF* 13.10.1.1.

N-acetylcysteine amino acid derivative see acetylcysteine.

Naloxone opioid receptor antagonist *Dose* 0.4–2.0mg IV/IM/SC, repeat after 2min if needed (max 10mg) *Indication* opioid reversal during OD/overtreatment *Caution* pregnancy, physical dependence on opioids, cardiovascular disease *SE* N+V, hypotension *BNF* Emergency treatment of poisoning.

Narcan® opioid receptor antagonist Narcan® is a brand name for naloxone that is no longer used. See naloxone for opioid overdose or reversal of narcosis.

Nefopam centrally-acting non-opioid analgesic *Dose* 30–60mg/8h PO (max 90mg/8h PO) *Indication* moderate pain *CI* convulsive disorders *Caution* pregnancy, breastfeeding, hepatic or renal impairment, elderly, urinary retention *SE* N+V, nervousness, urinary retention, dry mouth, lightheadedness, may colour urine pink *BNF* 4.7.1.

Nicorandil potassium channel activator *Dose* 5–10mg/12h PO (max 30mg/12h in divided doses) *Indication* angina prophylaxis and treatment (not 1st line) *CI* breastfeeding, hypotension, LVF with low filling pressures *Caution* pregnancy, hypovolaemia, acute pulmonary oedema, MI *SE* headache, flushing, GI disturbance *BNF* 2.6.3.

Nifedipine see calcium-channel blockers.

Nitrofurantoin antibiotic *Dose* 50–100mg/6h PO; take with food *Indication* urinary tract infections *CI* pregnancy, breastfeeding, renal impairment, G6PD deficiency, infants <3mth, acute porphyria *Caution* hepatic impairment, anaemia, DM, electrolyte imbalance, vitamin B_{12}/folate deficiency, lung disease *SE* anorexia, GI disturbance, acute and chronic pulmonary reactions *BNF* 5.1.13.

Nurofen® NSAID see ibuprofen.

Nystatin polyene antifungal *Dose* 100 000 units (1ml)/6h PO; topical gel PRN *Indication* candidiasis; oral, skin *Caution* GI absorbance minimal *SE* GI disturbance (at high doses), oral irritation, rash *BNF* 12.3.2.

Omeprazole proton pump inhibitor *Dose* 10–40mg/24h PO; IV preparation available for endoscopically proven bleeding ulcers (consult *BNF*/local guidelines) *Indication* prophylaxis and treatment of peptic ulcers, GORD, *H. pylori* eradication *Caution* hepatic impairment (no more than 20mg/24h), can mask gastric cancer *SE* GI disturbance, headache, dizziness *Interaction* proton pump inhibitors may reduce effectiveness of clopidogrel *BNF* 1.3.5.

Ondansetron see antiemetics (5HT$_3$ receptor antagonist).

Oral morphine opioid *Dose* oral solution 5–20mg/4h PO; tablets: 5–20mg/4h PO; 12h slow release preparations: 10–30mg/12h PO, adjust to response (larger dose tablets available; seek senior/specialist advice) *Indication* severe pain, chronic pain *CI* acute respiratory depression, paralytic ileus, raised ICP/head trauma, comatose patients, phaeochromocytoma *Caution* pregnancy (especially delivery), COPD, asthma, arrhythmias, renal impairment, hepatic impairment *SE* N+V, constipation, respiratory depression, dry mouth *Info* co-prescribe laxatives if using opioids for >24h *BNF* 4.7.2.

Oramorph® opioid see oral morphine.

Oseltamivir (Tamiflu®) antiviral *Dose* treatment of influenza 75mg/12h PO for 5d; prevention of influenza 75mg/24h PO for 10d *Indication* treatment of influenza if started within 48h of the onset of symptoms, post-exposure prophylaxis of influenza *Caution* renal impairment, pregnancy and breastfeeding (use only if potential benefit outweighs risk (eg during a pandemic)) *SE* GI disturbances, headache, arrhythmias, convulsions, thrombocytopenia *BNF* 5.3.4.

Oxybutynin antimuscarinic *Dose* 5mg/8–12h PO, increase if required (max 20mg/24h in divided doses); modified release preparations also available *Indication* detrusor instability; urinary frequency, urgency and incontinence *CI* pregnancy, breastfeeding, bladder outflow/ GI obstruction, myasthenia gravis *Caution* hepatic or renal impairment, prostatic hyperplasia, autonomic neuropathy *SE* antimuscarinic effects, GI disturbance *BNF* 7.4.2.

Oxycodone opioid *Dose* 5mg/4–6h PO (max 400mg/24h); 1–10mg/4h IV/SC titrated to effect *Indication* pain; moderate to severe *CI* acute respiratory depression, paralytic ileus, chronic constipation, acute abdomen, raised ICP/head trauma, hepatic or renal impairment if severe, acute porphyria, cor pulmonale, comatose patients *Caution* pregnancy, COPD, asthma, arrhythmias, renal impairment, hepatic impairment *SE* N+V, constipation, respiratory depression, dry mouth *Info* 2mg PO ≃1mg IV *Info* co-prescribe laxatives if using opioids for >24h *BNF* 4.7.2.

OxyContin® opioid see oxycodone.

OxyNorm® **opioid** see oxycodone.

Oxytetracycline tetracycline antibiotic *Dose* 250–500mg/6h PO *Indication* acne vulgaris, rosacea *CI* pregnancy, breastfeeding, renal impairment, age <12yr (irreversibly stains growing teeth and bones) *Caution* myasthenia gravis may worsen, exacerbates SLE *SE* GI disturbance including, dysphagia/oesophageal irritation *Interaction* decreased absorption with dairy products, decreases effects of oral contraceptive pill, mildly increases effects of warfarin *BNF* 5.1.3.

Pabrinex® see thiamine.

Pantoprazole proton pump inhibitor *Dose* 20–80mg/24h PO; IV preparation available for endoscopically proven bleeding ulcers (consult *BNF*/local guidelines) *Indication* prophylaxis and treatment of peptic ulcers, GORD, *H. pylori* eradication *Caution* hepatic impairment (max 20mg/24h), renal impairment (max oral dose 40mg/24h), can mask gastric cancer *SE* GI disturbance, headache, dizziness *Interaction* proton pump inhibitors may reduce effectiveness of clopidogrel *BNF* 1.3.5.

Paracetamol simple analgesic *Dose* 0.5–1g/4–6h PO/IV (max 4g/24h in divided doses) *Indication* pain; mild to moderate, pyrexia *Caution* alcohol dependence, hepatic impairment *SE* rare; rash, hypoglycaemia, blood disorders, hepatic impairment *Interaction* prolonged use can potentiate warfarin *BNF* 4.7.1.

Paroxetine selective serotonin re-uptake inhibitor *Dose* 20–40mg/24h PO (max 50–60/24h) *Indication* major depression, obsessive-compulsive disorder, panic disorder, post-traumatic stress disorder *Caution* pregnancy, epilepsy, cardiac disease, DM *SE* GI disturbance, anorexia, weight loss, ↓Na^+, agitation; increased incidence of antimuscarinic, extrapyramidal and withdrawal effects compared with fluoxetine *BNF* 4.3.3.

Penicillin G beta-lactam see benzylpenicillin.

Penicillin V beta-lactam see phenoxymethylpenicillin.

Pentasa® **aminosalicylate** see mesalazine.

Peppermint oil antispasmodic *Dose* 1–2 capsules/8h PO before meals *Indication* abdominal colic and distension especially in IBS *Caution* sensitivity to menthol *SE* heartburn, perianal irritation *BNF* 1.2.

Perindopril see ACEi.

Pethidine opioid *Dose* 25–100mg/4h SC/IM; 25–50mg/4h slow IV *Indication* pain; moderate to severe, obstetric, post-op *CI* acute respiratory depression, paralytic ileus, raised ICP/head trauma, comatose patients *Caution* pregnancy (especially delivery), COPD, asthma, arrhythmias, renal impairment, hepatic impairment *SE* N+V, less constipation than morphine, respiratory depression, dry mouth *BNF* 4.7.2.

Phenobarbital barbiturate Dose <u>epilepsy (not 1st line):</u> 60–180mg/24h PO at night; <u>status epilepticus:</u> 10mg/kg at max 100mg/min (max 1g) IV (see **BNF** 4.8.2) **Indication** epilepsy, status epilepticus **CI** pregnancy, breastfeeding, hepatic impairment **Caution** renal impairment, acute porphyria **SE** respiratory depression, hypotension, sedation **BNF** 4.8.1.

Monitoring phenobarbital	*Trough* 60–180micromol/l (15–40mg/l); *toxic* >180micromol/l (>40mg/l)

Phenoxymethylepenicillin (penicillin V) beta-lactam Dose 0.5–1g/6h PO **Indication** oral infections, post-splenectomy (prophylaxis) **CI** penicillin allergy **Caution** history of allergy **SE** diarrhoea **Interaction** decrease effects of oral contraceptive pill, allopurinol increases risk of rash **BNF** 5.1.1.1.

Phenytoin antiepileptic Dose <u>epilepsy:</u> 3–4mg/kg/24h PO increased gradually as necessary; <u>status epilepticus:</u> loading dose = 20mg/kg IV at no more than 50mg/min with ECG monitoring, maintenance = 100mg/6–8h thereafter IV (see **BNF** 4.8.2); monitor level (see box) **Indication** epilepsy, status epilepticus **CI** pregnancy, breastfeeding, sinus hypotension **Caution** hepatic impairment, avoid abrupt withdrawal, acute porphyria; monitor blood count **SE** drowsiness, cerebellar effects, hypotension, arrhythmias, purple glove syndrome, blood disorders; <u>chronic use:</u> coarse facies, hirsutism, gum hypertrophy **Info** as drug highly protein bound, may need to adjust monitored levels for low albumin (consult pharmacist) **BNF** 4.8.1.

Monitoring phenytoin	*Trough* 40–80micromol/l (10–20mg/l); *toxic* >80micromol/l (>20mg/l); *signs of toxicity* ataxia, nystagmus, dysarthria, diplopia

Phosphate enema see laxatives.

Phytomenadione vitamin K₁ Dose 1–10mg/STAT PO/IV depending upon indication—consult *BNF* and/or d/w haematologist **Indication** bleeding and/or over-anticoagulation with warfarin **Caution** pregnancy, give IV slowly **BNF** 9.6.6.

Picolax® see laxatives.

Piperacillin with tazobactam beta-lactam with tazobactam Dose 4.5g/6–8h IV **Indication** severe infection, infection in neutropenic patients (in combination with aminoglycoside) **CI** penicillin allergy **Caution** pregnancy, breastfeeding, renal impairment, history of penicillin allergy **SE** diarrhoea **BNF** 5.1.1.4.

Piriton® antihistamine (H₁-antagonist) see chlorphenamine.

Plavix® antiplatelet see clopidogrel.

Potassium oral supplement potassium salt *Dose* potassium chloride: 2–4g/24h PO (two tablets/8–12h) *Indication* potassium loss *CI* serum potassium >5mmol/l *Caution* renal impairment, elderly, intestinal strictures, history of peptic ulcer *SE* GI disturbance, upper GI ulceration *Info* check serum Mg^{2+} as this is also likely to be low in $\downarrow K^+$ *BNF* 9.2.1.1.

Pravastatin HMG CoA reductase inhibitor see statin.

Prednisolone corticosteroid *Dose* <u>initially:</u> 10–20mg/24h mane PO though often 30–40mg/24 PO in severe disease (up to 60mg/24h); <u>maintenance:</u> 2.5–15mg/24h PO *Indication* suppression of inflammatory and allergic disorders (eg IBD, asthma, COPD), immunosuppression *CI* systemic infection without antibiotic cover *Caution* adrenal suppression *SE* peptic ulceration, Cushing's syndrome, DM, osteoporosis *Interaction* duration of action decreased by rifampicin, carbamazepine, phenytoin; duration of action increased by erythromycin, ketoconazole, ciclosporin *Info* consider bone and GI protection strategies when using long-term corticosteroids; see 📖 p177 *BNF* 6.3.2.

Pregabalin antiepileptic *Dose* <u>epilepsy:</u> 25mg/12h PO increased every 7d by 50mg to 100–150mg/8–12h (max 600mg/24h in divided doses) <u>pain/anxiety:</u> 75mg/12h increased every 3–7d up to max 600mg/24h in divided doses *Indication* epilepsy, neuropathic pain, generalised anxiety disorder *CI* pregnancy, breastfeeding *Caution* renal impairment, severe congestive heart failure, avoid abrupt withdrawal *SE* GI disturbance, dry mouth, dizziness, drowsiness *BNF* 4.8.1.

Prochlorperazine phenothiazine see antiemetics.

Procyclidine anticholinergic *Dose* 2.5mg/8h PO increased every 3d up to max 30mg/24h in divided doses; <u>acute dystonia:</u> 5–10mg IM/IV *Indication* parkinsonism; drug-induced extrapyramidal symptoms *CI* urinary retention, glaucoma, myasthenia gravis *Caution* pregnancy, breastfeeding, hepatic or renal impairment, cardiovascular disease, prostatic hyperplasia, tardive dyskinesia *SE* antimuscarinic effects *BNF* 4.9.2.

Propranolol see beta-blockers.

Protamine heparin antagonist *Dose* 1mg IV neutralises 80–100units heparin IV in last 15min (max 50mg at rate <5mg/min); 1mg IV neutralises 100units heparin SC (max 50mg at rate <5mg/min) *Indication* heparin OD, bleeding in patient on heparin therapy *Caution* risk of allergy increased post-vasectomy, or in infertile men, fish allergy *SE* GI disturbance, flushing, hypotension, dyspnoea *Info* Protamine can also be used to help reverse the effects of LMWH but it is much less effective at this than for heparin *BNF* 2.8.3.

Prozac® **selective serotonin re-uptake inhibitor** see fluoxetine.

Pulmicort® **corticosteroid** see budesonide.

Quinine plant alkaloid *Dose* <u>nocturnal leg cramps</u> 200–300mg/24h (nocte) PO; <u>treatment of malaria</u> see *BNF* 5.4.1 *Indication* nocturnal leg cramps, treatment and prophylaxis of malaria *CI* haemoglobinuria, myasthenia gravis, optic neuritis, tinnitus *Caution* pregnancy (teratogenic in 1st trimester), breastfeeding, hepatic or renal impairment, cardiac disease (AF, conduction defects, heart block), elderly, G6PD deficiency *SE* cinchonism (tinnitus, headache, hot and flushed skin, nausea, abdominal pain, rashes, visual disturbances (including temporary blindness), confusion), acute renal failure, photosensitivity *BNF* 5.4.1 and 10.2.2.

Ramipril see ACEi.

Ranitidine antihistamine (H_2-antagonist) *Dose* 150mg/12h PO; IV preparation available (see *BNF*) *Indication* peptic ulcers, GORD *Caution* pregnancy, breastfeeding, renal impairment, acute porphyria, may mask symptoms of gastric cancer *SE* GI upset, confusion, fatigue *BNF* 1.3.1.

Reteplase plasminogen activator see fibrinolytic.

Rifampicin antibiotic *Dose* <u>tuberculosis:</u> consult *BNF*; <u>meningitis prophylaxis:</u> 600mg/12h PO for 2d; <u>other serious infections:</u> 600mg/12h IV (usually after microbiology advice) *Indication* tuberculosis, *N. meningitidis*/*H. influenza* meningitis prophylaxis, serious staphylococcal infections *CI* jaundice *Caution* pregnancy, hepatic or renal impairment, alcohol dependence, acute porphyria *SE* GI disturbance, headache, drowsiness, hepatotoxicity, turns body secretions orange *Interaction* induces p450, decreases effects of warfarin *BNF* 5.1.9.

Rosuvastatin HMG CoA reductase inhibitor see statin.

(r)tPA plasminogen activator see fibrinolytic.

Salbutamol β_2 agonist *Dose* <u>chronic airways disease</u> 100–200micrograms aerosol/200–400micrograms powder INH PRN (max 400–800micrograms/24h in divided doses); 2.5–5mg/4h NEB; <u>status asthmaticus</u> 2.5–5mg/PRN NEB; 250micrograms/STAT (diluted to 50micrograms/ml) slow IV, followed by maintenance infusion of 3–20micrograms/min (3–24ml/h of the 50micrograms/ml solution), titrated to heart-rate *Indication* asthma; chronic and acute, other reversible airway obstruction eg COPD, ↑K^+ *Caution* cardiovascular disease, DM, hyperthyroidism *SE* fine tremor, nervous tension, headache, palpitation, muscle cramps *BNF* 3.1.1.1.

Salmeterol long-acting β_2 agonist *Dose* 50–100micrograms/12h INH *Indication* chronic asthma, reversible airway obstruction *Caution* cardiovascular disease, DM, hyperthyroidism *SE* fine tremor, nervous tension, headache, palpitation, muscle cramps *BNF* 3.1.1.1.

Sando-K® potassium salt see potassium oral supplement.

Senna see laxatives.

Seretide® long-acting β_2 agonist with corticosteroid *Dose* 25–50micrograms salmeterol with 50–500micrograms fluticasone/12–24h INH (depends upon inhaler device, see *BNF*) *Indication* asthma (see 📖 p273) *Caution* cardiovascular disease, DM, hyperthyroidism, TB *SE* fine tremor, nervous tension, headache, palpitation, muscle cramps, oral candidiasis, hoarse voice, paradoxical bronchospasm (rare) *Interaction* see salmeterol and fluticasone *BNF* 3.2.

Sertraline selective serotonin re-uptake inhibitors *Dose* 50mg/24h PO increased by 50mg increments at intervals of at least 1wk until desired effect (max 200mg/24h) *Indication* depression, OCD, panic disorder *CI* hepatic or renal impairment, active mania *Caution* pregnancy, epilepsy, cardiac disease, DM *SE* GI disturbance, anorexia, weight loss *Interaction* MAOI within 2wk, inhibits p450 enzymes *BNF* 4.3.3.

Sevredol® opioid see oral morphine.

Simvastatin HMG CoA reductase inhibitor see statin.

Slow-K® potassium salt see potassium oral supplement.

Sodium valproate antiepileptic see valproate.

Sotalol see beta-blockers.

Spironolactone potassium-sparing diuretic (aldosterone antagonist) *Dose* 100–200mg/24h PO (max 400mg/24h) *Indication* oedema/ascites in cirrhosis/malignancy, nephritic syndrome, congestive heart failure *CI* pregnancy, breastfeeding, hyperkalaemia, hyponatraemia, Addison's disease *Caution* renal impairment, porphyria *SE* GI disturbance, impotence, gynaecomastia, menstrual irregularities *Interaction* increases digoxin and lithium levels; risk of ↑K^+ when used with ACEi or AT II receptor antagonists *BNF* 2.2.3.

Statins HMG CoA reductase inhibitor *Dose* see Table 5.18 *Indications* dyslipidaemias, primary and secondary prevention of cardiovascular disease (irrespective of serum cholesterol) *Caution* pregnancy, breastfeeding, hypothyroidism, hepatic impairment, high alcohol intake, *SE* myalgia, myositis (in severe cases rhabdomyolysis), GI disturbance, pancreatitis, altered LFTs (rarely hepatitis/jaundice) *Interaction* avoid concomitant use of macrolide antibiotics and amiodarone (possible increased risk of myopathy) *BNF* 2.12.

Table 5.18 Statins *BNF* 2.12

Atorvastatin	*Dose* initially 10mg/24h PO up to max 80mg/24h PO
Fluvastatin	*Dose* initially 20mg/24h PO up to max 80mg/24h PO
Pravastatin	*Dose* initially 10mg/24h PO up to max 40mg/24h PO
Rosuvastatin	*Dose* initially 5mg/24h PO up to max 40mg/24h PO
Simvastatin	*Dose* initially 10mg/24h PO up to max 80mg/24h PO

Stemetil® phenothiazine see antiemetic.

Streptokinase plasminogen activator see fibrinolytic.

Sulfasalazine aminosalicylate Dose <u>Maintenance:</u> 500mg/6h PO; <u>Acute:</u> 1–2g/6h PO until remission; PR preparations also available **Indication** rheumatoid arthritis, ulcerative colitis, Crohn's disease **CI** sulfonamide sensitivity **Caution** pregnancy, breastfeeding, renal impairment, G6DP deficiency **SE** GI disturbance, blood disorders, hepatotoxicity, discoloured bodily fluids **BNF** 1.5.1.

Sulphonylureas Dose see Table 5.19 **Indications** type 2 DM **CI** ketoacidosis **Caution** pregnancy, breastfeeding, hepatic or renal impairment, porphyria; should not be first-line agents in obese patients as will encourage further weight gain **SE** N+V, diarrhoea, constipation, hyponatraemia, hypoglycaemia, hepatic dysfunction, weight gain **Info** hypoglycaemia resulting from sulphonylureas can persist for many hours and must always be treated in hospital; sulphonylureas should not be given on the day of surgery due to the risk of hypoglycaemia **BNF** 6.1.2.1.

Table 5.19 *Sulphonylureas* **BNF** *6.1.2.1*

Glibenclamide	**Dose 5mg** (2.5–15mg) 24h PO mane **Info** long acting; use cautiously in the elderly
Gliclazide	**Dose 40–80mg** (40–160mg) usually 24h PO mane (max 320mg) **Info** medium acting
Glipizide	**Dose 2.5–5mg** (2.5–15mg) usually 24h PO mane (max 20mg) **Info** short acting
Tolbutamide	**Dose 0.5–1.5g** (0.5–2g) divided throughout the day PO with meals **Info** medium acting

Symbicort® long-acting β₂ agonist with corticosteroid Dose 6–12micrograms formoterol with 100–400micrograms budesonide/12–24h INH (depends upon inhaler device, see *BNF*) **Indication** asthma (see 📖 p273), COPD **Caution** cardiovascular disease, DM, hyperthyroidism, TB **SE** fine tremor, nervous tension, headache, palpitation, muscle cramps, oral candidiasis, hoarse voice, paradoxical bronchospasm (rare) **Interaction** see salmeterol and fluticasone **BNF** 3.2.

Synacthen® synthetic corticotrophin (ACTH) see tetracosactide.

Tamiflu® antiviral see oseltamivir.

Tamoxifen oestrogen receptor antagonist Dose <u>breast cancer</u> 20mg/24h PO; for other indications consult *BNF* **Indication** oestrogen receptor-positive breast cancer, anovulatory infertility **CI** pregnancy **Caution** breastfeeding, increased risk of thromboembolism, occasional cystic ovarian swellings in pre-menopausal women **SE** hot flushes, vaginal discharge/bleeding, menstrual suppression, GI disturbance **Interaction** increases effects of warfarin **BNF** 8.3.4.1.

Tamsulosin α_1 **antagonist** *Dose* 400micrograms/24h PO *Indication* benign prostatic hyperplasia *CI* breastfeeding, hypotension, hepatic impairment *Caution* renal impairment *SE* postural hypotension, headache, dizziness, urinary incontinence *Interaction* increases effects of antihypertensives *BNF* 7.4.1.

Tazocin® **beta-lactam with tazobactam** see piperacillin.

Tegretol® **antiepileptic** see carbamazepine.

Teicoplanin glycopeptide antibiotic see vancomycin.

Temazepam benzodiazepine *Dose* 10–20mg/24h PO at bedtime or pre-operative; dependency common (max 4wk course) *Indication* insomnia, pre-operative anxiety *CI* respiratory depression, sleep apnoea, unstable myasthenia gravis, hepatic impairment *Caution* pregnancy, breastfeeding, history of drug abuse, respiratory disease, muscle weakness, renal impairment *SE* drowsiness, confusion, muscle weakness *BNF* 4.1.1/15.1.4.1.

Tenecteplase plasminogen activator see fibrinolytic.

Terbutaline β_2 **agonist** *Dose* 500micrograms/6h INH; 5–10mg/6–12h NEB; oral preparations are also available, consult *BNF* *Indication* asthma and other reversible airway obstruction *Caution* cardiovascular disease, DM, hyperthyroidism *SE* fine tremor, nervous tension, headache, palpitation, muscle cramps *BNF* 3.1.1.1.

Tetanus vaccine and immunoglobulin see 📖 p437.

Tetracosactide (Synacthen®) synthetic corticotrophin (ACTH) *Dose* 250micrograms IV/IM *Indication* diagnosis of Addison's disease *Caution* pregnancy, breastfeeding, allergic disorders *SE* Cushing's syndrome, DM, osteoporosis *Info* blood should be sampled for cortisol pre-dose and again at 30min post Synacthen® dose (consultant local guidelines) *BNF* 6.5.1.

Tetracycline tetracycline antibiotic *Dose* 250–500mg/6h PO *Indication* infection, acne vulgaris *CI* pregnancy, breastfeeding, renal impairment, age <12y (irreversibly stains growing teeth and bones) *Caution* myasthenia gravis may worsen, exacerbates SLE *SE* GI disturbance including, dysphagia/oesophageal irritation *Interaction* decreased absorption with milk, decreases effects of oral contraceptive pill, mildly increases effects of warfarin *BNF* 5.1.3.

Theophylline methylxanthine Dose 200–500mg/12h PO (depending upon preparation, consult *BNF*) **Indication** severe asthma/COPD (see BTS guidelines) **CI** acute porphyria **Caution** cardiac disease, epilepsy, hyperthyroidism, peptic ulcer disease **SE** tachycardia, palpitation, GI disturbance **Info** theophylline is only available as an oral preparation; aminophylline consists of theophylline and ethylenediamine which simply improves the drug's solubility allowing IV administration **BNF** 3.1.3.

Monitoring theophylline	Toxic >20mg/l (>110micromol/l); signs of toxicity arrhythmia, anxiety, tremor, convulsions (OHAM3 □ p731)

Thiamine vitamin B$_1$ Dose <u>oral</u> 25–100mg/24h or 200–300mg/24h PO depending on severity (consult *BNF*); <u>parenteral</u> 2–3 pairs of ampoules/8h IV (Pabrinex®) (consult local guidelines) **Indication** nutritional deficiency, especially alcoholism **Caution** reports of anaphylaxis with parenteral preparations **BNF** 9.6.2.

Thyroxine thyroid hormone (T$_4$) see levothyroxine.

Tinzaparin low-molecular-weight heparin Dose depends upon indication, consult *BNF* **Indication** DVT/PE prophylaxis and treatment **CI** breastfeeding, bleeding disorders, thrombocytopenia, severe hypertension, recent trauma **Caution** hyperkalaemia, hepatic or renal impairment **SE** haemorrhage, thrombocytopenia, hyperkalaemia **Interaction** NSAIDs increase bleeding risk, effects increased by GTN **BNF** 2.8.1.

Tiotropium antimuscarinic (anti-M$_3$) Dose 18micrograms/24h INH; solution for inhalation also available (see *BNF*) **Indication** maintenance treatment of COPD **Caution** renal impairment, glaucoma, prostatic hypertrophy, cardiac rhythm disorders **SE** minimal antimuscarinic effects **BNF** 3.1.2.

Tirofiban glycoprotein IIb/IIIa inhibitor Dose <u>initially:</u> 400nanograms/kg/min for 30min IV <u>then:</u> 100nanograms/kg/min IV for at least 48h (max 108h treatment) **Indication** prevention of MI in unstable angina/NSTEMI patients **CI** breastfeeding, abnormal bleeding/cerebrovascular accident within 30d, history of haemorrhagic stroke, severe hypertension, intracranial disease **Caution** pregnancy, hepatic or renal impairment, increased risk of bleeding, surgery or major trauma within 3mth **SE** bleeding, reversible thrombocytopenia **BNF** 2.9.

Topical corticosteroids *Dose* consult *BNF*; guidance on applying topical steroids can be found on 📖 p178 *Indications* inflammatory conditions of the skin, eg eczema, contact dermatitis amongst others *CI* untreated bacterial, fungal, or viral skin lesions, rosacea, perioral dermatitis, widespread plaque psoriasis *Caution* use lowest potency agent possible (Table 5.20) for shortest duration of time to limit side effects *SE* local thinning of the skin, worsening local infection, striae and telangiectasia, acne, depigmentation, hypertrichosis; systemic rarely adrenal suppression, Cushing's syndrome *Info* topical steroids should only be commenced after seeking specialist advice (either following a dermatology review or after consideration by registrar). The decision to stop potent topical steroids should be taken as seriously – always be mindful of the potential for a patient to develop an Addison crisis after stopping long-term potent topical steroids *BNF* 13.4.

Table 5.20 *Topical corticosteroid potencies* **BNF 13.4**

Potency	Examples
Mild	Hydrocortisone 0.1–2.5%, Dioderm®, Mildison®, Synalar 1 in 10 dilution®
Moderately potent	Betnovate-RD®, Eumovate®, Haelan®, Modrasone®, Synalar 1 in 4 dilution®, Ultralanum Plain®
Potent	Beclometasone dipropionate 0.025%, Betamethasone valerate 0.1%, Betacap®, Betesil®, Bettamousse®, Betnovate®, Cutivate®, Diprosone®, Elocon®, hydrocortisone butyrate, Locoid®, Locoid Crelo®, Metosyn®, Nerisone®, Synalar®
Very potent	Clarelux®, Dermovate®, Etrivex®, Nerisone Forte®

Tramadol opioid *Dose* 50–100mg/4h PO/IM/IV (max 600mg/24h in divided doses) *Indication* pain *CI* acute respiratory depression, paralytic ileus, raised ICP/head trauma, comatose patients, acute porphyria, uncontrolled epilepsy *Caution* pregnancy (especially delivery), breastfeeding, COPD, asthma, arrhythmias, hepatic or renal impairment *SE* N+V constipation, respiratory depression, dry mouth *Interaction* MAOI within 2wk *Info* co-prescribe laxatives if using opioids for >24h *BNF* 4.7.2.

Trimethoprim antibiotic *Dose* acute infection: 200mg/12h PO; prophylaxis: 100mg/24h PO at night *Indication* urinary tract infections *CI* blood dyscrasias *Caution* pregnancy, breastfeeding, renal impairment, folate deficiency *SE* GI disturbance, rash, hyperkalaemia *Interaction* increases phenytoin levels, increases risk of arrhythmias with amiodarone *BNF* 5.1.8.

Valproate antiepileptic Dose 300mg/12h PO increasing by 200mg every 3d (max 2.5g/24h in divided doses) **Indication** epilepsy: all forms **CI** family history of hepatic dysfunction, acute porphyria **Caution** pregnancy, breastfeeding, hepatic or renal impairment, blood disorders (bleeding risk), SLE, pancreatitis **SE** GI disturbance, sedation, headache, cerebellar effects, hepatotoxicity, blood disorders **Interaction** effects decreased by antimalarials, antidepressants, antipsychotics and antiepileptics **BNF** 4.8.1.

Monitoring valproate	*Trough* 350–700micromol/l (50–100mg/l); *toxic* >1260micromol/l (>180mg/l)

Valsartan see **AT II antagonists**.

Vancomycin glycopeptide antibiotic Dose 125mg/6h PO; 1–1.5g/12h IV; some centres use continuous infusions of vancomycin (consult local guidelines) **Indication** serious Gram +ve infections: endocarditis, MRSA, antibiotic associated colitis **Caution** pregnancy, breastfeeding, renal impairment, avoid rapid infusion, history of deafness, inflammatory bowel disease **SE** nephrotoxicity, ototoxicity, blood disorders, rash (red man syndrome) **Interaction** increased nephrotoxicity with ciclosporin, increased ototoxicity with loop diuretics **BNF** 5.1.7.

Monitoring vancomycin	Usually before 3rd or 4th dose (check local guidelines) *trough* 10–15mg/l; *toxicity* can occur within therapeutic range

Venlafaxine serotonin and noradrenaline re-uptake inhibitor Dose initially 37.5mg/12h, increase if necessary at intervals of >2wks to 75mg/12h (max 375mg per 24h) **Indication** major depression, generalised anxiety disorder **CI** breastfeeding, high risk of cardiac arrhythmia, uncontrolled hypertension **Caution** pregnancy, hepatic or renal impairment, heart disease, epilepsy, history of mania, glaucoma **SE** GI disturbance, hypertension, palpitation, dizziness, drowsiness **Interaction** MAOIs within 2wk, increased risk of bleeding with aspirin/NSAIDs, CNS toxicity with selegiline, mildly increases effects of warfarin **BNF** 4.3.4.

Ventolin® β_2 **agonist** see salbutamol.

Verapamil see **calcium-channel blockers**.

Vitamin K see **phytomenadione**.

Warfarin coumarin Dose <u>loading:</u> see 📖 p407; <u>maintenance:</u> typically 1–5mg/24h PO dictated by the patient's INR (though higher doses and dosing on alternative days are not uncommon) **Indication** prophylaxis of thromboembolism (atrial fibrillation, mechanical heart valves etc), treatment of venous thrombosis or pulmonary embolism **CI** pregnancy, peptic ulcers, severe hypertension, bacterial endocarditis **Caution** breastfeeding, hepatic or renal impairment, conditions in which risk of bleeding is increased (eg GI bleeding, peptic ulcer, recent surgery, recent ischaemic stroke, postpartum, bacterial endocarditis), uncontrolled hypertension recent **SE** haemorrhage, rash, alopecia **Interaction** avoid cranberry juice (↑anticoagulant effect) **Info** warfarin is available in tablets of 0.5mg (white), 1mg (brown), 3mg (blue), and 5mg (pink) but check which tablets are stocked locally **BNF** 2.8.2.

Zolpidem non-benzodiazepine hypnotic Dose 10mg/24h PO at night **Indication** short-term treatment of insomnia **CI** breastfeeding, severe hepatic impairment, psychotic illness, neuromuscular respiratory weakness, unstable myasthenia gravis, respiratory failure, sleep apnoea **Caution** pregnancy, hepatic or renal impairment, muscle weakness, history of drug abuse **SE** taste disturbance, GI disturbance, headache **BNF** 4.1.1.

Zopiclone non-benzodiazepine hypnotic Dose 3.75–7.5mg/24h PO at night **Indication** short-term treatment of insomnia **CI** breastfeeding, severe hepatic impairment, neuromuscular respiratory weakness, unstable myasthenia gravis, respiratory failure, sleep apnoea **Caution** pregnancy, hepatic or renal impairment, muscle weakness, history of drug abuse **SE** taste disturbance, GI disturbance, headache **BNF** 4.1.1.

Zoton® **proton pump inhibitor** see lansoprazole.

Zyban® **treatment of nicotine dependence** see bupropion.

Chapter 6

Resuscitation

Early warning scores

Early detection of the 'unwell' patient has repeatedly been shown to improve outcome. Identification of such patients allows suitable changes in management, including early involvement of critical care teams or transfer to critical care areas (HDU/ICU) where necessary.

Identification of the 'at-risk' patient relies on measurement of simple physiological parameters, which generally deteriorate as the patient becomes more unwell; these include RR, HR, BP, O_2 saturation, level of consciousness, and temp. Remember that the sick patient might not always look that unwell from the bottom of the bed.

Scoring of these parameters can be carried out in many ways and is usually undertaken by nursing staff. Considerable variation still exists in the format of scoring systems in use in individual hospitals, and in the actions that are triggered when certain thresholds are reached. A national project to standardise these approaches into a single 'National Early Warning Score' (NEWS) is being led by the Royal College of Physicians.[1] Their scoring system is shown in Table 6.1. Normal observations are awarded a score of 0, whilst abnormal observations attract higher scores. The values for each physiological parameter are added together. If this total score reaches a 'threshold' value (≥5, or any individual parameter scoring 3), the nursing staff should increase frequency of observations and alert a doctor to review the patient, depending on local policy/guidelines.

Trends in physiological parameters are often more useful than one-off observations. Some patients may have abnormal scores even when they seem relatively 'well' because of compensatory mechanisms. For these patients, higher thresholds may be agreed by senior doctors, but bear in mind that they are also likely to deteriorate much more quickly.

Patients who should be monitored by such scores include:
- Emergency admissions
- Unstable patients
- Elderly patients
- Patients with pre-existing disease (cardiovascular, respiratory, DM)
- Patients who are failing to respond to treatment
- Patients who have returned from ICU/HDU
- Post-operative patients.

ALERT™

Acute Life-threatening Events: Recognition and Treatment
This is an evolving course that aims to guide people in early recognition of the unwell patient and in their immediate resuscitation. This course complements the Immediate Life Support (ILS) and Advanced Life Support (ALS) courses (📖 p228). Further information can be found at ⌁www.alert-course.com

---

[1] ⌁www.rcplondon.ac.uk/resources/national-early-warning-score-news See also NICE guidelines at ⌁guidance.nice.org.uk/CG50

PHYSIOLOGICAL PARAMETERS	3	2	1	0	1	2	3
Respiration Rate	≤8		9 - 11	12 - 20		21 - 24	≥25
Oxygen Saturations	≤91	92 - 93	94 - 95	≥96			
Any Supplemental Oxygen		Yes		No			
Temperature	≤35.0		35.1 - 36.0	36.1 - 38.0	38.1 - 39.0	≥39.1	
Systolic BP	≤90	91 - 100	101 - 110	111 - 219			≥220
Heart Rate	≤40		41 - 50	51 - 90	91 - 110	111 - 130	≥131
Level of Consciousness				A			V, P, or U

ᵃThe NEWS initiative flowed from the Royal College of Physicians' NEWSDIG, and was jointly developed and funded in collaboration with the Royal College of Physicians, Royal College of Nursing, National Outreach Forum and NHS Training for Innovation.

Table 6.1 National Early Warning Score (NEWS). A total score ≥5, or any individual parameter scoring 3 should prompt urgent review by a doctor. Reproduced from Royal College of Physicians. *National Early Warning Score (NEWS): Standardising the assessment of acute-illness severity in the NHS. Report of a working party.* London: RCP, 2012.

Peri-arrest

Airway	Check airway is patent; consider manoeuvres/adjuncts with C-spine control in trauma
Breathing	If no respiratory effort – **CALL ARREST TEAM**
Circulation	If no palpable pulse – **CALL ARREST TEAM**
Disability	If GCS ≤8 – **CALL ANAESTHETIST**

Airway – if irreversibly obstructed CALL ARREST TEAM
- **Look** inside the mouth, remove obvious objects/dentures
- Wide-bore suction under direct vision if secretions present
- **Listen** airway impaired if stridor, snoring, gurgling or no air entry
- Jaw thrust/head tilt/chin lift with cervical spine control in trauma
- **Oropharyngeal** or **nasopharyngeal** airway as tolerated
- If still impaired **CALL ARREST TEAM**.

Breathing – if poor or absent respiratory effort CALL ARREST TEAM
- **Look** for chest expansion (does R = L?), fogging of mask
- **Listen** to chest for air entry (does R = L?)
- **Feel** for expansion and percussion (does R = L?)
- **Non-rebreather** (trauma) mask and 15l/min O_2 initially in all patients
- **Bag** and mask if poor or absent breathing effort
- **Monitor** O_2 sats and RR
- **Think** tension pneumothorax.

Circulation – if no pulse CALL ARREST TEAM
- **Look** for pallor, cyanosis, distended neck veins
- **Feel** for a central pulse (carotid/femoral) – rate and rhythm
- **Monitor** defibrillator ECG leads and BP
- **Venous access**, send bloods if time allows
- **12-lead ECG**
- Call for **senior help** early if patient deteriorating.

Disability – if GCS ≤8 or falling CALL ANAESTHETIST
- Assess **GCS** (📖 p338) and check glucose
- **Look** for pupil reflexes and unusual posture
- **Feel** for tone in all four limbs and plantar reflexes.

Exposure
- **Remove** all clothing, check temp
- **Look** all over body including perineum and back for rash or injuries
- **Cover** patient with a blanket.

Common causes			
Arrhythmia	📖 p248	Hypoxia	📖 p271
Myocardial infarction	📖 p244	Pulmonary oedema	📖 p272
Hypovolaemia	📖 p379	Pulmonary embolism	📖 p278
Sepsis (UTI/pneumonia)	📖 p480	Metabolic (↑↓K^+)	📖 p384
Hypoglycaemia	📖 p322	(Tension) pneumothorax	📖 p279

In-hospital resuscitation

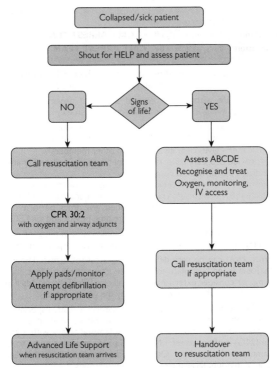

Fig. 6.1 In-hospital resuscitation algorithm; 2010 guidelines.
Reproduced with the kind permission of the Resuscitation Council (UK).

Signs of life	
Regular respiratory effort	Purposeful movement
Coughing	Speaking
Opening eyes	

Advanced Life Support (ALS)

Airway	Check airway is patent; consider manoeuvres/adjuncts with C-spine control in trauma
Breathing	If no respiratory effort – **CALL ARREST TEAM**
Circulation	If no palpable pulse – **CALL ARREST TEAM**

Basic life support should be initiated and the cardiac arrest team called as soon as cardiac or respiratory arrest is identified.

Advanced life support is centred around a 'universal algorithm' (Fig. 6.2) which is taught on a standardised course offered by most hospitals.

The cardiac arrest team usually consists of a team leader (medical StR), F1, anaesthetist, CCU nurse and senior hospital nurse:

- Team leader – gives clear instructions to other members
- F1 – provide BLS, cannulate, take arterial blood, defibrillate if trained, give drugs, perform chest compressions
- Anaesthetist – airway and breathing, they may choose to bag-and-mask ventilate the patient, insert a laryngeal mask or intubate (📖 p542)
- Nurses – provide BLS, defibrillate if trained, give drugs, perform chest compressions, record observations, note time points, and take ECGs.

Needle-stick injuries (📖 p106) are commonest in times of emergency. Have the sharps box nearby and never leave sharps on the bed.

Cannulation can be very difficult during a cardiac arrest. The antecubital fossa is the best place to look first; alternatively try feet, hands, forearms, or consider external jugular if all else fails. Take bloods if you are successful, but don't allow this to delay the giving of drugs.

Blood tests are occasionally useful in cardiac arrests, especially K^+ which can often be measured by arterial blood gas machines. Use a blood gas syringe to obtain a sample (the femoral artery with a green needle (21G) is often easiest – NAVY, 📖 p516) and ask a nurse to take the sample to the machine. Other blood tests depend on the clinical scenario; if in doubt fill all the common blood bottles.

Defibrillation is taught on specific courses (eg ILS, ALS) and must not be undertaken unless trained. The use of automated external defibrillators or AEDs (📖 p532) is becoming routine.

Cardiac arrest drugs are now prepared in pre-filled syringes: adrenaline (epinephrine) 1mg in 10ml (1:10,000), atropine (several preparations available), amiodarone 300mg in 10ml. Always give a large flush (20ml saline) after each dose to encourage it into the central circulation. See 📖 inside back cover for further emergency drug doses.

Cardiac arrest trolleys are found in most areas of the hospital. Know where they are for your wards. Ask the ward sister if you can open the trolley and have a good look at the equipment within it as they differ between hospitals. They are often arranged so the top drawer contains Airway equipment, the second contains Breathing equipment, the third contains Circulation equipment and the lower drawer contains the drugs and fluids. You'll seldom need anything that isn't on the trolley.

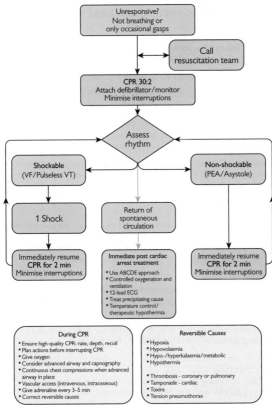

Fig. 6.2 Adult Advanced Life Support algorithm; 2010 guidelines.
Reproduced with the kind permission of the Resuscitation Council (UK).

Arrest equipment and tests

Airway

Jaw thrust Pull the jaw forward with your index and middle fingers at the angle of each mandible. Pull hard enough to make your fingers ache.

Head tilt Gently extend the neck, avoid if C-spine injury risk.

Chin lift Pull the chin up with two fingers, avoid if C-spine injury risk.

Oropharyngeal airway (Guedel) A rigid, curved plastic tube; choose the size that reaches the angle of the mouth from the tragus of the ear. Insert upside down to avoid pushing the tongue back, then rotate 180° when inside the mouth (do not insert upside down in children).

Nasopharyngeal airway A flexible, curved plastic tube, not to be used with significant head injury. Choose the size that will easily pass through the nose (size 6–7mm in most adults); insert by lubricating and pushing horizontally into the patient's nostril (not upwards). Use a safety pin through the end to prevent the tube being lost.

Suction Cover the hole on the side of a wide-bore suction catheter to cause suction at the tip. Secretions in the parts of the oropharynx that can be seen directly can be cleared. A thinner catheter can be used to clear secretions in the airway of an intubated patient.

Breathing

Non-rebreather mask (trauma mask) A plastic mask with a floppy bag attached; used in acutely ill patients to give ~80% O_2 with a 15l/min flow rate.

Standard mask (Hudson mask) A plastic mask that connects directly to O_2 tubing; delivers ~50% O_2 with a 15l/min flow rate.

Venturi A mask that connects to the O_2 tubing via a piece of coloured plastic, delivering either 24%, 28%, 35%, 40%, or 60% O_2. Adjust the flow rate according to the instructions on the coloured plastic connector, eg 4l/min with the 28% Venturi connection.

Bag and mask (Ambu bag) A self-inflating bag and valve that allows you to force O_2 into an inadequately ventilating patient. Attach the O_2 tubing to the bag with a 15l/min flow rate then seal the mask over the patient's nose and mouth. Easiest with two people; one person stands at the head to get a firm seal with both hands whilst the other squeezes the bag. The mask can be removed to attach the bag to an ETT or LMA (📖 p544).

Pulse oximeter Plastic clip with a red light that measures blood O_2 saturations. Clip onto the patient's index finger. Do not rely on the reading unless there is an even trace on the monitor and the patient has a pulse; use on the different arm from the BP cuff.

Nebuliser This is a 3cm-high cylinder that attaches beneath a mask. The cylinder is made of two halves that can be untwisted so that the fluid to be nebulised can be inserted. The nebuliser can be connected to a pump or directly to an O_2 or medical air supply.

Circulation

Defibrillation (📖 p532) Successful defibrillation requires ECG monitoring to identify a shockable rhythm, and delivery of current through electrodes attached to the chest wall. Previously, monitoring was performed using ECG leads: red to right shoulder, yellow to left shoulder and green to apex (📖 p528). Separate paddles were applied to deliver current. Most NHS trusts now use hands-free adhesive defibrillation electrodes which are safer and also double as monitoring leads (📖 p533).

Only defibrillate if you have been trained:

- Check the adhesive electrodes are correctly applied to the chest
- Switch the defibrillator to 'monitor' mode
- If a shockable rhythm is identified, select required defibrillation energy using the circular dial, then charge defibrillator using 'charge' button
- Tell staff to stand clear and stand clear yourself - try to minimise the interruption of chest compressions which should continue until the latest possible moment
- Check the O_2, staff and you are clear (O_2, top, middle, bottom, self)
- Check the rhythm is still shockable then press the 'shock' button to deliver the charge. Resume CPR, without pausing to check rhythm.

Blood pressure Attach the cuff to the patient's left arm so it is out of the way and leave in place. If it does not work or is not believable (eg irregular or tachyarrhythmia) then obtain a manual reading.

Venous access Ideally a brown/grey venflon in each antecubital fossa; however, get the best available (biggest and most central). Remember to take bloods but don't let this delay giving drugs.

Disability

Glucose Use a spot of blood from the venous sample or a skin prick to get a capillary sample; clean skin first with water to avoid false readings.

Examination GCS, pupil size and reactivity to light, posture, tone of all four limbs, plantar reflexes.

Exposure

Get all the patient's clothes off; have a low threshold for cutting them off. Inspect the patient's entire body for clues as to the cause of the arrest, eg rashes, injuries. Measure temp. Remember to cover the patient with a blanket to prevent hypothermia and for dignity.

Other investigations

Arterial blood gas Attempts to sample radial artery blood in a patient in extremis may be futile and waste valuable time. Instead, attach a green (21G) needle to a blood gas syringe, feel for the femoral pulse (½ to ⅔ between superior iliac spine and pubic symphysis) and insert the needle vertically until you get blood. Press hard after removal. Even if the sample is venous it can still offer useful information.

Femoral stab (📖 p516) If no blood has been taken you can insert a green needle into the femoral vein which is medial to the artery (NAVY). Feel for the artery then aim about 1cm medially. If you hit the artery take 20ml of blood anyway and send for arterial blood gas and normal blood tests, but press hard after removal.

ECG Attach the leads as shown on 📖 p529.

CXR Alert the radiographer early so that they can bring the X-ray machine for a portable CXR.

Advanced Trauma Life Support (ATLS)

ATLS is designed to quickly and safely stabilise the injured patient. The purpose of ATLS is not to provide definitive care of all injuries, but to recognise the immediate threats to life and to address these. As with ALS, in ATLS the patient's care is delivered by a team which will consist of a leader and various members. Details of how to undertake an ATLS course are given in the box.

The primary survey allows a rapid assessment and relevant management to be undertaken. If a life-threatening issue is found this must be treated before moving on to the next step of the primary survey. The primary survey is as follows: Airway with cervical spine protection; Breathing: ventilation and oxygenation; Circulation with haemorrhage control; Disability: brief neurological examination; Exposure/Environment; Reassess patient's ABCDE and consider need for patient transfer.

The secondary survey follows once all life-threatening issues have been identified and dealt with; the secondary survey is a top-to-toe examination looking for secondary injuries which are unlikely to be immediately life-threatening. The secondary survey is as follows: AMPLE history (**A**llergies, **M**edications, **P**ast medical history, **L**ast meal, **E**vents leading to presentation) and mechanism of injury; Head and maxillofacial; Cervical spine and neck; Chest; Abdomen; Perineum/rectum/vagina; Musculoskeletal; Neurologic; Adjuncts to the secondary survey.

ATLS and the F1 doctor it is highly unlikely the foundation doctor will be the first person to attend to a major trauma patient, though ATLS can be applied in principle to any patient who has sustained an injury. Having a logical, step-wise approach to injured patients minimises the risk of missing life-threatening complications or injuries which subsequently may become debilitating if left unrecognised and untreated.

> ### ATLS course
>
> In the UK, ATLS courses are coordinated by the Royal College of Surgeons. The course is currently 3 days long, and details of where and when courses are run can be obtained from the College (see 🕮 p600 for contact details). There is usually a long waiting list for places as this is a popular course; the cost for the 3-day course is around £600.

Paediatric Basic Life Support

Airway	Check airway is patent; consider manoeuvres/adjuncts
Breathing	If poor respiratory effort – **CALL ARREST TEAM**
Circulation	If HR <60bpm – **CALL ARREST TEAM**
Disability	If unresponsive to voice – **CALL ARREST TEAM**

▶▶Call the **arrest team** if severely unwell; call **senior help** early (Fig. 6.3).

Airway – if irreversibly obstructed CALL ARREST TEAM
- Airway manoeuvres: (**head tilt**), **chin lift**, **jaw thrust** (see Table 6.2)
- Oropharyngeal or nasopharyngeal airway if responding only to pain
- If still impaired **CALL ARREST TEAM**.

If you suspect **epiglottitis** (stridor, drooling, septic) do not look in the mouth, but give O_2 call your senior help urgently and an anaesthetist and ENT surgeon.

Breathing – if poor or absent respiratory effort CALL ARREST TEAM
- **Bag and mask** with 15l/min O_2 if poor or absent breathing effort
- **Non-rebreather mask** and 15l/min O_2 in all other patients
- **Monitor** pulse oximeter
- **Effort** stridor, wheeze, RR, intercostal recession, grunting, accessory muscle use (head bobbing in infants), nasal flaring
- **Efficacy** chest expansion, air entry (does R=L?), O_2 sats
- **Effects** HR, pallor, cyanosis (late sign), agitation, drowsiness.

Circulation – if HR absent or <60bpm and unresponsive CALL ARREST TEAM
- Start **CPR** if HR absent or <60bpm and unresponsive
- **Monitor** defibrillator ECG leads
- **Status** HR + rhythm, pulse volume, cap refill (≤2s normal), BP
- **Effects** RR, mottled/pale/cold skin, urine output, agitation, drowsiness
- **Venous access** (consider intraosseous) check glucose and send blds
- **Consider fluid bolus** (20ml/kg IV 0.9% saline STAT) if shocked
- **Exclude heart failure** ↑JVP, gallop rhythm, crepitations, large liver.

Disability – if unresponsive to voice CALL ARREST TEAM
- Assess **AVPU** (**A**lert, responds to **V**oice, responds to **P**ain, **U**nresponsive); check **glucose** if not already done
- **Look** for pupil size and reflexes; assess posture and tone
- See 📖 p346 for **seizures**.

Exposure
- **Look** all over body for rashes, check temp, cover with a blanket.

Life-threatening causes

- Croup (exclude epiglottitis)
- Inhaled foreign body
- Bronchiolitis
- Asthma
- Dehydration (DKA)
- Sepsis, meningitis, pneumonia
- Anaphylaxis
- Heart failure (especially infants)

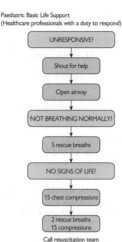

Paediatric Basic Life Support
(Healthcare professionals with a duty to respond)

UNRESPONSIVE?

↓

Shout for help

↓

Open airway

↓

NOT BREATHING NORMALLY?

↓

5 rescue breaths

↓

NO SIGNS OF LIFE?

↓

15 chest compressions

↓

2 rescue breaths
15 compressions

Call resuscitation team

Fig. 6.3 Paediatric Basic Life Support algorithm; 2010 guidelines.
Reproduced with the kind permission of the Resuscitation Council (UK).

Table 6.2 *Main age-related differences in paediatric life support*

Feature	Infant <1yr	Child >1yr	Post-puberty
Airway position	Neutral	Slightly extended	Slightly extended
Breaths	Mouth and nose	Mouth, ±nose	Mouth only
Pulse	Brachial	Carotid	Carotid
CPR position	1 finger above xiphisternum	1 finger above xiphisternum	2 fingers above xiphisternum
For CPR use	1 finger	1 or 2 hands	2 hands
Compressions:breaths	15:2	15:2	15:2

Common emergency drug doses
- **Fluid bolus** 20ml/kg 0.9% saline IV
- **Glucose** 2ml/kg 10% glucose IV
- **Adrenaline (arrest)** 0.1ml/kg 1:10,000 IV
- **Adrenaline (anaphylaxis)** 0.01ml/kg 1:1,000 IM.
- **Diazepam** 0.5mg/kg PR
- **Lorazepam** 0.1mg/kg IV
- **Ceftriaxone** 80mg/kg IV

Table 6.3 *Normal range for observations by age*

Age	RR (/min)	HR (/min)	Systolic BP (mmHg)
<1yr	30–40	110–160	70–90
2–5yr	20–30	95–140	80–100
6–12yr	12–20	80–120	90–110
>12yr	12–16	60–100	100–120

Newborn Life Support (NLS)

> If no improvement after 2min (earlier if you are concerned) of resuscitation then fast bleep a senior or **CALL THE NEONATAL ARREST TEAM** (Fig. 6.4).

Preparation
- Put non-sterile gloves on
- Turn on the heater and place warm towels on the resuscitaire
- Turn on O_2/air and check pressure, set PIP/PEEP to 30/10cmH$_2$O for term babies
- Turn on suction and check it works
- Get the laryngoscope and size 3.5 and 4.0 (term babies) ETT ready
- Check gestation, estimated birth weight and history.

Drying
- Post-delivery **start the clock** and place the baby on the resuscitaire
- **Dry** vigorously with a warm towel and cover
- Babies <30/40 gestation should be placed directly in a plastic bag.

> **Meconium delivery** if the baby is not breathing suck out meconium from the mouth and beneath the vocal cords under direct vision with a laryngoscope before drying; if the baby breathes then stop and resuscitate as usual.

Airway and breathing
- **Assess** RR and HR, if either impaired and not improving:
  - place the baby's head in the **neutral position**
  - place **Neopuff** over nose and mouth, jaw thrust; **give 5 inflation breaths**:
  - cover the Neopuff hole for 2–3s then uncover for 2–3s
  - look for **chest movement**, improved HR, colour
- If unsuccessful reposition head and give a further **5 inflation breaths**
- If unsuccessful *CALL ARREST TEAM* and consider intubation
- **Look for** oropharynx obstruction and consider a Guedel airway
- **Continue** Neopuff breaths at lower pressures (eg 20/5, 1s on 1s off).

Circulation – if HR <100bpm after breaths CALL ARREST TEAM
- **Assess** the HR by gripping the umbilicus or listening to the heart
- Start **CPR** if HR <60bpm/absent despite inflation breaths:
  - grip round the chest and use both thumbs over lower sternum
  - aim for a rate of 120 (twice a second)
  - ratio of 3:1 compressions to breaths
- Attempt to get **IV access** eg umbilical venous catheter, check glucose.

Drugs – if needed CALL ARREST TEAM
- **Adrenaline** 0.1–0.3ml/kg of 1:10,000 IV if HR not improving
- **Na$^+$ bicarbonate** 4.2% 2–4ml/kg IV if acidotic and not improving
- **Glucose** 10% 2.5ml/kg IV if hypoglycaemic
- **0.9% saline** 10ml/kg IV if large blood loss suspected.

Life-threatening causes

• Prematurity	• Meconium aspiration
• Hypoxia	• Congenital abnormality

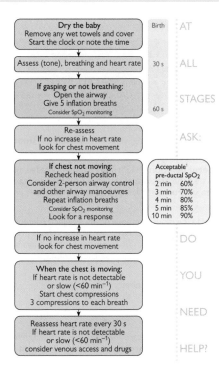

Fig. 6.4 Newborn Life Support algorithm; 2010 guidelines.
Reproduced with the kind permission of the Resuscitation Council (UK).

[1] Dawson J.A., Kamlin C.O., Vento M., et al. (2010). Defining the reference range for oxygen saturation for infants after birth. *Pediatrics* **125**:e1340–7.

Obstetric arrest

Airway	Check airway is patent; consider manoeuvres/adjuncts
Breathing	If no respiratory effort – **CALL ARREST TEAM**
Circulation	If no palpable pulse – **CALL ARREST TEAM**
Disability	If GCS ≤8 – **CALL OBSTETRIC ARREST TEAM**

Staff
- Standard arrest team along with **obstetrician** and **neonatologist**.

Position
- **Left lateral position** (>15°) using a Cardiff Wedge, pillows or your knees to take the pressure of the uterus off the vena cava and aorta
- **Push the uterus** to the left and up to further relieve pressure.

Airway
- **Look** inside the mouth, remove obvious objects/dentures
- Wide-bore **suction** under direct vision if secretions present
- **Jaw thrust**/head tilt/chin lift; **laryngeal mask** if available
- **Early intubation** to prevent gastric aspiration.

Breathing
- **Look/listen/feel** for respiratory effort
- **Bag and mask** if poor or absent respiratory effort
- **Monitor** O_2 sats and RR.

Circulation
- **Feel** for a central pulse (carotid/femoral) – HR and rhythm
- Mid-sternal **chest compression** (30:2) if pulse absent
- **Arrhythmias** – use a defibrillator/drugs as usual (□ p532)
- **Venous access**, send bloods and give IV fluids STAT
- **Monitor** defibrillator ECG leads and BP.

Disability
- **Assess** GCS and check **glucose**
- **Look/feel** for pupil reflexes, limb tone and plantar reflexes.

Surgery
- **Emergency Caesarean** if resuscitation is not successful by 5min:
  - improves maternal chest compliance and venous return
- The **mother's needs** take priority in all decisions.

Causes of obstetric arrest, see also □ p226

Haemorrhage/ hypovolaemia	□ p478	Pre-eclampsia/ eclampsia	□ p504
Excess magnesium sulphate	□ OHCM9 p693	Pulmonary embolism	□ p278
Acute coronary syndrome	□ p243	Amniotic fluid embolism	□ OHCM9 p89
Aortic dissection	□ p247	Stroke	□ p351

Cardiovascular

Chest pain emergency

Airway	Check airway is patent; consider manoeuvres/adjuncts
Breathing	If no respiratory effort – **CALL ARREST TEAM**
Circulation	If no palpable pulse – **CALL ARREST TEAM**

▶▶Call for **senior help** early if patient unwell or deteriorating.
- **Sit patient up**
- **15l/min O$_2$** if SOB or sats <94%
- **Monitor** pulse oximeter, BP, defibrillator ECG leads if unwell
- Obtain a full set of **observations** including **BP** in both arms and **ECG**
- Take brief **history** if possible/check **notes**/ask ward staff
- **Examine patient**: condensed CVS, RS, abdo exam
- Establish **likely causes** and rule out **serious causes**:
  - consider **percutaneous coronary intervention (PCI)** or **thrombolysis** (📖 p536)
  - consider giving **aspirin** 300mg PO STAT
  - consider **needle decompression** (📖 p279)
- **Initiate further treatment**, including analgesia, see following pages
- **Venous access**, take bloods:
  - FBC, U+E, LFT, CRP, glucose, cardiac markers, D-dimer
- Request urgent **CXR**, portable if too unwell
- Call for **senior help** if no improvement or worsening
- Repeat **ECG** after 20min if no improvement
- **Reassess**, starting with A, B, C …

Life-threatening causes

- Myocardial infarction
- (Tension) pneumothorax
- Acute coronary syndrome
- Pericardial effusion/cardiac tamponade
- Aortic dissection
- Pulmonary embolism
- Sickle-cell crisis

Chest pain

> *Worrying features* ↑↓HR, ↓BP, ↑RR, ↓GCS, sudden onset, sweating, nausea, vomiting, pain radiating to jaw, left arm or back, ECG changes.

Think about *common* myocardial infarction, acute coronary syndromes, angina, pulmonary embolism, musculoskeletal, pneumonia, pneumothorax (tension or simple), pericarditis, reflux and peptic ulcer disease; *uncommon* aortic dissection, cardiac tamponade, sickle-cell crisis (Table 7.1).

Ask about site of onset and radiation, quality (heavy, aching, sharp, tearing), intensity (scale of 1–10), time of onset, duration, associated symptoms (sweating, nausea, palpitations, breathlessness), exacerbating/relieving factors (breathing, position, exertion, eating), recent trauma/exertion, similarity to previous episodes; *PMH* cardiac or respiratory problems, DM, GORD; *DH* cardiac or respiratory medications, antacids; *FH* IHD, premature cardiac death; *SH* smoking, exercise tolerance.

Risk factors
- *IHD* ↑BP, ↑cholesterol, FH, smoking, obesity, DM, previous IHD
- *PE/DVT* previous PE/DVT, immobility, ↑oestrogens, recent surgery, FH, pregnancy, hypercoagulable states, smoking, long distance travel
- *GI* known GORD (📖 p294), known peptic ulcer, alcohol binge.

Obs HR, BP (both arms), RR, sats, temp.

Look for pulse rate/rhythm/volume, sweating, pallor, dyspnoea, cyanosis, ↑JVP, asymmetric chest expansion/percussion/breath sounds, chest wall tenderness, mediastinal shift, tracheal tug, swollen ankles, calf pain/swelling/erythema.

Investigations *ECG* (📖 p528/572 for procedure/interpretation); *blds* FBC, U+E, LFT, D-dimer, cardiac markers;[1] consider *ABG* taken on O_2 if patient acutely unwell (📖 p522/584 for procedure/interpretation); *CXR* if you suspect a tension pneumothorax clinically perform immediate needle decompression (📖 p279), otherwise request a portable CXR if the patient is severely ill (poorer image quality) or standard CXR (📖 p582 for interpretation); *urgent echo/CT* if large proximal PE or aortic root dissection suspected (discuss with cardiologist on-call).

Treatment 15l/min O_2 in everyone initially. Consider IV opioids (and an antiemetic) if pain is severe.

Diagnoses to exclude If you are unable to confirm a diagnosis immediately, consider life-threatening causes and investigate until excluded:
- *Cardiac ischaemia*: abnormal ECG, typical history, ↑cardiac markers[1]
- *PE*: ↓sats, abnormal ECG, clinical risk (📖 p278), ↑D-dimer, CT-PA
- *Pneumothorax*: mediastinal shift, ↓breath sounds, review CXR
- *Aortic dissection*: evidence of shock, left and right systolic BP differ by >15mmHg, mediastinal widening on CXR, abnormal CT/echo.

Contact cardiology/medical registrar on-call for advice if necessary.

---

[1] Various cardiac markers rise at different times, so check locally which you should send and at what time-point after onset of chest pain (📖 p243).

Table 7.1 *Common causes of chest pain*

	History	Examination	Investigations
▶▶ACS (STEMI)	Sudden onset pain, radiating to left arm/jaw, >20min, breathlessness, sweating, nausea	Dyspnoea, ±arrhythmia, sweating, non-tender	ST elevation or new LBBB, ↑cardiac markers. Cardiac markers are not needed to make the diagnosis of STEMI
▶▶ACS (NSTEMI)	Sudden onset pain, radiating to left arm/jaw, >20min, breathlessness, sweating, nausea	Dyspnoea, ±arrhythmia, sweating, non-tender	ST depression, T wave inversion; ↑troponin
▶▶ACS (Unstable angina)	Anginal pain at rest or with ↑frequency, severity or duration	Dyspnoea, ±arrhythmia, sweating, non-tender	ST depression, T wave inversion, troponin not elevated
Angina (stable)	Exertional pain, radiating to left arm/jaw, <20min, breathlessness, ↓by rest/GTN	Dyspnoea, tachycardia, non-tender, may be normal after pain resolves	Transient ECG changes, troponin not elevated, +ve stress ECG, + coronary angiography
Pericarditis	History of viral-like illness, pleuritic pain, ↑on lying, ↓sitting forwards	Pericardial rub, otherwise normal CVS and RS examinations	Saddle-shaped ST segments on most ECG leads, ↑CRP/ESR
▶▶Aortic dissection	Sudden onset severe interscapular pain, tearing in nature, breathlessness. Limb weakness/numbness	Tachycardia, ↓BP, difference in brachial pulses and pressures, ↑RR. Limb weakness or paraesthesia	Widened mediastinum on CXR, aortic dilatation on echo/CT, aortic leak on angiogram
Pulmonary embolism	Breathlessness, PE risk factors (🕮 p278), may have pleuritic chest pain and haemoptysis	Often normal, may have evidence of DVT (swollen red leg), tachycardia, dyspnoea, ↓BP	ABG: PaO_2↔/↓, CO_2↓, clear CXR, ↑D-dimer, sinus tachycardia, $S_1Q_3T_3$ (rare), thrombus on echo
Pneumothorax	Sudden onset pleuritic pain ±trauma; tall and thin; COPD	Mediastinal shift, unequal air entry and expansion, hyperresonance	Pleura separated from ribs on CXR, other investigations often normal
Pneumonia	Cough, productive with coloured sputum, pleuritic pain, feels unwell	Febrile, asymmetrical air entry, coarse creps (often unilateral), dull to percussion	↑WCC/↑NØ/↑CRP, consolidation on CXR (🕮 p582)
Musculoskeletal chest pain	Lifting, impact injury, may be pleuritic, worse on palpation or movement	Tender (presence does not exclude other causes), respiratory examination normal	ECG to exclude cardiac cause, normal CXR
Oesophageal reflux or spasm	Previous indigestion/reflux, known hiatus hernia, ↓by antacids	May have upper abdo tenderness, normal CVS and RS examinations	ECG to exclude cardiac cause, normal CXR, trial of antacids

▶▶**Acute coronary syndromes (ACS)** (OHCM9 📖 p112)

ACS is a general term referring to presentations of varying severities of myocardial ischaemia (Tables 7.2 and 7.3). The aim is to allow a prospective rather than a retrospective diagnosis to be made and so improve both acute management and subsequent patient outcome.

Table 7.2 *Acute coronary syndrome (ACS) classification in patients with typical cardiac-sounding chest pain lasting >20min*

ECG findings	Troponin (12h post-pain)	Diagnosis
ST elevation or new LBBB	Not needed to make a diagnosis, but will be ↑	STEMI (📖 p244)
Ischaemia (other than ST elevation), though may be normal	Trop T ≥0.1ng/ml or Trop I ≥1ng/ml	NSTEMI (📖 p245)
	Trop T <0.1ng/ml or Trop I <1ng/ml	Unstable angina (📖 p246)

Table 7.3 *Serum cardiac markers in suspected ACS*
The term 'cardiac enzymes' is incorrect when referring to the troponins as these are structural/regulatory proteins and have no enzymatic activity

Troponins (I or T)	Identification of these in the blood is highly suggestive of myocardial injury, though they can be raised in PE, renal failure, septicaemia and following tachyarrhythmias (but CK is seldom concurrently raised in these conditions). Detection is usually possible 6h after myocardial injury and levels remain elevated for up to 14d. Troponins are also used as a prognostic indicator in NSTEMI/UA (📖 p245)
Creatine kinase (CK)	Enzyme found in all muscle and released in muscle cell lysis; not specific for cardiac muscle. Peaks within 24h post-MI and usually returns to normal within 48–72h, so useful in detecting further infarction in patients with pain 3–14 days post MI (Fig. 7.1)
CK-MB	Cardiac isomer of CK enzyme, so more specific than total CK. Rises and falls in similar fashion to total CK
AST LDH	These were once used to retrospectively aid in the diagnosis of acute MI but have been superseded in recent years

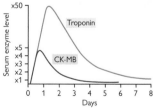

Fig. 7.1 Typical changes in cardiac markers following an acute myocardial infarction.

▶▶STEMI (ST Elevation MI)¹ (OHCM9 📖 p114)

Worrying signs features of LV failure, cardiac dysrhythmia.

Symptoms central, crushing, heavy chest pain (≥20min), ±radiating to left arm/jaw, shortness of breath, nausea, sweating, palpitations, anxiety.

Risk factors smoking, obesity, DM, ↑BP, ↑cholesterol, FH, previous IHD.

Signs tachycardia, cool and sweaty ('clammy'), ±LV failure or hypotension.

Investigations **ECG** ST elevation (>1mm in 2 or more contiguous limb leads or >2mm in chest leads) or new LBBB; subsequent Q waves (commonly) ±T wave inversion (Fig. 7.2); **CXR** cardiomegaly, signs of LV failure; **cardiac markers** will be raised but treatment should not be withheld as ECG findings and history alone are sufficient to make the diagnosis.

Acute treatment The goal is for rapid reperfusion by percutaneous coronary intervention (PCI) in those presenting within 12h of symptom onset so **seek senior help.** O_2 (15l/min), aspirin (300mg), clopidogrel (300mg), diamorphine (2.5–5mg IV), antiemetic (📖 p185), GTN (two puffs SL/5min until pain free; infusion if ongoing pain after 3 SL doses, provided not hypotensive, 📖 p201). Where PCI is not available within 3h, consider fibrinolysis (📖 p536). β-blockade (eg bisoprolol 10mg/PO STAT) limits infarct size and ↓mortality, but avoid use in COPD, hypotension and overt failure. Careful glycaemic control (eg insulin sliding scale 📖 p327) may improve outcomes.²

Secondary prophylaxis ↓modifiable risk factors (smoking, obesity, DM, ↑BP, ↑cholesterol), β-blockade, statin, anti-platelets (aspirin indefinitely, clopidogrel for 1 year), ACEi, symptom management (nitrates, Ca^{2+} channel antagonists).

Complications dysrhythmias (AV block, bradycardia, VF/VT), LVF, valve prolapse, ventricular septal rupture, ventricular aneurysm formation, pericarditis, Dressler's syndrome (OHAM3 📖 p32), recurrent pain.

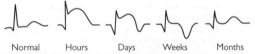

Normal   Hours   Days   Weeks   Months

Fig. 7.2 Typical sequential ECG changes following an acute STEMI.

Care after myocardial infarction (OHCM9 📖 p114)

- Bed rest for 48h with continuous ECG monitoring
- Daily 12-lead ECG and thorough clinical examination of CVS/RS
- Thromboembolism prophylaxis (📖 p406)
- β-blockade unless contraindicated
- ACEi/angiotensin II receptor antagonist
- Statin
- Discuss modifiable risk factors and arrange cardiac rehabilitation
- Primary PCI patients are at lower risk of complications and have shorter stays; thrombolysis patients will require risk stratification and consideration for in-patient angiography.
- Consider electrophysiological studies in those with new dysrhythmias
- Review in out-patients at 5wk and 3mth for symptoms and to check lipids+BP

¹ NICE guidelines available at ᐸℍguidance.nice.org.uk/CG167
² Evidence low quality and conflicting. NICE review available at ᐸℍguidance.nice.org.uk/CG130

▶▶NSTEMI (Non-ST Elevation MI)[1] (OHAM3 📖 p44)

Diagnosis and intervention are often less 'dramatic' than for STEMI, requiring recognition of evolving ECG changes; however, 1yr survival is poorer.

Worrying signs features of LV failure, cardiac dysrhythmia.

Symptoms, risk factors, and signs overlap with STEMI; patients typically tend to be older, with more co-morbidities.

Investigations **ECG** ST depression, inverted T waves; subsequent evolution of changes ±T wave inversion; **CXR** cardiomegaly, signs of LV failure; **cardiac markers** differentiate from UA by elevated troponin, taken according to local protocols (typically on presentation and 12h after worst pain).

Acute treatment O_2 (15l/min), aspirin (300mg), clopidogrel (300mg), diamorphine (2.5–5mg IV), antiemetic (📖 p185), GTN (two puffs SL/5min until pain free; infusion if ongoing pain after 3 SL doses, provided not hypotensive, 📖 p201) Anticoagulation with fondaparinux (📖 p407).[2] β-blockade (eg bisoprolol 10mg STAT) but beware use in patients with COPD, hypotension or overt failure. Risk stratify (see below) and involve CCU+cardiologist early for high-risk patients for consideration of prompt catheterisation and glycoprotein IIb/IIIa inhibitors.

Secondary prophylaxis and complications are broadly the same as in STEMI, though complications are less common.

Risk stratification in ACS

Estimation of the risk of death in ACS allows individualised assessment of the risks and benefits of interventions and careful targeting of resources to those patients who stand to benefit the most. A number of validated scoring algorithms have been developed from major clinical trial data. These include the pioneering *Thrombolysis In Myocardial Infarction* (TIMI) risk score[3] still widely used in many hospitals. However, many such trials had restricted entry criteria, leading to under-representation of patients with renal or heart failure. The *Global Registry of Acute Coronary Events* (GRACE) algorithms were developed from a multinational registry (94 hospitals, 14 countries, and 22,645 patients) involving patients with all subtypes of ACS (STEMI, NSTEMI, and UA).[4] Risk scores may be calculated on admission (to predict in hospital and 6mth mortality) or on discharge (to predict 6mth mortality). A free online calculator is available at ⁿ̂ www.outcomes-umassmed.org/grace

High-risk patients will need a CCU bed, and consideration for glycoprotein IIb/IIIa inhibitors and urgent catheterisation (within 96h).

Low/intermediate-risk require observation to ensure pain free, then further stratification using exercise ECG, coronary calcium scoring or stress imaging (echo or perfusion imaging) to determine need for catheterisation.

[3] Antman, E.M. *et al. JAMA* 2000 **284**:835 available free online at ⁿ̂ jama.ama-assn.org/cgi/content/full/284/7/835 See also the excellent collection of resources available free at ⁿ̂ www.timi.org

[4] Granger, C.B. *et al. Arch Intern Med* 2003 **163**:2345 available free online at ⁿ̂ archinte.ama-assn.org/cgi/content/full/163/19/2345

[1] NICE guidelines available at ⁿ̂ guidance.nice.org.uk/CG94

[2] Use unfractionated heparin infusion if angiography is planned within 24h, or if significant bleeding risk (consider in frail elderly, active/recent bleeding complications, significant renal impairment or those with extreme low body mass).

▶▶Unstable angina (OHAM3 📖 p44)

Diagnosis is based upon typical history in the presence of ECG changes, but without subsequent elevation of cardiac markers.

Worrying signs features of LV failure, cardiac dysrhythmia.

Symptoms, risk factors, and signs overlap with other forms of ACS; typically episodes of angina occurring on minimal provocation or at rest, with poor response to GTN; more frequent and more severe than patient's 'usual' angina; few symptoms or signs between episodes of pain.

Investigations **ECG** ST depression, flat or inverted T waves with dynamic changes over time, signs of previous MI; ***cardiac markers*** not elevated.

Acute treatment as for NSTEMI (📖 p245); analgesia (morphine, GTN), antiplatelet agents (aspirin, clopidogrel), limit ischaemia (β-blockade) and disrupt thrombus (fondaparinux). Risk stratify, further management and secondary prophylaxis as for NSTEMI (📖 p245).

Stable angina[1] (OHCM9 📖 p110)

Frequently encountered in primary care, retrosternal chest discomfort occurring predictably upon exertion and relieved by rest and nitrates.

Symptoms central, heavy chest pain (lasting <20min) radiating to left arm and jaw, precipitated by exertion and relieved by rest or rapidly by GTN (<5min), shortness of breath, nausea, sweating, palpitations.

Risk factors common for IHD; see ACS above; severe aortic stenosis.

Signs tachycardia, cool and sweaty ('clammy'), pallor. Normal after episode.

Investigations **ECG** transient ST depression during pain; flat or inverted T waves; signs of previous MI; ***cardiac markers*** are not elevated (if elevated this is NSTEMI). If diagnostic uncertainty, further assessment should be guided by assessment of the likelihood of IHD based upon age, sex, presence of risk factors and nature of pain.[2]

Acute treatment pain relief with rest and GTN is characteristic. If pain lasting >20min, investigate and treat as for NSTEMI/UA.

Primary prophylaxis assessment and reduction of modifiable risk factors (smoking, obesity, DM, BP, cholesterol), statin, anti-platelets, ACEi, symptom management (nitrates, β-blockade, Ca^{2+} channel antagonists, nicorandil).

Angina with normal coronaries?

Throughout your career, you will encounter numerous patients with atypical chest pain who require basic investigations to exclude serious pathology and subsequent reassurance. However, some patients experience convincing ischaemic heart pain, despite angiographically normal coronary arteries. Consider:

- Prinzmetal's angina: spontaneous coronary artery vasospasm
- Cocaine-induced vasospasm: give GTN ±benzodiazepines; can lead to MI
- 'Microvascular angina' eg coronary syndrome X in postmenopausal women with evidence of perfusion deficits on dynamic imaging.

---

[1] NICE guidelines available at 🔗guidance.nice.org.uk/CG126

[2] See NICE guidelines at 🔗guidance.nice.org.uk/CG95 for risk stratification table and a discussion of appropriate tests. In short, if the likelihood of angina is >90%, treat without further investigation; if likelihood 60–90%, consider coronary angiography; if likelihood 30–60% or unsuitable for angiography, offer functional imaging (stress echo or perfusion imaging); if likelihood 10–30%, perform CT coronary calcium scoring dynamic and proceed to CT coronary angiography if score >0; if likelihood <10%, reconsider other causes. Exercise ECG, though widely available, is limited by lower sensitivity and specificity than other tests, and should not be a 1st-line test in patients without known IHD.

▶▶Aortic dissection (OHCM9 📖 p656 or OHAM3 📖 p142)

Symptoms sudden onset severe chest pain, anterior or interscapular, tearing in nature, dizziness, breathlessness, sweating, neurological deficits.

Risk factors smoking, obesity, DM, ↑BP, ↑cholesterol, FH, previous IHD.

Signs unequal radial pulses, tachycardia, hypotension/hypertension, difference in brachial pressures of ≥15mmHg, aortic regurgitation, pleural effusion (L>R), neurological deficits from carotid artery dissection.

Investigations **ECG** may be normal or show LV strain/ischaemia (📖 p572); **CXR** classically widened mediastinum >8cm (rarely seen), irregularity of aortic knuckle and small left pleural effusion can develop from blood tracking down; **echo** may show aortic root leak, aortic valve regurgitation or pericardial effusion. Also consider MRI/CT/conventional angiography.

Acute treatment **seek senior help.** If **hypotensive**, treat as shock (📖 p476). O₂ (15l/min), two large-bore cannulae, X-match 6 units, analgesia (IV opioids). If **hypertensive** aim to keep systolic BP <100mmHg (📖 p265).

Further treatment surgery (for type A: involves the ascending aorta) or conservative management (for type B: involves descending aorta only).

Musculoskeletal chest pain

Symptoms localised chest wall pain, worse on movement and/or breathing, recent trauma or exertion (eg lifting).

Signs focal tenderness, erythema, absence of other signs in CVS or RS.

Investigations only investigate if you cannot satisfy yourself of the diagnosis on clinical grounds; **ECG** normal (no ischaemia/MI); **CXR** normal (no pneumothorax); **D-dimer** normal and low probability PE (📖 p278).

Acute treatment reassurance and simple analgesia (📖 p86).

Chronic treatment should settle within 2wk, prevention from further injury (no more heavy lifting for a few weeks), adequate regular analgesia to allow activities of daily living to be carried out and to allow deep inspiration and coughing (to prevent chest infection), stop smoking.

Pericarditis (OHAM3 📖 p150)

Symptoms pleuritic chest pain, worse on lying flat and deep inspiration, relieved by sitting forwards, recent viral illnesses.

Signs may be no abnormalities, ±pericardial rub.

Investigations **ECG** saddle-shaped ST segments in most leads (see Fig. 7.3); **blds** ↑WCC and inflammatory markers, ±↑viral titres; **echo** ±pericardial effusion.

Acute treatment reassurance and analgesia; paracetamol, NSAIDs.

Chronic treatment should settle within 2–4wk; recurrence common.

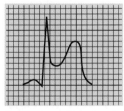

Fig. 7.3 Typical saddle-shaped ST segment seen in pericarditis.

Tachyarrhythmia emergency

Airway	Check airway is patent; consider manoeuvres/adjuncts
Breathing	If no respiratory effort – **CALL ARREST TEAM**
Circulation	If no palpable pulse – **CALL ARREST TEAM**

▶▶Call for **senior help** early if patient 'unstable' (Fig. 7.4):

Signs of an unstable patient include:

- Reduced conscious level
- Systolic BP <90mmHg
- Chest pain
- Heart failure

- **Sit patient** up unless hypotensive, then lay flat with legs elevated
- **15l/min** O$_2$ if SOB or sats <94%
- **Monitor** pulse oximeter, BP, defibrillator ECG leads if unwell
- Request full set of **observations** and **ECG**
- Take brief **history** if possible/check notes/ask ward staff
- **Examine patient**: condensed CVS, RS, ± abdo exam
- Establish **likely causes** and rule out **serious causes**
- **Initiate further treatment**, see 📖 p249
- **Venous access**, take bloods:
  - FBC, U+E, D-dimer, cardiac markers, TFT
- Consider requesting urgent **CXR**, portable if too unwell
- Call for **senior help**
- **Reassess**, starting with A, B, C …

Life-threatening causes

- Ventricular tachycardia (VT) or ventricular fibrillation (VF)
- Torsades de pointes
- Supraventricular tachycardia with haemodynamic compromise
- Fast atrial fibrillation/flutter with haemodynamic compromise
- Sinus tachycardia
  - secondary to shock, including PE
  - iatrogenic (drugs)

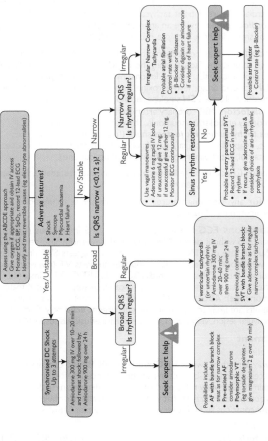

Fig. 7.4 Adult tachycardia (with a pulse) algorithm; 2010 guidelines.
Reproduced with the kind permission of the Resuscitation Council (UK).

Tachyarrhythmias

Worrying features ↓GCS, ↓BP (sys <90mmHg), chest pain, heart failure.

Think about *common* sinus tachycardia, fast ventricular rate in AF, supraventricular tachycardia (SVT), atrial flutter; *uncommon* ventricular tachycardia (VT), re-entrant tachycardia (eg Wolff–Parkinson–White); *non-cardiac causes* beware an appropriate tachycardic response to eg sepsis or shock, in those with pre-existing conduction defects.

Ask about onset, associated symptoms (chest pain, shortness of breath, dizziness, palpitations, facial flushing, headache), previous episodes; *PMH* cardiac problems (IHD, valvular lesions, hypertension), thyroid disease, DM; *DH* cardiac drugs, levothyroxine, salbutamol, anticholinergics, caffeine, nicotine, allergies; *SH* smoking, alcohol, recreational drug use.

- **AF risk factors** ↑BP, coronary artery and valvular heart disease, pulmonary embolism, pneumonia, thyrotoxicosis, alcohol, sepsis.
- **Sinus tachycardia risk factors** shock (hypovolaemic, cardiogenic, septic, anaphylactic, spinal), pain/anxiety, fever, drugs (levothyroxine, salbutamol, anticholinergics, caffeine, nicotine, cocaine).

Obs pulse (check apical pulse since radial can underestimate), BP, cap refill, RR, O_2 sats, GCS, temp.

Look for any 'worrying features' classify arrhythmia as 'unstable'; see Fig. 7.4 algorithm (📖 p249).

Investigations *ECG* P waves before each QRS imply sinus rhythm, irregular QRS without clear P waves implies AF, saw-tooth baseline implies atrial flutter, rate of ≥140 (narrow complexes) suggests SVT (including flutter with block), broad regular complexes suggests VT (always check for a pulse) (Tables 7.4 and 7.5); *blds* FBC, U+E, TFT, CRP, D-dimer (if PE suspected), cardiac markers, others as indicated by suspicion (eg X-match if haemorrhage); *ABG* and *CXR* only once treatment has been initiated or if results are likely to alter management; *urgent echo* only if large PE, acute valvular lesion, very poor LV or pericardial effusion is suspected.

Treatment

In all patients
- **A**irway, **B**reathing (with O_2), **C**irculation (HR, BP and capillary refill)
- IV access (two large-bore cannula in both antecubital fossa)
- Obtain ECG or view trace on defibrillator to decide on rhythm
- If hypotensive or dizzy lay flat with legs up – Call senior help
- If semi-conscious lay in recovery position – Call senior/ARREST TEAM.

Specific arrhythmias
- **Sinus tachycardia** establish cause of sinus tachycardia, ?shock (📖 p476)
- **AF** is the patient normally in AF or is this new onset? (📖 p252)
- **SVT** usually time to call for help and get drugs ready (📖 p253)
- **VT no pulse:** ▶▶call ARREST TEAM and start BLS/ALS (📖 p226)
- **VT with pulse:** if haemodynamically stable, attempt chemical cardioversion (eg amiodarone 📖 p184); if fails or if unstable, will need DC cardioversion (📖 p532), under anaesthetic unless unconscious.

Table 7.4 *ECG features of tachyarrhythmias*

	Rate	Regular	P waves	Broad/narrow
Sinus tachycardia	>100	✓	✓	Narrow (unless BBB)[1]
Fast AF	>100	✗	✗	Narrow (unless BBB)[1]
SVT	≥140	✓	✓ or ✗	Narrow (unless BBB)[1]
VT (with pulse)	≥150	✓	✗	Broad
VT (pulseless)	As for 'VT with pulse'; always perform a pulse-check (carotid)			
VF	Chaotic irregular electrical activity; never has a pulse			

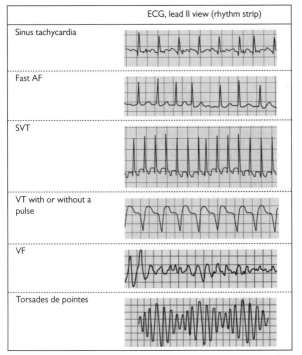

	ECG, lead II view (rhythm strip)
Sinus tachycardia	
Fast AF	
SVT	
VT with or without a pulse	
VF	
Torsades de pointes	

Fig. 7.5 Typical appearance of various tachyarrhythmias.

[1] An electrical impulse arising above the atrioventricular node, but then conducted into the ventricles through a diseased conduction pathway (as in BBB) will result in a broad complex tachycardia which can be hard to differentiate from VT. 'Concordance', in which the QRS 'direction' in all precordial leads is consistent, and occasional narrow complex 'capture beats' suggest VT, but the diagnosis is often not straightforward. **If in doubt, treat as VT.**

Atrial fibrillation (AF)[1] (OHAM3 📖 p72)

Worrying signs heart failure, hypotension, ↓GCS or chest pain.

Symptoms palpitations, shortness of breath, dizziness ±chest pains.

Risk factors previous AF, ↑BP, IHD, valvular heart disease, PE, pneumonia, thyrotoxicosis, alcohol (acute excess, chronic use or withdrawal), dilated cardiomyopathy, ↑age, acute illness.

Signs irregularly irregular pulse, hypotension if cardiovascular compromise, signs of concurrent/precipitant disease (pneumonia, thyrotoxicosis).

Investigations **ECG** absent P waves, irregularly irregular QRS complexes; **blds** FBC (↑WCC), U+E, TFT, alcohol, ±D-dimer (PE), troponin (if concern that ischaemic episode responsible); **CXR** heart size, pulmonary oedema, pneumonia; **echo** LV dilatation/impairment, valvular lesion.

Treatment

- *Haemodynamic compromise* seek immediate senior help. Treat shock (📖 p476); O$_2$, IV access, DC cardioversion; if unsuccessful, amiodarone IV ±further cardioversion. Chronic AF very unlikely to cause compromise: do not shock, but consider other causes of compromise, eg sepsis
- **Haemodynamically stable** treatment options include:
  - **Conservative:** if AF is likely new in onset and patient has obvious underlying precipitant (eg electrolyte disturbance, sepsis) then appropriate treatment of precipitant may be all that is required to resolve AF so long as patient remains monitored and stable
  - **Rate control:** control of tachycardia reduces myocardial metabolic demands. Effective means include β-blockade (📖 p188) or a rate-limiting calcium-channel blocker (diltiazem is better tolerated than verapamil). Digoxin can be added in where these are insufficient, but should not be used as a first-line therapy except in the sedentary elderly (📖 p196); this approach is especially useful in those who are unlikely to revert to sinus rhythm (older patients, established AF, dilated left atrium, mitral valve disease)
  - **Rhythm control:** younger patients and those with new presentations of AF, may be suitable for attempted cardioversion. If the patient is not known to have IHD, use PO/IV flecainide, otherwise use IV amiodarone (given via a central line). DC cardioversion under sedation may also be used. Maintenance of sinus rhythm after successful cardioversion, or less rapid cardioversion, may be achieved using β-blockade, escalated to sotalol, flecainide or amiodarone if this is not tolerated or fails (do not use sotalol or flecainide in those with structural heart disease). These agents also help maintain sinus rhythm in paroxysmal AF
- **Anticoagulation** In all patients in whom a rate control strategy is adopted, consider oral anticoagulation therapy (📖 p406) versus use of aspirin 75mg/24h PO, based upon a stroke risk assessment.[2] Full anticoagulation should be achieved for 4wk before and after any form of planned cardioversion, unless onset of AF is definitely within previous 48h, or trans-oesophageal echo demonstrates no thrombus in left atrium.

Complications thromboembolic disease (eg ischaemic stroke). Drug side-effects (amiodarone, warfarin, β-blockers, digoxin etc).

[1] NICE guidelines available at ⏚guidance.nice.uk/CG36

[2] eg CHADS$_2$ risk score—1 point each for presence of CHF, HTN, Age>75, DM; 2 points if prior TIA or stroke. A cumulative score of 2 predicts a 4% annual stroke risk, and is generally taken as a cut off for starting oral anticoagulation therapy. Gage, B.F. *et al. JAMA* 2001 **285**:2864 available free at ⏚jama.ama-assn.org/cgi/content/full/285/22/2864

Atrial flutter (OHAM3 📖 p78)

'Saw tooth' flutter waves reflecting atrial activity with ventricular response rate characteristically around 150bpm. Management is similar to AF, but cardioversion rates much lower. May require ablation.

Supraventricular tachycardia (SVT) (OHAM3 📖 p68)

Worrying signs heart failure, hypotension, ↓GCS or chest pain.

Symptoms palpitations, shortness of breath, dizziness ±chest pains.

Risk factors previous SVT, structural cardiac anomaly, alcohol, ↑T_4.

Signs tachycardia, anxiety, hypotension if haemodynamic compromise.

Investigations **ECG** narrow complex tachycardia (unless concurrent BBB) with P waves (which may merge into QRS and so be difficult to see), regular QRS complexes, rate usually ≥140; **further investigations** only required if diagnosis in question, otherwise initiate treatment as below.

Acute treatment O_2, large-bore IV access (antecubital fossa). Monitor rhythm on defibrillator:

- **Vagal manoeuvres** (📖 p531)
- **Chemical** (📖 p531)

Chronic treatment if recurrent, seek cardiology advice as may require electrophysiological testing of cardiac conduction pathways.

Complications hypotension, ischaemia, heart failure in individuals with existing cardiac disease, deterioration into more sinister arrhythmia.

Wolff–Parkinson–White syndrome (WPW) (OHAM3 📖 p80)

Aetiology This is a re-entrant tachycardia which results from an accessory conduction pathway between the atria and the ventricles (bundle of Kent). It classically appears as a short PR interval and a δ/delta wave (shown by arrow in Fig. 7.6).

Treatment Avoid digoxin and verapamil. Refer to a cardiologist for consideration of electrophysiology studies and ablation of accessory pathway.

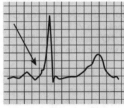

Fig. 7.6 δ wave in WPW.

Table 7.5 *Anti-dysrhythmics commonly used in tachyarrhythmias*

▶▶These drugs should only be used after discussion with a senior	
Amiodarone (should be given via a central vein, but can be given peripherally in an emergency)	**Loading dose** 300mg/over 60min IVI via central line followed by 900mg/over 24h IVI via central line OR 200mg/8h PO for 1wk then 200mg/12h PO for 1wk then **Maintenance dose** 200mg/24h PO
Verapamil (avoid if pt on β-blockers)	5mg/over 2min IV; further 0.5–1mg doses every 5min until target rate achieved (total maximum 20mg) OR 40–120mg/8h PO
Flecainide (avoid if pt has IHD)	2mg/kg/over 10min IV (maximum 150mg) OR 100–200mg/12h PO

Patient must be in a monitored bed during administration of these agents.

Ventricular tachycardia (VT) (OHAM3 📖 p62)
Worrying signs heart failure, hypotension, ↓GCS, chest pain or absent pulse (pulseless VT).

Symptoms palpitations, dizziness, shortness of breath ±chest pain, arrest.

Risk factors IHD, trauma, hypoxia, acidosis, long QT.

Signs tachycardia, anxiety, pallor, hypotension, ↓GCS, shock.

Investigations **ECG** broad complex tachycardia, absence of P waves, rate usually >150; **blds** check urgent U+E (especially K^+) and Mg^{2+}; **other investigations** should be directed by clinical situation though cardioversion is main priority at this stage.

Acute treatment – call senior help
- ▶▶*Pulseless VT:* Call ARREST TEAM, commence BLS/ALS (📖 p228) after pre-cordial thump (if witnessed and monitored arrest)
- *VT with a pulse:* O_2, large-bore IV cannula in antecubital fossa; restoration of sinus rhythm with either drugs (eg sotalol, amiodarone) or DC cardioversion (under sedation unless unconscious)
- *Possible SVT with bundle branch block or VT:* treat as VT.

Chronic treatment may need drug therapy to maintain sinus rhythm, electrophysiological studies/ablation or implantable cardioverter/defibrillator (OHAM3 📖 p62).

Complications may deteriorate into VF or other dysrhythmia.

Torsades de pointes (OHAM3 📖 p64)
Looks like VF but has a rotating axis (📖 p251). Develops on background of ↑QT interval. Give Mg^{2+} sulphate 2g/IV (8mmol) over 15min (dilute in small volume eg 50ml of 0.9% saline) ±overdrive pacing.

Table 7.6 *Causes of prolonged QT interval*

$QTc = QT/\sqrt{(RR\ interval)}$ – this allows correction of the QT interval for heart rate and is usually calculated automatically on an ECG trace.
Normal QTc values are gender-specific; values <430ms (♂) and <450ms (♀) are considered normal; values >450ms (♂) and >470ms (♀) are abnormal; values in between these are borderline. There is a dose-response relationship between risk of cardiac death and prolongation of QTc.[1]

Congenital	Romano–Ward syndrome (AD), Jervell, Lange–Nielsen syndrome (AR, associated with deafness)
Drugs	Anti-dysrhythmics (amiodarone, sotalol, quinidine), Psychoactives (thioridazine, haloperidol, fluoxetine), Antihistamines (terfenadine, loratadine), Antimicrobials (erythromycin, clarithromycin, fluconazole)
Electrolyte disturbance	↑/↓K^+, ↓Mg^{2+}, ↓Ca^{2+}
Severe bradycardia	Complete heart block, sinus bradycardia
IHD	Ischaemia, myocarditis
Intracranial bleed	Subarachnoid haemorrhage

[1] Straus, M. *et al. J Am Coll Cardiol.* 2006 **47**:362 available free online.

Bradyarrhythmia emergency

Airway	Check airway is patent; consider manoeuvres/adjuncts
Breathing	If no respiratory effort – **CALL ARREST TEAM**
Circulation	If no palpable pulse – **CALL ARREST TEAM**

▶▶Call for **senior help** early if patient has 'adverse features' (Fig. 7.7):

Adverse features include:

- Systolic BP <90mmHg
- Syncope
- Ischaemic chest pain
- Heart failure

- **Sit patient up** unless hypotensive/dizzy, then lay flat with legs elevated
- **15l/min O$_2$** if SOB or sats <94%
- **Monitor** pulse oximeter, BP, defibrillator's ECG leads if very unwell
- Request full set of **observations** and **ECG** with long **rhythm strip**
- Take brief **history** if possible/check **notes**/ask ward staff
- **Examine patient**: condensed CVS, RS, abdo exam
- Establish **likely causes** and rule out **serious causes**
- Consider **IV atropine**, 500micrograms, repeat at 2–3min intervals (max 3mg)
- **Initiate further treatment**, including transcutaneous pacing, see following pages
- **Venous access**, take bloods:
  - FBC, U+E, LFT, cardiac markers, TFT
- Consider requesting urgent **CXR**, portable if too unwell
- Call for **senior help**.
- **Reassess**, starting with A, B, C …

Life-threatening causes

- Complete (3rd degree) heart block (±following MI)
- Möbitz type II
- Pauses >3s on ECG
- Hypoxia in children

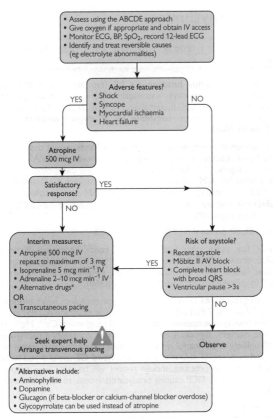

Fig. 7.7 Adult bradycardia algorithm; 2010 guidelines.
Reproduced with the kind permission of the Resuscitation Council (UK).

Bradyarrhythmias

Worrying features systolic BP <90mmHg, HR <40bpm, heart failure, ventricular arrhythmia.

Think about *sinus bradycardia* MI (typically inferior MI) drugs (including digoxin toxicity), vasovagal, ↓T_4, hypothermia, Cushing's reflex (bradycardia and hypertension 2° to ↑ICP), sleep, anorexia nervosa, physical fitness; **complete or 3rd-degree atrioventricular (AV) heart block.**

Ask about dizziness, postural dizziness, fits/faints, weight change, visual disturbance, nausea, vomiting; **PMH** cardiac disease (IHD/AF), thyroid disease/surgery, DM, head injury or intracranial pathology, glaucoma, eating disorder; **DH** cardiac medications (β-blockers, Ca^{2+} antagonists, amiodarone, digoxin), eye drops (β-blockers); **SH** exercise tolerance.

• **IHD risk factors** ↑BP, ↑cholesterol, FH, smoking, obesity, DM, previous angina/MI.

Obs HR, BP, postural BP, RR, sats, temp, GCS.

Look for pulse rate/rhythm/volume, pallor, shortness of breath, ↓GCS, drowsy, ↑JVP (cannon waves in 3rd-degree AV block), signs of cardiac failure (↑JVP, pulmonary oedema, swollen ankles), features of ↑ICP (papilloedema, focal neurology – 🕮 p360).

Investigations *ECG* sinus bradycardia or complete heart block (see Table 7.7 and Fig. 7.8), evidence of ischaemia or infarction (🕮 p572) or of digoxin toxicity (see opposite); *blds* FBC, U+E, glucose, Ca^{2+}, Mg^{2+}, TFT, cardiac markers, digoxin level, coagulation (if considering pacing-wire); *CXR* unlikely to be helpful in the immediate setting, but may reveal heart size and evidence of pulmonary oedema; *head CT* useful if you suspect raised intracranial pressure, though patient will be *in extremis* (about to cone, 🕮 p338) if ↑ICP causing bradycardia (speak to on-call neurosurgeon).

Treatment
• **A**irway, **B**reathing (with O_2) and monitor **C**irculation
• If either ↓GCS or ↓BP (<90mmHg systolic), ▶▶call senior help/ ARREST TEAM
• IV cannula and take bloods
• Consider giving IV atropine if systolic BP <90mmHg (500micrograms at 2–3min intervals to a maximum of 3mg)
• Check ECG to exclude myocardial infarction and to identify heart block or extreme sinus bradycardia or very slow atrial fibrillation.

Table 7.7 *ECG features of bradyarrhythmias and types of heart block*

Sinus bradycardia	P waves precede each QRS, rate <60
1st-degree AV block	P–R interval >5 small squares (>0.2s)
Möbitz I (Wenkebach)	P–R interval lengthens from beat to beat, until failure of AV conduction, then pattern restarts
Möbitz II	Intermittent P waves fail to conduct to ventricles, but P–R interval does not lengthen, unlike Möbitz type I; typically 2:1 (P waves:QRS complexes): Ratios of 3:1 and above are considered high-grade AV block
3rd-degree AV block	Complete dissociation between P waves and QRS complexes, which will be broad as a result
Digoxin effect/ toxicity	Down-sloping ST segment (reversed tick), inverted T waves; often present even when drug is at non-toxic levels
Rate controlled AF	No P waves; irregularly irregular rhythm

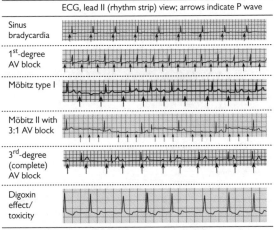

Fig. 7.8 Typical appearances of various bradyarrhythmias and types of heart block.

Sinus bradycardia (OHAM3 📖 p82)

Worrying signs features of heart failure, hypotension, ↓GCS.

Symptoms asymptomatic, dizziness (±on standing), recurrent falls, palpitations, shortness of breath, symptoms of ↑ICP, hypothermia or ↓T$_4$.

Signs orthostatic ↓BP, hypothermia, evidence of ↑ICP (📖 p360).

Investigations **ECG** QRS complex will be preceded by a P wave, rate <60, QRS will be narrow unless BBB; exclude ischaemia/infarction; **blds** FBC, U+E, Ca^{2+}, Mg^{2+}, TFT, cardiac markers, coagulation (if considering pacing-wire); **CXR** unlikely to be helpful in immediate resuscitation phase.

Acute treatment if symptomatic (dizzy or GCS <15) or systolic <90mmHg, monitor heart rate on defibrillator, lay flat with legs elevated (as long as ↑ICP not suspected). O$_2$, secure IV access and take bloods. If worrying signs present, ▶▶Call senior help/ARREST TEAM. Titrate 500micrograms atropine IV every 2–3min (to a maximum of 3mg) followed by a large flush, until HR improves. Identify and correct precipitant. Consider external pacing/pacing-wire via central line (📖 p534); a rhythmical precordial thump (percussion pacing) can be used *in extremis* when an external pacing machine is not immediately available.

Chronic treatment consider 24h tape; frequent symptomatic episodes of bradycardia or pauses are sign of sick sinus syndrome (📖 p261) and may need a permanent pacemaker (OHCM9 📖 p126).

Complications severe bradycardia and high vagal tone can deteriorate into asystole so prompt treatment is required. Remember to talk continually to the patient and/or check for a pulse since pulseless electrical activity (PEA) is common and the ECG trace may not change.

Vasovagal attacks

Sudden reflex bradycardia from unopposed parasympathetic inhibition upon heart rate is common. Often brief loss of consciousness, preceded by eg lightheadedness, visual disturbance, nausea or sweating. Recovery of consciousness is prompt – consider other diagnoses if not. Typical precipitants are listed.

Fear and pain (including needles)

Post-micturition (especially in older men)

Nausea and vomiting

Dilatation of anal sphincter and cervix (during surgery)

Pulling of extra-ocular muscles/pressure on eye (during ophthalmic surgery)

↑Intra-abdominal pressure (during laparoscopic surgery, straining on the toilet)

Drugs which can precipitate bradycardia

β-blockers	Reports of bradycardia even from β-blocking eye drops
Digoxin	Rhythm likely to be AF, but may be sinus if reverted
Ca^{2+} antagonists	Verapamil and diltiazem slow heart rate
Amiodarone	Can cause conduction defects and bradycardia
α-agonists	Phenylephrine is mainly used by anaesthetists and can cause reflex bradycardia by increasing peripheral vascular resistance

Complete (3rd-degree) heart block (OHAM3 📖 p86)

Worrying signs features of heart failure, hypotension, ↓GCS.

Symptoms asymptomatic, dizziness (±on standing), palpitations, shortness of breath, ±chest pain.

Causes frequently underlying ischaemic damage (typically after inferior MI); also post-cardiac surgery, drug-induced (β-blockers, Ca^{2+} channel blockers), amyloid, sarcoid, myeloma, infective (Chagas, Lyme).

Signs ↓BP (and potentially ↓GCS), cannon waves in ↑JVP (due to asynchronous contraction of the right atria against a closed tricuspid valve), signs of heart failure, features of underlying disease.

Investigations **ECG** complete dissociation of P waves from QRS complexes; narrow QRS implies proximal lesion (may respond to atropine), broad QRS implies distal lesion (less likely to respond to atropine); look for evidence of myocardial infarction; **blds** FBC, U+E, Ca^{2+}, Mg^{2+}, TFT, cardiac markers, coagulation (if considering pacing-wire); **CXR** unlikely to be helpful in immediate resuscitation phase.

Acute treatment if symptomatic (dizzy or GCS <15) or systolic <90mmHg, monitor heart rate on defibrillator, lay flat with legs elevated. O_2 supplementation, secure IV access and take bloods. ▶▶Call senior help/ARREST TEAM. Titrate 500micrograms atropine IV every 2–3min (to a maximum of 3mg), followed by a large flush, until HR improves. Identify and correct precipitant. Consider external pacing/pacing-wire via central line (📖 p534); a rhythmical precordial thump (percussion pacing) can be used *in extremis* when an external pacing machine is not immediately available.

Chronic treatment likely to need permanent pacemaker (OHCM9 📖 p126) and/or correction of precipitant.

Complications severe bradycardia and high vagal tone can deteriorate into asystole so prompt treatment is required. Remember to talk continually to the patient and/or check for a pulse since pulseless electrical activity (PEA) is common and the ECG trace may not change.

Sick sinus syndrome

Dysfunction of the sinoatrial node often precipitated by ischaemia/fibrosis. Results in bradycardia (±arrest), sinoatrial block or SVT with alternating bradycardia/asystole (tachy-brady syndrome). Needs pacing if symptomatic.

Other types of heart block (OHAM3 📖 p86)

1st-degree AV block and Möbitz I do not require treatment unless the patient is symptomatic or there is a reversible cause (usually drugs).

Möbitz II and high-grade AV block may deteriorate into complete heart block and may require temporary/permanent pacing, especially when associated with an ACS or general anaesthesia – seek cardiology advice.

Hypertension emergency

Airway	Check airway is patent; consider manoeuvres/adjuncts
Breathing	If no respiratory effort – **CALL ARREST TEAM**
Circulation	If no palpable pulse – **CALL ARREST TEAM**
Disability	If GCS <8 – **CALL ANAESTHETIST**

▶▶Call for **senior help** early if patient deteriorating.

If **systolic >200** or **diastolic >120**:
- **Sit patient up**
- **15l/min O$_2$** if SOB or sats <94%
- **Monitor** pulse oximeter, BP, defibrillator ECG leads if unwell
- Request full set of **observations** and ECG
- Take brief **history** if possible/check notes/ask ward staff
- **Examine patient**: condensed RS, CVS, abdo and eye examination
- Rule out serious causes and establish **likely causes**
  - Review history and previous observations: is hypertension new?
- **Do not** give STAT dose of antihypertensive without senior review
- **Initiate further treatment**, see 📖 p264
- **Venous access**, take bloods:
  - FBC, U+E, cardiac markers, TFT, glucose, cortisol
- Consider requesting urgent **CXR**, portable if too unwell
- Urinalysis and β-hCG (in women of child-bearing age)
- Call for **senior help** for advice
- Re-assess, starting with A, B, C …

Life-threatening causes

- Pre-eclampsia/eclampsia
- Malignant hypertension >200/120
- Hypertensive encephalopathy
- Phaeochromocytoma
- Thyrotoxic storm
- Cushing's reflex (raised ICP).

Hypertension (systolic >140 or diastolic >90)

Worrying features altered mental status, seizures, retinal haemorrhages, acute renal failure, chest pain.
Is this a hypertensive crisis? If any of above, or acute ↑BP >200 systolic or >120 diastolic (🕮 p262).

Think about *life-threatening* hypertensive crisis (acute ↑BP, typically >200 systolic or >120 diastolic; 🕮 p265), pre-eclampsia; *other* anxiety, pain, primary (essential) or secondary hypertension (including thyroid storm and phaeochromocytoma).

Ask about The majority of patients will be asymptomatic, but consider possibility of end organ damage (visual symptoms, headache, chest/back pains, haematuria) or **secondary causes** (see Table 7.8) *PMH* previous hypertension, Cushing's syndrome, acromegaly, Conn's syndrome, phaeochromocytoma, coarctation, thyroid disease, DM, renal artery stenosis; *DH* cardiac and antihypertensive medications, steroids, contraceptive pill, levothyroxine/carbimazole, MAOI, antipsychotics, recreational drugs (cocaine, amphetamines); *FH* hypertension, endocrine disease, polycystic kidney disease; *SH* exercise tolerance, smoking.

Obs HR, BP (both arms with correct sized cuff), sats, temp, GCS, repeat BP after a period of prone relaxation.

Look for *signs of precipitating disease* radiofemoral delay, striae, central obesity, large hands/feet/face, tremor, exophthalmos, proximal myopathy, gravid uterus, renal bruits/polycystic kidneys; *signs of end-organ damage* fundoscopy (papilloedema, hypertensive retinopathy), displaced apex beat of S₄ (suggest left ventricular hypertrophy), haematuria.

Table 7.8 *Key secondary causes of hypertension*

	Features	Investigations	Ref
Renal disease or renal artery stenosis	Renal failure, abnormal urine dipstick, FH may be relevant, renal bruit	Urine microscopy, renal Doppler USS, autoantibodies ±renal biopsy	🕮 p373
Phaeochromocytoma	Sweating, labile hypertension, palpitations	Plasma metanephrines; 24h urinary catecholamines +VMA	🕮 p333
Thyroid dysfunction	Cold/heat intolerance, sweating, lack of energy	TFTs	🕮 p334
Acromegaly	Headache, visual field disturbance, change in facial features	IGF-1 and pituitary hormone levels	🕮 p331
Cushing's syndrome	Centripetal obesity, skin thinning, weakness	Urinary free cortisol; dexamethasone suppression test	🕮 p332

Other causes include pregnancy (gestational, pre-eclampsia/eclampsia), Conn's syndrome (🕮 p333), hyperparathyroidism (🕮 p389), scleroderma, coarctation of the aorta, drugs (steroids, MAOI, OCP) and obstructive sleep apnoea.

Investigations *BP* ensure correct sized cuff and repeat manually; a new diagnosis of hypertension should be confirmed with ambulatory or home BP monitoring; *ECG* features of LVH (📖 p573); *blds* FBC, U+E, glucose, cholesterol, TFT; *urine* blood, protein, β-hCG; *CXR* unhelpful in immediate setting, but will show heart size and aortic contours. Consider investigations for secondary causes, especially if BP >180/110 (see Table 7.8).

Treatment Offer lifestyle advice (smoking cessation, regular exercise, reduce alcohol and caffeine intake, balanced low-salt diet). Identify and treat modifiable risk factors (DM and dyslipidaemia). Recommend pharmacological therapy if appropriate, based upon BP and risk factors (see box).

Hypertension: Who and How to treat[1]

Pharmacological therapy for hypertension should be initiated in:
- All patients with BP >160/100, aiming for BP <140/90 in those aged <80 and BP <150/90 in those aged >80
- Patients with type 2 DM, aiming for BP <140/80, or <130/80 if evidence of end-organ damage (microalbuminuria or eGFR<60ml/min, retinopathy, or history of TIA/CVA)
- Patients with type 1 DM, aiming for BP <135/80, or <130/80 if microalbuminuria or retinopathy
- Patients aged <80 with BP >140/90 and existing evidence of cardiovascular disease or end-organ damage, or a predicted 10yr risk of cardiovascular disease >20%, aiming for BP <140/90.

Choice of antihypertensive for non-diabetic patients should be guided by Fig. 7.9 and patient tolerability. Calcium-channel blockers (C) (or thiazide-type diuretics D, if C not suitable) represent the best first choice drug for most patients. Limited data from younger patient groups suggest that ACE-inhibitors or angiotensin receptor blockers (A) have better blood pressure lowering effects.

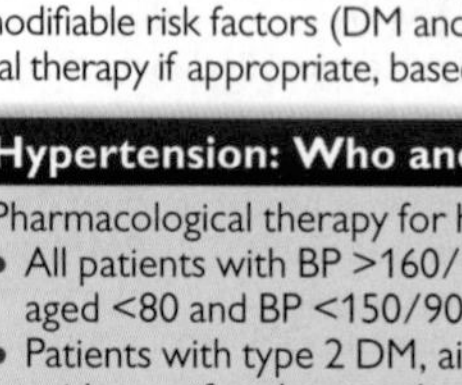

Fig. 7.9 Treating hypertension.

- β-blockers are less effective than other classes at reducing cardiovascular events, especially stroke. Their use is as an additive treatment, or to avoid polypharmacy in patients with other indications for a β-blocker (eg angina).
- For patients with DM, ACEi are the preferred first-line anti-hypertensive agents. Exceptions include patients with type 1 DM without nephropathy (D preferred) or female patients who may become pregnant (C preferred).

Follow-up If treatment initiated or altered in hospital, ensure GP knows what investigations have been undertaken, their results, and what the therapeutic plan is. Once BP control is acceptable, patients should have annual GP follow-up to review BP, lifestyle and medication. **Complications** end-organ damage, malignant hypertension.

[1] NICE guidelines available at ⬦**guidance.nice.org.uk/CG127** Thresholds and targets given in the box are based upon clinic measurements, but note that improved home monitoring equipment availability has led to increased emphasis on diagnosis and monitoring of hypertension in the patient's usual surroundings with slightly lower target values as per guidance.

Hypertensive crises (OHAM3 📖 p132)

Elevation of BP >200/120 is a hypertensive emergency when accompanied by evidence of end-organ damage (see Table 7.9) or hypertensive urgency in the absence of end-organ damage.

Symptoms and signs ↑BP, often acute, in presence of end-organ damage (see Table 7.9).

Table 7.9 *End-organ damage in hypertension*

Organ	Symptoms/signs	Investigations
CNS	↓GCS, headache, confusion, vomiting, new motor weakness, seizures, coma	CT head may show subarachnoid or intracranial haemorrhage; hypertensive encephalopathy occurs with cerebral oedema following loss of vascular autoregulation
Eyes	Headache, visual disturbance	Fundoscopy shows retinal haemorrhages ±papilloedema; often coexists with damage elsewhere
Heart	Chest pain, orthopnoea	ECG changes, elevated cardiac markers. pulmonary oedema on CXR
Aorta	Sudden tearing chest pain radiating to back; collapse	Echo or CT may reveal aortic dissection (📖 p247)
Kidneys	Haematuria, lethargy, anorexia	Rapidly worsening renal function; proteinuria, red cell casts on urine microscopy

Investigations see Table 7.9. Always confirm blood pressure yourself, using correct sized cuff. Consider secondary causes (see Table 7.8). Request formal ophthalmic assessment if suspect retinal disease.

Diagnosis relies on a compatible history, often with previously comparatively normal BP, and presence or absence of end-organ damage

Acute treatment in the absence of end-organ damage, oral therapy with a calcium-channel blocker or ACE-inhibitor should be instigated. If end-organ damage is present, admit patient to a monitored area (HDU/ICU), with close monitoring of BP, ECG, neurological state, and fluid balance (consider arterial line, central line, catheterisation). Rapid reduction in BP can be dangerous, resulting in cerebral hypoperfusion and is only necessary in an acute MI or aortic dissection. Otherwise, aim to reduce diastolic BP to 100mmHg or by 25% (whichever value is higher) over 24h (see Tables 7.10 and 7.11 for treatment options). Patients with early features of end-organ damage may be commenced on oral therapy, though more severe organ damage may require treatment with IV agents. If no evidence of LVF use labetalol; if LVF present commence furosemide (20–50mg IV) ±hydralazine. Consider ACEi to counteract high circulating levels of renin. Nitroprusside and hydralazine are still used as adjuncts in severe crises under expert guidance.

Chronic treatment BP needs checking regularly once discharged from hospital. Ensure GP knows what investigations have been undertaken, their results and what the therapeutic plan/target BP is.

> **BP control in acute CVA**
>
> In acute ischaemic stroke, cerebral autoregulation is impaired and aggressive lowering of BP results in hypoperfusion and poor outcomes. ▶▶Seek expert help. Generally, only treat if BP>220/120 or clear evidence of end-organ damage. Suitable agents include IV labetalol.

Table 7.10 *Oral antihypertensives for acute management of hypertensive crises (OHAM3 ⬚ p137)*

Drug	Dose	Comment
Atenolol	50–100mg/24h PO	Many β-blockers available. Contraindicated in asthma, peripheral vascular disease, DM
Amlodipine	5–10mg/24 PO	Ca^{2+} channel blocker; 1st line in elderly and when β-blocker contraindicated
Hydralazine	25–50mg/8h PO	Vasodilator. Safe in pregnancy
Nifedipine	10–20mg/8h PO	Avoid sublingual as rapidly drops BP. OK to use in conjunction with β-blocker (avoid verapamil or diltiazem with β-blockers)

Table 7.11 *IV antihypertensives for acute management of hypertensive crises (OHAM3 ⬚ p136)*
Patient must be in HDU/ICU, ideally with invasive BP monitoring. Intravenous therapy can result in rapid falls in BP so drugs must be titrated cautiously

Drug	Dose	Comment
Isoket® 0.05%[1] (0.5mg/ml)	2–10ml/h IVI (1–5mg/h)	Venodilates. Useful in LVF/angina. Easy for nurses to set up infusion. Drug of choice
GTN	1–10mg/h IVI	Venodilates. Useful in LVF and angina
Hydralazine	5–10mg/20min IVI	Vasodilates, can cause compensatory rise in heart rate; use with a β-blocker
Labetalol	20–80mg/10min IVI	Used in eg aortic dissection. Avoid in LVF
Nitroprusside	0.25–8micrograms/kg/min IVI	Rapid onset. Useful in LVF or hypertensive encephalopathy. Rarely used now: toxic cyanide metabolites may accumulate causing sweating, ↑HR, ↑RR, and ↓pH

[1] Isosorbide dinitrate: available as 25ml 0.1% solution (25mg in 25ml).

Heart failure[1]

Failure of the heart as a pump leads to well-recognised signs and symptoms with significant morbidity and mortality; rapidly growing prevalence.

Symptoms shortness of breath, orthopnoea, PND, ↓exercise tolerance, wheeze, ankle swelling, anorexia, nocturia.

Causes multiple factors may combine to reduce cardiac contractility and filling efficiency: ischaemia (post-MI), cardiomyopathy, dysrhythmia (eg AF), hypertension, valvular dysfunction, infections (eg HIV), infiltrative disease (eg amyloid, sarcoid), chemotherapy; also consider excess demands (eg hyperthyroidism, Paget's disease).

Signs cachexia, ↑RR, ↑HR, ↑JVP, displaced apex beat, ventricular heave, cardiac murmur (if valvular disease), 3rd heart sound, bibasilar crepitations, dependent oedema (typically ankles but check sacrum if bed-bound).

Investigations **ECG** no specific features but check for dysrhythmias or conduction blocks; **blds** FBC (exclude anaemia), U+E (?renal hypoperfusion), TFTs, fasting lipids and glucose, BNP (secreted by the failing ventricle – normal levels unlikely in untreated heart failure); **CXR** cardiomegaly, pulmonary oedema, pleural effusions, upper lobe diversion, Kerley B lines; **echo** will show valvular pathology, wall motion abnormalities and estimate left ventricular ejection fraction (LVEF). Heart failure with preserved LVEF (see box) may show evidence of ventricular hypertrophy and altered filling by Doppler flow across mitral valve.

Acute treatment of pulmonary oedema in acute decompensation (📖 p282).

Chronic treatment Support smoking cessation and a graded exercise programme. In failure with reduced LVEF, ACEi and β-blockers[2] both reduce mortality and morbidity and should be first-line therapy; if intolerant of ACEi, try ARB. 2nd-line options include cautious addition of an aldosterone antagonist, or combination hydralazine/nitrate (especially in those of African or Caribbean origin). Loop diuretics are useful for symptomatic management (with cautious addition of a thiazide if resistant). Consider aspirin ±statin if ischaemic heart disease. Those refractory to medical therapy with LVEF ≤35% and QRS prolongation may benefit from cardiac resynchronisation therapy with a biventricular pacemaker.

Heart failure with preserved ejection fraction

Much understanding in heart failure comes from the study of patients with clear echocardiographic evidence of inadequate left ventricular contraction. However, the signs and symptoms of heart failure frequently manifest in those with 'preserved LVEF'. Many of these patients will have raised left ventricular filling pressures with ventricular stiffening, reducing filling efficiency in diastole. This population is more likely to be older, female and hypertensive (a demographic rapidly increasing in size) but poorly represented in clinical trials. Despite good theoretical backing, little or no evidence of mortality benefit exists for ACEi, ARBs, β-blockers, or calcium channel blockers, whilst diuretics should be used with caution (since acute reductions in filling pressures may worsen failure). Management should involve close attention to correction of dysrhythmias and comorbid conditions, as well as control of blood pressure, and careful fluid balance.

---

[1] NICE guidelines available at 🔗guidance.nice.org.uk/CG108
[2] Avoid β-blockers in COPD. Few β-blockers are licensed for heart failure (eg bisoprolol, carvedilol, and nebivolol): Patients already on a β-blocker for another indication may need to switch.

Respiratory

Breathlessness and low sats emergency

Airway	Check airway is patent; consider manoeuvres/adjuncts
Breathing	If no respiratory effort – **CALL ARREST TEAM**
Circulation	If no palpable pulse – **CALL ARREST TEAM**

▶▶Call for **senior help** early if patient deteriorating.
- **Sit patient up**
- **15l/min O$_2$** in all patients if acutely unwell
- **Monitor** pulse oximeter, BP, defibrillator's ECG leads if unwell
- Obtain a full set of **observations** including temp
- Take brief **history** if possible/check **notes**/ask ward staff
- **Examine patient**: condensed RS, CVS, ± abdo exam
- Establish likely causes and rule out serious causes
- Initiate **further treatment**, see 🕮 p271
- **Venous access**, take bloods:
  - FBC, U+E, LFT, CRP, bld cultures, D-dimer, cardiac markers
- **Arterial blood gas**, but don't leave the patient alone
- **ECG** to exclude arrhythmias and acute MI
- Request urgent **CXR**, portable if too unwell
- Call for **senior help**
- Reassess, starting with A, B, C …
- In COPD/known CO$_2$ retention, **rapidly titrate down O$_2$** to lowest flow to maintain normal sats for this patient (usually 88–92%). Beware of CO$_2$ retention and have a low threshold for **repeat ABG**.

Life-threatening causes

- Asthma/COPD
- Pulmonary oedema (LVF)
- (Tension) pneumothorax
- MI/arrhythmia

- Pneumonia
- Pulmonary embolism (PE)
- Pleural effusion
- Anaphylaxis/airway obstruction

Breathlessness and low sats

Worrying features RR >30, sats <92%, systolic <100mmHg, chest pain, confusion, inability to complete sentences, exhaustion, tachy/bradycardia.

Think about *life-threatening* see Table 8.1 📖 p272; *most likely* COPD/asthma, pneumonia, pulmonary oedema (LVF), PE, MI; *other* pneumothorax, pleural effusion, arrhythmia, acute respiratory distress syndrome (ARDS), sepsis, metabolic acidosis, anaemia, pain, panic, foreign body/aspiration; *chronic* COPD, lung cancer, bronchiectasis, fibrosing alveolitis, TB.

Ask about speed of onset, cough, sputum (quantity, colour), haemoptysis, chest pain (related to movement, pleuritic), chest trauma, palpitations, dizziness, difficulty lying flat, recent travel, weight loss; *PMH* cardiac or respiratory problems, malignancy, TB; *DH* inhalers, home nebulisers, home O_2, cardiac medication, allergies; *SH* smoking, pets, exercise tolerance, previous and current occupation.

- *PE risk factors* recent surgery/immobility/fracture/travel, oestrogen (pregnancy, HRT, the pill), malignancy, previous PE/DVT, thrombophilia, varicose veins, obesity, central lines.

Obs temp, RR (11–20 is normal), BP, HR, sats (should be >94%[1]), O_2 requirements (improving or worsening?).

Look for ability to speak full sentences, confusion, cyanosis, CO_2 tremor, clubbing, rashes, itching, swollen lips/eyes, raised JVP, tracheal shift and tug, use of accessory muscles, abnormal percussion, unequal air entry, crackles, stridor, wheeze, bronchial breathing, swollen/red/hot/tender legs, swelling of ankles, cold peripheries.

Investigations *PEFR* if asthma suspected (may be too ill); *blds* FBC, U+E, LFT, CRP, D-dimer (if PE suspected), cardiac markers, blood cultures; *sputum* (may need physio or saline nebs to help) inspect and send for M,C+S; AFBs if TB risk; *ABG* (📖 p584), keep on O_2 if acutely SOB; *ECG* (📖 p572); *CXR* (📖 p582); portable if unwell, though image quality may be poor; *spirometry* should be done once the patient has been stabilised to help confirm the diagnosis (📖 p586).

Treatment Sit all patients up and give 15l/min O_2 – this saves lives. This can be reduced later since CO_2 retention in COPD takes a while to develop. Check sats and ECG in all patients:
- *Stridor* – call an anaesthetist (📖 p284)
- *Wheeze* – give nebuliser (📖 p273) eg salbutamol 5mg ± ipratropium 500micrograms STAT (drive by oxygen or air as appropriate)
- *Unilateral resonance, reduced air entry ±tracheal deviation and shock* – consider tension pneumothorax and treat urgently (📖 p279)
- *Asymmetrical crackles, ↓air entry* – consider pneumonia (📖 p276)
- *Symmetrical crackles, ↓air entry, ↑JVP* – consider LVF (📖 p282)
- *Normal examination* – consider PE, cardiac and systemic causes.

[1] Patients with chronic lung disease may normally have sats <92%. 88–92% is a better target. See BTS guidelines on emergency use of oxygen in adults at www.brit-thoracic.org.uk

Table 8.1 *Common causes of breathlessness*

	History	Examination	Investigations
COPD	Known respiratory problems, usually smoker, productive cough worse than usual	±wheeze/crackles, ±cyanosed/pursed-lip breathing, look for infection and pneumothorax	CXR hyperexpanded, flat diaphragms; exclude pneumonia and pneumothorax
Asthma	Known asthma, recent exposure to cold air, allergens or drugs (NSAIDS, β-blockers)	Wheeze ±crackles, look for signs of infection or pneumothorax	↓PEFR; CXR; exclude pneumonia and pneumothorax
Pneumonia	Productive cough, green sputum, feels unwell ± pleuritic pain	Febrile, asymmetrical air entry, crackles, bronchial breath sounds ±↓percussion	↑WCC/NØ/CRP, consolidation or blunted angles on CXR (🕮 p582)
Pulmonary embolism	PE risk factors, leg pain, ± pleuritic chest pain and haemoptysis	↑JVP, ↑HR (may be only sign); may have evidence of DVT; can be severely shocked	↓PaCO₂ ±hypoxia on ABGs, ↑D-dimer, CXR often normal
Pulmonary oedema	Known cardiac problems, orthopnoea, swollen legs	↑JVP, symmetrical fine crackles, pink frothy sputum, dependent oedema, cold peripheries	Cardiomegaly + fluid overload on CXR (🕮 p582), ECG may show ischaemia or previous MI
Pneumo-thorax	Sudden onset pleuritic chest pain ±trauma. Underlying lung disease and previous episodes or tall, thin, male	Unequal air entry and expansion, hyperresonant ±displaced trachea (late)	Needle decompression of tension pneumothorax; CXR shows pleura separated from ribs
Pleural effusion	Gradual onset breathlessness, ±pleuritic chest pain	Reduced expansion, stony dull base	Effusion on CXR
ARDS	Concurrent severe illness	Hypoxic	New bilateral infiltrates on CXR
Anaemia/ MI/ arrhythmias	Chest pain, palpitations, dizziness, tiredness	Irregular or fast pulse, shocked, pale	Abnormal ECG (🕮 p572), ↓Hb, ↑cardiac markers
▶▶ Anaphylaxis	Sudden onset, itching, swelling, urticarial rash, new drugs/food	Stridor, ±wheeze, shock, swollen lips and eyes, blanching rash	IM adrenaline, IV steroids (🕮 p470); acute and convalescent serum tryptase

Asthma[1] (OHAM3 📖 p178)

Common, chronic inflammatory airway disorder characterised by airway hypersensitivity resulting in episodic obstruction, wheeze and dyspnoea.

Symptoms episodic breathlessness, dyspnoea and wheeze, night or morning cough, excess sputum; triggers may include exercise, NSAIDs, β-blockers, allergens, cold; family or personal Hx of atopy (hayfever, eczema, asthma).

Signs wheeze, prolonged expiration, tachypnoea, hyperinflated chest.

Investigations **PEFR** reduced in acute setting compared with best or predicted based upon age/height,[1] or diurnal variation as out-patient; **ABG** normal or ↓PaO_2 with a ↓$PaCO_2$ due to hyperventilation ▶▶beware normal/rising CO_2 ?Pt tiring; **CXR** hyperexpanded, exclude pneumonia and pneumothorax; **spirometry** ↓FEV_1, ↓FEV_1:FVC ratio.

Acute exacerbation sit up and give 15l/min O_2. Salbutamol 5mg NEB ±ipratropium 500micrograms NEB and prednisolone 40mg PO (or hydrocortisone 200mg IV). Drive the nebuliser mask from O_2 supply, not air. Repeat salbutamol 2.5mg nebs every 10–15min and reassess PEFR and sats frequently. Antibiotics if evidence of infection.

▶▶Severe	Incomplete sentences, PEFR <50% of best, HR >110, RR >25
▶▶Life-threatening	PEFR <33% of best, silent chest, sats <92%, PaO_2 <8kPa, normal $PaCO_2$, poor respiratory effort, exhaustion, cyanosis, altered GCS, arrhythmia
▶▶Near-fatal	CO_2 retention – call ICU

Beware those with previous ICU admissions

- **No improvement** Call for **senior help**. Consider:
  - **ICU** input/assessment
  - **Aminophylline** 5mg/kg IV bolus over 20min unless the patient is on oral aminophylline or theophylline
  - **Mg^{2+} sulfate** 2g (8mmol) IV over 20min
- **Improving** admit those in whom PEFR<75% predicted after 1h therapy; gradually reduce supplemental O_2 and step from nebs back to inhalers over several days; always check inhaler technique and ensure follow-up plan in place before discharge.

Chronic treatment (OHCM9 📖 p174) Stepwise management (see Table 8.2) aiming for minimum treatment resulting in symptom control; monitor PEFR; always check inhaler technique before escalation; consider allergen testing; smoking cessation; oral steroids for exacerbations.

Table 8.2 *Simplified stepwise management of asthma[1]*

	Step 1	Step 2	Step 3*	Step 4	Step 5
Oral steroids					✓
High-dose steroid inhaler			✓	✓	✓
Long-acting β-agonist			✓	✓	✓
Low-dose steroid inhaler		✓	✓		
Salbutamol/terbutaline	✓	✓	✓	✓	✓

* Either low-dose steroid inhaler and long-acting β-agonist or high-dose steroid inhaler.

[1] BTS Asthma guidelines available at ⚲www.brit-thoracic.org.uk/guidelines/asthma-guidelines. **aspx** These include tables to predict PEFR where not known.

COPD[1] (OHAM3 📖 p186)

Relatively fixed airflow obstruction due to loss of elastic recoil in alveoli (emphysema) and narrowing of airways with excess secretions (bronchitis)
Worrying signs ↓GCS, rising CO_2.

Symptoms breathlessness, cough, ↑sputum, tight chest, confusion, ↓exercise tolerance. NB ↓index of suspicion in (ex-)smoker.

Signs wheeze, cyanosis, barrel-chested, poor expansion, tachypnoea.

Investigations **ABG** often deranged in COPD, compare with previous samples and pay close attention to FiO_2; repeat after 30min in seriously ill patients; **CXR** hyperexpanded, flat diaphragm (look for evidence of infection, pneumothorax or bullae); **spirometry** (see 📖 p586) ↓FEV_1, ↓FEV_1:FVC ratio (<70%).

Acute exacerbation sit the patient up and give the minimum amount of O_2 to maintain sats ≥88% (aim for PaO_2 ~8kPa). Give salbutamol 5mg ±ipratropium 500micrograms nebs (drive by air, leaving nasal O_2 cannulae on under mask if necessary) and prednisolone 30mg PO (or hydrocortisone 200mg IV). Sputum for M,C+S. Get an ABG and CXR (portable if unwell). Use ABG results and clinical observations to guide further management:

- **Normal ABG** (for them) continue current O_2 and give regular nebs
- **Worsening hypoxaemia** ↑FiO_2, repeat ABG <30min, watch for confusion which should prompt a repeat ABG sooner; consider NIV (see box)
- **↑CO_2 retention or ↓GCS** request senior help **urgently**; consider:
  - **ICU** input/assessment
  - **aminophylline** 5mg/kg IV bolus over 20min unless the patient is on oral aminophylline or theophylline
  - **NIV** (see box).

Antibiotics consider prescribing antibiotics (eg doxycycline 200mg PO loading then 100mg/24h PO or amoxicillin 500mg/8h PO) if the patient has increased SOB, fevers, worsening cough, purulent sputum, or focal changes on CXR.

Chronic treatment (OHCM9 📖 p176) Smoking cessation and graded exercise are vital. Stepwise therapy with inhalers (see Table 8.3) is based upon inhaled short-acting β-agonist or anti-cholinergic, then inhaled long-acting agents, then adding inhaled steroid before oral theophylline. If still breathless despite maximal inhaler therapy give home nebulisers. If PaO_2 consistently ≤7.3kPa (or ≤8kPa with additional risk factors) long-term O_2 therapy aiming for a minimum of 15h/d confers survival advantage.

Complications exacerbations, infection, cor pulmonale, pneumothorax, respiratory failure, lung cancer (beware haemoptysis and weight loss).

Non-invasive ventilation (NIV)

These are machines that assist ventilation through a tightly fitting mask rather than tracheal intubation. Bi-level positive airway pressure (BiPAP) used in COPD patients with a pH ≤7.35 and CO_2 ≥6.0kPa who have failed to respond to initial medical therapy reduces mortality and length of admission. Patients who need NIV are usually allocated specialist beds on the respiratory ward or on HDU/ICU. Continuous positive airway pressure (CPAP) is *not* a type of NIV since it does not help with the mechanics of ventilation (📖 p282).

---

[1] NICE guidelines available at 🖰guidance.nice.org.uk/CG101

Table 8.3 Common inhalers for COPD and asthma

Type of drug	Colour	Medication	Trade
Short-acting β-agonist	Blue	Salbutamol	Ventolin®
	Blue	Terbutaline	Bricanyl®
Inhaled steroids	Brown	Beclometasone	Qvar®
	Brown	Budesonide	Pulmicort®
	Orange	Fluticasone	Flixotide®
Short-acting anticholinergic	White + green	Ipratropium	Atrovent®
Short-acting β-agonist and anticholinergic	White + orange	Salbutamol and ipratropium	–
Inhaled steroids with long-acting β-agonist	Red	Budesonide and formoterol	Symbicort®
	Purple	Fluticasone and salmeterol	Seretide®
Long-acting β-agonist	Green	Salmeterol	Serevent®
Long-acting anticholinergic	Grey	Tiotropium	Spiriva®

Pulmonary rehabilitation

There is good evidence[1] that patients with chronic lung disease who take part in a pulmonary rehabilitation programme see increased exercise tolerance and improved well-being. These programmes do not reverse the pathological process or improve spirometry measurements.

Most hospitals and general practices have access to such programmes, and patients generally take part in a structured programme for 8–12wk. Exercise is encouraged which becomes progressively more strenuous. Diet and other lifestyle advice are also usually covered.

Once discharged from the programme, patients are encouraged to continue the exercises they have learnt, either as part of their daily lives at home or at leisure centres.

The British Lung Foundation can be contacted to find local programmes; 03000 030 555.

[1] Summarised at ⏣www.brit-thoracic.org.uk/guidelines-and-quality-standards/pulmonary-rehabilitation-guideline/

Online respiratory resources

British Thoracic Society	www.brit-thoracic.org.uk
British Lung Foundation	www.lunguk.org
Thorax (journal)[2]	thorax.bmj.com
Cochrane library	www.thecochranelibrary.com

[2] Subscription required, but many NHS organisations will grant access via ATHENS.

Pneumonia[1] (OHAM3 📖 p166)

Worrying signs CURB-65 score ≥3 (📖 Severity, p276).

Symptoms cough, increased sputum (coloured), pleuritic chest pain, breathless, haemoptysis, fever, unwell, confusion, anorexia.

Signs ↑temp, ↑RR, ↑HR, ↓sats, unequal air entry, reduced expansion, dull percussion, bronchial breathing.

Severity the CURB-65 criteria (see Fig. 8.1) are a validated set of variables that support (but do not replace) clinical judgement in community acquired pneumonia on whether to admit.[2] In the out-patient setting, omit urea to get a CRB-65 score; patients scoring 0 (and possibly 1–2) are suitable for home treatment.

Investigations **blds** ↑WCC, ↑NØ, ↑CRP; **bld cultures** if CURB-65 ≥2; **sputum cultures** if CURB-65 ≥3 (or CURB-65=2 and not had antibiotics); **urine** if CURB-65 ≥2 test for pneumococcal antigen; if CURB-65 ≥3 or clinical suspicion, test for legionella antigen; **ABG** ↓PaO$_2$ (±↓PaCO$_2$ due to hyperventilation but not if tiring or COPD); **CXR** on hospital admission may show focal consolidation; repeat at 6wk if ongoing symptoms or high risk for malignancy.

Treatment sit up and give O$_2$ as required. Give antibiotics according to local policy or see 📖 p179 for empirical treatment. Look for dehydration and consider IV fluids. Most patients who require IV antibiotics can safely be switched to PO therapy by day 3;[3] if symptoms not resolving by this time, repeat CRP and CXR to exclude pleural effusion/empyema.

Complications empyema, respiratory failure, sepsis, confusion.

Hospital acquired pneumonia Pneumonia developing ≥48h after admission and not felt to have been incubating at time of admission. Causative organisms will include Gram –ve bacilli (eg *Pseudomonas* or *Klebsiella* species, *E. coli.*) as well as *S. pneumoniae* and *S. aureus* (including MRSA). Symptoms and signs can be severe, particularly in frail patients with other comorbidities, and lung necrosis and cavitation may develop. Empirical antibiotic selection should be guided by local policy ±discussion with a microbiologist.

Aspiration pneumonia Aspiration of gastric contents refluxing up the oesophagus and down the trachea may lead to a sterile chemical pneumonitis. Alternatively, oropharyngeal bacteria may be aspirated causing a bacterial pneumonia. **Risk factors** include ↓GCS (eg sepsis, anaesthesia, seizures), oesophageal pathology (eg strictures, neoplasia), neurological disability (eg dementia, MS, Parkinson's disease) or iatrogenic interventions (eg NG tube, OGD, bronchoscopy). At-risk patients can be identified by bedside swallow evaluation (📖 p352). Care is supportive, with O$_2$ supplementation, suctioning of secretions and attention to prevention of further aspiration (involve SALT). Empirical antibiotics can be of benefit if bacterial pneumonia suspected (eg persistent fever, purulent sputum) – eg co-amoxiclav 625mg/8h PO or 1.2g/8h IV with metronidazole 400mg/8h PO or 500mg/8h IV.

[1] British Thoracic Society guidelines for the management of community acquired pneumonia in adults available at: ⬠**www.brit-thoracic.org.uk/guidelines-and-quality-standards/community-acquired-pneumonia-in-adults-guideline/**

[2] Lim, W.S. *et al. Thorax* 2003 **58:**377 full-text available free at: ⬠**www.ncbi.nlm.nih.gov/pmc/articles/PMC1746657**

[3] Oosterheert, J.J. *et al. BMJ* 2006 **333:**1193 full-text available free at: ⬠**www.ncbi.nlm.nih.gov/pmc/articles/PMC1693658**

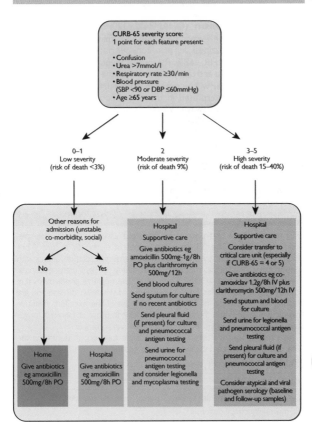

Fig. 8.1 Severity assessment and investigations in community acquired pneumonia. Adapted by permission from BMJ Publishing Group Limited. British Thoracic Society guidelines for the management of community acquired pneumonia in adults: update 2009, Lim, W.S. et al. Thorax 2009 **64** (Suppl 3):iii1.

Pulmonary embolism[1] (OHAM3 📖 p120)

Symptoms often none except breathlessness; may have pleuritic chest pain, haemoptysis, dizziness, leg pain; consider risk factors in Table 8.4.

Signs ↑JVP, ↑RR, ↑HR, ↓BP, RV heave, hypotension, pleural rub, ±pyrexia. Tachycardia and tachypnoea may be the only clinical signs.

Investigations **D-dimer** will be raised in many situations, whilst a normal D-dimer must be interpreted in the clinical context (see box); **ECG** ↑HR, RBBB, inverted T waves V1–V4 or $S_1Q_3T_3$; **ABG** ↓CO_2, ± ↓O_2 (if large); **CT-PA** is the definitive imaging modality, though **V/Q scan** may be used eg in those with renal failure.

Acute treatment sit up (unless ↓BP) and give 15l/min O_2. If life-threatening seek immediate senior support, arrange an urgent CT-PA ±echo and consider thrombolysis. Otherwise parenteral anticoagulation (📖 p399) eg enoxaparin 1.5mg/kg/24h SC and pain relief; IV fluids if ↓BP.

Chronic treatment generally oral anticoagulation (📖 p406) eg warfarin (INR 2–3) for at least 3mth.[2]

Clinical risk assessment for PE

PEs are common and potentially fatal, but associated with non-specific clinical signs. The CT-PA offers excellent diagnostic accuracy but exposes your patient to 3.6 years of background radiation, along with nephrotoxic IV contrast medium, whilst taking up significant resources. So can D-dimer testing help? Remember, the negative predictive value of any test is determined by the prevalence of whatever disease you are testing for: The value of D-dimer testing lies in the excellent negative predictive value when the risk of a PE is low. In those at high risk, negative D-dimer levels do not provide sufficient reassurance.

The Wells score for PE is a clinically reliable method of identifying the risk of PE, and hence deciding on further testing

Table 8.4 *Wells score for pulmonary embolism*[3]

Clinical feature	Points
Signs/symptoms of DVT (leg swelling & pain on deep vein palpation)	3
PE most likely clinical diagnosis	3
HR >100	1.5
>3d immobilisation or surgery in past 4wk	1.5
Previous DVT/PE	1.5
Haemoptysis	1
Malignancy (current treatment or treatment in past 6mth or palliative)	1

- Those scoring ≤4 are low risk: Test for D-dimers.[3] If elevated, proceed to CT-PA; if negative, then consider alternative diagnoses
- Those scoring >4 are high risk: Proceed to CT-PA testing (with LMWH if scan cannot be performed immediately)

[3] In pregnancy D-dimer testing is uninterpretable. If clinical suspicion, then a Doppler U/S of leg veins is the safest initial investigation–treat if DVT seen. If this is negative, a half-dose V/Q scan provides an acceptable balance of diagnostic utility with radiation exposure. The risk of CT-PA is not to the foetus (which can be shielded) but to proliferating maternal breast tissue.

[1] NICE guidelines available at ⌐guidance.nice.org.uk/CG144
[2] 3mth may suffice if low risk (eg 1st PE with identified risk factor now removed); if higher risk (recurrent or unprovoked PEs, or thrombophilia) treatment may need to be long term.

Spontaneous pneumothorax (OHAM3 📖 p204)[1]

May occur apparently spontaneously (primary) or in the presence of underlying lung disease or injury (secondary).

Risk factors **primary** tall, thin, male; Marfan's; recent central line, pleural aspiration or chest drain; **secondary** COPD, asthma, infection, trauma, mechanical ventilation.

Symptoms breathlessness ±chest pain.

Signs hyper-resonant and reduced air entry on affected side, tachypnoea, may have tracheal deviation or fractured ribs.

Investigations **CXR** lung markings not extending to the peripheries, line of pleura seen away from the periphery.

Treatment sit up and give 15l/min O_2. Chest drain/aspiration as directed by BTS guidelines (📖 p280). In essence, primary pneumothoraces can potentially be discharged, whilst secondary pneumothoraces require admission and either aspiration (📖 p538) or, more usually, drainage (📖 p540).

▶▶Tension pneumothorax

If air trapped in the pleural space is under positive pressure (eg following penetrating trauma or mechanical ventilation) then mediastinal shift may occur, compressing the contralateral lung and reducing venous return. The patient may be hypotensive, tachycardic, tachypnoeic, with unilateral hyperresonance and reduced air entry; ↑JVP and may have tracheal deviation. This is an emergency, it will rapidly worsen if not treated. Sit up and give 15l/min O_2. Treat prior to CXR. Insert a large cannula (orange/grey) into the 2nd intercostal space, midclavicular line. Listen for a hiss and leave it *in situ*; insert a chest drain on the same side. If there is no hiss, leave the cannula *in situ* and consider placing a 2nd cannula or consider alternative diagnoses; a chest drain is usually still required to prevent a tension pneumothorax accumulating.

Pleural effusion (OHAM3 📖 p216)[1]

Excessive fluid within the pleural space reflects an imbalance between hydrostatic and oncotic pressures within the pleural vasculature, and/or disruption to lymphatic drainage.

Causes may be divided into those causing **transudates** (where pleural fluid protein <25g/l – tend to be bilateral) pulmonary oedema, cirrhosis, nephrotic syndrome, hypothyroidism, intestinal malabsoprtion/failure and **exudates** (protein >35g/l – may be unilateral or bilateral) malignancy, infection, vasculitides, rheumatoid; if purulent and pH <7.2, this is **empyema** reflecting infection.

Light's criteria help differentiate, especially when protein >25g/l but <35g/l. Consider the effusion an exudate if pleural protein:serum protein >0.5, pleural LDH:serum LDH >0.6 or pleural LDH >2/3 of upper limit of normal serum value.

Symptoms may be breathless with pleuritic chest pain.

Signs stony dull to percussion with reduced air entry, tachypnoea.

Investigations **CXR** loss of costophrenic angle with a meniscus, 📖 p582.

Treatment sit up and give 15l/min O_2. Investigate the cause; if the effusion is large, pleural aspiration (see 📖 p538) may relieve symptoms and aid diagnosis (draining >1.5l/24h may cause pulmonary oedema).

[1] British Thoracic Society guidelines available at ⌁**www.brit-thoracic.org.uk/guidelines-and-quality-standards/pleural-disease-guideline/**

Algorithms for the treatment of spontaneous pneumothorax

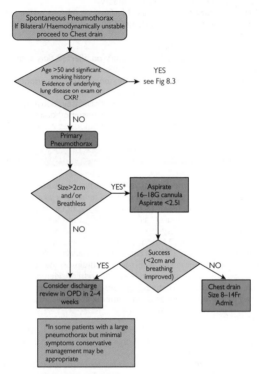

Fig. 8.2 Treating spontaneous pneumothorax in patients over 50 with no significant smoking history or evidence of underlying lung disease. Adapted by permission from BMJ Publishing Group Ltd, Management of spontaneous pneumothorax: British Thoracic Society pleural disease guideline 2010, MacDuff, A. *et al. Thorax* 2010 **65** (Suppl 2):ii18.

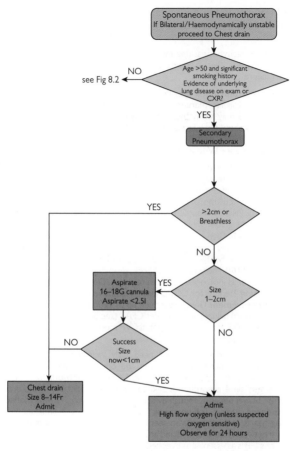

Fig. 8.3 Treating pneumothorax in patients over 50 with significant smoking history or evidence of underlying lung disease. Adapted by permission from BMJ Publishing Group Ltd, Management of spontaneous pneumothorax: British Thoracic Society pleural disease guideline 2010, MacDuff, A. *et al. Thorax* 2010 **65** (Suppl 2):ii18.

Pulmonary oedema (OHAM3 📖 p87)

Symptoms dyspnoea, orthopnea, paroxysmal nocturnal dyspnoea, frothy sputum; coexistent dependent oedema or previous heart disease.

Signs ↑JVP, tachypnoea, fine inspiratory basal crackles, wheeze, pitting cold hands and feet; oedema (ankles and/or sacrum) suggests right heart failure.

Investigations **blds** (look specifically for anaemia, infection or MI): FBC, U+E, CRP, cardiac markers; BNP (normal levels unlikely in cardiac failure); **ABG** may show hypoxia; **ECG** exclude arrhythmias and acute STEMI, may show old infarcts, LV hypertrophy or strain (📖 p572); **CXR** cardiomegaly (not if AP projection), signs of pulmonary oedema (📖 p582); **echo** poor LV function/ejection fraction.

Acute treatment sit up and give 15l/min O_2. If the attack is life-threatening call an intensivist early as CPAP and ICU may be required. Otherwise monitor HR, BP, RR, and O_2 sats whilst giving furosemide 40–120mg IV ±diamorphine (repeat every 5min up to 5mg max, watch RR) 1mg boluses IV (repeat up to 5mg, watch RR). If further treatment is required, be guided by blood pressure:

- **Systolic >100** Give 2 sprays of sublingual GTN followed by an IV nitrate infusion (eg GTN starting at 4mg/h and increasing by 2mg/h every 10min, aiming to keep systolic >100; usual range 4–10mg/h; see 📖 p201)
- **Systolic <100** The patient is in shock, probably cardiogenic. Get senior help as inotropes are often required. Do not give nitrates
- **Wheezing** Treat as for COPD alongside above treatment
- **No improvement** Give furosemide up to 120mg total (more if chronic renal failure) and consider CPAP (see below). Insert a urinary catheter to monitor urine output, ±CVP monitoring. Request senior help. Consider HDU/ICU.

Once stabilised, the patient will need daily weights ±fluid restriction. Document LV function with an echo and optimise treatment of heart failure (📖 p267). Oral bumetanide may be preferred to oral furosemide for diuresis since absorption is said to be more predictable in the presence of bowel oedema, though evidence for this is lacking. Always monitor U+E during diuresis: The heart-sink patients are those with simultaneously failing hearts and kidneys who seem fated to spend their last days alternating between fluid overload and acute renal failure – close liaison with the patient's GP is as essential as ever here.

Continuous positive airway pressure (CPAP)

Application of positive airway pressure throughout all phases of the respiratory cycle limits alveolar and small airway collapse, though the patient must still initiate a breath and have sufficient muscular power to inhale and exhale. Pursed-lip breathing has a similar effect, and is often observed in patients with chronic lung disease. CPAP is often used in the acute treatment of pulmonary oedema or the chronic treatment of sleep apnoea (may use nasal CPAP).

SVC obstruction (OHCM9 📖 p526)

Symptoms breathlessness, orthopnoea, facial/arm swelling, headache.

Signs facial plethora (redness), facial oedema, engorged veins, stridor.

Pemberton's test elevating the arms over the head for 1min results in increased facial plethora and ↑JVP.

Investigations **CXR/CT** mediastinal mass, tracheal deviation; ***venogram*** venous congestion distal to lesion; ***other*** sputum cytology for atypical cells.

Treatment Seek senior input early. Sit up and give 15l/min O$_2$. Dexamethasone 4mg/6h PO/IV. Consider diuretics to decrease venous return and relieve SVC pressure (eg furosemide 40mg/12h PO). Otherwise symptomatic treatment whilst arranging for tissue diagnosis.

Acute respiratory distress syndrome (ARDS) (OHAM3 📖 p198)

Acute onset respiratory failure due to diffuse alveolar injury following a pulmonary insult (eg pneumonia, gastric aspiration) or systemic insult (shock, pancreatitis, sepsis). Characterised by the acute development of bilateral pulmonary infiltrates and severe hypoxaemia in the absence of evidence for cardiogenic pulmonary oedema.

Symptoms breathlessness, often multiorgan failure.

Signs hypoxic, signs of respiratory distress and underlying condition.

Investigations **CXR** bilateral infiltrates.

Treatment sit up and give 15l/min O$_2$. Refer to HDU/ICU and treat underlying cause. Often requires ventilation.

Stridor in a conscious adult patient

Airway	Acute stridor – **CALL ANAESTHETIST AND ENT URGENTLY**
Breathing	If poor respiratory effort – **CALL ARREST TEAM**
Circulation	If no palpable pulse – **CALL ARREST TEAM**

▶▶Call for **senior anaesthetics** and **ENT help** immediately.
- **Do not** attempt to look in the mouth/examine the neck
- If **choking**, follow algorithm in Fig. 8.4
- Avoid **disturbing/upsetting** the patient in any way
- Let the **patient sit** in whatever position they choose
- Offer **supplemental O₂** to all patients
- **Fast bleep** senior anaesthetist
- **Fast bleep** senior ENT
- **Adrenaline (epinephrine) nebs** (5ml of 1:1000 with O₂)
- **Monitor** pulse oximeter ±defibrillator's ECG leads if unwell
- Check **temp**
- Take brief **history** from relatives/ward staff or check notes
- **Look for** swelling, rashes, itching (**?anaphylaxis**)
- Consider **serious causes** (below)
- Await **anaesthetic** and **ENT** input
- Request urgent portable **CXR**
- Call for **senior** help
- **Reassess**, starting with A, B, C …

Life-threatening causes

• Infection (epiglottitis, abscess)	• Foreign body
• Tumour	• Post-op
• Trauma	• Anaphylaxis

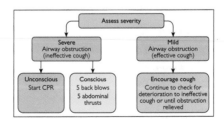

Fig. 8.4 Adult choking treatment algorithm, 2010 guidelines.
Reproduced with the kind permission of the Resuscitation Council (UK).

Cough

Causes of coughs

Acute	URTI, post-viral, post-nasal drip (allergy), pneumonia, LVF, PE
Chronic	Asthma, COPD, bronchitis, bronchiectasis, smoking, post-nasal drip, oesophageal reflux, pneumonia, TB, parasites, interstitial lung disease, heart failure, ACE inhibitors, lung cancer, sarcoid, sinusitis, cystic fibrosis, habitual
Bloody	Massive bronchiectasis, lung cancer, infection (including TB and aspergilloma), trauma, AV malformations; other bronchitis, PE, LVF, mitral stenosis, aortic aneurysm, vasculitides, parasites

Usually, the cause of coughing is obvious. However, chronic, unexplained coughing with a normal CXR and the absence of infective features requires a considered approach. Is there diurnal or seasonal variation in coughing (cough-variant asthma might be investigated with a PEFR diary, lung function testing, and a trial of inhaled steroids)? Is there a history suggestive of gastro-oesophageal reflux (consider a trial of PPI)? Does the onset of a dry cough follow the introduction of an ACE inhibitor (consider using an AT II receptor blocker)? Or is there a sensation of mucus accumulation at the back of the throat (consider chronic/allergic rhinitis and 'post-nasal drip' and a trial of nasal steroids or antihistamines)?

Haemoptysis coughing up blood, ≥400ml is considered 'massive'.
Management FBC, U+E, LFT, clotting, G+S, sputum C+S and cytology, ABG, ECG, CXR. Sit up, 15l/min O$_2$. Codeine 60mg PO (may ↓cough)
if massive: good IV access (≥green), monitor HR and BP, immediate referral to respiratory team for bronchoscopy ±CT thorax.

Bronchiectasis[1] (OHCM9 📖 p166)

Abnormal and permanent distortion of the medium sized airways caused by destruction of the elastic tissue of the bronchial walls.

Causes cystic fibrosis, infection (pneumonia, TB, HIV), tumours, immunodeficiency, allergic bronchopulmonary aspergillosis, foreign bodies, rheumatoid arthritis, idiopathic.

Symptoms chronic cough with purulent sputum ±haemoptysis, halitosis.

Signs clubbing, coarse inspiratory crepitations ±wheeze.

Investigations FBC, immunoglobulins, aspergillus serology; blood or sweat test (for **_CF_**); **_sputum_** C+S; **_CXR_** thickened bronchial outline (tramline and ring shadows) ±fibrotic changes; **_CT thorax_** bronchial dilatation; **_bronchoscopy_** to exclude other diagnoses.

Acute treatment O$_2$ ±BiPAP as required, ±bronchodilators ±corticosteroids. Typical recurrent infections include *Pseudomonas* (consult local antibiotic guidelines). Chest physiotherapy to mobilise secretions.

Chronic treatment postural drainage (chest physio), inhaled/nebulised bronchodilators/corticosteroids/antibiotics, surgery may be considered; consider prophylactic, rotating antibiotics.

Complications recurrent pneumonia, pseudomonal infection, massive haemoptysis, cor pulmonale.

---

[1] British Thoracic Society guidelines available at ⏚**www.brit-thoracic.org.uk/guidelines-and-quality-standards/bronchiectasis-guideline/**

Chapter 9

Gastroenterology

Abdominal pain emergency

Airway	Check airway is patent; consider manoeuvres/adjuncts
Breathing	If no respiratory effort – **CALL ARREST TEAM**
Circulation	If no palpable pulse – **CALL ARREST TEAM**

▶▶Call for **senior help** early if patient deteriorating.
- **15l/min O$_2$** if SOB or sats <94%
- **Monitor** BP, pulse oximeter, defibrillator's ECG leads if unwell
- Obtain a full set of **observations**, are they haemodynamically stable?
- Take brief **history** if possible/check **notes**/ask ward staff
- **Examine patient**: condensed RS, CVS, abdo, ±wound exam
- Consider **serious causes** (see box) and treat if present
- Initiate **further treatment**, see 🕮 p289
- **Venous access**, take bloods:
  - FBC, U+E, LFT, amylase, CRP, clotting, X-match 4 units, bld cultures
- Give IV **fluids** if hypovolaemic or shocked (🕮 p476)
- **Analgesia** as appropriate
- **Arterial blood gas**, but don't leave the patient alone
- **Erect CXR** (portable if unwell) and consider **plain AXR**
- **ECG**
- **Urine dipstick** and β-**hCG** (all pre-menopausal women), ± catheter
- Keep patient **NBM** if likely to need theatre
- Call for **senior help**
- **Reassess**, starting with A, B, C …

Life-threatening causes and emergencies

- Perforation
- Bowel infarction/ischaemia
- Bowel obstruction
- Acute pancreatitis
- Acute cholangitis
- Appendicitis
- Leaking abdominal aortic aneurysm (AAA)
- Strangulated hernia
- Testicular or ovarian torsion
- Ruptured ectopic pregnancy
- Referred pain (MI, aortic dissection)

Abdominal pain

> *Worrying features* sudden onset, ↑HR, ↓BP, ↓GCS, massive distension, peritonism, expansile mass, persistent vomiting, haematemesis, massive PR bleeding; *if life-threatening, see* 📖 *p288.*

Think about pain by anatomical structure, see Fig. 9.1; ***common*** gastroenteritis, peptic ulcer, gastro-oesophageal reflux disease (GORD), constipation, inflammatory bowel disease (IBD), irritable bowel syndrome (IBS), diverticular disease, adhesions, mesenteric adenitis, renal colic, UTI/pyelonephritis, urinary retention, biliary colic/sepsis, pancreatitis, bleeding AAA, incarcerated hernia, ischaemic bowel; ***obs/gynae*** ectopic pregnancy, ovarian cyst, ovarian torsion, PID, endometriosis, labour; ***other*** trauma, MI, pneumonia, sickle-cell crises, DKA, psoas abscess, porphyria. See Table 9.1.

Ask about nature of pain (constant, colicky, changes with eating/vomiting/bowels), duration, onset, frequency, severity, radiation to the back, dysphagia, dyspepsia, abdominal swelling, nausea and vomiting, stool colour, change in bowel habit, urinary symptoms, weight loss, breathlessness, rashes, lumps, chest pain, recent surgery, last period; ***PMH*** DM, IBD, IHD, jaundice, gallstones, pancreatitis, previous abdo surgery; ***DH*** NSAIDs; ***SH*** alcohol.

Obs temp, HR, BP, RR, sats, finger-prick glucose, urine output.

Look for jaundice, sweating, pallor, pulse volume, clubbing, leuconychia (white nails), lymphadenopathy (Virchow's node), abdominal scars, distension, ascites, visible peristalsis, tenderness, peritonitis (tenderness with guarding, rebound or rigidity), loin tenderness, hepatomegaly, splenomegaly, masses (?expansile/pulsatile), check hernial orifices, examine external genitalia (♂: testicular vs. epididymal tenderness), femoral pulses, bowel sounds, lung air entry; ***PR*** perianal skin tags, fissures, warts; tenderness, masses, prostate hypertrophy, stool, check glove for blood, mucus, melaena and stool colour.

Investigations *urine* dipstick, β-*hCG* in all pre-menopausal women of reproductive age, MSU; *blds* FBC, U+E, LFT, amylase, Ca^{2+}, glucose, ±cardiac markers, venous lactate, clotting, bld cultures if pyrexial; *ABG* if unwell; *ECG* to exclude MI; *erect CXR* to exclude perforation; *plain AXR* to exclude bowel obstruction or *KUB* for renal colic; *USS* especially if hepatobiliary cause suspected; *CT abdo* discuss with senior.

Treatment Give all patients O_2, analgesia ±antiemetics; insert a urinary catheter if unwell. Keep NBM until urgent surgery is ruled out.

- ***Shocked*** IV fluids ▶▶urgent senior review
- ***Peritonitic*** with IV fluids, IV antibiotics ▶▶urgent senior review
- ***>50yr in severe pain*** ?AAA, IV fluids ▶▶urgent senior review
- ***Abdo pain and vomiting*** consider obstruction, IV fluids, NG tube, AXR (📖 p588) ▶▶urgent senior review
- ***GI bleed*** resuscitate with IV fluids (📖 p298) ▶▶urgent senior review.

Table 9.1 Common causes of abdominal pain

	History	Examination	Investigations
▶▶Perforation	Rapid onset, severe abdominal pain	Peritonitis, ± bowel sounds	Gas under diaphragm, acidotic
Bowel obstruction	Pain, distension, nausea, vomiting, constipation	Distension, tenderness, tinkling bowel sounds	Dilated loops of bowel on AXR
Bowel ischaemia/infarction	Sudden onset, severe pain, previous arterial disease, ±AF	Shock, generalised tenderness	↑WCC, ↑lactate/acidotic, ±AF or previous MI on ECG
Appendicitis	RIF pain (initially periumbilical), anorexia, nausea, vomiting	Slight temp, RIF tenderness, ±peritonitic	↑WCC, ↑CRP
Strangulated hernia	Sudden onset pain, previous hernia	Tender hernial mass	Needs urgent surgery
GORD/peptic ulcer	Dyspepsia, heartburn, anorexia, NSAIDs	Epigastric tenderness	Consider need for OGD
Gastroenteritis	Rapid onset, vomiting, diarrhoea	↑temp, epigastric tenderness, no peritonitis	↑WCC, ↑CRP
Inflammatory bowel disease	Weight loss, mouth ulcers, PR blood±mucus, diarrhoea	Tender±mass ±peritonitis	↑WCC, ↑CRP, ↑plts, oedematous bowel on AXR, lesions on colonoscopy
Diverticular disease	Pain, diarrhoea, constipation, PR bleeding	Tenderness, ±peritonitis	↑WCC, ↑CRP, diverticulae on colonoscopy
▶▶Acute pancreatitis	Constant epigastric pain radiating to back, vomiting, anorexia, ↑alcohol or gallstones	Shock, epigastric tenderness, ↓bowel sounds	↑↑↑amylase, ↑WCC, ↑CRP, ↑glucose, ↓Ca²⁺
▶▶Abdominal aortic aneurysm (AAA)	Abdominal and back pain, collapse, prev heart disease/↑BP, age >50yr, ♂	Expansile mass, unwell, often ↓BP, ↓leg pulses	Urgent USS (bedside if possible); immediate surgery if leaking
Renal colic	Sudden severe colicky flank pain, radiates to groin, nausea/vomiting	Sweating, restless, loin tenderness	60% of stones visible on KUB; >99% on non-contrast CT
Hepatobiliary disease	Constant or colicky RUQ pain, gallstone	RUQ tenderness, ±jaundice	Deranged LFTs; dilated CBD on USS
Obs/gynae disease	Lower abdo pain, PV bleeding, irregular/absent periods	Lower abdo tenderness, PV exam abnormal	β-hCG +ve, lesions seen on USS
▶▶Testicular torsion	Sudden onset severe unilateral groin pain	Tender testicle, ±swelling	Urgent surgery

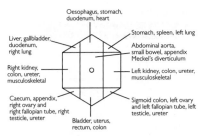

Fig. 9.1 Abdominal organs and pain, by region.

Causes of abdominal pain in this section and elsewhere			
Bowel			
Adhesions/ischaemia	📖 p293	Appendicitis	📖 p293
Diverticular disease	📖 p295	Dyspepsia/peptic ulcers	📖 p294
Gastroenteritis	📖 p307	Hernias	📖 p292
Inflammatory bowel disease	📖 p309	Irritable bowel syndrome	📖 p308
Obstruction	📖 p292	Perforation	📖 p291
Hepatopancreatobiliary			
Biliary colic/cholecystitis	📖 p295	Hepatitis	📖 p315
Pancreatitis (acute/chronic)	📖 p296		
Genitourinary			
Ectopic pregnancy	📖 p498	Endometriosis	📖 p500
Ovarian cyst	📖 p500	Pelvic inflammatory disease	📖 p500
Testicular torsion	📖 p463		
Other			
Abdominal aortic aneurysm	📖 p474	Renal colic	📖 p296

▶▶**Perforation** (OHCM9 📖 p608)

Causes peptic ulcer, appendicitis, diverticulitis, inflammatory bowel disease, bowel obstruction, GI cancer, gallbladder.

Symptoms acute abdominal pain worse on coughing or moving; **PMH** peptic ulcer, cancer, IBD; **DH** NSAIDs; **SH** alcohol.

Signs ↑HR, ±↓BP, ↑RR, peritonism (abdo tenderness, guarding, rebound, rigidity), reduced or absent bowel sounds.

Investigations **blds** ↑WCC, ↓Hb, ↑amylase, ↑lactate; **CXR** erect film shows air under the diaphragm, ±obstruction on **AXR**; **ABG** acidosis.

Management **seek senior review;** resuscitate with IV fluids, 15l/min O₂, good IV access (large ×2), analgesia (eg morphine 5–10mg IV with cyclizine 50mg/8h IV), NBM and urgent X-match 4 units: IV antibiotics (eg co-amox-iclav 1.2g/8h IV) insert NG tube and urinary catheter, consider emergency CT once stable, prepare for emergency laparotomy (📖 p112).

Bowel obstruction (OHCM9 📖 p612)

Causes of intestinal obstruction	
Outside the bowel	Adhesions, hernias, masses, volvulus
Within the bowel wall	Tumours, IBD, diverticular disease, infarction, congenital atresia, Hirschsprung's disease
Inside the bowel lumen	Impacted faeces, FB, intussusception, strictures, polyps, gallstones
Paralytic ileus (pseudo-obstruction)	Post-op, electrolyte imbalance, uraemia, DM, anticholinergic drugs

Symptoms vomiting (may be faeculant), colicky abdo pain, pain may improve with vomiting, constipation (±absolute – no flatus or stool), bloating, anorexia, recent surgery.

Signs ↑HR ±↓BP, ↑RR, distended abdomen, absent or tinkling bowel sounds, peritonitis, scars from previous surgery, hernias.

Investigations **blds** mild ↑WCC and ↑amylase ±acidosis; **AXR** look for dilated bowel (?small or large) or volvulus (📖 p588); erect **CXR** ?free air.

Management may need fluid resuscitation and analgesia, treat according to the type and location of the obstruction:

- **Strangulated** constant severe pain in an ill patient with peritonitis (acute abdomen); can be small or large bowel. This will require urgent surgery especially if caused by a hernia
- **Small bowel** early vomiting with late constipation, usually caused by hernias, adhesions or Crohn's. Treat conservatively with NBM, an NG tube and IV fluids (📖 p380) – often referred to as drip and suck – until the obstruction resolves; surgery if patient deteriorates. K^+ is often lost into the bowel and needs to be replaced in fluids (eg 20mmol/l)
- **Large bowel** early absolute constipation with late vomiting, usually caused by tumours, diverticulitis, volvulus (sigmoid or caecal) or faeces. IV fluids, NBM and refer to a senior surgeon. Urgent surgery may be required if the caecum is >10cm across on AXR otherwise a CT, colonoscopy or water-soluble contrast enema may be requested to investigate the cause. Surgery is usually required except for:
  - sigmoid volvulus – sigmoidoscopy and flatus tube insertion
  - faecal obstruction – laxative enemas (📖 p205)
  - colonic stenting – may be offered for tumour palliation
- **Paralytic ileus** loss of bowel motility can mimic the signs and symptoms of a mechanical blockage. It is a response of the bowel to inflammation locally (eg surgery) or adjacently (eg pancreatitis). The main distinguishing feature is the relative lack of abdo pain, although the pathology responsible for the ileus may cause abdo pain itself. USS abdo, contrast enema or CT may be required to exclude mechanical obstruction. Treat conservatively with NBM, NG tube, IV fluids (📖 p380) until the underlying pathology improves. Check and correct electrolyte abnormalities, including K^+ and Mg^{2+} both of which may need to be replaced.

Complications strangulation, bowel infarction, bowel perforation, ↓K^+, hypovolaemia.

Adhesions

Causes previous surgery, abdominal sepsis, IBD, cancer, endometriosis.

Symptoms and signs chronic intermittent abdominal pain and tenderness, may develop bowel obstruction (distension, vomiting, constipation).

Management analgesia and stool softeners; may need operative division of adhesions, but this may lead to new adhesions forming.

Bowel ischaemia/infarction (OHCM9 📖 p622)

Symptoms unwell, sudden onset severe constant abdominal pain, PR blood; **PMH** AF, MI, polycythaemia.

Signs ↑HR (?irregular), ±↓BP, ↑RR, ↑temp, cold extremities, generalised tenderness but few specific signs.

Investigations **blds** ↑WCC, ↑amylase, metabolic/lactic acidosis; **sigmoidoscopy** ±biopsy may show pale, ulcerated mucosa.

Management NBM, resuscitate with IV fluids; analgesia, IV ABx (eg co-amoxiclav 1.2g/8h IV), consider anticoagulation with IV heparin (📖 p406), surgical resection is often necessary. Very poor prognosis – clarify premorbid state and consider ICU care as appropriate.

Appendicitis (OHCM9 📖 p610)

A common diagnostic challenge[1] – complications can be severe if left untreated, but 15–40% of appendicectomy specimens are normal. Can occur in any age group; classical cases are easy enough to spot, variable anatomy and extremes of age can make presentation atypical.

Differential UTI, diverticulitis, gastroenteritis, mesenteric adenitis, perforated ulcer, IBD, diverticulitis; **gynae** ectopic pregnancy, ovarian torsion, ruptured ovarian cyst, salpingitis.

Symptoms central, abdominal colicky pain worsening over 1–2d then developing into constant RIF pain (sensitivity and specificity of ~80%[2]), worse on moving, anorexia, nausea, vomiting, may have constipation, diarrhoea, dysuria, oliguria (all non-specific and common).

Signs ↑temp, ↑HR, ±↓BP, RIF tenderness ± guarding/rebound/rigidity, RIF pain on palpating LIF (Rovsing's sign), PR tender on right (there is no evidence that this has diagnostic utility in adults, but failure to perform PR still considered negligent).

Investigations ↑WCC, neutrophilia>75%, ↑CRP (a useful triad with negative predictive value >97% in adults, but beware children and elderly); bld cultures (if pyrexial), G+S; US and contrast-enhanced CT reduce laparotomy rates, but this must be balanced against risks of radiation exposure and local resources.

Management surgery – NBM, IV fluids, analgesia, IV ABx (eg co-amoxiclav 1.2g/8h IV). Laparoscopic approaches reduce scarring, post-operative pain, recovery time and incidence of wound infections, but require more operative time and higher skill levels than open appendicectomy. If peritonitic send for immediate surgery, otherwise reassess regularly whilst awaiting surgery. If diagnostic uncertainty a short period of safe observation ± imaging can be informative.

---

[1] And hence an all too common source of tension between ED staff and junior surgical doctors - try to avoid becoming part of this seemingly perpetual cliché when your turn comes.

[2] See Yeh, B. *Ann Emerg Med* 2008 **52**:301, for an excellent review of the clinical utility of signs and symptoms in adult appendicitis; available free at: www.annemergmed.com/article/S0196-0644(07)01732-5/fulltext

Dyspepsia[1] (OHCM9 📖 p242)

Any persistent symptom referable to the upper GI tract. This will include patients with peptic ulcer disease, gastro-oesophageal reflux disease, oesophagitis, and rare upper GI malignancies, as well as those without significant endoscopic changes. Aim to identify those at risk of significant pathology, and control symptoms in those without.

Symptoms burning retrosternal or epigastric pain, worse on bending and lying, waterbrash (excess saliva), acid reflux, nausea, vomiting, nocturnal cough, symptoms improved by antacids; symptom patterns are poorly predictive of endoscopic findings.

Signs epigastric tenderness (no peritonitis), rarely epigastric mass.

Common risk factors smoking, alcohol, obesity, pregnancy, hiatus hernia, medications (bisphosphonates, calcium antagonists, nitrates, corticosteroids, NSAIDs).

Investigations urgent endoscopy if 'red flag' symptoms (chronic GI bleeding/iron deficiency anaemia, unintentional weight loss, progressive dysphagia, persistent vomiting, epigastric mass) or ≥55yr and persistent/unexplained dyspepsia. Else test and treat for *H. pylori* (see box). Some reserve testing for those who fail empirical treatment with 1mth full dose PPI. Consider low-dose maintenance or as-required PPI for those who respond. If symptoms persist, consider endoscopy or 24h ambulatory pH monitoring.

Management **lifestyle advice** weight loss, smoking cessation, alcohol reduction, avoid foods/drugs which exacerbate symptoms, especially NSAIDs.

- *GORD* antacids (📖 p184) PRN if mild; full dose PPI for 1–2mth, then low dose or PRN PPI; H_2 receptor blockers (eg ranitidine) less effective than PPI, but individual patients may respond better; surgical fundoplication (rarely) if severe
- *Oesophagitis* as for GORD; frequency of surveillance if Barrett's oesophagus detected requires specialist guidance
- *Peptic ulcer* 1–2mth full dose PPI. 95% of duodenal and 80% of gastric ulcers are related to *H. pylori*, therefore ensure eradication (see box). Gastric ulcers are also associated with malignancy, therefore repeat endoscopy at 6wk to confirm healing. If symptom recurrence, retest, since eradication may require different or prolonged antibiotics, and re-infection can occur
- *Gastric/oesophageal malignancy* urgent multidisciplinary team referral for surgery/palliation.

H. pylori infection and eradication

- ^{13}C-urea breath testing reliably detects infection or confirms eradication and is widely used in secondary care; faecal antigen tests are used in primary care
- CLO tests require a biopsy taken at OGD and rely upon pH indicator changes
- A 'wash-out' period of 2wk off PPI is needed for these tests; serological tests are less reliable, but can be used in a patient on a PPI
- Treatment is with triple therapy for 1wk, eg lansoprazole 30mg/12h PO, amoxicillin 1g/12h PO, clarithromycin 500mg/12h PO **BNF** 1.3
- Regimens containing metronidazole may increase resistance and may be better reserved for 2nd-line therapy
- 2wk courses increase eradication rates by 10%, but are not cost-effective.

---

[1] NICE guidelines available at ⬚guidance.nice.org.uk/CG17

Diverticular disease (OHCM9 📖 p630)

Diverticulosis = diverticulae (out pouchings) in the large bowel.

Diverticulitis = inflammation of diverticulae; acutely symptomatic.

Symptoms abdominal pain/cramps (usually left sided, improves with bowel opening), irregular bowel habit, flatus, bloating, PR bleeding.

Signs ↑temp, ↑HR, ±↓BP, LIF tenderness, ±peritonitis, distension.

Investigations **blds** ↑WCC, ↑CRP; *CT/colonoscopy* for indirect/direct visualisation.

Management **diverticulosis** high-fibre diet, antispasmodics (eg mebeverine), laxatives (eg senna, 📖 p205); **diverticulitis** NBM, analgesia, fluids and ABx (eg co-amoxiclav 1.2g/8h IV).

Complications obstruction, perforation, abscess, adhesions, strictures, fistula, PR bleeding (usually painless).

Renal colic (OHCM9 📖 p640)

Always consider other causes of abdominal pain, including AAA, especially if no previous renal stone disease.

Symptoms acute onset severe unilateral colicky pain radiating from loin to groin, nausea and vomiting, sweating, haematuria, dysuria, strangury (frequent, painful passage of small volumes of urine with sensation of incomplete emptying); iliac fossa or suprapubic pain suggests another pathology.

Signs ↑HR, sweating, patient restless and in severe pain, usually no tenderness on palpation unless superimposed infection.

Investigations **urine** Hb on dipstick (~90% cases), nitrates suggest UTI, β-*hCG* if ♀; *blds* FBC, U+E, Ca^{2+}, urate; *KUB* detects 60% stones, *CT* >99%.

Management analgesia (NSAID first, then opioids), if <5mm should pass spontaneously. If evidence of infection give IV ABx (check local policy). If evidence of infection or hydronephrosis refer urgently to urologist for nephrostomy or stent.

Complications pyelonephritis, renal dysfunction.

Biliary colic

Contraction of the gallbladder or cystic duct around gallstones.

Symptoms recurrent colicky or constant RUQ/epigastric pain (especially on eating fatty foods), nausea, vomiting, bloating.

Signs RUQ tenderness, non-peritonitic, not jaundiced.

Results **blds** normal; *USS* gallstones.

Management analgesia, dietary advice and elective cholecystectomy.

Complications passage of stone into common bile duct may cause cholestatic jaundice, cholangitis or acute pancreatitis.

Acute cholecystitis

Gallbladder inflammation eg 2° to cystic duct occlusion by gallstone.

Symptoms continuous RUQ/epigastric pain, unwell, vomiting.

Signs ↑temp, RUQ tenderness and peritonitis, Murphy's sign (pain and cessation of deep inspiration during palpation in RUQ, not present on LUQ).

Results **blds** ↑WCC, ↑CRP; *USS* gallstones and thickened gallbladder.

Management NBM, analgesia, ABx (eg co-amoxiclav 1.2g/8h IV); consider urgent cholecystectomy vs. interval procedure. ERCP if distal CBD stone.

▶▶**Acute pancreatitis**[1] (OHCM9 📖 p638)

Varies from a mild self-limiting illness to severe and life-threatening.

Causes 'I GET SMASHED': **i**diopathic, **g**allstones (50%), **e**thanol (25%), **t**rauma, **s**teroids, **m**umps, **a**utoimmune, **s**corpion bites (rare),[2] **h**yperlipidaemia, **h**ypercalcaemia, **h**ypothermia, **E**RCP, **d**rugs (eg thiazide diuretics).

Symptoms constant severe epigastric pain radiating to the back, improved with sitting forward, nausea, vomiting, anorexia.

Signs ↑HR, ±↓BP, ↑temp, cold extremities, epigastric tenderness with peritonitis, abdominal distension, ↓bowel sounds, mild jaundice, Cullen's (bruised umbilicus) or Grey–Turner's (bruised flanks) sign.

Results **blds** ↓Hb, ↑WCC, ↑↑↑lipase (or amylase),[3] ↑glucose, ↓Ca^{2+}, deranged clotting (±DIC), LFT; **USS** ?gallstones; **CT** if diagnosis in doubt.

Management IV fluid resuscitation, O$_2$, analgesia, urinary catheter, NBM, NG tube. If severe (Table 9.2) involve ICU and plan ERCP if gallstone aetiology. Monitor fluid balance, obs, glucose. Daily U+E, FBC, CRP; prophylactic LMWH (📖 p406).

Complications DIC, renal failure, respiratory failure, haemorrhage, thrombosis, sepsis (infected necrosis), pseudocysts, abscess, chronic pancreatitis.

Table 9.2 *Modified Glasgow score for predicting acute pancreatitis severity*

Variable	Criteria	
Age	>55yr	In 1974 **Ranson** developed a scoring system, validated for use in alcohol-induced acute pancreatitis; this remains widely used. The **modified Ranson** criteria (1979) have been validated for gallstone related disease. In 1984, Blamey et al.[4] at the Royal Infirmary in **Glasgow** modified 8 of the 11 Ranson criteria and validated these for prognostic use in both alcohol and gallstone induced acute pancreatitis.
PaO$_2$	<8.0kPa	
WCC	>15 x 10^9/l	
Ca^{2+} (uncorr.)	<2mmol/l	
Glucose	>10mmol/l	
ALT	>100u/l	
LDH	>600u/l	
Urea	>16mmol/l	
Albumin	<32g/l	

Score 1 point for each parameter present on admission or within the first 48h. A score of ≥3 predicts an episode of severe pancreatitis and should prompt ICU/HDU referral.

[4] Original article available free at www.ncbi.nlm.nih.gov/pmc/articles/PMC1420197

Chronic pancreatitis (OHCM9 📖 p280)

Causes usually alcohol, but can be due to gallstones (which may also cause recurrent pancreatitis), familial, cystic fibrosis, hyperparathyroidism, ↑Ca^{2+}.

Symptoms general malaise, anorexia, weight loss, recurrent epigastric pain radiating to back, steatorrhoea, bloating, DM.

Signs cachexia, epigastric tenderness.

Investigations **blds** glucose (?DM, 📖 p328); **stool** ↓elastase; **USS** (±endoscopic), **CT**.

Management analgesia, advise to stop drinking alcohol; **diet** refer to dietician: low fat, high calorie, high protein with fat-soluble vitamin supplements; **pancreatic enzymes** eg Creon® before eating; **surgery** coeliac-plexus block, stenting of the pancreatic duct, pancreatectomy.

[1] British Gastroenterology Society guidelines available at 🔗gut.bmj.com/content/54/suppl_3/iii1.full
[2] Case series available free at 🔗www.ncbi.nlm.nih.gov/pmc/articles/PMC1700547
[3] Lipase slightly more specific. Overall trend in relation to pain is more important than absolute values.

GI bleeding emergency

Airway	Check airway is patent; consider manoeuvres/adjuncts
Breathing	If no respiratory effort – **CALL ARREST TEAM**
Circulation	If no palpable pulse – **CALL ARREST TEAM**

▶▶Call for **senior help** early if patient deteriorating.
- Lay the patient **on their side** if vomiting
- **15l/min O₂** if SOB or sats <94%
- **Monitor** pulse oximeter, BP, defibrillator's ECG leads if unwell
- Obtain a full set of **observations** including temp
- Two good (large) sites of **venous access**, take bloods:
  - FBC, U+E, LFT, clotting, urgent 4 unit X-match
- **0.9% saline** 1l IV
- Take brief **history** if possible/check **notes**/ask ward staff
- **Examine patient:** condensed CVS, RS and abdo exam
- **Correct clotting** abnormalities if present (📖 p404)
- **Arterial blood gas**, but don't leave the patient alone
- Initiate **further treatment**, see following sections
- Consider **serious causes** (see box) and treat if present
- Seniors may consider giving terlipressin 2mg IV over 5min if **gastro-oesophageal varices** suspected (📖 p300)

If bleeding is severe and the patient haemodynamically unstable:
- Call for **senior help**
- Give **O–ve blood**, request X-matched units
- Contact the on-call endoscopist and alert **surgeons**
- *Reassess*, starting with A, B, C …

Life-threatening causes

• Peptic ulcer	• Gastro-oesophageal varices
• Vascular malformations	• Upper GI malignancy

Acute upper GI bleeds[1] (OHAM3 📖 p224)

Worrying features ↓GCS, ↑HR, ↓BP, postural BP drop, ↓urine output, frank haematemesis, frank PR blood, chest pain, coagulopathy, liver disease.

Think about *common* peptic ulcer (NSAIDs, H. pylori), Mallory–Weiss tear, gastro-oesophageal varices, oesophagitis, swallowed blood (eg epistaxis); *other* oesophageal or gastric cancer, vascular malformations, underlying coagulopathy (Table 9.4).

Ask about colour, quantity, mixed in or throughout vomit, frequency, onset, stool colour and consistency (those on iron may have black stool but it should not be tarry), chest pain, abdominal pain, dysphagia, dizziness, fainting, sweating, SOB, weight loss; **PMH** coagulopathy, liver problems (?varices), peptic ulcers; **DH** NSAIDs, anticoagulants, steroids; **SH** alcohol.

Obs Pay special attention for ↑HR, ↓BP; check postural BP, GCS.

Look for continued bleeding, colour of vomit, cold extremities, sweating, pulse volume, bruises, other bleeding (nose, mouth), abdominal tenderness±peritonitis, masses, signs of chronic liver disease (📖 p313); **PR** fresh blood/melaena.

Investigations **blds** FBC, U+E, LFT, clotting, G+S or 2-4 unit X-match; low platelets may indicate hypersplenism (?2° to portal hypertension/chronic liver disease); ↑↑urea (out of proportion to ↑creatinine); check for coagulopathy; **ECG** ?ischaemia; **OGD** allows diagnosis and definitive treatment only *after* adequate resuscitation; timing guided by clinical assessment of severity: Risk scoring can be useful in this regard (Table 9.3), but does not replace clinical judgement. Discuss all potential major bleeds with seniors and an endoscopist at an early stage.

Table 9.3 *Rockall risk scoring system for GI bleeds*

Clinical information allows initial risk stratification, to which endoscopic findings (in italics) are added for complete assessment. ≤2 = low risk

Feature	0	1	2	3
Age	<60yr	60–79yr	≥80yr	
Shock: systolic BP and HR	>100mmHg <100/min	>100/min	<100mmHg	
Comorbidity	Nil major	Heart failure, IHD	Renal/liver failure	Metastatic disease
Diagnosis	*Mallory–Weiss/none*	*All other*	*Upper GI malignancy*	
Bleeding on OGD	*Nil recent*		*Recent*	

The Rockall score was developed to predict risk of death or rebleeding based upon the complete score calculated after endoscopy (eg will occur in 11% of those with Rockall=3). ▶▶Suspicion of rebleeding requires urgent discussion with the endoscopist and surgeon on call ±interventional radiology. As an alternative, the Blatchford score was developed to predict those not requiring intervention based upon admission parameters, marginally outperforming the Rockall score in this regard. It is somewhat more complex and less widely used (online calculators available eg ⌀www.mdcalc.com). NICE has managed to end up recommending the use of both scores.

[1] NICE guidelines available at ⌀guidance.nice.org.uk/CG141

Table 9.4 *Common causes of upper GI bleeding*

	History	Examination	Investigation
Peptic ulcers	Epigastric/chest pain, heartburn, melaena, previous ulcers, NSAIDs, alcohol	Epigastric tenderness, may be peritonitic if perforated	Ulcer on OGD, CLO test may be +ve
Oesophagitis/ gastritis	Heartburn, NSAIDs, alcohol, hiatus hernia	Epigastric tenderness	Inflammation/ erosions on OGD
Gastro-oesophageal varices	Frank haematemesis previous liver disease, alcohol	Epigastric tenderness, signs of chronic liver disease	↑PT, deranged LFT, varices on OGD
Mallory–Weiss tear	Forceful vomiting precedes bloodstaining	Epigastric tenderness	Tear seen on OGD if not resolving

Management NBM until OGD, O₂, two large-bore cannulae. IV fluids ± blood,[1] regular obs (HR, BP, postural BP, urine output); consider catheterisation, CVC line and HDU/ICU:

- **Blood transfusion** is often vital and lifesaving. However, over-transfusion is also associated with increased mortality and rebleeding.[1] Assess each patient carefully and discuss transfusion targets with a senior
- **PPIs** reduce rebleeding, need for surgery and mortality, but only when given *after* endoscopy to high-risk patients (bolus then 72h infusion)
- **Mallory–Weiss tears** (OHAM3 📖 p234) occur after repeated forceful vomiting, often after alcohol excess. Bright red blood appears as streaks or mixed with vomit. Bleeding often resolves spontaneously
- **Clotting abnormalities** (📖 p404) consider: platelet transfusion if active bleeding and plts <50×10⁹/l; FFP if PT/APTT >1.5 x control; Prothrombin complex concentrate if on warfarin
- **H. pylori** (📖 p294) test and eradicate if positive.

▶▶**Gastro-oesophageal varices** (OHAM3 📖p232)
Symptoms of chronic liver failure (📖 p313); known liver disease, excess alcohol; varices are asymptomatic until they bleed.
Signs of chronic liver failure (📖 p313).
Investigations varices seen on OGD.
Acute bleed resuscitate according to 📖 p298 then:

- **Terlipressin** 2mg/over 5min IV if not already given
- **Antibiotics** cirrhotic patients have ↓immune function; spontaneous bacterial infections are associated with ↑mortality (eg Tazocin® 4.5g/8h IV)
- **OGD** (urgent) for banding (oesophageal) or sclerotherapy (gastric)
- **Bleeding still uncontrolled** consider a Sengstaken–Blakemore tube and transjugular intrahepatic portosystemic shunting (TIPS)

Once bleeding controlled Terlipressin 1–2mg/6h over 5min IV, for up to 5d; treat cause of liver failure; ↓risk of recurrent bleeding by ↓portal pressure (by TIPS or propranolol 40–80mg/12h PO) or further banding.

What about other drugs?

Once haemostasis is achieved, continuation of aspirin where previously indicated (under PPI cover) is associated with reduced mortality (albeit at a higher risk of rebleeding).[2] NSAIDs should be stopped and alternative analgesics prescribed. Data for other antiplatelet drugs and anticoagulants are more complex and each case will need careful discussion between the relevant specialists.
[2] Sung J.J.Y. et al. *Ann Intern Med.* 2010 **152**:1 (subscription required – check ATHENS).

---

[1] Villanueva C. et al. *NEJM* 2013 **368**:11 free at ⟲www.nejm.org/doi/full/10.1056/NEJMoa1211801

Acute lower GI bleeds

Worrying features continuous bright-red PR bleeding, ↑HR, ↓BP, postural drop, dizziness, ↓GCS, abdominal pain, weight loss, vomiting.

Think about *common* polyps, diverticular disease, angiodysplasia, haemorrhoids, IBD, colon cancer, upper GI bleed (🕮 p299); *other* aortoenteric fistulae, ischaemic colitis, radiation proctitis, Meckel's diverticulum.

Ask about onset, quantity, colour (red, black, clots), type of blood (fresh, mixed with stool, streaks on toilet paper), abdominal pain, vomiting (colour), pain on opening bowels, straining, change in bowel habit, anorexia, weight loss, dizziness, SOB; *PMH* previous bleeding, diverticular disease, IBD, peptic ulcer, liver disease, AAA; *DH* NSAIDs, anticoagulants, steroids, iron; *FH* IBD, bowel cancer; *SH* alcohol.

Obs HR, BP, postural BP, GCS, RR, sats.

Look for pale and cold extremities, sweating, pulse volume, bruises, other sources of bleeding (nose, mouth), abdominal tenderness ±peritonism, masses, signs of chronic liver disease (🕮 p313); *PR* blood, melaena, palpable mass, haemorrhoids. See Table 9.5.

Investigations *blds* FBC, clotting, U+E, LFT, G+S or X-match 2 units; *ABG* only if unwell; *OGD* to exclude upper GI bleed, urgent if shocked; *ECG* if age >50yr; *sigmoidoscopy/colonoscopy* for investigation, biopsy and treatment; may require *mesenteric angiography* or *capsule enteroscopy* if bleeding source cannot be identified.

Management lower GI bleeding is traditionally managed by surgeons whilst upper GI bleeding is usually a medical condition. Although ~85% lower GI bleeds will settle with conservative management, always beware the brisk upper GI bleed presenting as PR bleeding.

• *Diagnosis* it is rarely possible to tell the cause of significant lower GI bleeds from history and examination alone, investigations are essential
• *Fresh blood on toilet paper* or streaking stool only and patient well: Treat as haemorrhoids/anal fissure, but arrange follow-up flexible sigmoidoscopy to rule out bowel cancer
• *Mild bleeding* (no evidence of shock) should usually settle with conservative management. Consider early discharge and follow-up
• *Moderate bleeding* (postural drop, ↑HR) secure IV access and fluid resuscitate ± blood until haemodynamically stable, catheterise, hourly fluid balance, senior review, may need urgent OGD if possibility of upper GI source
• ▶▶*Severe bleeding* (fresh bleeding/clots, ↓BP) resuscitate according to 🕮 p298, transfuse, call senior, on-call endoscopist and surgical registrar. ~15% of patients with acute, severe PR bleeding will have an upper GI bleeding source identified on OGD. For the remainder, options include colonoscopic haemostasis, radiological embolisation, or surgical resection.

Table 9.5 *Common causes of lower GI bleeding*

	History	Examination	Investigation
Upper GI bleed	Haematemesis, fresh PR bleeding, clots or melaena, epigastric pain	Liver disease, epigastric tenderness, PR blood or melaena	↓Hb, ↑urea, lesion on OGD
GI cancer or polyps	Change in bowel habit, weight loss, abdominal pain	PR blood or melaena, mucus, palpable mass	↓Hb±↓MCV, lesion on sigmoidoscopy or colonoscopy
Inflammatory bowel disease	Abdominal pain, diarrhoea, weight loss, mouth ulcers	↑temp, abdo tender ±peritonitic, PR blood, mucus, melaena	↓Hb, ↑WCC, ↑CRP, lesions on sigmoidoscopy or colonoscopy
Diverticular disease	Abdominal pain, fever, change in bowel habit	Tenderness, ±peritonism, PR blood, mucus	↓Hb, diverticulae on colonoscopy
Bowel ischaemia	Abdo pain, previous arterial disease	Shock, generalised tenderness	↑WCC, acidotic, ±AF or previous MI on ECG
Angiodysplasia or radiation proctitis	Recurrent fresh PR blood, old age, previous pelvic radiotherapy	PR blood or melaena	↓Hb, lesions on colonoscopy, consider argon plasma coagulation
Haemorrhoids	Painless, fresh red blood on toilet paper, perianal itch, constipation	Often not palpable on PR, perianal tags, may have rectal prolapse	Lesions seen on proctoscopy
Anal fissure	Pain on defecating, fresh blood on toilet paper, constipation	Posterior/anterior PR tear, perianal tags, tenderness	Proctoscopy to visualise lesions

Chronic gastrointestinal blood loss

Causes oesophagitis, gastric erosions, gastritis, peptic ulcer, gastric/bowel cancer, polyps, IBD, angiodysplasia, GI lymphoma.

Symptoms anorexia, weight loss, tired, change in bowel habit, melaena, vague intermittent abdo pain.

Signs pale/anaemic, cachexic, mild abdo tenderness; **PR** blood, mass.

Investigations **stool** faecal occult blood (FOB), ova, cysts and parasites; **blds** FBC (↓Hb, ↓MCV[1]), iron, ferritin, B₁₂, folate, U+E, LFT; **OGD** ±**colonoscopy**; may need a video **capsule endoscopy** or small bowel **CT/MRI** if small bowel disease suspected.

Treatment investigate and treat the cause, treat anaemia with ferrous sulfate 200mg/8h PO, consider admission for transfusion if Hb <80g/L or if symptomatic with anaemia.

---

[1] Those with a simultaneous iron deficiency and B₁₂ and/or folate deficieny may have a normal or raised MCV; in this instance, significant variation in red cell size will be reflected in an increased red cell distribution width (RDW).

Colorectal polyps (OHCM9 📖 p618)

A common finding at colonoscopy; their importance lies in the premalignant potential of adenomatous polyps.

Causes vast majority sporadic; rare familial syndromes.

Symptoms often none; intermittent abdo pain, altered bowel habit, blood or melaena in stool, tenesmus, weight loss.

Signs **PR** palpable mass if very distal, blood, mucus.

Investigations ↓Hb, lesion on **colonoscopy**.

Treatment polypectomy (send for histology), multiple polyps may need colonic resection or regular colonoscopy follow-up.[1]

Haemorrhoids (OHCM9 📖 p634)

Dilated and displaced perianal vascular tissue (anal cushions).

Symptoms recurrent fresh red blood on toilet paper or streaking stools ±pain or pruritus ani (anal itch), constipation.

Risk factors constipation with straining, multiple vaginal deliveries.

Signs not palpable unless prolapsed; **PR** blood, otherwise normal.

Investigations **proctoscopy** to visualise haemorrhoids, **sigmoidoscopy** to identify other pathology (eg malignancy).

Treatment high-fibre diet, topical Anusol®, injection of sclerosants, band ligation, coagulation, cryotherapy, may need haemorrhoidectomy.

Strangulated haemorrhoids painful, tender mass, unable to sit down, treat with ice packs, stool softeners, regular analgesia and bed rest. Once stable, inject piles and consider elective haemorrhoidectomy.

Anal fissure (OHCM9 📖 p632)

Symptoms new onset extreme pain±fresh red blood on opening bowels, history of constipation and straining (beware Crohn's and cancer).

Signs anal tear visible posteriorly on the anal margin (10% anterior), perianal ulcers, fistulae; **PR** may be impossible due to pain.

Investigations **sigmoidoscopy** if suspicious of pathology once pain controlled.

Treatment conservative high-fibre diet; 5% lidocaine ointment, 0.2–0.3% GTN ointment, botox injection all marginally better than placebo;[2] internal sphincterotomy cure rate 95%.

Angiodysplasia (OHCM9 📖 p630)

Submucosal arteriovenous malformation, often ascending colon.

Symptoms elderly, recurrent blood in the stool, abdo pain is rare.

Signs may be normal, pallor; **PR** blood or melaena.

Investigations faecal occult blood, **colonoscopy**, **mesenteric angiography**.

Treatment angiographic embolisation if active bleeding; argon plasma coagulation (endoscopic); rarely resection; treat anaemia, eg ferrous sulphate.

Causes of rectal bleeding covered elsewhere			
Inflammatory bowel disease	📖 p309	Upper GI bleed	📖 p299
Bowel ischaemia	📖 p293	Diverticular disease	📖 p295
		Infective diarrhoea	📖 p307

---

[1] The British Society of Gastroenterology guidelines for colonoscopic follow-up are at ⌐www. bsg.org.uk/images/stories/docs/clinical/guidelines/endoscopy/ccs_10.pdf

[2] For a useful meta-analysis, see ⌐http://summaries.cochrane.org/CD003431

Nausea and vomiting

Worrying features ↑HR, ↑/↓BP, ↓GCS, severe pain (head, chest, abdomen), head injury, constipation, blood/coffee grounds, purpuric rash.

Think about *life-threatening* raised intracranial pressure (ICP), meningitis, MI, bowel obstruction, acute abdomen, DKA; *common* post-op, pain, drug induced (opioids), gastroenteritis, other infection, alcohol; *other* gastroparesis, paralytic ileus, pregnancy, electrolyte imbalance (Ca^{2+}, Na^+), migraine, labyrinthitis, Ménière's, chemotherapy, Addison's, eating disorder (Table 9.6).

Ask about frequency, timing, relation to food or medications, colour, blood, coffee grounds, melaena, dizziness, diarrhoea, constipation, flatus, pain, headaches, head trauma, visual problems, pregnancy; *PMH* previous surgery, migraines, DM; *DH* opioids, chemotherapy, digoxin; *SH* alcohol.

Obs temp, fluid balance, HR, BP, blood glucose, GCS, stool chart.

Look for and assess volume status (🕮 p380), SOB, distended/tender/peritonitic abdomen, tinkling bowel sounds, hernias, surgical scars, mouth ulcers, neck stiffness, rash, photophobia, papilloedema.

Investigations vomiting without the worrying features usually does not require urgent investigation. If recurrent, check U+E for dehydration or electrolyte imbalance and *AXR* if bowel obstruction suspected. Otherwise investigate according to related symptoms. Consider: *blds* FBC, U+E, LFT, glucose, amylase, Ca^{2+}, Mg^{2+}; *CXR* aspiration; *ABG* if acutely unwell; *CT brain* if head trauma (🕮 p438); gastric emptying studies if suspect gastroparesis.

Treatment Investigate and treat underlying disease; vomiting is distressing – so see 🕮 p185 for pharmacology and selection of appropriate antiemetics.

Table 9.6 *Common causes of nausea and vomiting*

	History	Examination	Investigations
Raised ICP/ meningitis	Headache, blurred vision, dizzy, feels ill, drowsy	Febrile, stiff neck, photophobia, rash, low GCS	↑WCC/NØ/CRP, abnormal CT brain or CSF results
Bowel obstruction or ileus	Colicky pain, absolute constipation, brown vomit	Distended tender abdomen, tinkling bowel sounds	Distended bowel loops on AXR, (🕮 p588)
Acute abdomen	Severe abdo pain	Tender, rigid, guarding, rebound	Pneumoperitoneum on CXR
Upper GI bleed	Blood/coffee-ground vomit	Tender abdomen, PR melaena	↓Hb, ↑urea
Gastro-enteritis	Diarrhoea, feels better after vomiting	Febrile, epigastric tenderness, not peritonitic	↑WBC, ↑LØ or NØ, positive stool culture
Labyrinthitis	Dizziness predominant, tinnitus	Unable to stand	Acute investigations normal (🕮 p363)
Migraine	Visual aura, headache	Photophobia, visual field defects	Acute investigations normal
Hyperemesis gravidarum	♀ usually between 7–12/40	Normal; palpable uterus	β-hCG+ TFTs often ↑, ↑urea if dehydrated
Drug induced	Many medications can induce vomiting, particularly opioids, chemotherapy and digoxin toxicity		

Diarrhoea

Worrying features ↑HR, ↓BP, low urine output, PR blood, weight loss, abdo pain.

Think about *acute* gastroenteritis, antibiotics, laxatives, drugs, pseudomembranous colitis (see 🔲 p308), overflow diarrhoea (2° to constipation), post-chemotherapy, bowel ischaemia; *chronic* IBD, IBS, colorectal cancer, diverticular disease, alcoholism, malabsorption disorders (eg coeliac, chronic pancreatitis), thyrotoxicosis, bowel resection, parasitic/fungal infections, autonomic neuropathy, carcinoid, Addison's disease (Table 9.7).

Traveller's diarrhoea E. coli, Salmonella, Shigella, Campylobacter spp., giardiasis, amoebic dysentery, cholera, tropical sprue.

Ask about normal bowel habit and frequency, onset/frequency of diarrhoea, recent constipation, stool character (floating, greasy, bloody, mucus), colour, abdominal pain, pain relief on opening bowels, nausea, vomiting, flatus, fluid intake, weight loss, mouth ulcers; *PMH* colorectal cancer, IBD, diverticular disease, IBS, surgery; *DH* recent ABx, immunosuppression; *SH* travel abroad, other household members affected/sick contacts, occupation (food, healthcare), alcohol.

Medications causing diarrhoea: antibiotics, laxatives, colchicine, digoxin, iron, NSAIDs, ranitidine, thiazide diuretics, propranolol, PPIs.

Obs temp, HR, BP, postural BP, RR, sats, fluid balance, stool chart.

Look for volume status (🔲 p380), cachexia, mouth ulcers, clubbing, jaundice, rashes, pale conjunctiva, thyroid mass, abdomen tenderness ±peritonitis, masses, distension, surgical scars; *PR* pain, masses, stool colour, consistency; may reveal a rectum loaded with faeces suggesting overflow diarrhoea, particularly in the elderly, immobile patient with poor diet and recent constipation – treat as constipation (🔲 p310).

Investigations *stool* M,C+S x3, *C. difficile* toxin, ova, cysts and parasites; *blds* FBC, U+E, glucose, LFT, Ca²⁺, TFT, CRP, B₁₂, folate, iron studies, anti tissue transglutaminase (TTG) antibodies, bld cultures; *AXR* obstruction, mucosal oedema, faecal impaction; *sigmoidoscopy* if not improving (or within 24h if known IBD/likely flare); *colonoscopy* if cancer suspected.

General management of diarrhoea

- *Conservative* increase fluid intake, review drugs (consider alternatives without GI side effects); start stool chart – this will often be kept more accurately on a busy ward if you educate patients to complete it themselves
- *Infective* isolation and barrier nurse if infective source thought possible, ABx if systemically unwell
- *Medical* anti-motility agents should be avoided in infective diarrhoea, IBD or pseudomembranous colitis.

Table 9.7 *Common causes of diarrhoea*

	History	Examination	Investigation
Gastroenteritis	Sudden onset, ±vomiting, abdominal cramps	↑temp, sweating, abdo tenderness	↑WCC, ↑CRP, +ve microbiology on stool sample
Inflammatory bowel disease	Crampy abdo pain, weight loss, blood in stool, mouth ulcers	Abdo tenderness, ±peritonitis, PR blood/mucus, eye/skin/joint manifestations	↑WCC, ↑CRP; mucosal oedema or megacolon on AXR; lesions seen on sigmoidoscopy
Irritable bowel syndrome	Bloating, abdominal cramps, relieved by defecation	Abdo tenderness, non-peritonitic	Diagnosis of exclusion; normal investigations
Malabsorption disorders	Weight loss, pale greasy stools, tired, anaemia	Pale, abdo tenderness, oedema, bloating, PR pale stool	↓Hb, ↓albumin, ↓Ca²⁺ ±anti-TTG or endomysial antibodies
Bowel cancer	Abdo pain, weight loss, fresh blood or melaena	PR blood or melaena, mucus/palpable mass	↓Hb, ↓MCV, lesion on colonoscopy
Diverticular disease	LIF pain, PR bleeding	LIF tenderness, ±peritonitis	↑WCC, ↑CRP, diverticulae on colonoscopy
Pseudo-membranous colitis	Recent antibiotics (days/weeks), crampy abdo pain, green watery stool	↑temp, abdo tenderness, PR green, foul smelling, ±blood	↑WCC, ↑CRP, *C. diff.* toxin +ve; AXR may show toxic dilatation
Overflow diarrhoea	Constipation, poor mobility, abdominal pain	Abdo distension and tenderness, PR palpable stool	AXR may show faecal loading

Infective gastroenteritis (OHCM9 □ p390)

Diarrhoea, accompanied by nausea, vomiting ±abdominal pain; in most cases due to viruses (including norovirus) but other infectious agents important.

Symptoms rapid onset, recent vomiting and/or diarrhoea, patient may implicate a certain food, feels unwell, crampy abdominal pain, flu-like symptoms, pyrexia; other members of household/contacts affected.

Appearance of stool blood 2° colonic ulceration (typical for *Campylobacter* or *Shigella* spp.); watery 'rice' stool suggests cholera.

Signs ↑temp, ↑HR, dehydrated, flushing, sweating, abdominal tenderness, general malaise; *PR* tender, peri-anal erythema.

Investigations **stool culture** result may take ≥48h; *C. diff.* toxin assays and norovirus PCR where clinical suspicion; **blds** ↑WCC, ↑CRP, ↑urea; if prolonged, consider **sigmoidoscopy** and discuss with microbiology.

Treatment Admit if clinical concern or not meeting fluid needs orally; isolation/barrier nursing with rigorous hand-washing by nurses, doctors and visitors; push oral fluids ±oral rehydration solutions, antiemetics (□ p185); IV fluids if not tolerating oral fluids. Surprisingly few indications for antibiotics, even after identification of a causative bacterium – always discuss with microbiology. Some causes are notifiable (□ p487).

Pseudomembranous colitis

Overgrowth of *Clostridium difficile*, often following antibiotic use. Difficult to treat, with a high mortality in vulnerable groups, always remember this condition when tempted to start antibiotics on scanty evidence.

Symptoms usually 3–9d after antibiotic therapy (can be 24h–6wk), rapid onset of high-quantity green, foul-smelling stool, crampy abdo pain.

Investigations **blds** ↑↑WCC, ↓K⁺; **stool** *C. difficile* toxin, M,C+S.

Treatment stop unnecessary antibiotics; isolate and barrier nurse, rehydrate with PO/IV fluids and correct electrolyte abnormalities, metronidazole 400mg/8h PO and/or vancomycin 125mg/6h PO (oral route targets GI tract). Can use IV metronidazole and PR vancomycin as per ID advice.

Complications toxic megacolon, perforation, high risk of spread to other patients via hands of healthcare workers; spores not killed by alcohol gels.

Irritable bowel syndrome – IBS[1] (OHCM9 📖 p276)

Consider in those with >6mth abdo pain, bloating or altered bowel habit.

Diagnostic criteria central/lower abdo pain or discomfort, this is relieved by defecation **or** associated with altered bowel frequency/stool form, **and** is accompanied by at least 2 of: bloating, passage of mucus, altered stool passage (eg straining, urgency), symptoms worse on/after eating.

Red flags that should prompt urgent consideration of other diagnoses include unintentional weight loss, rectal bleeding, age >60, family history of bowel or ovarian cancer.

Signs often normal or generalised abdo tenderness; exclude a pelvic mass.

Investigations If fits diagnostic criteria and no red flags, exclude other pathology by checking for normal FBC, ESR, CRP, anti-endomysial antibodies; further tests only if suspicion this is *not* IBS (eg TFT, sigmoidoscopy, colonoscopy, OGD, parasites). CA125 if ♀ with persistent bloating/pain.

Treatment[2] reassure and explain; basic lifestyle, exercise and dietary advice including attention to regular meals and non-caffeinated drinks, with limited intake of foods high in insoluble fibre (eg bran); consider dietician referral; mebeverine 135mg/8h PO, loperamide or Fybogel® according to symptoms, amitriptyline 10mg OD or SSRIs (2nd line) can have visceral analgesic effect.

Malabsorption disorders (OHCM9 📖 p280)

Impaired absorption of nutrients owing to a wide range of GI pathology.

Causes coeliac disease, chronic pancreatitis, tropical sprue, cystic fibrosis, small bowel/gastric resection, bacterial overgrowth, IBD.

Symptoms diarrhoea±steatorrhoea, weight loss, tiredness, SOB, dizziness, bruising, swelling, vomiting, gluten intolerance, abdo pain.

Signs cachexia, pale, dehydrated, mouth ulcers, sore tongue, abdo tenderness, oedema, bruises.

Investigations **blds** ↓Hb, ↓MCV, ↓Ca²⁺, ↓albumin, ↓iron, ↓folate, ↑PT; +ve anti-endomysial antibodies sensitive for coeliac disease but **duodenal biopsy** gold standard; **stool** elastase for assessment of pancreatic function; **hydrogen breath test** for small bowel bacterial overgrowth.

Treatment refer to dietician and gastroenterologist, may need nutrient ±pancreatic supplements, gluten-free diet (coeliac).

[1] See 🖰www.romecriteria.org for diagnostic resources
[2] 🖰NICE guidelines available at 🖰guidance.nice.org.uk/CG61

Inflammatory bowel disease – IBD[1]

Ulcerative colitis (OHCM9 📖 p272), Crohn's disease (OHCM9 📖 p274).
Symptoms recurrent diarrhoea ±blood ±mucus associated with abdo pain, malaise, tiredness, anorexia and weight loss.
Signs ↑temp, ↑HR ±↓BP, pale, abdo pain ±peritonism, palpable abdo mass, abdo swelling (toxic megacolon), malnourished; fistulae ±fissures in Crohn's (Table 9.8).

> *Extra-intestinal signs* mouth ulcers*, erythema nodosum*, pyoderma gangrenosum*, conjunctivitis*, episcleritis*, iritis*, acute arthropathy*, clubbing, sacroiliitis, ankylosing spondylitis, fatty liver, primary sclerosing cholangitis, cholangiocarcinoma.
>
> *related to disease activity

Investigations **blds** ↑WCC, ↑CRP, ↓albumin (as a marker of inflammation, not nutrition), ↓K+ (diarrhoeal losses), ↓Ca^{2+}, ↓iron, ↓folate, ↓B$_{12}$ (terminal ileal disease), bld cultures; **stool cultures** vital in ruling out infective causes of exacerbation including *C. difficile*; **AXR** mucosal oedema, toxic megacolon >6cm, faecal residue suggests uninvolved mucosa; **sigmoidoscopy ± colonoscopy** shows characteristic appearances/ulceration and allows biopsy; **CT** if concern of abscess and if surgery being considered.
Complications toxic megacolon, bowel obstruction, perforation, malabsorption, fistulae, fissures, strictures, malignancy.

Table 9.8 *Differentiating between ulcerative colitis and Crohn's*

Feature	Ulcerative colitis (UC)	Crohn's
Symptoms	Diarrhoea and PR blood/mucus prominent	Diarrhoea, abdo pain and weight loss prominent
GI involvement	Colon only, extending proximally from rectum to variable extent	Anywhere along GI tract, most commonly terminal ileum
Sigmoidoscopy	Inflamed mucosa, continuous lesions	Inflamed, thickened mucosa, skip lesions
Histology	Mucosal and submucosal inflammation, crypt abscesses, reduced goblet cells	Inflammation extends beyond the submucosa, granulomas present

Treatment depends upon disease severity. Rehydrate and correct electrolyte imbalances; avoid antimotility/antispasmodic agents. Systemically well patients with mild-moderate disease (<6 stools/day) should start oral ±rectal steroids (eg prednisolone 30–40mg/day PO). In UC oral±rectal mesalazine (eg Pentasa® 1g/12h PO) should be added. More severe disease requires IV steroids (eg hydrocortisone 100mg/6h IV), as well as antibiotics until infectious causes ruled out (eg co-amoxiclav 1.2g/8h IV). Monitor the patient closely (daily abdo exam, bloods ±AXR) and involve surgeons early. Elemental diet, immunosuppressive drugs (eg azathioprine) and biological agents (eg infliximab) may also be used.
Surgery is indicated as an emergency procedure in cases of perforation or massive haemorrhage. Urgent surgery is performed in UC for toxic megacolon or failure to respond to maximal medical therapy after 5–7d; delaying beyond this risks poor operative results. Surgery in Crohn's is never curative and associated with high recurrence and complication rates, but is indicated for obstruction, abscesses, and fistulae.

---

[1] See www.ecco-ibd.eu for a range of European guidelines.

Constipation

> *Worrying features* abdominal pain, distension, nausea/vomiting, ↑HR, ↓BP, absent/tinkling bowel sounds, weight loss, PR bleeding.

Think about *serious* bowel obstruction, bowel/ovarian cancer; *common* medications, poor diet, paralytic ileus, dehydration, functional disorders; *other* anal fissure/stricture, pelvic mass, spinal injury, hypothyroid (Table 9.9).

Ask about abdo pain, nausea, vomiting, date bowels last opened, normal bowel habit and frequency, stool consistency and colour, blood in stools, pain on opening bowels, straining, bloating, flatus, fluid intake, weight loss, tenesmus, recent surgery; ♀: periods, discharge; **PMH** IBD, diverticulosis, hernias, previous surgery, colon cancer, hypothyroidism; **DH** (see box) **SH** mobility, diet.

> **Medications causing constipation**: opioids, iron supplements, non-magnesium antacids, calcium-channel blockers, psychotropic drugs, anticholinergics, chronic laxative use (may lead to the development of a dilated atonic colon).

Obs temp, HR, BP, fluid balance.

Look for volume status (🕮 p380), tenderness ± peritonism, distension, masses, absent/tinkling bowel sounds, hernias, scars; **PR** anal fissures, rectal masses, faecal impaction, melaena/blood.

Investigations *blds* FBC, U+E, TFT, Ca^{2+}; **AXR** to exclude obstruction **sigmoidoscopy** ±biopsy if sub-acute onset; **colonoscopy** if cancer suspected.

> ### General management of constipation
>
> - **Conservative** increase fluid intake, high-fibre diet, review drugs: consider alternatives without GI side effects; start stool chart – this will often be kept more accurately if you educate patients to complete it themselves
> - **Medical** see 🕮 p205 for detailed laxative prescribing information; mild symptoms respond to senna or lactulose; more severe symptoms may require sodium docusate or Movicol®; glycerol suppositories will soften impacted stool, whilst phosphate enemas or Picolax® bowel prep should be reserved for when other measures fail
> - **Surgical disimpaction** scooping hard faeces from the rectum is a seriously unpleasant point of last resort for everyone concerned.

Table 9.9 *Common causes of constipation*

	History	Examination	Investigation
Bowel obstruction	Pain, distension, nausea, vomiting, constipation	Distension, tenderness, absent/ tinkling bowel sounds	Dilated loops of bowel on AXR
Paralytic ileus	Absence of flatus, recent operation	Distended abdomen, absent bowel sounds	Distended bowel loops on AXR, ↓K⁺
Bowel cancer	Abdo pain, weight loss, fresh blood or melaena	PR blood or melaena, mucus/palpable mass	↓Hb, lesion on sigmoidoscopy/ colonoscopy
Ano-rectal pathology	Fresh red blood on toilet paper, ±pain	Perianal tags, may have a tear or tenderness	Proctoscopy or sigmoidoscopy
Poor diet	Anorexia (eg post-op), low-fibre diet	Cachexia	↓Hb, ↓MCV, ↓Ca²⁺
Drugs	See 'Medications causing constipation' box		

Poor diet

A surprising number of in-patients fail to achieve adequate nutrition, with major impacts on wound healing, recovery, and physical condition. Try to recognise this and involve dieticians where appropriate, whilst avoiding prolonged NBM periods where possible. Markers for nutritional adequacy are problematic, but end of the bed assessment is useful. Where constipation is a feature, encourage to aim for regular high-fibre meals, with good fluid intake and regular physical activity.

Hints and tips

- Prescribe prophylactic laxatives for patients at risk of developing constipation (eg when prescribing opioids, post-op)
- Exclude obstruction before prescribing a laxative
- Lactulose is poorly tolerated by many patients and is associated with abdominal pain and bloating
- Reassess regularly for resolution of constipation – do not put off doing a rectal examination
- Consider malignancy in all patients >40yr presenting with altered bowel habit.

Causes of constipation covered elsewhere

Anal fissures/haemorrhoids	📖 p303	Bowel obstruction	📖 p292
Inflammatory bowel disease	📖 p309	Polyps	📖 p303
Irritable bowel syndrome	📖 p308		

Liver failure emergency

Airway	Check airway is patent; consider manoeuvres/adjuncts
Breathing	If no respiratory effort – **CALL ARREST TEAM**
Circulation	If no palpable pulse – **CALL ARREST TEAM**
Disability	If GCS ≤8 – **CALL ANAESTHETIST**

Altered mental state or coagulopathy in the presence of jaundice.
▶▶Call for **senior help** early if patient deteriorating.

Airway
- **Look** inside the mouth, wide-bore **suction** if secretions present
- **Jaw thrust**/head tilt/chin lift; **oro/nasopharyngeal** airway if tolerated.

Breathing
- **15l/min** O_2 if SOB or sats <94%
- **Monitor** O_2 sats and RR.

Circulation
- **Venous access**, take bloods:
  - FBC, U+E, LFT, PT/APTT, CRP, glucose, amylase, Ca^{2+}, Mg^{2+}, PO_4^{3-}, bld cultures, paracetamol levels, viral serology
- Start **IV fluids** 1l of 5% glucose over 4–6h
- **Monitor** HR, ECG, BP.

Disability
- Check blood **glucose** treat if <3.5mmol/l (📖 p322)
- **Check** GCS, pupil reflexes, limb tone, plantar responses.

Exposure
- Check **temp**
- Ask ward staff for a brief **history** or check notes:
  - previous liver disease, likely causes
- **Examine** patient brief RS, CVS, abdo and neuro exam:
  - signs of chronic liver disease
- **ECG**, **ABG** and urgent portable **CXR**
- **Stabilise** and treat, see 📖 p313
- Call for **senior help** and arrange transfer to HDU/ICU
- **Reassess**, starting with A, B, C …

Causes of liver failure

Acute liver failure	Paracetamol overdose, drugs, toxins, viral hepatitis, autoimmune hepatitis, ischaemic hepatitis (heart failure and shock), Budd–Chiari
Decompensated chronic liver disease	Alcohol excess, malignancy, GI bleeds, metabolic disturbances, sedatives, portal vein thrombosis, acute illness, surgery, infection (eg spontaneous bacterial peritonitis)

Liver failure

Worrying features Ascites, hepatic flap, altered mental state and jaundice are cardinal features of decompensation in liver disease; also beware active bleeding, renal failure, ↑HR, ↓BP.

Think about *emergencies* acute liver failure, decompensated chronic liver disease, hepatic encephalopathy; *acute liver failure* paracetamol overdose (□ p495), viral hepatitis (A, B, C, E, CMV, EMV), pregnancy, medications (see below), toxins (eg poisonous mushrooms), vascular (eg Budd–Chiari), sepsis, Weil's disease, abscess; *chronic liver failure* alcohol, medications (see below), idiopathic, autoimmune, hepatitis (B±D, C), malignancy, Wilson's disease, haemochromatosis, $α_1$-antitrypsin deficiency.

> **Drug-induced hepatotoxicity**[1] may result in response to a large number of drugs, ranging from mild elevations in LFTs to fulminant hepatic failure. Paracetamol, NSAIDs, ACE inhibitors, erythromycin, fluconazole and statins commonly cause hepatocellular injury (ALT >2x upper limit normal with normal/minimally ↑ALP). Chlorpromazine, oestrogens, ciprofloxacin, isoniazid, phenytoin, erythromycin and co-amoxiclav can all cause cholestasis (↑ALP, with or without associated hepatocellular damage). Always ask about recreational drugs (eg cocaine, mushrooms) and over the counter or herbal medications.
> [1] Useful review article available free at ⌐⋄www.ncbi.nlm.nih.gov/pmc/articles/PMC2773872

Ask about tiredness, jaundice (+onset), abdo pain, drowsiness ± confusion, bruising, bleeding (skin, nose, bowel, urine), distension, ankle swelling, vomiting, rashes, recent infections (sore throat), weight loss, hair loss, darkening skin; *PMH* previous jaundice, gallstones, blood transfusions; *DH* see box above; *FH* liver disease, recent jaundice; *SH* alcohol, IVDU, tattoos, piercings, foreign travel, sexual activity.

Obs temp, HR, BP, RR, O_2 sats, GCS, blood glucose, urine output.

Look for volume status □ p380; *acute liver failure* drowsiness, confusion, slurred speech, jaundice, flapping tremor (asterixis), poor co-ordination, bruising, foetor hepaticus (sweet, faecal smelling breath), abdominal tenderness, hepatomegaly, ascites; *chronic liver disease* cachexia, palmar erythema, clubbing, xanthelasma, spider naevi, caput medusa, gynaecomastia, muscle wasting, splenomegaly, genital atrophy, track marks (IVDU), pneumonia/chronic lung disease, darkened skin.

Investigations These are aimed at establishing the extent and possible cause of liver damage, and finding a possible cause of any decompensation, especially intercurrent infection *urine* MSU; *blds* FBC, clotting, iron, ferritin, U+E, LFT, hepatitis serology (A, B+C), EBV and CMV serology, caeruloplasmin (if <50yr), autoimmune screen (antimitochondrial, antinuclear and anti-smooth muscle antibodies, □ p593), bld cultures; *urgent USS abdo* looking for parenchymal mass(es), dilated ducts or portal vein thrombosis; *urgent ascitic tap* (□ p550) and white cell count to check for spontaneous bacterial peritonitis (□ p316).

▶▶**Acute liver failure** (OHAM3 📖 p268)
Acute encephalopathy, coagulopathy and jaundice without previous cirrhosis (Table 9.10).

Table 9.10 *Types of acute liver failure*

Liver failure <7d of disease onset	Hyperacute fulminant hepatic failure
Liver failure 1–4wk of disease onset	Acute fulminant hepatic failure
Liver failure 4–12wk of disease onset	Subacute fulminant hepatic failure
Liver failure 12–26wk of disease onset	Late-onset hepatic failure

Symptoms bruising/bleeding, drowsy±confusion, abdo pain.

Signs drowsiness, confusion, slurred speech, jaundice, flapping tremor (asterixis), poor co-ordination, bruising, hepatomegaly, ascites.

Investigations initiate liver screen as detailed (📖 p313) **blds** ↑PT/APTT, ↑↑ALT, ↑ALP, ↑bilirubin, ↑ammonia, ↑WCC, ↓glucose, ↓Mg^{2+}, ↓PO_4^{3-}; **ABG** respiratory alkalosis, metabolic acidosis (poor prognosis); **USS** masses, echogenicity, portal vein flow.

Treatment discuss with a senior early, often needs ICU/HDU with invasive monitoring, and may need transfer to a specialist liver centre, where may be considered for transplantation. Monitor blood glucose every 2h; insert a catheter and monitor fluid balance.
- ↑**PT** give one-off dose of vitamin K 10mg IV:
  - always discuss with a senior; PT prolongation is used to monitor disease progress; FFP may be indicated if the patient is bleeding or needs an invasive procedure
- **Stop** aspirin, NSAIDs and hepatotoxic drugs (📖 p313); check all drugs in *BNF*
- **Antibiotic** prophylaxis in all patients (eg cefotaxime) ± antifungals
- **Daily bloods** (FBC, U+E, LFT, PT[1])
- **Lactulose** 10–20ml/8h PO in all patients (helps remove ammonia)
- **Close monitoring** of cardiovascular status and blood glucose; if need IV fluids, avoid Na+ if chronic liver disease/ascites.

Complications renal failure (hepatorenal syndrome), respiratory failure (ARDS), cerebral oedema, bleeding, sepsis, ↓glucose, ↑Na^+, ↓K^+.

Vascular liver disease
Diagnosed by Doppler USS; these diseases can cause hepatic jaundice or acute liver failure, often treated by anticoagulation or endovascular methods.
- **Budd–Chiari** hepatic vein obstruction
- **Portal vein** obstruction (pain and deranged LFTs; jaundice only if other causes of liver disease coexist)
- **Liver ischaemia** due to hypotension and/or hepatic artery stenosis. Typically causes massive ALT rise.

---

[1] Strictly, the INR is specific for warfarin therapy; the pattern abnormal clotting in liver disease is different and more reliably reported as PT and APTT prolongation.

Glandular fever (infectious mononucleosis, Epstein–Barr virus, EBV)
Symptoms usually young (10–30yr), sore throat >1wk, fever, lethargy, malaise, rash, lumps in the neck, anorexia.
Signs red tonsils ±white exudate, tender lymphadenopathy, splenomegaly, rash (especially with amoxicillin/ampicillin), palatal petechiae, jaundice.
Investigations **blds** ↑lymphocytes (atypical on film), ↑ALT, +ve Monospot/Paul Bunnell, +ve IgM for EBV.
Management rest, rehydration, analgesia, gargle with warm saline/aspirin, avoid amoxicillin/ampicillin, avoid alcohol, consider short course of oral steroids if very severe (eg hepatic encephalopathy).
Complications hepatitis, liver failure, thrombocytopenia, splenic rupture, haemolysis, encephalitis.

Acute viral hepatitis (OHCM9 📖 p406)
Causes hepatitis A,B,C and E, cytomegalovirus (CMV) and EBV.
Symptoms jaundice, rash, diarrhoea, abdo pain, flu-like symptoms (eg fever, malaise, anorexia, fatigue, nausea, vomiting, arthralgia, sore throat).
Signs may have no signs, ↑temp, urticarial rash, jaundice, hepatomegaly, splenomegaly, lymphadenopathy.
Investigations **blds** ↑WCC, ↑bilirubin, ↑ALT ±↑PT, +ve hepatitis serology (Table 9.11).
Management avoid alcohol, supportive treatment, monitor for progression to acute liver failure (📖 p314) which may need interferon-α.
Complications natural history varies widely depending upon virus and host; risks include acute liver failure or chronic disease.

Chronic viral hepatitis (OHCM9 📖 p406)
Hepatitis >6mth, *caused by* hepatitis B (±D) and C.
Symptoms and signs usually asymptomatic, signs of chronic liver disease.
Investigations **blds** deranged LFT ±↑PT; abnormal viral serology (Table 9.11); **USS** liver may be suggestive of cirrhosis.
Treatment avoid alcohol, consider referral to a hepatologist for specific antiviral treatment (eg interferon-α or ribavirin).[1]
Complications cirrhosis (20%), hepatocellular carcinoma (esp HBV).

Table 9.11 *Serology in hepatitis B*

Surface antigen (HBsAg)	Active virus replication – acute or chronic disease
Anti-core (Anti-HBc) IgM	Acute infection
Anti-core (Anti-HBc) IgG	Chronic infection (or previous infection if HBsAg –ve)
'e' antigen (HBeAg)	High infectivity
Anti-e (Anti-HBe)	Low infectivity

In chronic hepatitis B infection, HBeAg negativity is associated with immune control of the virus and low/undetectable viral DNA. Beware, however, the subset of patients in whom the virus develops a *precore mutation* leading to absent production of HBeAg, despite loss of immune control and rising viral DNA titres. These patients are at high risk for disease complications.

[1] See 🔍www.bsg.org.uk/clinical-guidelines/liver/index.html for treatment guidance.

Decompensated chronic liver failure (OHCM9 📖 p260)

Cirrhosis is the final common histological pathway for a variety of liver diseases; problems relate to synthetic function (coagulopathy, ascites 2° to hypoalbuminaemia), decreased detoxification (encephalopathy), or portal hypertension (variceal bleeding).

Symptoms and *signs* as for acute liver failure (📖 p314) but look for stigmata of chronic liver disease: spider angioma, palmar erythema, gynaecomastia.

Investigations **measure severity**: LFTs, U+E and clotting profile; **establish underlying cause**: hepatitis serology, immunoglobulins, liver autoantibodies, ferritin, α_1-antitrypsin, ceruloplasmin, USS, liver biopsy; **identify precipitant of decompensation**: FBC, bld cultures, ascitic tap, OGD.

Treatment requires hepatology input and transplant assessment; deal with upper GI bleeding (📖 p299), treat sepsis, support alcohol cessation, lactulose (to reduce ammonia levels).

Ascites low-salt diet, daily weights, spironolactone 100mg/24h PO increasing dose every 48h to 400mg/24h ±furosemide; ascitic tap for diagnosis (📖 p550) and to exclude spontaneous bacterial peritonitis; may need long-term antibiotics, therapeutic paracentesis or TIPS if recurrent.

Complications high mortality, portal hypertension, bleeding varices, encephalopathy, hepatocellular carcinoma.

Spontaneous bacterial peritonitis

Symptoms abdominal pain in the presence of ascites, associated with fever.
Signs fever, ↑HR ±↓BP, abdo tenderness ±peritonitis.
Investigations **blds** ↑WCC, ↑CRP; **ascitic tap** >250 white cells/mm³ or identification of organisms (📖 p550).
Treatment prompt IV antibiotics: (eg Tazocin® 4.5g/8h IV).

Autoimmune liver disease (OHCM9 📖 p266)

Causes primary biliary cirrhosis (📖 p319), primary sclerosing cholangitis (📖 p319), autoimmune hepatitis (type I and II – see below); primary biliary cirrhosis and type I autoimmune hepatitis may overlap.

Symptoms often asymptomatic, may have fever, malaise, rash, joint pain or symptoms of chronic liver disease.

Signs of chronic liver disease.

Investigations **blds** deranged LFT ±↑PT, +ve autoantibodies (Table 9.12); **USS** and liver biopsy.

Treatment **autoimmune hepatitis** prednisolone 30mg/24h PO initially then azathioprine; **other diseases** see 📖 p319.

Complications acute liver failure, cirrhosis, hepatocellular carcinoma.

Table 9.12 *Autoantibodies in autoimmune liver disease*

Primary biliary cirrhosis (~80% ♀)	Anti-mitochondrial (AMA) present in 95% and 98% specific
Primary sclerosing cholangitis (~70% ♀, ~80% IBD)	Anti-smooth muscle (SMA), antinuclear (ANA), p-ANCA
Autoimmune hepatitis type I (80% ♀)	Anti-smooth muscle (SMA), antinuclear (ANA)
Autoimmune hepatitis type II (mainly children; 90% ♀)	Anti-liver/kidney microsomal type 1 (LKM1)

Haemochromatosis (OHCM9 📖 p262)
Autosomal-recessive disease causing excess iron accumulation.
Symptoms fatigue, lethargy, arthralgia, hyperpigmentation, DM.
Signs hepatomegaly, signs of chronic liver disease, cardiac failure or conduction defects, hypogonadism ±impotence, tanned skin.
Investigations **blds** ↑transferrin saturation (>60% in ♂ and >50% in ♀ highly specific, but false negatives esp. in younger ♀), ↑ALT, ↑glucose, genetic testing (2 common mutations account for 70% of Caucasian patients); *ECG* cardiomyopathy or conduction delays; *liver biopsy* (diagnosis, severity).
Treatment venesection (1 unit/wk) until ferritin normalises then every 3–6mth; transferrin saturation or genetic screening of relatives.

α₁-antitrypsin deficiency (OHCM9 📖 p264)
Genetic disease with complex inheritance causing liver and lung damage.
Symptoms breathlessness, liver failure, family history.
Signs emphysema, signs of chronic liver disease.
Investigations **blds** ↓α₁-antitrypsin levels, genetic testing; *liver biopsy*.
Treatment stop smoking, may need liver transplant, COPD treatment.

Wilson's disease (OHCM9 📖 p269)
Autosomal-recessive disease; copper accumulates in the liver and CNS.
Symptoms tremor, slurred speech, abnormal movements, clumsiness, depression, personality change, psychosis, liver failure, family history.
Signs Kaiser–Fleischer rings in eyes, signs of liver failure.
Investigations **blds** ↓caeruloplasmin, ↓total serum copper, ↑serum free copper, genetic testing; *urine* ↑24h copper excretion (especially if a dose of penicillamine is given); copper on *liver biopsy*.
Treatment lifelong penicillamine, may need liver transplant, screen relatives.

Weil's disease (leptospirosis)
Bacterial infection typically transmitted via exposure of skin cuts or mucous membranes to water contaminated with rat urine.
Symptoms recent contact with dirty water, high fever, malaise, anorexia, fatigue, nausea, vomiting, arthralgia, pharyngitis, conjunctival oedema, neck stiffness, photophobia, jaundice, bleeding and kidney failure.
Signs acute liver failure, meningism, bruising, tender RUQ, myocarditis.
Investigations **urine** dipstick haematuria, culture; **blds** ↓Hb (haemolytic), ↑urea, ↑creatinine, ↑bilirubin, ↑ALT, serology.
Treatment doxycycline 100mg/12h PO or benzylpenicillin 600mg/6h IV and supportive care of renal/liver failure.

Predicting outcomes in chronic liver disease is of considerable importance, not least in prioritising use of organs for transplantation. The 'Child' scoring system originated in 1964 from attempts by Child and Turcotte to assess operative risks for cirrhotic patients undergoing porto-systemic shunt surgery. Later modifications to include albumin and INR led to the 'Child–Turcotte–Pugh' score which is still widely used. With the advent of liver transplantation more precise stratification of patients with advanced disease was needed: For the NHS transplantation programme, the UKELD (UK end-stage liver disease) score is calculated from serum Na⁺, creatinine, bilirubin and INR.
The original description of the UKELD score (Neuberger, J. et al., Gut 2008 **57**:252) is available online at ⏚gut.bmj.com/content/57/2/252.abstract (subscription required, but many NHS trusts provide access through ATHENS). Online calculators for the Child score are widely available (eg ⏚www.mdcalc. com). Information on the NHS transplantation programme, including liver transplants and a UKELD calculator is available at ⏚www.organdonation.nhs.uk

Jaundice

Worrying features ↑HR, ↓BP, drowsiness, ↓GCS, bleeding, slurred speech, poor coordination, tremor/flap, renal failure, weight loss.

Think about
- **Pre-hepatic** haemolysis, malaria.
- **Hepatic** paracetamol overdose, viral hepatitis, alcohol, chronic liver disease, Gilbert's syndrome, pregnancy, medications (📖 p319), toxins (eg poisonous fungi), vascular disease (eg ischaemia, Budd–Chiari), sepsis.
- **Cholestatic** choledocholithiasis, ascending cholangitis, pancreatic cancer, cholangiocarcinoma, primary biliary cirrhosis, 1° sclerosing cholangitis.

Ask about tiredness, jaundice (+onset), abdo pain, itching, dark urine, pale stools, drowsiness, confusion, bruising, bleeding (skin, nose, bowel, urine), bloating, vomiting, rashes, recent infections (sore throat), weight loss, generalised aching, hair loss, darkening skin, joint pain; **PMH** previous jaundice, gallstones, breathing problems, blood transfusions; **DH** paracetamol and medications (📖 p319); **FH** liver disease, recent jaundice; **SH** alcohol, IVDU, tattoos, piercings, foreign travel, sexual activity (?abroad).

Obs temp, RR, HR, BP, urine output, O_2 sats, glucose, GCS.

Look for volume status (📖 p380), bruising, evidence of bleeding, drowsiness, confusion:
- **Pre-hepatic** splenomegaly, pale conjunctiva, breathlessness
- **Hepatic** signs of acute or chronic liver failure (📖 p313)
- **Cholestatic** abdominal tenderness ±peritonism, Charcot's triad (fever, jaundice and RUQ pain = cholangitis), palpable gallbladder, cachexia.

Initial investigations *urine* MSU, bilirubin, urobilinogen; *blds* FBC, reticulocytes and LDH (both elevated in haemolysis), blood film, clotting, U+E, LFT (total and conjugated bilirubin), amylase, lipase, paracetamol levels, hepatitis, EBV and CMV serology, bld cultures; *urgent USS abdo* (?dilated bile ducts, cirrhosis, pancreatic mass, metastases). See Table 9.13.

Table 9.13 *Laboratory investigation of jaundice*

	Urine	Liver tests	Other tests
Pre-hepatic jaundice	Urobilinogen	↑unconjugated bilirubin	↓Hb, ↔MCV, ↓haptoglobin, ↑reticulocytes
Hepatic jaundice	Urobilinogen	↑mixed bilirubin, ↑ALT/AST	May have positive hepatitis serology or ↑paracetamol levels
Cholestasis	Bilirubin, dark urine	↑conjugated bilirubin, ↑ALP, ↑γGT	Dilated ducts on USS
Cholangitis	Bilirubin, dark urine	↑conjugated bilirubin, ↑ALP, ↑γGT	↑WCC, ↑CRP, dilated biliary ducts

---

Causes of jaundice covered elsewhere

Haemolysis   📖 p394   Liver failure   📖 p313

Gilbert's syndrome
Benign autosomal recessive disease causing mild, self-resolving unconjugated hyperbilirubinaemia typically during acute illness.

Choledocholithiasis
Gallstone in common bile duct, causing obstructive jaundice.
Risk factors ♀, pregnancy, DM, obesity, age.
Symptoms often none, preceding biliary colic, dark urine, pale stool.
Signs jaundice, mild RUQ tenderness.
*Investigations **bld*** ↑ALP, ↑bilirubin; *USS* dilated bile ducts.
Treatment maintain hydration, exclude pancreatitis and cholangitis, prophylactic antibiotics (eg co-amoxiclav 1.2g/8h IV); ERCP permits diagnosis and stone removal; cholecystectomy usually deferred until jaundice resolved.
Complications pancreatitis, cholangitis, hepatitis, clotting defects.

Cholangitis
Infection of the bile duct with Charcot's triad: fever, jaundice, RUQ pain.
Symptoms unwell, abdo pain, rigors, jaundice.
Signs ↑temp, ↑HR ±↓BP, RUQ tenderness (Murphy's +ve).
*Investigations **bld*** ↑WCC, ↑CRP, ↑bilirubin; *USS* ?duct dilatation, stones.
Treatment eg co-amoxiclav 1.2g/8h IV; may need an urgent ERCP if gallstones are in the common bile duct.

Primary biliary cirrhosis (OHCM9 ⊞ p266)
Chronic, progressive autoimmune destruction of interlobular bile ducts.
Symptoms and signs fatigue, pruritus, cholestatic jaundice, cirrhosis.
*Investigations **bld*** ↑ALP, ↑γGT ±↑bilirubin, ↑IgM, anti-mitochondrial antibodies (⊞ p316); *USS* ±liver biopsy for staging.
Treatment ursodeoxycholic acid (helps symptoms and delays progression); colestyramine 4–8g/24h PO for itching; monitor for signs of decompensation and screen for osteoporosis (DEXA); in advanced disease immunosuppression (eg methotrexate, steroids); replace fat-soluble vitamins (A, D, E, K); refer for liver transplant assessment.

Primary sclerosing cholangitis (OHCM9 ⊞ p267)
Inflammation and fibrosis of intra- and extrahepatic bile ducts.
Symptoms and signs chronic biliary obstruction leading to cirrhosis; IBD present in ~80%, of which ~90% UC, but course of IBD not related to PSC.
*Investigations **bld*** ↑ALP, ±↑bilirubin, ↑immunoglobulin levels, anti-smooth muscle antibodies (SMA), antinuclear antibodies (ANA), p-ANCA, HLA-A1, B8 or DR3; *ERCP* multiple strictures; fibrosis on liver **biopsy**.
Treatment trials of immunosuppressive agents have proven disappointing; ursodeoxycholic acid can help symptoms; screen for osteoporosis (DEXA) and monitor for cholangiocarcinoma (~1% per annum); transplantation key, but disease recurs in 15% post transplant.

Cholangiocarcinoma (OHCM9 ⊞ p270)
Adenocarcinoma (90%) or squamous cell carcinoma of intra- and extrahepatic biliary epithelium; strong relationship with IBD and PSC.
Symptoms and signs jaundice, pruritus, weight loss, dull RUQ ache.
Courvoisier's law an enlarged gallbladder in the presence of jaundice is not caused by gallstones (suggests pancreatic or biliary cancer).
*Investigations **bld*** ↑ALP, ↑bilirubin, CA19.9; *USS, MRCP, ERCP* ± biopsy.
Treatment surgery (10–40%); else palliate: chemotherapy, ERCP + stenting.

Endocrinology

Hypoglycaemia emergency

Airway	Check airway is patent; consider manoeuvres/adjuncts
Breathing	If no respiratory effort – **CALL ARREST TEAM**
Circulation	If no palpable pulse – **CALL ARREST TEAM**
Disability	If GCS ≤8 – **CALL ANAESTHETIST**

▶▶Call for **senior help** early if patient deteriorating.
- Blood glucose is normally >3.5mmol/l
- Poorly controlled diabetics can have symptoms of hypoglycaemia with a glucose >3.5mmol/l.

Coma or low GCS with low glucose

- Protect airway
- **15l/min O₂** if SOB or sats <94%
- Establish **venous access** unless already present
- Give **IV glucose** STAT (100ml of 20% or 200ml of 10%)
- For large insulin overdoses give 1mg **glucagon** SC/IM/IV
- Begin to follow **emergency protocol** on 🔲 p338 (low GCS)
- If hypoglycaemia is responsible, GCS should return to 15 in <10min
- Start **1l 10% glucose/4–8h IV**, adjust rate to keep glucose >5mmol/l
- **Monitor finger-prick glucose** every 30min–1h until patient stable
- Attempt to determine the **cause** of the hypoglycaemia
- Call for **senior help**
- **Reassess**, starting with A, B, C; if no improvement see 🔲 p338.

GCS 15/15 with low glucose

- Give at least 120ml Lucozade® or a single dose of **glucose** gel (**GlucoGel®**) orally (this will only last up to an hour, so give a sandwich too)
- **Monitor finger-prick glucose** 1–2h until stable, aim for >5mmol/l
- For persistent hypoglycaemia give **1l 10% glucose/6–8h IV**
- Attempt to determine the **cause** of the hypoglycaemia.

Life-threatening causes

- Insulin overdose
- Oral hypoglycaemia overdose
- Sepsis
- Alcohol excess
- Acute liver failure

Hypoglycaemia

Worrying features ↓GCS, recurrent episodes, loss of awareness,[1] non-diabetic.

Think about *most likely* excess insulin or oral hypoglycaemics in a diabetic or accidental dose in non-diabetic, alcohol; *other* dumping syndrome (DM or post-gastric surgery), liver failure, adrenal failure (Addison's), pituitary insufficiency, sepsis, insulinoma, other neoplasia, malaria.

Ask about sweating, hunger, exercise, recent food, previous hypos and awareness,[1] usual blood sugars, seizures, weight loss, tiredness, anxiety, palpitations; **PMH** DM, gastric surgery, liver or endocrine disease; **DH** insulin dose, oral hypoglycaemic dose, compliance; **SH** alcohol.

Obs HR, BP, RR, temp, GCS, recent and current blood glucose.

Look for pale, sweating, tremor, slurred speech, focal neurology (can be severe, eg hemiplegia), ↓GCS, abdo scars (injection sites, lipodystrophy), pigmented scars, jaundice, spider naevi, hepatomegaly.

Investigations *finger-prick glucose* – if the result is unexpected ask for a repeat on a different machine and send a blood sample in a fluoride oxalate (📖 p517) tube for a laboratory glucose result. If **not known to be diabetic** send samples for FBC, U+E, LFT, glucose, insulin and C-peptide prior to correcting hypoglycaemia, but do not let this delay your treatment. *Further investigations* hypoglycaemia is very rare in an otherwise healthy non-diabetic patient in the absence of alcohol. Consider 'other' causes listed above. For suspected insulinoma, the investigation of choice is glucose, insulin and C-peptide levels in a 72h observed fast. Gut hormones may also be requested. See OHCM9 📖 p206.

Treatment follow treatment for 'Hypoglycaemia emergency' (📖 p322).
DM A single episode of mild hypoglycaemia should not prompt a change of medication. If the patient is having regular hypos then consider a dose reduction, especially if lack of awareness of hypoglycaemic episodes. Try to establish any diurnal pattern of hypos, then reduce appropriate insulin dose by 20%; consult *BNF* to reduce the doses of oral hypoglycaemics. Ensure the patient is aware of the sick day rules (📖 p329).
Alcohol hypoglycaemia following alcohol will not reoccur after correction in the absence of further alcohol consumption. Once the patient's blood sugars are stable they can be discharged.
Dumping syndrome fast passage of food into the small intestine (following gastric surgery or in severe diabetic autonomic neuropathy) can cause fluid shifts and rapid glucose absorption. Excessive insulin secretion results in rebound hypoglycaemia 1–3h after a meal. A diet low in glucose and high in fibre will improve the symptoms.
Neoplasia if suspected, arrange appropriate imaging and referral

Addison's/pituitary failure	📖 p332/331
Sepsis	📖 p480
Acute liver failure	📖 p314

[1] Loss of early autonomic symptoms warning of mild hypoglycaemia (eg tremor, sweating) seen in those with longstanding DM and frequent hypoglycaemic episodes.

Hyperglycaemia emergency

Airway	Check airway is patent; consider manoeuvres/adjuncts
Breathing	If no respiratory effort – **CALL ARREST TEAM**
Circulation	If no palpable pulse – **CALL ARREST TEAM**
Disability	If GCS ≤12 – **CALL ANAESTHETIST**

▶▶Call for **senior help** early if patient deteriorating.

Diabetic ketoacidosis (DKA) – see 📖 **p326**
- **15l/min O₂** if SOB or sats <94%
- Call for **senior help**
- Establish **venous access**, take bloods:
  - FBC, U+E, glucose, osmolality, HCO₃⁻, bld cultures
- Check BP:
  - if SBP<90mmHg, give **500ml 0.9% saline IV** over 10–15min then recheck; if SBP<90, give further **500ml 0.9% saline IV** over 10–15min and call ICU/critical care teams.
  - if SBP ≥90, give **1l 0.9% saline IV** over 60min
- Check **finger-prick glucose and ketones** (dipstick **urine** for ketones if capillary testing unavailable)
- Start a **fixed rate insulin infusion of 0.1unit/kg/h IV** (use 50 units human soluble insulin eg Actrapid® in 50ml 0.9% saline)
- **Venous blood gas**; if pH <7.1 call ICU/critical care team
- **Monitor** glucose and ketones hourly, and venous HCO₃⁻ and K⁺ at 60 min and 2hrly thereafter; remember K⁺ will fall unless replaced
- Further management, 📖 p326; ECG, CXR, MSU to **determine cause**
- **Reassess**, starting with A, B, C …

Consider HDU admission in DKA for:

- Heart or kidney failure
- GCS <12, Sats <92%
- SBP <90
- Young people, elderly, comorbidities or pregnant
- Ketones >6mmol/l, HCO₃⁻ <5mmol/l, pH <7.1
- K⁺ <3.5mmol/l, anion gap >16 📖 p585

Hyperosmolar non-ketotic state (HONK) – see 📖 **p326**
- **15l/min O₂** if SOB or sats <94%
- Call for **senior help**
- Establish **venous access**, take bloods:
  - FBC, U+E, glucose, osmolality, bld cultures
- Give **1l 0.9% saline IV** over 30min
- Check **finger-prick glucose**
- Start a **sliding scale** if glucose still raised after 1h of fluids, see 📖 p326
- **Monitor** U+E and glucose
- Further management, 📖 p326; ECG, CXR, MSU to **determine cause**
- **Reassess**, starting with A, B, C …

Life-threatening precipitants of DKA/HONK

- Sepsis
- MI
- Trauma/surgery
- Other acute illness

Hyperglycaemia

Worrying features ↓GCS, ketonuria, acidosis, vomiting.

Think about *emergencies* diabetic ketoacidosis (DKA, 📖 p326), hyperosmolar non-ketotic state (HONK, 📖 p326); ***common*** after sugary food, steroids, non-compliance with diabetic treatment, infection or acute illness (in diabetics or severely unwell non-diabetics), new diagnosis of DM.

Ask about 'osmotic symptoms' (thirst, polyuria, frequency, urgency), tiredness, weight loss, vomiting, rashes, breathlessness, cough, sputum, chest pain, abdo pain, dysuria; ***PMH*** DM; ***DH*** insulin dose, oral hypoglycaemic dose, medication changes and compliance, steroids; ***SH*** alcohol.

Obs temp, RR, GCS, recent and current blood glucose, fluid balance.

Look for volume status (📖 p380), sweet-smelling breath (ketones): *signs of infection*: check skin thoroughly (including perineum and feet) for abscesses or rashes, look in mouth for dental infection, chest for poor air entry or creps, abdominal tenderness.

Investigations ***finger-prick glucose*** (±ketones if available and suspect DKA) repeat if result unexpected; ***urine dipstick*** ketones, evidence of infection (📖 p590); ***blds*** send if patient is unwell, has persistent hyperglycaemia (over 48h) or has urinary ketones (type 1 DM), request FBC, U+E, LFT, osmolality, pH/HCO_3^- (venous), blood cultures; ***ABG*** unnecessary unless concerns regarding respiratory status (venous pH adequate for DKA); ***ECG/CXR*** if treatment has been required.

Treatment a single episode of hyperglycaemia in an otherwise well patient is unlikely to suggest underlying pathology. DKA takes hours to days to develop whilst HONK takes days to weeks.

Type 1 diabetes Check finger-prick glucose (±ketones if available) and urine. Glucose is usually high in DKA but may be transiently normal soon after a dose of insulin. Assess volume status (📖 p380), check dipstick for ketonuria and check a venous blood gas for pH/HCO_3^- (normal venous pH or absence of urinary ketones excludes DKA). If hyperglycaemia persistent try to establish any diurnal pattern and ↑ appropriate insulin doses by 20% with close monitoring of blood glucose.

Type 2 diabetes Check finger-prick glucose and urine. The glucose must be raised for a diagnosis of HONK. If unwell follow the treatment plan for HONK initially. Otherwise monitor glucose levels every 6h for 48h, increase oral/IV fluid intake and reassess. DKA can occur in type 2 diabetics who require insulin but it is very unusual (even low levels of residual insulin production inhibit ketogenesis). For persistent hyperglycaemia increase the dose of hypoglycaemic medication or consider starting/increasing insulin with frequent finger-prick glucose checks.

Non-diabetic patients New diabetics often present with DKA/HONK; have a low threshold for starting treatment plans later in this section. *Other triggers* can include steroids, pregnancy and stress, eg severe illness or surgery.

Diabetic ketoacidosis (DKA)[1] (OHAM3 📖 p516)

Insulin deficiency resulting in hyperglycaemia and dehydration. Ketone body formation leads to acidosis and ketonuria. Typically seen following missed insulin treatments or infection in T1DM, or as a first presentation of T1DM.

- Diagnose based upon presence of hyperglycaemia (≥11mmol/l), acidosis (venous pH<7.3) and blood ketones ≥3mmol/l or ketonuria(≥2+). Stabilise the patient as shown on 📖 p324, then:
- Continue IV insulin infusion and fluid rehydration (see box)
- Monitor venous K^+, pH and HCO_3^- after 1h, 2h and then 2hrly using a venous sample on a gas analyser for rapid testing
- Monitor venous glucose and ketones hourly aiming for blood ketones to fall by >0.5 mmol/l/h and glucose by >3mmol/l/h
- If patient uses long-acting insulin continue at normal dose/time
- Continue insulin infusion until ketones <0.3mmol/l and pH>7.3. At this point convert to regular SC insulin if eating and drinking normally, else use a sliding scale (📖 p327).

> *DKA fluids* 0.9% saline is the most appropriate fluid replacement. A guide in adults would be to prescribe 1l over 1h, 1l over 2h, 1l over 2h and 1l over 4h. If systolic BP <90mmHg on admission an initial 500–1000ml bolus must be carefully given under senior supervision. Since excess fluid replacement can lead to cerebral oedema, reassess frequently for signs of overload (📖 p380), and tailor to volume status and patient weight. Add 40mmol/l KCl after the first litre of fluid if the plasma K^+ is 3.5–5.5mmol/l. Omit additional KCl if K^+ >5.5; if K^+ <3.5 seek senior review. Adding a 10% glucose infusion at 125ml/h if glucose <14mmol/l but do not stop saline.

Management tips in DKA/HONK

These patients require close monitoring. If severely ill, catheterise, consider admission to HDU or ICU and an arterial and/or central line. If obtunded or persistent vomiting, keep NBM and pass NG tube. Dehydration and ↓GCS predispose to thromboembolism: give prophylactic LMWH (📖 p406). Consider likely precipitants: poor compliance/incorrect insulin dose, alcohol, infections (may be asymptomatic – check blood cultures, MSU and CXR; low threshold for starting antibiotics), MI (check an ECG), CVA, surgery.

Hyperosmolar non-ketotic state (HONK) (OHAM3 📖 p524)

Severe, uncorrected hyperglycaemia leads to dehydration, but in the presence of residual insulin production in T2DM, ketoacidosis does not develop. Also referred to as hyperosmolar hyperglycaemic state (HHS). Diagnose based upon raised plasma osmolality[2] (typically >340 mOsmol/kg) with high glucose (typically >30mmol/l).

- Stabilise the patient as shown on the treatment plan, 📖 p324, then:
- Continue IV fluid replacement (eg at half the rate used in DKA)
- Monitor U+E, glucose and osmolality every 2h. Be aware that hyperglycaemia will drive redistribution of water into the extracellular fluid, lowering serum Na^+ concentrations ('spurious hyponatraemia')
- Convert to insulin/oral hypoglycaemics when glucose <12mmol/l.

---

[1] Joint British Diabetes Societies guidelines at ⏛www.diabetologists-abcd.org.uk/JBDS_DKA_Management.pdf

[2] Plasma osmolality may be estimated as 2x($[Na^+] + [K^+]$)+ urea + glucose whilst awaiting a formal lab measurement.

Sliding scales

These give strict monitoring and control of blood glucose levels. They are used in the treatment of HONK, for diabetic patients requiring insulin whose oral intake is significantly disrupted (eg NBM, severe vomiting or serious illness), and in critical illness, where good glycaemic control improves outcomes, eg post-MI or on ICU.

You need to prescribe both the insulin infusion and appropriate IV maintenance fluids on the infusions section of the drug card (Fig. 10.1). Use 0.9% saline or 5% glucose (with KCl as necessary), according to the blood glucose (use 0.9% saline if the glucose is running >11mmol/l).

Date	Route	Fluid	Additives	Vol	Rate	Signature
18.8.14	IV	0.9% saline	50units Actrapid 50ml		Sliding Scale	P Roluos
18.8.14	IV	5% glucose	20mmol KCl	1l	8h	P Roluos

Fig. 10.1 Prescribing insulin and fluids for a sliding scale.

Insulin	Date	Start time	Blood glucose (mmol/l)	Rate (ml/h)
Actrapid	18.8.14	13:45	<4	Stop – call doctor
Dose	Route		4–7	1
1unit/ml	IV		7.1–11	2
		Signature	11.1–20	4
		S Dixon	>20	7 – call doctor

Fig. 10.2 Example of sliding scale regimen (check local guidelines).

If the patient remains hyperglycaemic despite the sliding scale (Fig. 10.2) then check the infusion pump and cannula; if no problems found, prescribe a STAT bolus of short-acting insulin eg Actrapid® 4–6 units SC. If control still poor, increase infusion rates by 1.5–2-fold, and check venous pH (T1DM) or osmolality (T2DM). If the capillary blood glucose is <4mmol/l check that there is 5% glucose running, increase the fluid rate and/or glucose concentration (up to 10%); recheck glucose in 30min. If persistently <4mmol/l stop the sliding scale, and restart the infusion at half the doses once blood glucose >6mmol/l. If glucose <2, see 📖 p322. *Stop a sliding scale* once a patient is eating normally and able to resume normal diabetes medication. Give normal dose of SC insulin 30mins before stopping the scale, unless rapid acting (eg Novorapid®, Humalog®) in which case give at same time as stopping the scale.

Prescribing insulin

Most hospitals have separate drug cards for prescribing insulin. Always specify the insulin formulation, and avoid using the abbreviation 'U' for units (since this can be misread as a number). See Fig. 10.3 for an example.

Breakfast	Insulin	Dose (units)	Route	Start
	Novomix® 30	18	SC	18.8.14
Night	Insulin	Dose (units)	Route	Start
	Novomix® 30	10	SC	18.8.14

Fig. 10.3 Prescribing subcutaneous insulins.

Diabetes mellitus

Fasting plasma glucose ≥7.0mmol/l, or ≥11.1mmol/l 2h after a 75g oral glucose load (given in 300ml water as oral glucose tolerance test – OGTT).[1]

- **Type 1** autoimmune pancreatic β cell destruction, resulting in dependence on exogenous insulin; typically presents in children or young adults
- **Type 2** relative insulin hyposecretion or resistance to effects, requiring drugs to potentiate insulin secretion or effects, or exogenous insulin; typically occurs in adults, especially if overweight
- **Impaired glucose tolerance (IGT)** plasma glucose ≥7.8mmol/l after OGTT, but <11.1mmol/l; 20–50% progress to T2DM in 10yr
- **Impaired fasting glucose (IFG)** plasma glucose ≥6.1mmol/l after an overnight fast, but <7.0mmol/l; lower risk of developing T2DM
- **Gestational** any degree of glucose intolerance first detected during pregnancy (📖 p505); around 30% will progress to T2DM within 5yr.

Type 1 DM (OHCM9 📖 p198)

Symptoms tiredness, weight loss, thirst, polyuria, abdo pain, vomiting.

Signs sweet-smelling breath, shock, abdominal pain (all suggest DKA).

Investigations Glucose testing as above. Check venous HCO_3^- and pH and urine (ketones) to exclude DKA. If uncertainty about type of diabetes, positive islet cell or glutamic acid decarboxylase antibodies, or low C-peptide levels all suggest T1DM. Check HbA_{1C} (see box).

Treatment resuscitate and investigate for DKA; in the absence of DKA, a new diagnosis of T1DM does not necessitate admission, but the patient should be started on a suitable insulin regimen by an appropriately experienced individual (eg endocrine registrar or diabetes nurse specialist) with regular finger-prick glucose monitoring and prompt out-patient follow-up. For properties of some commonly used insulins, see 📖 p203. Chronic management – see 📖 p330.

HbA_{1c}

HbA_{1c} reflects non-enzymatic glycosylation of haemoglobin at a rate proportional to plasma glucose. Since erythrocytes (and hence haemoglobin) undergo slow but constant turnover, HbA_{1c} reflects plasma glucose control over the preceding 1–3 months and is a reliable predictor of diabetes complications. Target HbA_{1c} levels should be set with patient involvement, taking into account an individual's risk profile, as well as tolerability of therapy. In T2DM targets are generally around 48mmol/mol, whilst for T1DM <59mmol/mol is a better target given risks of recurrent hypoglycaemia.[2]

[2] ie ≈7.5% (T2DM) or <6.5% (T1DM). Since 2009 HbA_{1c} levels have been reported as mmol per mol (of haemoglobin without glucose attached) but previous units of % were reported in key trials, used in guidelines and permeate the consciousness of patients and clinicians alike.

[1] In the presence of diabetes symptoms, a random plasma glucose ≥11.1mmol/l may be considered diagnostic; in the absence of symptoms, all tests should be repeated on a separate occasion.

Type 2 DM (OHCM9 📖 p198)

Symptoms as for type 1, but can also present with diabetic complications, eg visual problems, neuropathy, CRF, MI, CVA, claudication.

Signs foot ulcers, infections, peripheral neuropathy, poor visual acuity and retinopathy, evidence of cardiovascular disease.

Investigations **blds** confirm diagnosis based upon plasma glucose testing ±OGTT (📖 p328), HbA$_{1c}$ (see 'HbA$_{1c}$' box), U+E, lipid profile; *ECG*

Treatment T2DM may initially be controlled by a healthy diet with minimal rapid-release carbohydrates (as found in sugary drinks or sweets) and weight loss. If medication required, uptitrate pharmacological agents before adding in insulin therapy (see Table 10.1). Chronic management – see 📖 p330.

Table 10.1 *Medications for glycaemic control in T2DM[1]*

Class	Examples	Comment
Biguanides	Metformin	1st line for obese; ↑glucose uptake and ↓appetite; avoid if any renal failure
Sulphonylureas	Gliclazide	Add to metformin (1st line if metformin not suitable); ↑insulin secretion, but causes weight gain
Insulin	Isophane (given SC)	Added if metformin+sulphonylurea insufficient, but add 2nd line agents instead if insulin unacceptable
Thiazolidinediones	Pioglitazone	2nd line if other drugs not tolerated or effective; ↓insulin resistance; avoid in heart failure
DPP-4 inhibitors	Sitagliptin, dapagliflozin	2nd line if other drugs not tolerated or effective; ↑insulin and ↓glucagon secretion
GLP-1 activators (given SC)	Exenatide, liraglutide	2nd line if other drugs not tolerated or effective, especially if ↑BMI; ↑insulin and ↓glucagon secretion
α-glucosidase inhibitors	Acarbose	3rd line where other oral drugs not tolerated; ↓carbohydrate absorption; causes flatulence

[1] NICE guidelines available at ⌁guidance.nice.org.uk/CG87

Sick day rules

Educate diabetic patients what to do if they are feeling unwell:
- Drink plenty of fluids
- If not eating try milk, soup, fruit juice or fizzy drinks instead
- Increase frequency of blood glucose monitoring to at least 4 times/day
- Seek medical attention if you cannot keep fluids down, becoming drowsy or confused, blood glucose <4mmol/l or persistently >20mmol/l
- **If on insulin:** this should never be stopped; hyperglycaemia can arise from intercurrent illness, regardless of calorie intake. Consider increasing insulin dose if blood glucose >13mmol/l even if unable to eat. Dipstick urine for ketones at least daily and seek medical attention if +ve
- **If on tablets:** continue regular diabetic medications providing calorie intake continues. Metformin may need to be stopped if becoming dehydrated: seek medical advice.

Long-term management of diabetes mellitus[1,2]

Diabetes mellitus is associated with macrovascular (IHD, CVA, PVD) and microvascular (CRF, nephropathy, neuropathy, retinopathy) complications. Large, long-term studies show reductions in complications with control of risk factors; these should be assessed at least annually in a formal review.

Education and lifestyle ensure understanding and motivation for glycaemic control (including self-monitoring, medication compliance, and diet), vascular risk factors and complications (physical activity, smoking cessation, foot care).

Glycaemic control measure HbA1c (every 2–6mth)and adjust therapy accordingly (see box, 📖 p328); consider revising target if tight control unacceptable to patient based upon individual risk profile.

BP aim for BP <140/80 (uncomplicated T2DM) or <135/80 (uncomplicated T1DM); if end-organ damage aim for BP <130/80 (📖 p263). Use an ACEi as 1st line in T2DM (plus diuretic or Ca^{2+} channel blocker if African-Caribbean descent); use a thiazide diuretic in T1DM (ACEi if nephropathy).

Lipids measure lipid profile and consider cardiovascular risk factors; in all T2DM age >40yr (except those judged to be very low risk) initiate statin therapy and assess response; in T1DM consider statin therapy in those with microalbuminuria, family history, age>35yr, or other high-risk features.

Nephropathy test early morning urine albumin:creatinine ratio; if ≥2 repeated measurements show microalbuminuria (♂: >2.5mg/mmol, ♀: >3.5mg/mmol), tighten BP control, initiate ACEi and consider renal referral.

Retinopathy arrange annual retinal photography and review by appropriately trained staff; sudden loss of vision, rubeosis iridis, pre-retinal or vitreous haemorrhage, or retinal detachment require emergency ophthalmology review; new vessel formation requires urgent referral; pre-proliferative retinopathy, significant maculopathy, or unexplained change in visual acuity require routine referral.

Footcare[3] assess for ulcers, peripheral pulses, sensory function, and foot deformity. If ulcers present, refer urgently to a specialist diabetic footcare team. Those with previous ulcers, absent pulses or impaired sensation require referral to a footcare team for frequent review.

Neuropathy assess for autonomic neuropathy in the form of unexplained vomiting (gastroparesis – consider trial of prokinetic agents, eg metoclopramide), erectile dysfunction (offer phosphodiesterase-5 inhibitor, eg sildenafil), nocturnal diarrhoea, bladder voiding problems, or orthostatic hypotension. *Neuropathic pain*[4] requires oral duloxetine as 1st line; if this fails, switch to or combine with pregabalin, or switch to amitriptyline. Refractory or severe pain may require opioid analgesia and specialist pain service referral.

Aspirin is used,[5] but not licensed, for primary prevention of vascular events. Risk of GI bleeding needs to be balanced against vascular risk. Consider aspirin in T1DM if on a statin, or in T2DM if age ≥50 (provided BP controlled to <145/90) or age<50 and significant cardiovascular risk factors.

Pneumovax® and yearly flu vaccines should be offered to all patients.

---

[1] For NICE guidelines on management of T1DM see ⁀ᐟguidance.nice.org.uk/CG15
[2] For NICE guidelines on management of T2DM, see ⁀ᐟguidance.nice.org.uk/CG87
[3] For NICE guidelines on footcare in T2DM, see ⁀ᐟguidance.nice.org.uk/CG10
[4] For NICE guidelines on neuropathic pain, see ⁀ᐟguidance.nice.org.uk/CG173
[5] Evidence and recommendations conflicting, see ⁀ᐟwww.ncbi.nlm.nih.gov/pmc/articles/PMC3513879

Pituitary axis

Hypopituitarism

Failure of secretion may affect one or more anterior pituitary hormones.

Causes damage to the hypothalamic–pituitary axis after surgery, irradiation, tumours, ischaemia, infection (eg meningitis) or infiltration (eg amyloidosis).

Symptoms and signs are specific to each hormone lost, eg growth hormone (GH) loss: weakness, malaise, ↓cardiac output, hypoglycaemia; gonadotrophin (LH, FSH) loss: amenorrhoea, ↓libido, erectile dysfunction; TSH loss: hypothyroidism (📖 p334); ACTH loss: adrenal insufficiency (📖 p332).

Investigations tests of pituitary function include LH, FSH, TSH, paired with target organ hormones: testosterone/oestradiol, T_4, cortisol and insulin-like growth factor-1 (IGF-1, a marker of growth hormone secretion). Dynamic testing (eg short Synacthen® test, 📖 p571) is also informative. Generally testing of pituitary function should be undertaken and interpreted with specialist advice.

Treatment identify and treat underlying cause; appropriate hormone replacement may be required eg hydrocortisone (📖 p202) or thyroxine (📖 p205). ▶▶*On the ward, the most important point is to ensure any patient with panhypopituitarism gets regular steroids (increased in acute illness and given IV if necessary) with early endocrinologist involvement (📖 p332).*

Diabetes insipidus

Failure of urine concentration due to loss of either ADH secretion (neurogenic) or renal response (nephrogenic).

Causes **neurogenic** idiopathic, brain tumour or metastases, head trauma, cranial surgery; **nephrogenic** drugs (eg lithium), CRF, post-obstructive uropathy, ↑Ca^{2+}, ↓K^+.

Symptoms polyuria, thirst (may be extreme).

Signs dilute urine, clinically dehydrated (📖 p380).

Investigations ↓urine osmolality (<400mOsmol/kg), ↑plasma osmolality and ↑Na^+. In the water deprivation test (fluid balance, weight, urine and plasma osmolality recorded over 8h without fluids) – failure to concentrate urine (>600mOsmol/kg) confirms DI. Desmopressin (an ADH analogue) is then given – the production of a concentrated urine at this point implies neurogenic DI; failure to concentrate implies nephrogenic DI.

Treatment identify and treat the cause. In neurogenic DI, intranasal desmopressin may be used regularly. In nephrogenic DI, bendroflumethiazide or NSAIDs may be used.

Acromegaly

Hypersecretion of GH from a pituitary tumour drives soft-tissue and skeletal growth resulting in characteristic facial and body features.

Symptoms and signs enlarged hands and feet, coarse facial features, prognathism, macroglossia; headache ±bitemporal hemianopia. Sweating, hypertension and hyperglycaemia are markers of disease activity.

Investigations IGF-1 levels reflect GH secretion; OGTT and other tests of pituitary function under specialist guidance; pituitary MRI.

Treatment Transsphenoidal resection of pituitary tumour where possible; medical therapy includes somastostatin analogues (eg octreotide).

Adrenal disease

Cushing's syndrome (OHCM9 📖 p216)

Excess of glucocorticoids (eg cortisol); 'Cushing's disease' when due to an ACTH-producing pituitary tumour. ACTH may also be produced ectopically, eg by small-cell lung cancers. Adrenal adenomas or carcinomas are ACTH-independent causes (and will suppress ACTH). A patient on steroids may become 'Cushingoid'.

Symptoms weight gain, depression, psychosis, tiredness, weakness, oligo- or amenorrhoea, hirsutism, impotence, infections, DM.

Signs central obesity (buffalo hump), moon-face, water retention, ↑BP, thin skin, striae, bruising, peripheral wasting; hyperpigmentation only in Cushing's disease or ectopic ACTH production.

Investigations ↑glucose, ↑24h urinary cortisol, plasma ACTH and 8am cortisol, dexamethasone suppression tests (OHCM9 📖 p217); imaging tests are problematic due to high rates of 'incidentalomas' on adrenal CT or pituitary MRI.

Treatment localise and remove source of cortisol, eg transsphenoidal resection of pituitary adenoma, adrenalectomy for adrenal adenoma. If surgical treatment fails or unsuitable (eg ectopic ACTH from metastatic lung cancer), suppress steroidogenesis, eg with ketoconazole or metyrapone. If iatrogenic cause, try to taper steroid dose (📖 p177). Consider bone protection with bisphosphonate and vitamin D; monitor for ↑glucose.

Complications osteoporosis, DM, infection, poor healing, infertility.

Adrenal insufficiency (OHCM9 📖 p218)

Adrenal deficiency, typically seen upon abrupt withdrawal of long-term steroid therapy; 1° adrenal (Addison's) disease includes autoimmune (commonest in UK), TB (commonest worldwide), metastases (eg lung, breast), Waterhouse–Friederichsen syndrome (sepsis and adrenal haemorrhage).

Symptoms tiredness, lethargy, weight loss, weakness, dizziness, depression, abdo pain, diarrhoea or constipation, vomiting, myalgia.

Signs vitiligo, postural hypotension, hyperpigmentation of creases, scars and mouth (buccal).

Investigations ↓Na⁺, ↑K⁺, ↑urea, may have abnormal FBC and LFT. If suspected perform short Synacthen® test: order 250micrograms Synacthen® from pharmacy, once this arrives send a blood sample for cortisol and ACTH levels, give the Synacthen® IM/IV (📖 p524); repeat cortisol levels in 30min. Addison's is excluded if initial, or 30min cortisol are >550nmol/l.

Treatment hydrocortisone 20mg PO OM and 10mg PO ON, may also need fludrocortisone (50–200micrograms PO OD) if electrolytes deranged or postural hypotension. If unwell, trauma or post-op double all steroid doses for at least 1wk. If vomiting, replace oral dose with hydrocortisone 100mg IM/IV and seek specialist advice.

Addisonian crisis shock, ↓GCS or hypoglycaemia in a patient with Addison's disease or stopping long-term steroid therapy. Resuscitate according to 📖 p472, send bloods for cortisol levels and give hydrocortisone (200mg IV STAT, then 100mg IV/8h) with broad-spectrum antibiotics (eg Tazocin® 4.5g IV); seek urgent endocrinologist advice.

Hyperaldersteronism (OHCM9 📖 p220)

Excess aldosterone secretion, resulting in Na^+ and water retention; typically from an adrenal adenoma (Conn's syndrome), or adrenal hyperplasia.

Symptoms thirst, polyuria, weakness, muscle spasms, headaches.

Signs hypertension (especially if refractory to multiple antihypertensive agents or young age of onset).

Investigations $\downarrow K^+$, normal or $\uparrow Na^+$, metabolic alkalosis; measure plasma renin and aldosterone together after 2h in sitting position (postural changes affect renin secretion). Ideally the patient should be off all antihypertensives apart from α-blockers. ↑Aldosterone with ↓renin supports the diagnosis; consider CT abdo (but beware 'incidentalomas': abnormal CT findings, such as a small adrenal mass of no clinical significance).

Treatment spironolactone 200–300mg/24h PO; if adenoma, surgical resection may be attempted after 4wk medical therapy once electrolytes and BP controlled.

Secondary hyperaldosteronism occurs when renal perfusion is decreased, leading to high renin secretion. Common causes include diuretics, heart failure, liver failure and renal artery stenosis. Features are similar, but aldosterone:renin ratio will not be high. Manage with spironolactone or ACEi.

Phaeochromocytoma (OHCM9 📖 p220)

Catecholamine (eg noradrenaline) production from tumours within the adrenal medulla, or more rarely extra-adrenal source. Consider in those with drug-resistant or young onset hypertension, or typical symptoms.

Symptoms episodic anxiety, sweating, facial flushing, chest tightness, breathlessness, tremor, palpitations, headaches, abdo pain, vomiting or diarrhoea.

Signs episodic hypertension.

Investigations glycosuria during attack; plasma metanephrine testing has high sensitivity, but lower specificity (hence useful in high-risk patients); in all others, 24h urine collection for creatinine, total catecholamines, vanillylmandelic acid (VMA), and metanephrines has a high specificity and acceptable sensitivity; CT abdomen to evaluate for tumour.

Treatment surgical resection of tumour can safely be performed only after adrenoreceptor blockade. α-blockers (eg phenoxybenzamine), are used before β-blockers (eg propranolol) to avoid hypertensive crisis of unopposed α-adrenoreceptor stimulation.

Thyroid disease

Hyperthyroidism

Hypermetabolic state driven by excess thyroxine.

Causes Graves' disease (50–60%; agonistic autoantibodies to TSH receptor), toxic multinodular goitre (15–20%), subacute thyroiditis (15%; self-limiting, with painful granulomatous infiltrates as de Quervain's thyroiditis, or painless lymphocytic infiltrates), toxic adenoma (5%), excess exogenous replacement, metastatic thyroid carcinoma, struma ovarii.

Symptoms weight loss, agitation, anxiety, psychosis, sweating, heat intolerance, diarrhoea, tremor, oligomenorrhoea.

Signs thin, ↑HR, irregular pulse, warm hands, tremor, goitre ±nodules, lid lag, lid retraction, muscle weakness; *specific to Graves' disease:* exophthalmos, ophthalmoplegia, pretibial myxoedema, thyroid acropachy.

Investigations TSH used as screening test – if ↓ then measure fT₄ (*free thyroxine*, ie active, not bound to plasma proteins); antithyroid peroxidase (TPO) antibodies positive in Graves' and other forms of thyroiditis (TSH receptor antibodies more specific for Graves' but not routinely measured); **ECG** to exclude AF; **USS** thyroid, or nuclear scintigraphy may help localise lesion and assess uptake.

Treatment symptom relief with propranolol 40mg/6h (or rate limiting calcium-channel blocker if asthmatic); suppress thyroid function using carbimazole in dose titrated to TFTs, or with thyroxine in 'block and replace' approach. Other options include radioiodine ablation or surgical resection.

Complications CCF, AF, ophthalmopathy, osteoporosis.

▶▶*Thyrotoxic storm* Caused by infection, severe illness, recent thyroid surgery or radioiodine. Tachycardia, ±AF, agitation, confusion or coma with ↑fT₄ or ↑T₃. Resuscitate as required (📖 p472) and get senior help. Propranolol (suppresses sympathetic response, blocks T4 to T3 conversion and alleviates symptoms), propylthiouracil (inhibits T3/T4 production and T4 to T3 conversion and hydrocortisone (reduces iodine uptake and inhibits T4 to T3 conversion) are the main treatments. Carbimazole (inhibits T3/T4 production) has a slower onset of action but may be preferred to propylthiouracil since it has a longer duration of action and is less hepatotoxic.

Hypothyroidism

Common and insidious; characterised by insufficient thyroxine release.

Causes Hashimoto's thyroiditis (autoimmune destruction), resolution stage of subacute thyroiditis, drugs (eg amiodarone, lithium), iatrogenic (post surgery or radioiodine), iodine deficiency (commonest worldwide).

Symptoms fatigue, lethargy, weight gain, hair loss, depression, confusion, dementia, cold intolerance, constipation, menorrhagia, infertility.

Signs obese, bradycardia, ↓temp, cold/dry hands, macroglossia, jaundice, pitting oedema, goitre, peripheral neuropathy, slow relaxing reflexes.

Investigations ↑TSH, ↓fT₄; +ve thyroid autoantibodies.

Treatment levothyroxine (T₄): 50micrograms/24h PO, gradually titrated up into range 50–150micrograms/24h based upon monthly TFTs until TSH in normal range; yearly TFT once stable. Beware of worsening underlying ischaemic heart disease: Consider propranolol 40mg/6h PO to prevent ↑HR.

Complications angina from treatment, myxoedema coma.

Subclinical thyroid disease

Patients with normal fT_4 and T_3 but ↑or↓TSH have subclinical thyroid disease. Although some will progress to frank hypo/hyperthyroidism, there is no management consensus. Recheck TFTs after 3mth; if TSH grossly ↑or↓ (eg >10 or <0.1mU/l) then consider thyroxine/ carbimazole or surveillance. ↓TSH and ↓fT_4 suggests 'sick euthy-roidism' in systemic illness – recheck after recovery.

Parathyroid disease – see 📖 p389.

Neurology and psychiatry

Coma and reduced GCS emergency

Airway	Check airway is patent; consider manoeuvres/adjuncts
Breathing	If no respiratory effort – **CALL ARREST TEAM**
Circulation	If no palpable pulse – **CALL ARREST TEAM**
Disability	If GCS ≤8 – **CALL ANAESTHETIST**

▶▶Call for **senior help** early if patient unwell or deteriorating.

Airway and C-spine
- Stabilise **cervical spine** if there is any risk of injury (eg fall)
- **Look** inside the mouth, remove obvious objects/dentures
- Wide-bore **suction** under direct vision if secretions present
- **Jaw thrust**/chin lift; **oro/nasopharyngeal** airway if tolerated.

Breathing
- **15l/min O₂** if SOB or sats <94%; beware if known COPD/CO₂ retainer
- If hypoxic see 📖 p270
- **Monitor** O₂ sats and RR
- **Bag and mask** ventilation if poor/absent respiratory effort.

Circulation
- **Venous access**, take bloods:
  - FBC, U+E, LFT, glucose, Ca²⁺, cardiac markers, clotting, G+S, bld cultures, paracetamol, salicylate and alcohol levels
- **ECG** and treat arrhythmias (tachy 📖 p248, brady 📖 p256)
- Start **IV fluids** if shocked
- **Monitor** HR, cardiac trace and BP.

Disability
- Check blood **glucose**
- Check **drug card** especially for opioids and benzodiazepines
- Control **seizures** (📖 p344)
- **Check** GCS, pupil reflexes, limb tone, plantar responses
  - **Look** for brainstem, lateralising or meningeal signs (see Table 11.1)
- Call **anaesthetist** for airway support if GCS ≤8.

Exposure
- Check **temp**
- **Look** over whole body for evidence of injury or rashes
- Ask ward staff for a brief **history** or check notes
- **Examine** patient brief RS, CVS, abdo and neuro exam
- **ABG**, but don't leave the patient alone
- Request urgent portable **CXR**
- **Stabilise** and treat, see following sections
- Call for **senior help**
- **Reassess**, starting with A, B, C …

Stabilisation
- Get **senior help**
- Treat **hypoxia** with O₂, airway aids, ± ventilation
- Treat **arrhythmias** and **hypotension** urgently
- Start broad-spectrum **antibiotics** if sepsis suspected (?meningitis)
- Treat simple **metabolic/intoxication** abnormalities:
  - **glucose <3.5mmol/l**, give 100ml of 20% glucose STAT
  - **glucose >20mmol/l**, 0.9% saline 1l IV STAT (consider DKA/HONK)
  - **opioids** (pinpoint pupils and ↓RR), naloxone 0.4mg IV/IM STAT
  - history of chronic **alcohol** excess, Pabrinex® 2 pairs IV over 10min
  - **benzodiazepine** overdose **alone**, flumazenil 200micrograms IV.

Hypoxia	📖 p271	Hypoglycaemia	📖 p323
Hypotension	📖 p473	Hyperglycaemia	📖 p325
Hypertension	📖 p263	Liver failure	📖 p313
Tachyarrhythmia	📖 p250	Metabolic	📖 p385
Bradyarrhythmia	📖 p258	Pyrexia	📖 p482
Meningitis	📖 p360	Overdose	📖 p493

Further management
- Check brainstem function (see Table 11.1):
  - **normal** stabilise the patient and get an urgent CT head
  - **gradual onset dysfunction** consider mannitol and urgent CT head
  - **rapid onset dysfunction** give mannitol, normalise PaCO₂ with ventilator and contact a neurosurgeon urgently; the patient's brain is probably herniating due to ↑intracranial pressure
- If **CT normal** consider LP to test for meningitis or encephalitis
- If **CT and LP normal** the cause is probably metabolic or intoxication.

Table 11.1 *Common causes of reduced GCS*

Cause	Signs
Intoxication	May have shallow, slow breathing, pinpoint pupils suggests opioids, ↑↑RR suggests salicylates
Brainstem dysfunction	**Eyes** dilated or slow reacting pupil (unilateral or bilateral), absent corneal reflex, eyes looking in different directions (III, IV, VI lesion), eyes fixed: doll's head movements (not drifting back to forwards gaze when neck rotated)
	Swallow water not swallowed spontaneously/no gag reflex
	Respiration apnoeas, gasping, irregular or Cheyne–Stokes breathing (alternating rapid breathing and apnoeas)
	Body increased tone and upgoing plantars unilaterally/bilaterally/crossed
Lateralising (cerebral dysfunction)	Facial asymmetry, asymmetrical tone and plantar responses
Meningism	Neck stiffness, photophobia, Kernig's sign, Brudzinski's sign, straight leg raise (📖 p132)

Coma and reduced GCS

Think about

- **No focal neurology** $\downarrow O_2$, $\uparrow CO_2$, hypotension, metabolic ($\uparrow/\downarrow$glucose, Na^+, Ca^{2+}, K^+; acidosis, alkalosis, renal failure, liver failure), overdose (alcohol, opioids, tricyclics, benzodiazepines), epilepsy/post-ictal, hypothermia, pyrexia, hypothyroid, malignant hypertension
- **Brainstem dysfunction or lateralising signs** CVA, tumour, abscess, haematoma, hypoglycaemia or rarely other metabolic abnormalities
- **Meningism** meningitis, encephalitis, subarachnoid haemorrhage.

Ask about (notes, relatives, nurses) speed of onset, headache, chest pain, palpitations, vomiting, seizures, weight loss; **PMH** cardiac, respiratory, DM, kidney, liver, psychiatric, stroke/TIA, seizures; **DH** elicit past medical history from medications, consider the possibility of overdose; **SH** alcohol, recreational drugs (overdose or withdrawal).

Obs GCS (Table 11.2), temp, BP, HR, O_2 sats, O_2 requirements, RR, pupil size.

> **Neuro obs** GCS, limb movements, pupil size and reactivity, HR, BP, RR, temp.

Look for *respiration* rate, depth, distress, added sounds, air entry on both sides; *pulse* rate and rhythm; *abdomen* rigidity, pulsatile mass, organomegaly; *neuro* pupil responses, papilloedema (late sign), limb tone, plantar reflexes; *skin* rashes, injection marks or trauma.

Investigations *blds* FBC, U+E, LFT, Ca^{2+}, glucose, cardiac markers, CRP, clotting, bld cultures, toxicology screen (paracetamol, salicylate, alcohol); **ABG** pH, $\downarrow O_2$ or $\downarrow\uparrow CO_2$; **ECG** arrhythmias; **CXR** evidence of aspiration; CT if the patient has focal neurology or there is no clear diagnosis then an urgent CT head is required, the patient may need to be intubated first; **LP** after a CT scan if CT normal.

Table 11.2 *GCS scoring (3/15 minimum)*

Eyes			Motor	
Eyes	Open spontaneously	**4**	Obeys commands	**6**
	Open to command	3	Localises pain	5
	Open to pain	2	Flexes/withdraws to pain	4
	No response	1	Abnormal flexion to pain	3
Voice	Talking and orientated	**5**	Extension to pain	2
	Confused/disorientated	4	No movement	1
	Inappropriate words	3		
	Incomprehensible sounds	2		
	No vocalisations	1		

Originally described in 1974 as a 14-point scale (omitting 'abnormal flexion') by neurosurgeons at the University of Glasgow for use in patients with head injuries, this revised scale is now widely used in acute medicine and trauma.

Acute confusion[1]

Delirium or **acute confusional state** is a common but easily missed diagnosis associated with increased morbidity and mortality. Delirium can affect any patient but is especially common in the hospitalised elderly, where it may be misdiagnosed as dementia (with which it may co-exist). Unlike dementia, delirium is often fluctuating, worse at certain times of day.[2]

> ## CAM: Confusion assessment method[3]
>
> This validated aid to the recognition of delirium requires the presence of:
> - Acute onset + fluctuating course <u>and</u> • Inattention (easily distractible)
>   *Both of the above must be present, together with either of:*
> - Disorganised thinking   <u>or</u>   • Altered level of consciousness

Think about *emergencies* $\downarrow O_2$, $\uparrow CO_2$, MI, CVA, intracranial bleed, meningitis, encephalitis; ***common*** sepsis, metabolic ($\downarrow$glucose, $\downarrow Na^+$), drug toxicity (opioids, benzodiazepines, post-GA), heart failure, head injury, alcohol withdrawal or intoxication, post-ictal, urinary retention, constipation, pain.

Ask about use direct questions to assess eg for pain; further history from the ward staff, relatives, notes or residential/nursing home: speed of onset, chest pain, cough, sputum, dysuria, frequency, incontinence, head injury, headache, photophobia, vomiting, dizziness; ***PMH*** DM, heart, lung, liver or kidney problems, epilepsy, dementia, psychiatric illness; ***DH*** benzodiazepines, antidepressants, opioids, steroids, NSAIDs, antiparkinsonian drugs; ***SH*** alcohol, recreational drugs, baseline mobility and state.

Obs GCS (Table 11.2), temp, HR, BP, RR, O_2 sats.

Look for *respiration* rate, depth, added sounds, cyanosis; *pulse* rate and rhythm; ***abdomen*** rigidity, palpable bladder; ***PR*** faecal impaction; ***neuro*** signs of head injury, pupil responses, neck stiffness, photophobia, focal neurology, plantar responses; ***AMT score*** (see Table 11.3).

Investigations *urine* dipstick, M,C+S; ***blds*** FBC, U+E, LFT, CRP, glucose, Ca^{2+}, consider cardiac markers, blood cultures, amylase, TFT, B_{12}, folate; ***ABG*** $\downarrow O_2$ $\pm\downarrow\uparrow CO_2$; ***ECG*** arrhythmias; ***CXR*** infection or aspiration; ***CT*** if focal neurology, head injury or non-resolving confusion; ***LP*** if CT normal.

Table 11.3 *Abbreviated Mental Test (AMT) score (≥ 8 is normal for an elderly patient)*

Age	1	Recognise two people (eg Dr, nurse)	1
Date of birth	1	Year World War Two ended (1945)	1
Current year	1	Who is on the throne (Elizabeth II)	1
Time (nearest hour)	1	Recall address: '42 West Street'	1
Name of hospital	1	Count backwards from 20 to 1	1

Management

- Nurse in a quiet, appropriately lit environment with close, supportive observation (relatives, 'special' nurse); avoid restraints
- Investigate and treat the cause; pain and infection are the most common
- Sedate only if patient or staff safety threatened; use oral route where possible (eg haloperidol 0.5–1mg PO/1–2mg IM every 1–2h, max 5mg/24h; if PMH Lewy body dementia, alcohol excess or Parkinson's, lorazepam 0.5–1mg PO/IM every 1–2h, max 3mg/24h).

---

[1] NICE guidelines available at ⏀guidance.nice.org.uk/CG103

[2] Typically 'out-of-hours', when you may be asked to review whilst on-call.

[3] Inouye, S.K. et al. Ann Intern Med. 1990 **113**:941 (requires subscription)

Dementia[1]

Progressive global cognitive impairment with normal consciousness.

Worrying features **rapid progression, <65yr.**

Think about *common* Alzheimer's, Lewy body disease, frontotemporal dementia (Pick's), vascular dementia, Parkinson's (late), normal pressure hydrocephalus, depression (pseudodementia), chronic subdural haematoma, Korsakoff's syndrome; *rare* HIV, CJD, syphilis, space-occupying lesions, hypothyroid, B_{12} deficiency, malnutrition.

Ask about age of onset, progression, memory (short and long term), personality, thinking, planning, judgement, language, visuospatial skills, concentration, social behaviour, confusion, wandering, falls, head injury, tremor, mood, sleep quality, delusions, hallucinations, hearing, sight; *PMH* seizures, CVA/TIA; *DH* regular medications, sleeping tablets, anticholinergics; *FH* dementia, neurological problems; *SH* effect on work, relationships and social abilities; independence with activities of daily living (ADLs – food, cleaning, washing, dressing, toilet); ability to manage finances; alcohol intake; try to build a picture of the domestic environment: Who is at home and what local support is available?

Obs GCS, HR, BP, glucose.

Look for Mini-Mental State Examination (📖 p343), Abbreviated Mental Test score (📖 p341); full systems exam with careful neurological exam including general appearance, tremor, gait, dysphasia, cog-wheeling.

Investigations *blds* FBC, ESR, U+E, LFT, Ca^{2+}, TFT, B_{12}, folate, consider HIV, VDRL/TPHA; *imaging*, CXR, CT/MRI brain; *ECG*; *LP*; *EEG*.

Management The aim of initial investigations is to rule out and treat any reversible causes; refer to a neurologist/psychogeriatrician for specialist diagnosis and management; use an MDT approach to ensure the patient has appropriate accommodation and support with ADLs.

Support organisations

High-quality advice and access to support for dementia sufferers and their carers is available from a number of organisations, including:
- Dementia UK (0845 257 9406 🖰www.dementiauk.org)
- Alzheimer's Society (0300 222 1122 🖰www.alzheimers.org.uk) [for England, Wales and Northern Ireland] or Alzheimer's Scotland (0808 808 3000 🖰www.alzscot.org) [for those in Scotland]
- Carers Direct (0808 802 0202 🖰www.nhs.uk/carersdirect) for telephone and online support and advice for carers
- Age UK (0800 169 6565 🖰www.ageuk.org.uk) for a wide range of advice and services in support of ageing people

---

[1] NICE guidelines available at 🖰guidance.nice.org.uk/CG42

Common types of dementia

Alzheimer's slowly progressive loss of memory, with later loss of language, executive or visuospatial functions; anticholinesterases (eg donepezil) may benefit in moderate disease.

Vascular impairment of memory and at least one other cognitive domain in the presence of vascular risk factors ±neuroimaging evidence of ischaemia; often co-exists with Alzheimer's.

Lewy body early loss of executive function, with hallucinations (especially visual) and fluctuating levels of consciousness; memory loss is a later feature.

Frontotemporal prominent and early language loss ±loss of social functioning/disinhibition; may present in younger age group.

Some potentially reversible causes of dementia

Sub-dural haematoma dementia ±focal neurology (eg limb weakness); more common in elderly, atrophic brains; often history of trauma; characteristic CT appearances; evacuate.

Normal pressure hydrocephalus dementia, gait disturbance and urinary incontinence with hydrocephalus on CT and normal CSF opening pressure; idiopathic (50%) or may occur after meningitis, trauma or subarachnoid haemorrhage; ventriculo-peritoneal shunt may improve symptoms.

Korsakoff's syndrome amnesia and confabulation seen in thiamine deficiency (eg alcoholism); may show very slow and limited improvement with thiamine replacement.

Mini-Mental State Examination (MMSE)[1]

Since its publication in 1975, the MMSE has become a widely used test of cognitive function and is commonly used in screening for, and assessing progression of dementia. In 2001, the authors transferred reproduction and distribution rights to a commercial organisation which has since aggressively asserted copyright claims. Nonetheless, the full test remains widely available to use in most hospitals.

The test consists of 30 questions which together test various components of a patient's mental state:

- orientation (in time, place and person)
- registration (ability to listen and recite, to obey commands)
- attention and arithmetic (counting backwards)
- recall (reciting a list of objects)
- language (naming objects, reciting an address, etc)
- executive function (copying a drawing)

The maximum score in the MMSE is 30, though ≥28 is regarded as 'normal'. Scores of 24–27 are borderline and <24 suggests dementia. Results are unreliable if the patient is delirious, has a sensory impairment, affective disorder or has not been taught to read and write in English.

An abbreviated (10-point) version is often used (□ p341) and correlates well with MMSE for those with very high or low scores; in the intermediate range and for tracking changes, MMSE is a more reliable test; there are also numerous other, less widely used tests of cognitive function.[2]

[1] Folstein, M.F. et al. *J Psychiatr Res* 1975 **12**:189 (requires subscription).
[2] Holsinger, T. et al. *JAMA* 2007 **297**:2391 (available free online at ⨀jama.ama-assn.org/cgi/content/full/297/21/2391)

Adult seizures emergency

Airway	Check airway is patent; consider manoeuvres/adjuncts
Breathing	If no respiratory effort – **CALL ARREST TEAM**
Circulation	If no palpable pulse – **CALL ARREST TEAM**
Disability	If GCS ≤8 – **CALL ANAESTHETIST**

▶▶Call for **senior help** if seizure >5min. All timings are from the start of the first fit; the clock only restarts once the patient has been fit-free >30mins.

0–5min

- Start **timing**; this is very important and easy to forget
- **15l/min O$_2$** in all patients
- Keep patient safe and put into **recovery position** if possible
- **Monitor** HR, O$_2$ sats, BP, cardiac trace, temp
- **Venous access** (after 3–4min). Take bloods:
  - FBC, U+E, LFT, Ca^{2+}, glucose, bld cultures, anticonvulsant levels
- **Check GLUCOSE**: if <3.5mmol/l give 100ml of 20% glucose STAT.

5–20min

- Call for **senior help** and attach a cardiac monitor
- **Consider** an airway adjunct but do not force teeth apart
- If IV access: **lorazepam** 4mg IV over 2min, repeat at 10min if no effect
- If no IV access: diazepam 10mg PR, repeat every 10min if no effect up to 30mg total
- Ask ward staff about **history**/check notes
- If alcoholism/malnourished give **Pabrinex**® 2 pairs IV over 10min if not already given this admission.

20–40min

- Call for **anaesthetist** and senior help
- If not taking phenytoin: **phenytoin** 20mg/kg IV at <50mg/min
- If taking phenytoin: phenobarbital 10mg/kg IV over 10min (max 1g)
- **Monitor** ECG, BP and temp.

>40min

- **Thiopental** or propofol on ICU/HDU
- Transfer to **ICU** for general anaesthetic and EEG monitoring.

Life-threatening causes

- Hypoxia/cardiac disease
- Hypoglycaemia
- Metabolic (↓Ca^{2+}, ↑↓Na$^+$)
- Trauma
- Meningitis, encephalitis, malaria
- ↑ICP and CVA
- Drug overdose
- Hypertension/eclampsia (pregnancy)

Paediatric seizures emergency

Airway	Check airway is patent; consider manoeuvres/adjuncts
Breathing	If no respiratory effort – **CALL ARREST TEAM**
Circulation	If no palpable pulse – **CALL ARREST TEAM**
Disability	If GCS ≤8 – **CALL ANAESTHETIST**

▶▶Call for **senior help** in all children having a seizure. All timings are from the start of the first fit; the clock only restarts with a fit-free period >30mins.

Step 1
- Start **timing**; this is very important and easy to forget
- Maintain **airway**, assess ABC, check pupil size, posture, neck stiffness, fontanelle, temp and for rashes
- **15l/min O_2** in all patients
- Check **GLUCOSE**: if <3.5mmol/l give 2ml/kg of 10% glucose STAT:
  - take 10ml of clotted blood and one fluoride bottle (📖 p520) prior to giving glucose, but don't let this delay treatment
- Keep patient safe, be alert for vomit occluding the airway
- **Monitor** HR, O_2 sats, BP, cardiac trace, temp
- **Venous access**, take bloods:
  - FBC, U+E, LFT, CRP, Ca^{2+}, Mg^{2+}, glucose, bld cultures, anticonvulsant levels (if on anticonvulsants), venous blood gas
- If IV access: further **lorazepam** 0.1mg/kg IV (max 4mg)
- If no IV access: diazepam 0.5mg/kg PR (max 10mg)
- Ask parents or ward staff about history/check notes.

Step 2 (10min after either lorazepam/diazepam)
- If IV access: further **lorazepam** 0.1mg/kg IV (max 4mg)
- If no IV access: paraldehyde 0.4ml/kg PR with 0.4ml/kg olive oil or 0.8ml/kg of a pre-prepared 50:50 solution (max 20ml of mixture).

Step 3 (10min after either lorazepam/paraldehyde)
- Call for **anaesthetist** and senior help
- **Paraldehyde** 0.4ml/kg PR as above unless already given
- If not on phenytoin: **phenytoin** 20mg/kg IV/IO at <50mg/min
- If on phenytoin: phenobarbital 20mg/kg IV/IO over 20min.

Step 4 (20min after either phenytoin/phenobarbital)
- Rapid sequence **intubation**
- **Consider** mannitol, pyridoxine, paracetamol, diclofenac.

Life-threatening causes

- Meningitis, encephalitis, malaria
- Hypoglycaemia
- Metabolic (↓Ca^{2+}, ↑↓Na^+)
- Trauma/non-accidental injury
- Hypoxia
- ↑ICP and CVA
- Drug overdose
- Hypertension

Seizures

Worrying features preceding headache or head injury, duration >5min, prolonged post-ictal phase, adult onset, recent depression (overdose).

Think about *life-threatening* see box (📖 p344); **most likely** idiopathic (>50%), epilepsy, alcohol withdrawal, hypoglycaemia, hypoxia, trauma; **other** kidney or liver failure, pseudoseizures, overdose (tricyclics, phenothiazines, amphetamines); **non-seizure** brief limb jerking during a faint, rigors, syncope, arrhythmias. See Table 11.4.

Ask about get a detailed description of the fit from anyone who witnessed the episode (see box); headache, antecedent head trauma, chest pain, palpitations, sob; pmh previous seizures, dm, alcoholism, cardiac, respiratory, renal or hepatic disease, pregnant; **DH** anticonvulsants, hypoglycaemics; **SH** alcohol intake, last drink, recreational drugs, recent travel; **FH** epilepsy.

Obs GCS, temp, glucose (recheck), BP, O_2 sats.

Look for sweating, tremor, head injury, tongue biting, neck stiffness, papilloedema, focal neurology, urinary or faecal incontinence, pregnancy, infection, limb trauma (eg posterior dislocation of shoulder).

Investigations *blds* FBC, U+E, LFT, glucose, Ca^{2+}, Mg^{2+}, blood cultures, anticonvulsant levels; **ABG** if hypoxia or metabolic upset suspected; **urine** consider drug screen, β-hCG if pre-menopausal ♀; **ECG** to exclude dysrhythmia; **CT** may show a focal lesion, ↑ICP, haemorrhage or infarction, perform as urgent if the patient has a persistent GCS <15 post-fit, focal neurology or if the seizure was <4d post-trauma; **MRI** is the neuroimaging of choice in suspected epilepsy; **LP** if meningitis or encephalitis suspected; **EEG** may help to exclude encephalitis or as out-patient investigation for epilepsy.

Treatment Stop the seizure using the treatment outlined on 📖 p344. Correct any metabolic upset (glucose, Mg^{2+}, Ca^{2+}, Na^+) and exclude life-threatening causes whilst trying to establish the cause. Secure airway if still fitting or GCS ≤8.

Describing a seizure

If witnessing a seizure, try to document:
- **Onset** position, activity, any warning, starting in one limb or all over, presence of tonic phase (arched back, muscle spasm)
- **During** loss of consciousness, limb movements, eye movements, jaw and lip movements, breathing, peripheral or central cyanosis, incontinence (urinary and faecal), duration, HR and rhythm
- **Afterwards** tongue trauma, sleepy, limb weakness (Todd's paresis, 📖 p348).

Table 11.4 *Common causes of transient loss of consciousness*

	History	Examination	Investigations
Epileptic seizure (p348)	Known epilepsy, may have aura, post-ictal confusion/weakness	Often normal, may have tongue or limb trauma	Often normal, may have focal lesion or metabolic cause
Alcohol withdrawal (p348)	Usually >50units/wk alcohol consumption, last drink >24h ago	Anxious, sweating, tachycardic, tremor ±liver disease	↑MCV and γGT; may have a mild anaemia
Pseudo-seizures/ psychogenic	Unusual features, short duration, memory of event	Responsive to pain, normal respiration, no injuries	Normal investigations
Rigors	Feels cold/hot, no LOC, coarse shaking, infection symptoms	Febrile, source of infection (eg UTI, pneumonia), no injury	↑WBC, NØ or LØ and CRP, +ve urine dipstick
Eclampsia (p504)	Pregnant, may be unaware	↑BP, palpable uterus	Proteinuria, foetal heart on Doppler
Transient arrhythmia/ Stokes–Adams	Palpitations, pale, sudden LOC ±limb jerking; rapid recovery with flushing	Evidence of cardiac disease, injury following fall, irregular/absent pulse during attack	Arrhythmia or heart block on ECG, 24h ECG and BP monitoring
Narcolepsy	Excessive daytime sleepiness, collapse, sleep paralysis ±hallucinations	Often normal; loss of postural muscle tone and tendon reflexes during attacks	HLA typing, sleep studies
Vasovagal syncope (p260)	Feels light-headed ±hot, then collapse while standing, ±fine limb jerking, ±urinary incontinence, rapid recovery, no post-ictal phase	Bradycardia and hypotension during episode, GCS 15/15 within min, no focal neurology	±postural drop (systolic drop of 20mmHg or more)

Assessing a 'first fit'

History Detailed account from a first-hand witness.

Investigations FBC, U+E, LFT, glucose, Ca^{2+}, Mg^{2+}, PO_4^{3-}, clotting, medication levels, urine and serum toxicology screen (including paracetamol and salicylate); CT to exclude structural causes (non-urgent, unless recent trauma or altered neurology); consider LP after CT only if infection suspected; MRI is the neurologist's imaging of choice in suspected epilepsy, but can be arranged from their clinic.

Management Admit only if GCS<15 or drowsy; discuss with senior doctor regarding suspicion of seizures and need to advise to stop driving (see p605, 1yr ban); do **not** start antiepileptic medication – this decision should be made by a neurologist in an urgent out-patient clinic ('first fit' clinic).

Causes of seizures elsewhere in this book

Raised ICP	p360	Hypertensive emergency	p262
Hypoglycaemia	p323	Hypoxia	p260
Hypocalcaemia	p388	Meningitis/encephalitis	p360
Hyper/hyponatraemia	p387/386	Eclampsia	p504

Epilepsy[1] (OHCM9 📖 p494)

The abnormal, unprovoked discharge of a group of neurons results in an epileptic seizure; *epilepsy* is the recurrence of ≥2 such seizures.

Symptoms depend upon where the misfiring neurons are located. Seizures may be classified based upon a careful history into:

- **Partial** seizures start in a focal area of the brain giving, eg stereotyped motor, sensory, or autonomic symptoms; further subcategorised as:
  - *simple partial seizure* with preserved consciousness
  - *complex partial seizure* with altered consciousness, eg temporal lobe epilepsy (altered mood, hallucinations, stereotyped movements)
  - *secondary generalised seizures* start focally with a partial seizure, and evolve to the widespread discharge of generalised seizures
- **Generalised** seizures involve both cerebral hemispheres and include:
  - *tonic–clonic* with LOC and initial muscle spasm of whole body (tonic) followed by jerking phase (clonic)
  - *absence* sudden stopping of activity with staring or eye rolling, lasts <45s, most common in children.

Signs ↓GCS, tongue trauma, limb weakness, incontinence, Todd's paresis (transient weakness following a seizure; mimics a TIA).

Investigations often normal; **MRI** and **EEG** (±provocation) may help with the diagnosis and seizure classification.

Treatment decisions regarding use, titration and cessation of antiepileptic medications should be taken by an epilepsy specialist, and involve the patient. When treating a patient with epilepsy, be aware that certain drugs can lower seizure thresholds (eg fluoroquinolones, cephalosporins, penicillins, pethidine, tricyclics, clozapine); seek advice from a pharmacist. Always ensure patients are able to take their antiepileptic medication (eg consider NG or IV preparations if NBM).

Alcohol withdrawal (OHAM3 📖 p414)

Symptoms 12–36h *post-alcohol*: anxiety, shaking, sweating, vomiting, tonic-clonic seizures; 3–4d *post-alcohol* delirium tremens may develop: coarse tremor, confusion, delusions, hallucinations (untreated mortality 15%).

Signs hypertension, tachycardia, pale, sweaty, tremor, hypoglycaemia; *delirium tremens*: pyrexia.

Investigations **blds** may have ↓Mg^{2+}, ↓PO_4^{3-} or ↓urea.

Treatment monitor patients with a significant alcohol history for withdrawal; prescribe a reducing dose of chlordiazepoxide (📖 p193); correct electrolyte abnormalities; give vitamin replacements PO (thiamine 25mg/24h and vitamin B (compound strong) one tablet/24h) or IV (Pabrinex® 2 pairs/8h IV for 5d; this is a high-potency combination of B and C vitamins that may sometimes cause anaphylaxis). Monitor BP and blood glucose. Withdrawal seizures are usually self-limiting, treat as 📖 p344 if required.

Complications seizures, coma, encephalopathy, hypoglycaemia.

Post-traumatic seizures

Seen in more severe traumatic brain injury, where antiepileptic drugs are often used prophylactically. Arrange an urgent CT scan if not already done; if haematoma seen (📖 p438), contact a neurosurgeon, otherwise hourly neuro obs and reassess if ↓GCS.

[1] NICE guidelines available at 🔗guidance.nice.org.uk/CG137

Neurodegenerative disorders

Parkinson's disease[1] (OHCM9 📖 p498)

Common neurological disorder (affects ~1% of >60yr). Cardinal features include resting tremor, rigidity and bradykinesia.

Symptoms and signs coarse resting tremor ('pill rolling', usually unilateral at onset); rigidity ('cog-wheeling'); stumbling, festinant gait; small hand-writing, depression, speech and swallowing problems; sensation normal.

Investigations clinical diagnosis; single photon emission *CT* (SPECT) if diagnostic uncertainty; exclude other causes of similar symptoms of 'Parkinsonism', eg drug induced (haloperidol).

Treatment Antiparkinsonian medications should be initiated and titrated by a specialist. Levodopa given together with a peripheral dopa-decarboxylase inhibitor (eg carbidopa) enhances dopaminergic transmission. Effectiveness reduces after some years, so start only when symptoms interfere with life. Problematic 'on-off' and 'end-of-dose' phenomena may require addition of a monoamine-oxidase-B inhibitor (eg selegiline) or a COMT-inhibitor (eg tolcapone). Dopamine agonists (eg ropinirole) give slightly less effective symptom control but have fewer side effects so may be preferred in early therapy. Medications need to be given at precise times which may require alteration of standard in-patient drug charts.

Complications depression, dementia (late stage): Parkinson's disease may have pathological overlap with Lewy body dementia (📖 p343) with movement and cognitive dysfunction coming at contrasting stages in each disease.

Parkinson's-plus syndromes share some features of Parkinson's (eg multi-system atrophy: Parkinson's plus autonomic and cerebellar dysfunction; progressive supranuclear palsy: Parkinson's plus impaired upwards gaze). These tend to be refractory to standard therapy.

Motor neuron disease[2]

Degenerative disease affecting upper and lower motor neurons.

Symptoms and signs slowly progressive painless weakness, with mixed UMN and LMN features (📖 p353) eg spasticity, fasciculations; later speech and swallowing difficulties leading to aspiration.

Investigations **EMG** fibrillation and fasciculations.

Treatment mostly symptomatic, life expectancy is usually 3–5yr.

Complications aspiration pneumonia, respiratory failure, spasticity.

Huntington's disease

Incurable inherited (autosomal dominant) disorder characterised by involuntary limb movements (chorea), dementia and behavioural disturbance (depression, psychoses). Onset at 30–50yr.

Friedreich's ataxia

Inherited (autosomal recessive) disorder characterised by progressive limb and gait ataxia, dysarthria, loss of proprioception, absent tendon reflexes in the legs, and extensor plantar responses. Inability to walk occurs ~15 years after disease onset. May also develop heart failure and DM. Supportive management.

[1] NICE guidelines available at ⌂guidance.nice.org.uk/CG35
[2] Resources for patients, carers and doctors at ⌂www.mndassociation.org

Stroke/CVA/TIA emergency

Airway	Check airway is patent; consider manoeuvres/adjuncts
Breathing	If no respiratory effort – **CALL ARREST TEAM**
Circulation	If no palpable pulse – **CALL ARREST TEAM**
Disability	If GCS ≤8 – **CALL ANAESTHETIST**

▶▶Call for **senior help** early. Pt may need immediate transfer to Hyperacute Stroke Unit (HASU).

If **GCS is reduced** see 🔲 p338.
- **15l/min O$_2$** if SOB or sats <94%
- Check blood **glucose**; treat if too low (🔲 p322) or high (🔲 p324)
- Check **temp**; treat if too low (blankets) or high (IV/PR paracetamol)
- **Monitor** O$_2$ sats, RR, HR, cardiac trace, temp and BP
- **Venous access**, take bloods:
  - FBC, ESR, U+E, LFT, lipids, glucose, cardiac markers, clotting, G+S
- **NBM** and start **IV fluids** for hydration (eg 0.9% saline at 100ml/h)
- **ECG** looking for atrial fibrillation or arrhythmia
- Take a focused **history** particularly:
  - when did the symptoms start (get an exact time)?
  - are symptoms worsening, static or improving?
  - intracranial pathology, clotting problems, bleeding (eg GI/ PV), pregnancy, recent trauma/invasive procedures/surgery/ thrombolysis
- **Examine** patient: RS, CVS, abdo and neuro exam:
  - document exact neurological deficits
- Request urgent **CT** scan
- Consider thrombolysis (see box) **OR** aspirin 300mg PO STAT after CT.
- **Reassess**, starting with A, B, C …

Consider thrombolysis with t-PA in CVA if:

- Age <80: ≤4.5 hours from start of symptoms (and possibly even if 4.5-6h from start of symptoms though benefits less)
- Age ≥80: ≤3 hours from start of symptoms
- Non-haemorrhagic stroke (excluded by CT)
- Significant symptoms and not improving.

Contraindications as for cardiac thrombolysis 🔲 p536.

Key differentials

Hypo/hyperglycaemia	🔲 p323	Other intracranial pathology	🔲 p353
Encephalitis/meningitis	🔲 p360	Seizure/Todd's paresis	🔲 p346
Overdose	🔲 p493	Severe liver/renal failure	🔲 p313/373
Bell's palsy	🔲 p355	Hypertensive encephalopathy	🔲 p265

Stroke[1]

Neurological disability due to sudden loss of perfusion of an area of brain.
Causes ischaemia (85%, eg AF, carotid stenosis) or haemorrhage (15%).
Symptoms sudden onset focal neurology though onset can be stuttering.
Signs Check for irregular heartbeat and carotid bruit. The Bamford stroke
classification (see Table 11.5) allows easy recognition of the area of
brain affected, as well as prognostication. **Posterior circulation strokes**
(POCS) affect the territory of the vertebrobasilar artery (occipital lobes,
brainstem and cerebellum). **Anterior circulation strokes** involve the
internal carotid artery territory, which supplies all the rest of brain. These
are further subcategorised as **Total anterior circulation stroke** (TACS),
Partial anterior circulation stroke (PACS), and **Lacunar stroke** (LACS)

Table 11.5 *Bamford stroke classification*[2]

TACS	All of:	Motor/sensory deficit in ≥2 of face, arm, leg Homonymous hemianopia[3] Higher cortical dysfunction[4]
PACS	Either: or: or:	2 out of 3 of TACS criteria met Higher cortical dysfunction alone Isolated motor deficit not meeting LACS criteria
LACS		Motor and/or sensory deficit affecting ≥2 of face, arm, leg No higher cortical dysfunction or hemianopia
POCS	Any of:	Ipsilateral cranial nerve palsy + contralateral motor/sensory deficit Bilateral motor/sensory deficit Disordered conjugate eye movement Cerebellar dysfunction Isolated hemianopia or cortical blindness

[2] Bamford, J. et al. Lancet 1991 **337**:1521 (subscription required).
[3] Loss of vision on the same side in both eyes (□ p133).
[4] Includes dysphasia, visuospatial problems, ↓GCS.

Prognosis LACS, PACS, and POCS have a similar prognosis with 15%
mortality by 1yr while 60% live independently; TACS carries a 1yr mortality
of 60% with only 5% living independently.
Investigations **blds** FBC, U+E, LFT, glucose, lipids, clotting; **ECG**; **CXR**;
CT head: urgent if within thrombolysis window, GCS persistently low,
on oral anticoagulants/known bleeding disorder, severe headache at
onset of stroke or evidence of ↑ICP; otherwise within 24h. Anterior
circulation strokes also require **echo**, **carotid Doppler** and **24h ECG**.
Treatment see emergency treatment □ p350; if the patient is a candidate
for thrombolysis,[5] move fast to ensure timely treatment. Otherwise, aspirin
300mg/24h PO/PR for 14d (provided no haemorrhage on CT). Assess
safety of swallow (□ p352); if concerns, keep NBM+IV fluids and request
SALT assessment. Monitor BP, but do not try to lower BP without discussing
with a senior (□ p264). Do not use LMWH in acute setting with haemorrhagic or ischaemic strokes (risk of haemorrhagic transformation). Do not
prescribe TEDS (high risk of pressure ulcers). Admit to stroke ward for
early mobilisation and rehabilitation with multidisciplinary team.
Complications aspiration pneumonia, dependent lifestyle, further CVA.

[1] NICE guidelines available at ⌨guidance.nice.org.uk/CG68
[5] See 'Consider thrombolysis' box and resources from the international stroke trial collabora-
tors, available free at ⌨www.dcn.ed.ac.uk/ist3

Transient ischaemic attack (TIA)

A transient episode of neurological dysfunction caused by focal brain ischaemia without infarction. Symptoms typically last less than an hour, but prolonged episodes can occur.

Symptoms/signs as for stroke but resolve completely (though classical definitions of TIA describe resolution within 24h, there is no precise time cutoff to distinguish ischaemia from infarction); note that a transient loss of consciousness, or 'dizzy turns' are unlikely to represent a TIA.

Management if <3h since symptoms began see 🕮 p350; use ABCD2 score to estimate risk of stroke (see Table 11.6) start aspirin 300mg/24h PO.

Table 11.6 *ABCD2 score to calculate 7d stroke risk*[1]

Age	≥60yr		1 point
BP	Systolic >140mmHg and/or diastolic ≥90mmHg		1 point
Clinical features	Unilateral weakness		2 points
	Speech disturbance without weakness		1 point
	Other signs		0 points
Duration	≥60min		2 points
	10–59min		1 point
	<10min		0 points
Diabetes	Yes		1 point
Total Score	**7d risk**	**Management**	
0–3	1.2%	Urgent out-patient 'TIA clinic' follow-up (1wk)	
4–5	5.9%	Discuss with stroke physician – likely to need	
6–7	11.7%	admission for urgent investigation	

[1] Johnston, S.C. *et al. Lancet* 2007 **369**:283 (subscription required).

CVA prevention the risk of further events after TIA or stroke can be reduced with close attention to risk factors. Medical management includes control of BP, cholesterol, and glycaemia. Antiplatelet therapy options include clopidogrel 75mg/24h PO, aspirin 75mg/24h and dipyridamole MR 200mg/12h PO: Current health-economic modelling favours the use of clopidogrel for those who have had a stroke, and aspirin/dipyridamole combination therapy after a TIA.[2] Encourage smoking cessation, healthy diet and moderate exercise. Carotid endarterectomy should be considered within 2wk if symptomatic carotid stenosis >70%.

Safe to swallow?

For any patient with ↓GCS or a suspected neurological disability, perform a simple test of a patient's safety to swallow by watching the patient attempt to drink 30ml of water while seated in an upright position. Monitor for:

- Delayed swallowing (>2s to initiate swallow)
- Drooling
- Cough during or within 1min of swallowing
- Dysphonia/'wet voice' after swallowing.

If any of these features are present, keep NBM+IV fluids and request a SALT assessment.

---

[2] NICE interpretation of study data; see 🕮guidance.nice.org.uk/TA210

Focal neurology

Worrying features ↓HR, ↑/↓BP, ↓GCS, severe headache, pyrexia, neck stiffness, photophobia, vomiting, papilloedema.

Think about try to establish an anatomical pattern to abnormalities that will narrow the differential diagnosis (see Table 11.7 📖 p354).

Ask about motor problems (weakness, gait disturbance); sensory disturbance (tingling, pain, numbness); features of cerebellar disease (clumsiness, dysphasia, gait disturbance); symptoms of cranial nerve and cerebrum involvement (double vision, blurred vision, vertigo, hearing loss, dysphasia, facial droop); establish speed of onset and signs of underlying disease (weight loss, fever, cough, photophobia, neck stiffness, rashes, behavioural change) or ↑ICP (headache, nausea, morning vomiting); *PMH* previous neurology, migraines, epilepsy, eye problems, recent infections, ↑BP, irregular heart, DM, psychiatric disorder *DH* focus to symptom pattern (eg if peripheral neuropathy, ask about isoniazid, metronidazole) *SH* alcohol, recreational drugs; *FH* nerve or muscle problems.

Obs BP, HR, GCS (see 📖 p338 if ↓), glucose.

Look for perform a complete neuro exam (📖 p132) including cerebellar signs; CVS exam for AF and carotid bruit.

Investigations these should be determined by the location of the lesion determined by clinical examination. *blds* FBC, U+E, Ca^{2+}, glucose, ESR, CRP, autoantibodies; *EMG and nerve conduction studies* can help peripheral neuropathy or myopathy; *CT/MRI* imaging and *LP*.

Urgent CT brainstem or cerebral (lateralising) signs, persistent ↓GCS, suspected subarachnoid haemorrhage (📖 p360), head injury (📖 p438).

Lesion location your aim is to determine which region of the nervous system is affected to help target further investigation and aid diagnosis. With motor symptoms there are three main areas:

• **Lower motor neuron (LMN)** peripheral nervous system; wasting, fasciculations, reduced reflexes and tone, forehead involved if CN VII
• **Upper motor neuron (UMN)** central nervous system; increased tone and reflexes with upgoing plantars, if facial weakness forehead spared
• **Mixed** consider motor neuron disease, multiple sclerosis, spinal cord compression (LMN signs at level of compression, UMN signs below), Friedreich's ataxia (UMN weakness with absent ankle and knee jerks), syphilis (taboparesis), subacute combined degeneration of the cord.

Sensory loss may map to a particular nerve, a nerve root (dermatome), or affect one side of the body up to the level of a significant lesion within the brain or spinal cord (sensory level). Alternatively, loss may be bilateral and distal ('glove and stocking') suggesting peripheral neuropathy (eg DM).

The combination of the anatomical pattern, timecourse and associated features should enable you to make a clinical diagnosis for most lesions.

Table 11.7 *Guide to localising neurological lesions*

	Motor power	Sensory	Reflexes and tone	Features	Common causes
Cerebrum	Hemiparesis	Hemisensory loss	↑[1]	Unilateral ±higher cortical dysfunction (eg dysphasia) ±hemianopia	Stroke (📖 p351), SOL (📖 p355), migraine
Cerebellum	Normal	Normal	Normal	Ataxia, nystagmus, slurred speech, intention tremor, past-pointing	POCS (📖 p351), SOL (📖 p355), MS (📖 p355), alcohol, phenytoin
Brainstem	Hemiparesis	Hemisensory loss	↑	Cranial nerve deficit on opposite side to motor/sensory signs	POCS (📖 p355), SOL (📖 p355), MS (📖 p355)
Myelopathy (spinal cord damage)	Bilateral weakness (fitting spinal level)	Bilateral paraesthesia (sensory level)	↑ below level may be ↓ at level	UMN signs below level of cord damage; may see LMN signs at level	Cord compression/central disc herniation (📖 p357), spinal stenosis (📖 p448), MS (📖 p355)
Radiculopathy (nerve root damage)	Unilateral weakness (fitting nerve root)	Unilateral paraesthesia or pain (fits nerve root)	Normal/↓	Shooting, stabbing pain, often worse on postural change or cough	Spinal stenosis (📖 p448); Disc prolapse, cauda equina syndrome (both 📖 p357)
Neuropathy	Weakness	Paraesthesia	Normal/↓	May be **mono**neuropathy (specific nerve) or **poly**neuropathy (multiple nerves—distal deficit > proximal)	**Mono:** trauma, compression, inflammation (eg Bell's palsy 📖 p355); **Poly:** several (📖 p355)
Neuromuscular junction	Fatigable weakness	Normal	Normal/↓	Bilateral; fatigue with repetitive effort	Myasthenia gravis (📖 p355) Lambert-Eaton (paraneoplastic)
Myopathy	Bilateral weakness (proximal > distal)	Normal	Normal/↓	Acquired form may be painful with ↑CK	Hereditary (eg muscular dystrophy); alcohol, inflammatory (eg polymyositis), statins, ↓T₄

[1] Acute intracranial pathology may present with ↓ tone and reflexes before the characteristic UMN signs develop.

Space-occupying lesion (OHCM9 📖 p502).
Causes tumour, aneurysm, abscess, subdural or extradural haematoma.
Symptoms focal neurology, seizures, behavioural change, early morning headache, vomiting, visual disturbance.
Signs focal neurology, papilloedema.
Investigations **CT**, **MRI** (brainstem/cerebellum); **LP** only if no ↑ICP.
Treatment for ↑ICP see 📖 p360, surgical removal of lesion.

Spinal stenosis spinal canal narrowing 2° eg osteoarthritis (spondylosis) causes radiculopathy or myelopathy; consider decompressive laminectomy.

Myasthenia gravis (OHCM9 📖 p516).
Symptoms weakness, diplopia, dysarthria; worse in evening than morning.
Signs muscle fatigability, especially on upward gaze, normal reflexes.
Investigations **blds** antibodies to ACh receptor; **EMG**; Tensilon® test (improvement with edrophonium); **CT** chest (15% will have thymoma).
Treatment anticholinesterase (eg pyridostigmine), immunosuppression; thymectomy (even if no thymoma); plasmapheresis in refractory cases.
Myasthenic crisis triggered by illness, surgery or drugs; severe fatigue may involve the diaphragm causing respiratory failure requiring ventilation; assess with spirometry (FVC). Requires immunosuppression±plasmapheresis.

Bell's palsy rapid onset mononeuropathy of facial nerve (VII); prednisolone (40mg/24h PO) started within 72h reduces symptoms; aciclovir *may* also help; protect affected eye (tape closed at night, artificial tears and sunglasses).

Polyneuropathies (OHCM9 📖 p508).
Causes **acute** Guillain–Barré (post-infectious; can rapidly progress to respiratory failure; regular spirometry (FVC) to assess; treat with IV immunoglobulins±ventilation if worsening); **subacute** drugs (eg isoniazid, metronidazole), toxins (eg lead), nutritional deficiency (eg vitamin B); **chronic** malignancy, paraproteinaemia (📖 p396), connective tissue disease, metabolic disorders (eg uraemia, DM, 📖 p328), hypothyroidism (📖 p334); **hereditary** eg Charcot–Marie–Tooth.
Symptoms/signs may be motor (distal weakness) and/or sensory (paraesthesia).
Investigations **blds** FBC, B_{12}, folate, U+E, LFT, glucose, TFT, ESR, serum electrophoresis, ANCA, ANA; **urine** dipstick; **CXR**; **nerve conduction studies**.
Treatment treat or remove the cause if possible.
Complications wounds, ulcers, joint abnormalities eg Charcot joint.

Multiple sclerosis[1] (OHCM9 📖 p500)
Inflammatory, demyelinating disease of the CNS, leading to multiple neurological deficits separated in time and location.
Symptoms patients will present variably with motor (weakness, clumsiness), sensory (visual disturbance, numbness) or autonomic deficits (incontinence).
Signs any focal neurology, including LMN and UMN signs; typically bilateral spastic limbs, visual disturbance, internuclear ophthalmoplegia.
Investigations areas of inflammation and demyelination on **MRI**; slowed nerve conduction; **LP** CSF electrophoresis may show oligoclonal bands.
Treatment **MDT approach** to preserve and support function; consider steroids in acute flares (avoid >3 courses/year); β-interferon or glatiramer acetate can reduce relapse frequency; antispasmodics (eg baclofen).
Complications contractures, pressure ulcers, recurrent UTIs, unsafe swallow.

---

[1] NICE guidelines available at ⌁guidance.nice.org.uk/CG8

Back pain (OHGP3 📖 p484)

Worrying features bladder/bowel changes, fever, weight loss, age <20yr or >55yr, steroids, thoracic pain, previous cancer, progressive neurological deficit, perianal anaesthesia, pulsatile abdominal mass.

Think about *serious* cord compression, cauda equina syndrome, metastases, myeloma, infection, fracture, aortic aneurysm; ***common*** mechanical back pain (see Table 11.8), renal colic.

Ask about trauma/lifting (mechanism), location of pain, duration, aggravating/relieving factors, radiation, pain in joints, pain or tingling in legs, leg weakness, bladder (retention or incontinence), faecal incontinence, altered sensation on passing stool, weight loss; *PMH* previous back/joint pain, neurological problems, osteoporosis, anaemia; *DH* steroids, analgesia; *FH* joint or back problems; *SH* occupation (lifting, prolonged sitting).

Look for scoliosis, kyphosis, bony or paraspinal tenderness; reduced range of movement (especially flexion), pain on straight leg raise (📖 p149); lower limb neurological deficit (motor, sensory, reflexes); expansile abdominal mass; *PR* ↓tone or sensation (sacral/saddle anaesthesia).

Investigations if you suspect mechanical back pain and worrying features are not present, no further investigation required; otherwise consider: *blds* FBC, ESR, CRP, Ca^{2+}, ALP, PSA; *CXR* ±spinal X-ray if post-trauma or risk of pathological fracture; *MRI* spine: as emergency if cord compression or cauda equina suspected, urgent if suspect malignancy, infection or fracture, routine if suspect inflammatory disorder; *DEXA*.[1]

Table 11.8 *Common causes of back pain*

	History	Examination	Investigations
▶▶Cord compression	Weakness, numbness (±pain) below lesion, incontinence	Dermatomal distribution; UMN below lesion, LMN at lesion	Emergency/Urgent MRI to look for lesion
▶▶Cauda equina syndrome	Leg weakness and pain (often bilateral), urinary and/or faecal incontinence	↓perianal sensation, ↓anal tone, ↓leg power, sensation and reflexes	Emergency/Urgent MRI to look for lesion
Mechanical back pain	Pain, worse on movement, brought on by lifting/trauma	Pain reproduced by straight leg raise, unilateral neurology	Rarely needed; MRI only if considering referral for fusion
Spondylitis	'Inflammatory type' pain,[2] joint pain, no trauma, family history	↓lumbar flexion, pain on squeezing pelvis; ±painful red eye (📖 p426)	RhF –ve, ↑ESR, sacroiliitis on X-ray
Vertebral collapse fracture	Sudden onset pain in an elderly patient	Central pain over a discrete vertebrae; reduced ROM	Fracture on X-ray (wedge-shaped vertebral body)

[2] Pointers to an inflammatory aetiology include: morning stiffness, pain that improves with exercise but not rest, alternating buttock pain, nocturnal pain during 2nd half of night only. Finding ≥2/4 of these should prompt a search for a spondyloarthropathy (eg ankylosing spondylitis, reactive arthritis, psoriatic or IBD associated arthritis).

[1] See 🖰**www.sheffield.ac.uk/FRAX/** – a WHO validated tool to assess fracture risk (and need for DEXA or osteoporosis treatment) in those without worrying features (📖 p437).

Mechanical back pain including disc prolapse[1,2]

Symptoms low back pain, worse on coughing/moving, may radiate to leg.
Signs pain on straight leg raise (📖 p149), tenderness next to the verte-brae; radiculopathic pain/numbness; normal sensation and tone on PR.
Investigations **MRI** spine only if progressive abnormal neurology or fea-tures of cord compression/cauda equina syndrome. See Table 11.9.
Treatment early mobilisation, avoid lifting, maintain good posture; analgesia (📖 p86, consider tricyclic or strong opioids if paracetamol, NSAIDs and weak opioid ineffective); diazepam 2mg/8h PO for muscular spasm; reassess urgently if bilateral symptoms or urinary/faecal incontinence.

Table 11.9 *Types of mechanical back pain*

'Sprain'	Muscular pain and spasm without neurology
Disc prolapse	'Slipped disc', may compress the nerve root causing a unilateral radiculopathy (eg sciatica)
Spondylosis	Degenerative changes of the spine eg osteoarthritis
Spondylolysis	Recurrent stress fracture leading to a defect (typically in L5)
Spondylolisthesis	Anterior displacement of a vertebra; may present in younger patients; conservative management; spinal fusion if severe
Lumbar spinal stenosis (📖 p448)	Narrowing of the spinal canal eg due to osteoarthritis, causes leg aching and heaviness on walking (spinal claudication)

▶▶Cord compression

Causes tumour, abscess/TB, trauma, haematoma, central disc prolapse.
Symptoms weakness and/or numbness of legs, continuous/shooting pains, urinary retention or incontinence, faecal incontinence.
Signs LMN signs at the level of the lesion, UMN signs below, normal above, sharp boundary of reduced sensation, spinal shock (📖 p481).
Investigations urgent **MRI** spine, look for cause.
Treatment catheterise; refer immediately to orthopaedics/neurosurgeons.
Complications weakness, reduced sensation, incontinence, impotence.

▶▶Cauda equina syndrome

Causes central disc prolapse, tumour, abscess/TB, haematoma, trauma.
Symptoms urinary incontinence or retention (may be painless), faecal incontinence, bilateral leg weakness and pain.
Signs bilateral reduced power (LMN) and sensation, reduced perianal (saddle) sensation, reduced anal tone, bilateral absent ankle reflexes.
Investigations urgent **MRI** spine.
Treatment catheterise; refer immediately to orthopaedics/neurosurgeons.
Complications weakness, reduced sensation, incontinence, impotence.

Vertebral collapse fracture

Causes trauma, osteoporosis, tumour.
Symptoms sudden onset back pain; may be mild trauma if pathological.
Signs central vertebral tenderness, reduced mobility.
Investigations spinal **X-ray**.
Treatment analgesia, assess ability to cope, treat osteoporosis (📖 p437).

---

[1] See ⬙www.bmj.com/content/326/7388/535.full for a brief, free and readable overview.
[2] NICE guidelines for persistent pain available at ⬙guidance.nice.org.uk/CG88

Headache[1]

> *Worrying features* ↓GCS, sudden onset, severe, recurrent vomiting, photophobia, rash, neck stiffness, focal neurology, seizures, papilloedema, ↓↑HR, ↓↑BP.

Think about *emergencies* intracranial haemorrhage (subarachnoid, subdural, extradural), meningitis, encephalitis, ↑intracranial pressure (ICP), temporal arteritis, acute glaucoma, hypertensive crisis; *common* dehydration, tension, infection, migraine, extracranial (sinuses, eyes, ears, teeth), trauma, post-LP, post-nitrates; *other* cluster, postcoital, hypoglycaemia, hyponatraemia. See Table 11.10.

Ask about severity, location, bilateral vs. unilateral, speed of onset, character, change with coughing, nausea and vomiting, visual changes (before or currently), trauma, seizures, rashes, neck pain, sweating; *PMH* previous headaches, migraines (and usual symptoms); *DH* nitrates, analgesics, antihypertensives; *SH* recent stressors.

Obs temp, GCS, glucose, HR, BP, fluid balance:
• **Cushing's reflex** is a late sign of ↑ICP: ↓HR and ↑BP.

Look for volume status (📖 p380); evidence of meningism: neck stiffness, photophobia, Kernig's sign (fully flex hip and passively extend knee, +ve if painful in head or neck); non-blanching rash (check whole body); red eye (📖 p426), visual disturbance or papilloedema; focal neurology; temporal artery tenderness and pulsatility; tenderness over sinuses; evidence of recent head trauma; dental hygiene, ear discharge.

Investigations in the absence of worrying features it is appropriate to give pain relief without investigations; otherwise secure IV access and send *blds* FBC, ESR, U+E, LFT, glucose, CRP, clotting and bld cultures; *ABG* especially if ↓GCS. Discuss with a senior whether a *CT head ±LP* are required (see 📖 p552); *EEG* may help diagnose encephalitis.

Treatment exclude emergencies and treat other causes with simple analgesia (📖 p86) and fluids if dehydrated (📖 p380); ask to be contacted if symptoms fail to improve or worsen:
• **New onset** GCS <15 (see 📖 p338)
• **New onset focal neurology** reevaluate for meningitis, encephalitis or ↑ICP (📖 p360): 15l/min O₂, consider ABx – call a senior urgently
• **Sudden (onset <2min), severe and constant** consider a subarachnoid (📖 p360): 15l/min O₂, lie flat – call a senior urgently
• **Unwell, deranged obs** always consider meningitis/sepsis (📖 p360), classic symptoms in <30%: 15l/min O₂, IV fluids, discuss ABx with senior
• **Red, painful eye, ↓acuity** acute glaucoma (📖 p427), urgent ophthalmology referral
• **Temporal tenderness** consider temporal arteritis (📖 p361)
• **Hypertensive** (BP >200/120mmHg) (📖 p262).

[1] NICE guidelines available at 🖰guidance.nice.org.uk/CG150

Table 11.10 *Common causes of headache*

	History	Examination	Investigations
Subarachnoid or warning bleed	Rapid onset, severe pain, vomiting, ↓GCS if severe	May be normal, neck stiffness, photophobia, focal neurology	Bleed seen on CT; xanthochromia in CSF
Subdural or extradural haematoma	Trauma, confusion, vomiting	↓/fluctuating GCS; may be signs of ↑ICP	Blood seen on CT
Meningitis ±septicaemia	Unwell, irritable, drowsy, feels ill ±rash	Febrile ±septic, neck stiffness, photophobia ±non-blanching rash	↑WCC, ↑CRP; CSF: neutrophilia ±↓glucose
Raised ICP	Vomiting, blurred vision, dizzy, drowsy, worse on coughing/bending, seizures	Pupillary abnormalities, focal neurology; *late signs*: papilloedema, Cushing's reflex	Abnormal CT: enlarged ventricles ±focal lesion
Encephalitis	Drowsy, confused, vomiting, seizures, preceding flu-like illness, non-specific symptoms	Pyrexia, ↓GCS, confusion, focal neurology, neck stiffness, photophobia	CT/MRI: oedema, temporal lobe changes; CSF: ↑LØ ± protein
Temporal arteritis	Age >55yr, visual disturbances, weight loss, polymyalgia, jaw pain	Tender, palpable, non-pulsatile temporal artery, tender scalp	↑CRP, ↑↑↑ESR with anaemia, ↑plts and ↑ALP
Migraine	Previous migraines, visual aura; unilateral, throbbing, nausea, ±vomiting	Photophobia, visual field defects, may have focal neurology	None
Cluster	Recurrent daily headaches, unilateral, 'stabbing'	Agitated, rhinorrhoea, lacrimation, sweating	None
Tension	Bilateral, band-like pressure, worse when stressed	Normal; occasional scalp tenderness	None
Sinusitis	Frontal pain, blocked/runny nose	Tender above or below eyes	May have ↑LØ, NØ or EØ
Trigeminal neuralgia	Frequent, brief 'stabbing' pains; unilateral in distribution of CN V; previous facial herpes zoster	Normal; may identify 'trigger point'	None
Exertional	Sudden, explosive bilateral pain typically on exercise or orgasm	May mimic migraine or SAH, but meningism absent	Consider CT/LP to rule out SAH
Acute glaucoma	Age >50yr, blurred vision, pain in one eye, often occurs at night	↓visual acuity, dilated, ±oval pupil, red around cornea, tender	↑intraocular pressure
Drug induced	Many medications can induce headaches, particularly nitrates, Ca²⁺ channel antagonists and metronidazole with alcohol		

Subdural haematoma	📖 p438	Extradural haematoma	📖 p438
Acute glaucoma	📖 p427	Sepsis	📖 p480

▶▶Subarachnoid haemorrhage (OHAM3 📖 p384)

Potentially devastating bleed (typically aneurysmal) into subarachnoid space.
Symptoms rapid onset (<2min), severe, continuous (>2h) headache; often occipital ('hit around back of head'), vomiting, dizziness; may have seizures.
Signs neck stiffness, drowsy, photophobia, focal neurology, ↓GCS.
Investigations urgent **CT** head; since this may miss small bleeds (20%), if CT normal, then **LP** (>12h after onset) for xanthochromia.
Treatment 15l/min O₂, analgesia (codeine 30mg PO or 5mg morphine IV) and anti-emetic, eg metoclopramide 10mg IV/IM. Refer urgently to neurosurgeon for endovascular coiling or neurosurgical clipping and consider transfer to ICU if ↓GCS. Lie the patient flat and advise not to get up or eat. Reassess often and request neuro obs. Nimodipine (60mg/4h PO) prevents vasospasm and improves outcome.[1] Keep systolic <130mmHg, using IV β-blockers, unless lethargic (suggests vasospasm; may require permissive hypertension). Focal neurology or ↓GCS carry a worse prognosis.
Complications cerebral ischaemia, rebleeding, hydrocephalus, death.

▶▶Meningitis (OHAM3 📖 p355, OHCM9 📖 p832)

Symptoms headache, neck pain, photophobia, seizures, unwell.
Signs ↑HR, ±↓BP, ↑temp, ↓GCS or abnormal mood, neck stiffness, ±rash, focal neurology.
Investigations treat first; **blds** ↑WCC, ↑CRP; **CT** then **LP** (📖 p552).
Treatment contact a senior; ceftriaxone 4g IV STAT if you have a clinical suspicion of bacterial meningitis. Resuscitate as needed (📖 p472). Contact public health regarding contact tracing (see also sepsis, 📖 p480).
Complications ↑ICP, hydrocephalus, focal neurology, seizures, death.

▶▶Encephalitis (OHAM3 📖 p362)

Brain inflammation, usually viral. Rare and easily missed in early stages.
Symptoms abnormal behaviour, seizures, drowsy, headache, neck pain.
Signs altered personality, ↓GCS, focal neurology, neck stiffness, ↑temp.
Investigations **CT** followed by **LP** (📖 p552), send CSF for viral PCR; **CT/MRI/EEG** may all show temporal lobe changes.
Treatment be guided by microbiology; eg aciclovir 10mg/kg/8h IV (10–14d).
Complications ↑ICP, seizures, death.

▶▶Raised intracranial pressure – ICP (OHAM3 📖 p372)

Causes CVA, tumours, trauma, infection (including abscess), cerebral oedema (eg post-hypoxia), electrolyte imbalance, idiopathic.
Symptoms headache and vomiting (worse in morning and coughing/bending over), tiredness, visual problems, seizures.
Signs ↓GCS, focal neurology; late signs include Cushing's reflex (↓HR, ↑BP) ±papilloedema.
Investigations urgent **CT** head to assess cause and severity.
Treatment elevate the head end of the bed to 30° and correct hypotension with 0.9% saline. Discuss with a senior before giving mannitol or dexamethasone (tumours only) to reduce the ICP. Involve a neurosurgeon/neurologist early.
Complications herniation of the brain ('coning').

▶▶Acute glaucoma (📖 p427), needs urgent ophthalmology review.

[1] Pickard, J.D. *et al. BMJ* 1989 **298**:636 available free at ⌐www.ncbi.nlm.nih.gov/pmc/articles/PMC1835889/

Temporal arteritis (OHAM3 📖 p644)

Symptoms headache, jaw pain on eating, visual problems, aching muscles.
Signs temporal artery and scalp tenderness, pulseless or nodular temporal artery.
Investigations **blds** ↑↑ESR (>50mm/h), ↑CRP, ↑plts, ↓Hb all suggestive; definitive diagnosis requires **biopsies** (multiple sites) in ≤1wk of starting therapy.
Treatment start 60mg/24h prednisolone PO and strong analgesia. Discuss with on-call surgeon/ENT to arrange urgent out-patient biopsy and liaise with ophthalmology to exclude visual complications; Doppler USS of the artery can be helpful. Out-patient rheumatology follow-up.
Complications blindness (10–50%), TIA/stroke.

Migraine (OHCM9 📖 p462)

Recurrent, pulsatile headaches with strong familial tendency. Suspect an alternative pathology if sudden onset, or >55yr with no previous migraines.
Symptoms throbbing headache, initially unilateral often with nausea ±vomiting, photophobia; 20% may experience a preceding aura (flashing lights, zigzag, visual loss).
Signs may mimic TIA (visual defects, focal neurology) *but* slower onset.
Investigations normal; perform **blds, CT, LP** as required to rule out alternative/coexistent pathology.
Treatment **abortive**: simple analgesia (see 📖 p86), ±anti-emetic, ±5HT$_1$ agonists (eg sumatriptan); **preventative**: β-blocker (eg propranolol), or antiepileptics (eg topiramate).

Sinusitis

Inflammation of the mucosa of the paranasal sinuses due to bacteria, viruses or fungi; may become chronic.
Symptoms blocked nose, nasal discharge, facial pain, unable to smell.
Signs tender over sinuses (above medial eyebrows, bridge of nose, below eyes), purulent nasal discharge, temp usually normal.
Treatment try a mixture of beclometasone nasal spray 2 sprays to each nostril/12h ±ephedrine nasal drops 1–2 drops in each nostril/6h (7d max) ± saline nebs 5ml/2–4h. If severe (eg purulent mucus, systemically unwell) prescribe amoxicillin 500mg/8h PO.
Complications local spread of infection, chronic sinusitis.

Cluster headaches

Recurrent, short-lived, severe, unilateral 'stabbing' headaches occurring up to several times/day (often in early morning). Patients become agitated during attacks, and may experience rhinorrhoea, lacrimation or facial sweating.
Treatment **abortive**: 5HT$_1$ agonists (eg sumatriptan nasal spray), 15l/min O$_2$; **preventative**: Ca^{2+} channel blockers (eg verapamil), lithium.

Post-dural puncture usually present within 4–5d of LP, epidural or spinal anaesthetic, (rarely up to 7d); lie patient flat, treat with analgesia and ↑fluid intake (especially caffeinated drinks). Contact anaesthetist if severe/persistent to consider epidural blood patch.

▶▶**Hypertensive crises** hypertension usually represents a response to the pain of headache and responds to treatment of the headache. However, BP>200/120mmHg may represent the cause of a headache (📖 p265).

Dizziness

Worrying features hypoxia, ↑HR, irregular HR, ↓BP, ↓glucose, chest pain, sudden onset, unable to stand.

Think about *vertigo* labyrinthitis, vestibular neuronitis, benign positional vertigo, trauma, ototoxic drugs, Ménière's, CVA, multiple sclerosis, acoustic neuroma; *imbalance* hypoglycaemia, alcohol intoxication, Wernicke's encephalopathy, CVA, cerebellar space-occupying lesion, intracranial infection, B₁₂ deficiency, normal pressure hydrocephalus, *syncope/presyncope* (🕮 p442).
Ask about see box; *PMH* previous dizziness, ↑BP, DM, MS, IHD; *DH* antihypertensives, diuretics, aminoglycosides, insulin, oral hypoglycaemics; *SH* alcohol.
Obs temp, HR, lying and standing BP, glucose, GCS.
Look for ability to stand, gait; Romberg's test (see box), change with position, cerebellar signs (DANISH – dysdiadochokinesia, ataxia, nystagmus, intention tremor and past pointing, slurred speech, hypotonia); focal neurology, examine ear using otoscope (effusion, perforation); irregular pulse.
Investigations the type of dizziness (vertigo, ataxia, postural, syncope) should be determined from history alone; if syncope is suspected, investigate for cardiogenic causes (🕮 p260); for vertigo and ataxia, acute investigation is rarely required; consider a *CT head* if a CVA or tumour is suspected or there are cerebellar signs; *audiometry* if vestibular features.

Key questions in 'dizziness'

The sensation of dizziness is difficult to describe ('giddy', 'funny do', 'muzzy headed') and reflects some critically different underlying pathologies; try to map your patient's symptoms onto a medical equivalent by asking about:

- *Loss of consciousness* suggests seizures (🕮 p346) or syncope (🕮 p260). The impending sense of loss of consciousness, often with a 'greying out' of vision, is described as presyncope; causes and management are similar to syncope
- *Postural symptoms* are worse on standing after a sedentary period; this suggests postural hypotension and should prompt a review of medications
- *Vertigo* is the sensation of the world moving or spinning about the patient and is worse on sudden head movements; this suggests a problem with the labyrinth, vestibular nerve or brainstem (🕮 p363)
- *Ataxia* is shown by the inability to stand or walk straight; patients may have problems with fine limb movements; this suggests problems with proprioception or cerebellar function (🕮 p363)

Always ask about onset, deterioration, hearing loss, tinnitus, nausea, vomiting.

Romberg's test[1]

The cerebellum normally receives information needed to keep us upright from 2 sensory systems: vision and proprioception (via the spinal dorsal columns). Normally, one system can compensate for loss of the other. With the eyes closed and the feet placed together, a patient who sways excessively or falls is 'Romberg +ve', having lost proprioception. With a cerebellar lesion, the patient will struggle to maintain posture even with the eyes open.

[1] Described by the pioneering C19th German neurologist Moritz Romberg, working amongst the destitute of Berlin with tabes dorsalis (tertiary neurosyphilis).

Vertigo (OHCS8 📖 p554)

> *Worrying features* focal neurology, multidirectional or non-fatiguing nystagmus.

Treat the sensation of vertigo whilst determining the underlying cause. Centrally acting antihistamines (eg cyclizine 50mg/8h PO) and phenothiazines (eg prochlorperazine 5mg/8h PO) are particularly effective; betahistine 16mg/8h PO may also be used.

Benign positional vertigo Sudden onset vertigo lasting seconds following specific head movements. Treated with Epley manoeuvre (a series of movements to dislodge the vestibular debris causing the symptoms OHCS8 📖 p555) and referral to physiotherapy for vestibular exercises.

Inner ear inflammation causes sudden onset vertigo, nystagmus and severe nausea without focal neurology. Reassure and treat as above.

- **Vestibular neuronitis** viral infection of the vestibular nerve; improves within 1–2wk but can take 2–3mth to fully resolve
- **Labyrinthitis** as for vestibular neuronitis with hearing loss or tinnitus.

Ménière's attacks of severe vertigo lasting several hours, with tinnitus and progressive low frequency hearing loss. Treat as above, and refer to ENT.

Motion sickness rarely encountered in hospital, however cinnarizine 30mg PO 2h before journey is effective.

> *Nystagmus* is found with many peripheral and central causes of vertigo. Causes include: stroke, MS, space occupying lesions, labyrinthitis, vestibular neuronitis, benign positional vertigo, trauma, drugs of abuse (alcohol, LSD, PCP, ketamine), medications (lithium, SSRIs, phenytoin), Ménière's, Wernicke's encephalopathy; congenital (rare).

Imbalance/ataxia

Ataxia can be differentiated from vertigo on history; there are two types:
- **Cerebellar** 'DANISH' signs (see earlier in this topic); unstable even with eyes open
- **Sensory** Romberg's +ve (see box), loss of proprioception, preservation of fine coordination; 'stamping' gait, spinal/neuropathy signs.

Cerebellar ataxia
Causes CVA, multiple sclerosis, alcohol toxicity, Wernicke's encephalopathy, phenytoin, B_{12} deficiency, normal pressure hydrocephalus, infection, space-occupying lesions, trauma, paraneoplastic.

Management MRI is the most useful diagnostic test (consider CT if acute onset), neurology referral, some underlying causes are treatable:
- **Wernicke's encephalopathy** thiamine (B_1) deficiency often as a result of chronic alcohol excess results in confusion, ataxia, ophthalmoplegia, and nystagmus; treated with thiamine (PO/IV, 📖 p218), as for Korsakoff's syndrome, to which it may progress if left untreated.

Sensory ataxia
Causes cervical spondylosis, MS, peripheral neuropathy, syringomyelia, spinal tumour, spinal infection, B_{12} deficiency, Friedreich's ataxia, syphilis.
Management urgent MRI if acute onset, otherwise consider tests for peripheral neuropathy (📖 p355), spinal X-rays, routine MRI, nerve conduction studies, neurology referral; often treated with B_{12}.

Aggressive behaviour emergency

Safety	• Stay between the aggressor and the exit
	• Get extra help from other staff and/or security
	• Consider phoning the police.

▶▶Call for **senior help/security** early if the situation is deteriorating.
- **Assess the safety** is anyone at acute risk?
- **Emergency sedation** if they are a risk to themselves or others[1]
  - lorazepam 1–2mg (1mg elderly/renal failure) PO/IM/IV STAT
  - haloperidol 5–10mg (2mg elderly) PO/IM/IV STAT
  - Can be used together or separately
- Try to **establish the precipitant** from staff/relatives
- Ask a **member of staff** who knows the patient to accompany you
- Invite the patient to **sit down** with you and discuss the problem
- **Listen** until they feel they have explained the problem
- **Assess** the patient for signs of psychosis or acute confusion – are they physiologically unwell, psychologically disturbed or merely angry
- **Apologise** and/or offer sympathy as appropriate
- **Address any concerns** raised by the patient
- **Ask** specifically about pain or worry
- Consider offering **oral sedation** or **analgesia**
- Attempt to **defuse the situation**
- If unsuccessful **contact a senior** for help.

Common causes

- Acute confusion (delirium) 🕮 p341
- Intoxication (drugs/alcohol)
- Psychosis due to an underlying psychiatric disorder 🕮 p365
- Anger/frustration/poor communication 🕮 p21
- Pain 🕮 p86
- Hypoxia 🕮 p270
- Hypoglycaemia 🕮 p323.

'Sectioning' and the Mental Health Act 2007

In England and Wales, this Act allows the hospitalisation of individuals who are believed to be affected by a mental illness that:
- Requires assessment or treatment *and*
- Is sufficiently serious to pose a threat to self or others *and*
- Requires hospitalisation to which they are unable/unwilling to consent.

If you feel this applies to your patient, speak to your seniors and the psychiatrist on call urgently. Critically, these powers only apply to detention for the purposes of assessment or treatment of mental illness and cannot be used to detain for treatment of physical illness. In this case, treatment decisions should be based upon an assessment of mental capacity (🕮 p28).

In Scotland and Northern Ireland, similar powers are granted under the Mental Health Act 2003 and Mental Health Order 1986 respectively.

---

[1] If a patient poses a risk to themselves or others any doctor can give emergency sedation, without the patient's consent and with restraint, under the Mental Capacity Act (2005).

Mood disturbance/psychosis

> *Worrying features* delusions, hallucinations, suicidal intent.

Think about *emergency* acutely suicidal; *psychosis* schizophrenia, depression, bipolar disorder, postpartum, substance abuse, alcoholism or withdrawal; *low mood* depression, bipolar disorder, anxiety disorder, personality disorder, eating disorder, seasonal affective disorder, postpartum, grief, alcoholism or withdrawal, substance abuse; *high mood* bipolar disorder, cyclothymia, substance abuse; *organic* endocrine (hypo/hyperthyroid, Cushing's, Addison's), neurological (CVA, dementia, MS, Parkinson's, head injury, brain tumour), infections (HIV, Lyme disease, EBV syphilis), inflammatory disease (eg rheumatoid, SLE), electrolyte imbalance (eg Na$^+$, Ca^{2+}), metabolic problems (eg porphyria, Wilson's), malnutrition, anaemia, paraneoplastic, medications (📖 p366). See Table 11.11.

Ask about (see psychiatric history 📖 p160) *medical* bowel habit, weight change, appetite, cold/heat intolerance, tremor, previous head trauma, changes in vision, headaches, unusual sensations, weakness, seizures, sleeping problems, sexually transmitted illnesses and risk, rashes, joint pain; *psychiatric* early morning waking, concentration, energy levels, lack of pleasure, appetite, recent stresses, mood, change in personality, suicidal ideation; *personal* childhood, education, employment, relationships; *forensic* previous criminal convictions, custodial sentences; *PMH* previous psychiatric problems or care, mania, suicide attempts, chronic illness; *DH* regular medications, alternative medicines; *FH* psychiatric problems, thyroid, liver or brain problems, occupations; *SH* who do they live with, family, friends, alcohol intake, smoking, illicit substance abuse.

Obs GCS, temp, HR, BP, RR, glucose.

Look for (see mental state examination 📖 p160) *medical* full systems exam and careful neurological exam including tremor, eye reflexes, papilloedema, tendon reflexes; *psychiatric* general appearance, signs of neglect or flamboyancy, unusual posture or movements, aggression, affect, speech (form and content), thought (form and content including delusions), perception including hallucinations, cognition (concentration, memory, orientation), risk (to self or others), insight.

Investigations it is important to consider organic causes of mental disturbance. *blds* consider: FBC, U+E, LFT, Ca^{2+}, TFT, ESR, ANA, B$_{12}$, folate, cortisol, HIV (📖 p490), EBV and Lyme disease serology, VDRL/ THPA; *urine* toxicology screen; *LP*, *EEG*, *CT/MRI* brain.

Management

- Is the patient manic, psychotic (delusions or hallucinations, 📖 p162) or acutely suicidal? If so they need urgent psychiatric referral
- Could there be an organic cause for their symptoms (see earlier in topic)?
- Is the patient already known to local community mental health team?
- For milder symptoms would their GP or the local crisis team be better placed to manage in community?

Table 11.11 *Common causes of mood disturbance and psychosis*

	History	Examination	Investigations
Depression	Low mood, tearful, loss of interests, sleep disturbance	Poor eye contact, neglect, low mood and affect, ±psychosis	Usually normal
Bipolar disorder	Mixture of low and high mood events	Signs of high or low mood, ±psychosis	Usually normal
Schizophrenia	Delusions, auditory hallucinations, apathy	Neglect, poverty of speech/thought	Usually normal
Anxiety	Worry, sweating, dizziness, palpitations	Fearful, tense or normal	Usually normal
Personality disorder	Longstanding difficulties	Evidence of self-harm, usually normal	Usually normal
Dementia	Problems with memory, concentration, cognition	Neglect, poor cognition with normal consciousness	May have abnormal CT/ MRI brain
Organic cause	Weight loss, seizures, rapid onset, visual hallucinations	Neurological signs, rashes, wasting	Usually abnormal

Bipolar disorder

Recurrent episodes of high mood, usually interspersed with episodes of low mood. High mood may be mania (impairs job or social life and may have psychotic features) or hypomania (no impairment to job or social life). DSM-5[1] classifies bipolar disorder as occurring after even a single episode of mania; ICD-10[1] classifies this as a manic episode, and reserves 'bipolar disorder' to describe recurrent episodes of mania, or mania with depressive episodes. Recurrent swings between mild depression and hypomania are called 'cyclothymia'.

Mania signs flamboyant dress/appearance, excess/rapid speech, easy distractibility, restless.

Investigations if first manic episode: **CT** head; **EEG**; **urine** toxicology.

Treatment consider admission based on severity of episode and risk to self (suicide or reputation), job, assets, relationships. Mania is treated acutely with antipsychotics (particularly olanzapine) and benzodiazepines. Antidepressants are used for depressive episodes but may precipitate mania. Preventive treatment is with lithium, carbamazepine, valproate, or lamotrigine.

Complications financial errors, criminal activity, unemployment, relationship breakdown, suicide.

Examples of medications with psychiatric side effects

NSAIDs, antihypertensives, β-blockers, digoxin, oral contraceptive pill, antiepileptics, corticosteroids, antibiotics, cytotoxics, levodopa, anticholinergics, sedatives

These may all affect mood, cognition or exacerbate underlying psychiatric disease

---

[1] See box 🕮 p161 for details of the DSM-5 and ICD-10 classification systems.

Depression[1]

Depression is low mood that is not usual and persists for over 2 weeks. It can be a symptom of other psychiatric disorders (eg bipolar disorder, personality disorders) or a disease in its own right.[2]

Symptoms low mood, low energy, feeling worthless or guilty, poor concentration, recurrent thoughts of suicide or death, low self-esteem, tearfulness, loss of interests, anhedonia; **somatic symptoms** weight/appetite loss, sleep problems (early morning wakening, insomnia or excess sleeping), loss of libido, psychomotor agitation or retardation, change in mood with time of day **psychotic symptoms** delusions, hallucinations.

Signs neglect, agitation, slowed speech or movement, poor eye contact.

Bereavement avoid diagnosing within 2mth of bereavement; be aware of cultural variation in grief reactions; features pointing to depression include prolonged, severe functional impairment or psychomotor retardation.

Investigations often none; consider an organic cause and investigate if suspected, otherwise initiate treatment and review if not working.

Treatment

- Psychotherapy usually cognitive–behavioural therapy (CBT) but interpersonal therapy (IPT) may also be effective; can be used with or without medications
- Antidepressants:
  - first line: selective serotonin re-uptake inhibitors (SSRIs) eg citalopram, fluoxetine
  - if a patient does not respond to SSRIs liaise with a psychiatrist about which medications to recommend; this may be second-line antidepressants, eg venlafaxine, mirtazapine or augmentation with lithium
- Electroconvulsive therapy (ECT) is considered if the patient is at high risk (eg not eating or drinking) and/or has failed to respond to medications.

Prognosis outcome is generally good with the following: young, somatic symptoms, reactive depression (due to a life-event) and acute onset.

Complications deliberate self-harm, unemployment, relationship breakdown, recurrence, suicide.

Starting an antidepressant medication

- Antidepressants generally start to work by 2–3wk but can take up to 6wk
- Suicide risk may increase over the first few weeks
- Antidepressants are generally well tolerated; side effects are usually mild
- Treatment should continue for at least 6mth after the symptoms have resolved
- Antidepressants should be gradually weaned rather than stopped abruptly.

---

[1] NICE guidelines available at ⌐guidance.nice.org.uk/CG90

[2] A depressive episode is classified by DSM-5 as minor or major and may be associated with somatic symptoms or psychotic symptoms; major depressive disorder is the recurrence of major depressive episodes without mania; ICD-10 use the terms mild, moderate and severe, adding recurrent if more than one episode without mania. See box 🕮 p161 for details of the DSM-5 and ICD-10 classification systems.

Schizophrenia[1]

A chronic illness characterised by psychotic symptoms lasting over a month. Acute presentations are often characterised by positive symptoms; negative symptoms can persist despite treatment.

Positive symptoms delusions, hallucinations (often auditory): see first-rank symptoms box. *Negative symptoms* blunted affect, apathy, loss of drive, social withdrawal, social inappropriateness, poverty of thought/speech, cognitive impairment.

Signs neglect, disorganised behaviour, paranoia.

Investigations **blds** FBC, U+E, LFT, Ca^{2+}, glucose, consider TFT, VDRL, cortisol; **urine** toxicology; **EEG**; **CT/MRI**.

Treatment all people with a first presentation should be urgently referred to a mental health team either in the community (eg crisis resolution or home treatment team) or in secondary care depending on the severity of episode (risk to self: suicide, job, assets, relationships and others).

Antipsychotic medications (neuroleptics) are the mainstay of acute and chronic treatment:

- **Atypical antipsychotics** have less extrapyramidal side effects and a better effect on negative symptoms eg amisulpride, olanzapine, risperidone, quetiapine, clozapine; these are the preferred treatment in newly diagnosed schizophrenia, and for those experiencing side effects or relapse on conventional antipsychotics
- **Conventional antipsychotics** eg chlorpromazine, haloperidol, trifluoperazine, flupentixol.

> **Clozapine** is a 3rd-line antipsychotic, used in treatment-resistant schizophrenia. It can cause potentially fatal agranulocytosis; monitor FBC weekly for the 1st 18wk of treatment, 2wkly for the next 34wk, and 4wkly thereafter.

Side effects of antipsychotics include sedation, anticholinergic effects (eg dry mouth, blurred vision, constipation), extrapyramidal side effects (eg parkinsonism) and tardive dyskinesia (late onset oral grimacing and upper limb writhing). Procyclidine may be used to reduce Parkinsonism.

Complications deliberate self-harm, unemployment, relationship breakdown, drug side effects, suicide.

First-rank symptoms[2]

Delusions	Passivity
Delusional perception	Passivity of thought, feelings or actions
Hallucinations	**Thought flow and possession**
Thought echo (audible thoughts)	Thought withdrawal
Third-person auditory hallucinations	Thought insertion
Running commentary	Thought broadcasting

In the absence of organic pathology, the presence of these features is suggestive, but not diagnostic of schizophrenia

---

[1] NICE guidelines available at ⌁**guidance.nice.org.uk/CG178**
[2] Originally described by Kurt Schneider, a leading German psychiatrist, in 1959.

Anxiety disorders/neuroses[1]

It is normal to have a degree of worry or fear. However if this causes distress or interferes with life then it is considered abnormal. There are several types of anxiety- and stress-related disorders:

- *Specific phobic* fear of a specific situation or object, eg flying, spiders
- *Social phobia* fear in social situations, eg public speaking
- *Panic attack* excessive fear without any obvious trigger; associated with symptoms of autonomic arousal, eg sweating, dizziness, nausea, palpitations, breathlessness; usually lasts <30min
- *Panic disorder* recurrent panic attacks with fear of having another
- *Generalised anxiety disorder* (GAD) excessive worry in everyday life
- *Obsessive–compulsive disorder* (OCD) obsessive thoughts, eg 'my hands are dirty' leading to compulsions, eg repetitive hand washing.

Symptoms worry, irritability, fear, avoidance of feared situations, checking, seeking reassurance, tight chest, shortness of breath, palpitations, 'butter-flies', tremor, tingling of fingers, aches, pain.

Signs tremor, ↑HR, ↑RR; be careful to exclude any organic causes of symptoms such as breathlessness, chest pain or palpitations.

Investigations consider FBC, U+E, LFT, Ca^{2+}, cardiac markers, TFT, glucose; urinary VMA; ECG to exclude organic causes of symptoms.

Treatment careful explanation of the cause of their problems; relaxation techniques, psychological therapies, eg CBT; medications, eg SSRIs; benzodi-azepine use should be avoided in panic disorder and used only for <4wks in GAD, as these have poor long-term benefits and carry a risk of dependence.

Relaxation techniques

- Breathing exercises (silently counting breaths up to 10)
- Visualisation techniques (imagining a place, colour, or image that is calming)
- Progressive muscle relaxation (tensing and relaxing muscle groups in turn)
- Relaxation CDs
- Yoga.

Personality disorders

Ingrained patterns of behaviour manifesting as abnormal and inflexible responses to a broad range of personal and social situations; the diagnosis is to be avoided in adolescents when the personality is still developing.

Classification DSM-V divides personality disorders into 3 clusters: type A (odd, eccentric; includes paranoid); type B (dramatic, emotional; includes antisocial and borderline); type C (anxious, fearful; includes dependent).

Investigations usually none, but they require careful assessment over mul-tiple occasions and the exclusion of other psychiatric diagnoses.

Treatment personality disorders are challenging to treat. Psychotherapies may be useful, including dialectical behaviour therapy, cognitive–analytical therapy, CBT, and psychodynamic psychotherapy. Antidepressants, mood stabilisers, and antipsychotics may also be used though the evidence of benefit is limited.

Complications suicide, self-harm, social isolation.

---

[1] NICE guidelines available at ⌐ guidance.nice.org.uk/CG113

Fluids and renal

Acute kidney injury[1]

Acute rise from baseline of serum urea and creatinine ±oliguria (Table 12.1);[1] there are three basic mechanisms:

- **Prerenal** hypoperfusion of kidney due to eg ↓BP, hypovolaemia, renal artery occlusion (mass, emboli)
- **Renal** intrinsic renal pathology eg glomerulonephritis, vasculitis, drugs
- **Obstruction** of outflow tract (ureter, bladder, urethra) by, eg enlarged prostate, single functioning kidney with calculi, pelvic mass or surgery.

Acute tubular necrosis refers to irreversible renal damage with nephron loss that may occur due to prerenal *or* renal triggers eg due to prolonged hypoperfusion or nephrotoxic drugs (NSAIDs, gentamicin, IV contrast).

▶▶Call for **senior help** early.

Table 12.1 *Features of different types of renal failure*

Prerenal hypoperfusion	Oliguria, urine osmolality >500mOsmol/kg, urine Na⁺ <20mmol/l[2]
Acute tubular necrosis	Oliguria/normal/polyuria, urine osmolality <350mOsmol/kg, urine Na⁺ >40mmol/l[2]
Renal	Oligo/anuria, haematuria, ↑BP
Obstruction	Oligo/anuria, hydronephrosis on USS; if urethral: painful anuria with palpable bladder
Chronic renal failure	Oliguria/normal/polyuria, previous ↑creatinine, ↓Hb, ↓Ca²⁺, ↑PO₄³⁻, small kidneys on USS, fatigue, nocturia

History previous renal or other medical problems, urine output, fluid intake, medications (?nephrotoxic), rashes, bleeding, lethargy, anorexia.

Examination volume status (🕮 p380), BP (compare to what is *normal for patient* from eg old obs charts), HR, JVP, basal creps, gallop rhythm, oedema, palpable bladder.

Investigations *urine* colour, hourly volume, dipstick, M,C+S, osmolality and Na⁺ (🕮 p590); *blds* FBC, U+E, LFT, CK, CRP, osmolality, ESR, clotting; *ABG* beware acidosis or ↑K⁺; *urgent ECG* ↑K⁺ causes flat P waves, wide QRS and tall, peaked T waves; *CXR*, *urinary tract USS*.

Treatment insert catheter (🕮 p546) to monitor output; assess for and treat causes and serious complications:

- **Obstructed** catheter will relieve urethral obstruction; ureteric obstruction may require nephrostomy or stenting
- **Shocked** ↑HR, ↓BP, absent JVP; fluid resuscitate (🕮 p472) ±inotropes
- **Overloaded** oedema, basal creps, ↑↑JVP; O₂, furosemide (🕮 p200), CXR
- **Hyperkalaemia** insulin/glucose, Ca²⁺ gluconate, salbutamol (🕮 p384).

Continue IV fluids unless overloaded (no KCl if ↑K⁺), stop nephrotoxic drugs (🕮 p172) – this includes ACEi/metformin even if CCF/DM; monitor urine output; consider HDU referral for CVP monitoring.

---

[1] May be defined as any of: ↑creatinine of ≥26 μmol/l in ≤48h, *or* ≥50% in 7d (if recent bloods unavailable consider baseline values plus clinical history); or ↓urine output <0.5 ml/kg/h for >6h (adults) or >8h (children); *or* ≥25% ↓eGFR in 7d (children only).NICE guidelines available at ⟨ᵖ guidance.nice.org.uk/CG169

[2] In prerenal states, the hypoperfused kidney attempts to conserve water and electrolytes, passing waste solutes as a maximally concentrated urine low in sodium. With tubular necrosis, concentrating ability is lost. Calculating the fractional excretion of sodium (FE_{Na}) corrects for dilution by relating sodium concentrations to creatinine (Cr): $FE_{Na} = (Urine_{Na}/Plasma_{Na})/(Urine_{Cr}/Plasma_{Cr}) \times 100$. $FE_{Na}>1\%$ supports a diagnosis of ATN.

Chronic renal failure[1]

Long-standing and irreversible reduction in GFR.

Causes DM, ↑BP, chronic urinary retention, glomerulonephritis, nephritis, pyelonephritis, polycystic kidneys, vasculitis.

Symptoms initially none; tiredness, weight loss, nausea.

Signs initially none, may have signs of causative disease eg DM.

Results ↑urea, ↑creatinine, ↓eGFR[2], ↓Hb, ↓Ca^{2+}, ↑PO_4^{3-}, persistent proteinuria and/or haematuria, abnormal/small kidneys on USS; biopsy sometimes necessary when cause unclear.

Treatment involves regular review by a nephrologist. Tight control of BP and DM, smoking cessation, ACEi and avoidance of nephrotoxins slows the progression to ESRF. Management of complications includes correction of anaemia with iron infusions ±erythropoietin, dietary modification and oral Ca^{2+} supplements/PO_4^{3-} binders to prevent ↓Ca^{2+}/↑PO_4^{3-}, control of secondary hyperparathyroidism with vitamin D analogues. As the patient nears chronic kidney disease stage 5 (CKD 5 – see Table 12.2), wishes and suitability for dialysis and transplantation should be discussed and necessary arrangements made (eg dialysis counselling, fistula creation).

Table 12.2 *Stages of CKD[3]*

eGFR (ml/min)	Stage
>90	1
60–89	2
45–59	3a
30-44	3b
15–29	4
<15	5 (ESRF)

[3] Reduction in eGFR needs to be sustained (eg ≥3 mth) and accompanied by evidence of renal disease (eg structural abnormalities, persistent haematuria, proteinuria or microalbuminuria)

Complications vascular disease, anaemia, ↓Ca^{2+}, renal osteodystrophy, ↑K^+, fluid overload, immune compromise, peripheral neuropathy.

Prescribing see 📖 p172; avoid nephrotoxic drugs (eg metformin, NSAIDs, gentamicin); reduce doses/frequency of renal excreted drugs (eg opioids, benzodiazepines, penicillins); see also 📖 p380 for fluids.

Radiology avoid IV contrast imaging except in emergency since this is nephrotoxic; discuss carefully with nephrology and radiology. Where essential, use IV hydration and monitor renal function closely.

Patients on dialysis

Approximately 15,000 UK patients are on haemodialysis, usually for 3–5h 3x/week via an arteriovenous (AV) fistula. Blood tests and BP measurements should never be made from a fistula arm. Placing fingers or a stethoscope bell gently over a fistula will confirm if a gentle buzz is felt or heard. A further 5000 UK patients use peritoneal dialysis via an abdominal (Tenckhoff) catheter. Peritoneal infections in these patients can be devastating; if septic, a sample of dialysate should be inspected (?turbid) and sent for cell count, Gram stain and culture; intraperitoneal antibiotics may be required. Always inform the renal team.

[1] NICE guidelines available at ⌁**guidance.nice.org.uk/CG73** See also the UK renal association website ⌁**www.renal.org/home.aspx** for useful educational material and links.

[2] There are various methods of giving an estimated GFR (eGFR). Most labs use variations on the formula developed by the Modification of Diet in Renal Disease (MDRD) study group which combine demographic data (age, sex, race) and serum chemistry (usually just creatinine). Original paper: Levey, A.S. et al. *Ann Intern Med.* 1999 **130**:461 available at ⌁**annals.org/article.aspx?articleid=712617** (subscription required – check ATHENS)

Haematuria

Worrying features weight loss, frank blood or clots (?malignancy); ↑BP, proteinuria (?nephritic syndrome 📖 p376).

Think about macroscopic UTI, tumours, stones; **microscopic with red cells** UTI, bladder, renal or prostate tumour, stones, recent catheterisation, glomerulonephritis/nephritic syndrome, endocarditis, clotting abnormality, sickle cell, TB, schistosomiasis, trauma, strenuous exercise, PV bleeding (📖 p496); **microscopic without red cells** (haemoglobinuria) haemolytic anaemia, myositis, rhabdomyolysis, trauma, ischaemia; **red discolouration** rifampicin, beetroot.

Ask about urine colour and volume, clots, dysuria, frequency, urgency, fever, abdominal pain, hesitancy, poor stream, recent trauma or catheterisation, weight loss, malaise, lethargy, menstruation; **PMH** kidney disease, stones, prostate disease, cancer, clotting disorders, sickle cell; **DH** nephrotoxic drugs (eg NSAIDs, gentamicin), rifampicin, anticoagulants.

Obs BP, HR, temp, fluid balance.

Look for ↑BP, haematuria and proteinuria suggest nephritic syndrome (📖 p376); inspect the urine; rashes, bruises, splinter haemorrhages, palpate for suprapubic or loin tenderness or masses; PR: enlarged prostate; PV bleeding.

Investigations urine dipstick may not distinguish red cells and haemoglobin, microscopy (for red cell or protein casts), culture; **blds** FBC, U+E, LFT, Ca^{2+}, ESR, CRP, clotting; consider G+S, autoantibodies (anti-GBM, ANCA, ANA, anti-DNA), complement, PSA, **USS** urinary tract.

Management *Macroscopic* (red/pink urine) resuscitate (📖 p478), if heavy consider inserting a three-lumen catheter for bladder wash-out, discuss with urology to exclude malignancy (IVU, cystoscopy, CT).
Microscopic (urine looks normal, red cells on microscopy):

• **With nitrites/white cells** treat as a UTI/pyelonephritis (📖 p484), check urine once infection has cleared to be sure haematuria has resolved
• **Without proteinuria** suggests urological tumour or stones (📖 p295), refer to urology (urgently if >50yr) for IVU/CT-KUB ±cystoscopy
• **With proteinuria** suggests glomerular pathology, refer to nephrology and check BP, urinary output, urine casts, autoantibodies, complement, urine protein:creatinine, 24h urine collection for protein, renal USS.

Haemoglobinuria haemolytic anaemia (📖 p394), rhabdomyolysis (see box).

Rhabdomyolysis

First described in crush victims during the Blitz, this involves muscle necrosis after crush injuries or after lying on a hard surface for prolonged periods (eg elderly patients who fall and are unable to get up). Myocyte contents are nephrotoxic and lead to renal failure with ↑↑↑CK (but normal troponins), with haemoglobinuria. Treatment is as for acute renal failure (📖 p372), with management of hyperkalaemia (📖 p384) ± surgical debridement.

Proteinuria

Worrying features ↑BP, oliguria, haematuria, ↑↑proteinuria, oedema.

Think about *transient* physical exertion, fever, UTI, vaginal discharge, recent ejaculation; *extra-renal causes* orthostatic, hypertension, CCF; *primary renal disease* glomerulonephritis; *multisystemic disease* vasculitis, lupus, endocarditis, myeloma, hepatitis C, pre-eclampsia.

Ask about recent exercise, vaginal discharge, pregnancy, dysuria, frequency, urgency, urine output, fever, haematuria, arthralgia or rash, malaise, lethargy, oedema, orthopnoea, recent URTI/tonsillitis; *PMH* kidney disease, ↑BP, heart disease, cholesterol, DM; *DH* nephrotoxic drugs (eg NSAIDS, gentamicin).

Obs BP, HR, RR, temp, fluid balance, blood glucose.

Look for evidence of the underlying pathology: oedema, basal creps, ↑JVP, suprapubic or loin tenderness, palpable kidneys or uterus, rashes/arthralgia, splinter haemorrhages.

Investigations *urine* dipstick (protein, blood, nitrites, leucocytes; repeat early in morning to exclude postural proteinuria), check β-hCG, microscopy (for casts), culture, electrophoresis, spot albumin:creatinine ratio – a more practical initial investigation than a 24h collection for protein (🕮 p591); *blds* FBC, U+E, LFT, triglycerides, ESR, CRP, autoantibodies (anti-GBM, ANCA, ANA, anti-DNA), complement, cryoglobulins, serum electrophoresis; *USS* kidneys/urinary tract.

Diagnosis and management
- **Fever/exercise/transient** repeat urine dipstick normal, no treatment
- **Orthostatic** age <30yr, no protein in early morning, no treatment
- **UTI** dysuria, frequency, urine nitrites/leucocytes, culture +ve (🕮 p484)
- **Pre-eclampsia** pregnancy, ↑BP ±oedema (🕮 p504)
- **Myeloma** >60yr, bone pain, urine Bence Jones, ↑Ca²⁺ (🕮 p389)
- **Nephrotic** oedema, ↓albumin, ↑triglycerides (🕮 p376)
- **DM** tight glycaemic and BP control, ACEi (🕮 p330).

Tumour lysis syndrome

The destruction of malignant cells during chemotherapy causes release of intracellular contents which may overwhelm renal elimination and extracellular buffers; the resulting metabolic derangement, together with the precipitation of uric acid crystals within the tubules, can cause acute renal failure. Risk factors include pre-existing renal impairment with high-grade tumours, lymphoma or leukaemia. Onset is generally within 3d of chemotherapy, with oliguria, muscle cramps, tingling, weakness, tetany and seizures. Blood tests will show ↑K^+, ↑PO_4^{3-}, ↓Ca^{2+}, ↑urate, ↑urea, ↑creatinine.

Treatment involves recognition of at-risk patients and prophylactic IV hydration and allopurinol started 24–48h prior to therapy with careful monitoring of electrolytes during therapy. If the syndrome still develops, attempt hyperhydration with IV fluids, allopurinol, bicarbonate, K^+ restriction and PO_4^{3-} binding under advice from the renal team. Dialysis may be necessary to prevent worsening renal failure, refractory hyperkalaemia and ultimately arrhythmias and cardiac arrest.

Glomerular disease

Nomenclature

To overcome those palpitations that you experienced as a student, remember that the wide range of primary and secondary pathologies affecting glomeruli, all share a limited repertoire of clinical manifestations (eg nephrotic syndrome). These pathological processes also share a limited repertoire of histological features and in the absence of a definitive diagnosis, nephrologists will often refer instead to the pattern seen on biopsy (eg membranous glomerulonephritis).

Glomerulonephritis

Inflammation of the glomeruli triggered by an immunologic mechanism results in tissue damage, often with proliferation of basement membrane, mesangial cells, or capillary endothelium. Some important histological types and associated causes and clinical features are listed in Table 12.3.

Table 12.3 *Classification of glomerulonephritis*

Biopsy	Presentation	Causes	Management
Minimal change (normal by light microscopy)	Nephrotic syndrome (commonest cause in children)	?T cell mediated podocyte damage	Majority steroid responsive; very few progress to ESRF
Membranous	Heavy proteinuria ± nephrotic syndrome	Idiopathic (70%); malignancy, connective tissue disease, drugs	1/3 stabilise with immunosuppression; 1/3 remit spontaneously; 1/3 progress to ESRF
Focal segmental glomerulo-sclerosis	Proteinuria ± nephrotic syndrome; CRF	Idiopathic; secondary causes include heroin abuse and HIV	Primary disease may respond to steroids but significant progression to ESRF; secondary disease managed with ACEi
Mesangio-proliferative	Haematuria (often <72h after URTI); nephritic syndrome	Idiopathic IgA deposition	Majority self-limiting but 20–40% progress to ESRF; ACEi ± steroids

Nephrotic syndrome

Defined as >3g proteinuria/24h with hypoalbuminaemia and oedema. Hypercholesterolaemia, ↓IgG and hypercoaguability may also feature. Causes include primary glomerulonephritis as above (typically minimal change or membranous disease) but also extra-renal causes including DM, anti-GBM disease, malaria, pre-eclampsia and drugs (eg gold, penicillamine, NSAIDs). Treatment is of the underlying cause along with diuretics, active treatment of infection, ± anticoagulants.

Nephritic syndrome

Characterised by ↑BP, oliguria and haematuria. This may classically be seen around 3wk after a streptococcal throat infection as a self-resolving glomerulonephritis, but is also associated with some much more aggressive pathologies including vasculitis and anti-GBM disease.

Urological disorders

▶▶**Acute urinary retention**

Causes enlarged prostate, post-operative, pain, anticholinergics, spinal pathology/MS (painless), pregnancy, constipation, UTI.

Symptoms suprapubic pain + urge to urinate, anuria/oliguria, delirium.

Signs palpable distended bladder (dull to percussion and tender), check leg power/reflexes and tone, perianal sensation and prostate on PR.

Investigations bladder scan if unsure or simply pass a catheter.

Management urgent catheterisation (🕮 p546), record residual volume of urine (normal bladder size is 400–500ml, consider acute-on-chronic retention if >1l); urine dipstick and send for M,C+S; stool chart ± laxatives; urgent MRI spine if new lower limb neurology and diminished perianal sensation/tone (🕮 p357). Beware post-obstructive diuresis: pay close attention to fluid balance and electrolytes. Once reversible precipitants addressed, attempt a trial without catheter (TWOC) with close monitoring for recurrence of retention. If this occurs, reinsert catheter and treat as chronic retention.

Complications acute renal failure, chronic obstruction.

Chronic urinary retention

Causes obstruction (prostate), DM, MS, dysfunctional bladder.

Symptoms incontinence, dribbling, poor stream, recurrent UTI.

Signs palpable distended bladder (usually non-tender), enlarged prostate.

Investigations **blds** FBC, U+E, PSA, Ca^{2+}, PO_4^{3-}.

Management do not catheterise unless in pain or anuric (acute on chronic retention); refer to urology to investigate cause; options include TURP, intermittent self-catheterisation, anti-androgens (eg finasteride) or alpha-blockers (eg tamsulosin).

Complications chronic renal failure, recurrent UTI.

Urinary incontinence

Types of incontinence:

- **Stress** leakage on exercise/coughing/laughing
- **Urge** severe and sudden urgency (often due to detrusor instability)
- **Overflow** urine volume exceeds bladder capacity (eg chronic retention)
- **Functional** restricted mobility so unable to get to toilet in time.

Causes UTI, detrusor instability, neurological problem (eg MS, DM), diuretics + reduced mobility; ♀: uterine prolapse, weak pelvic muscles, pelvic mass; ♂: post-prostate surgery.

Ask about urgency, frequency, leakage, dysuria, poor stream, haematuria, fluid intake (including caffeine consumption late in the day), effects on lifestyle, obstetric history and previous pelvic surgery or trauma, DM, chronic cough, faecal incontinence. If acute presentation with new leg weakness suspect spinal cord compression (🕮 p357).

Look for abdo/pelvic masses, prolapse (🕮 p156); assess leakage on coughing.

Investigations **urine** MSU, glucose, urinary diary, urodynamics studies. ♂: **blds** PSA (take prior to checking prostate size and nodularity by PR).

Treatment **general** weight loss, less caffeine, stop smoking, treat prolapse; **stress incontinence** fluid restriction, pelvic floor exercises, transvaginal tape; **detrusor instability** behavioural therapy (bladder drill), tolterodine 2mg/12h PO; **overflow** see 'Chronic urinary retention'; **functional** aid mobility.

Low urine output

Worrying features low urine output <0.5ml/kg/h (Table 12.4) sustained >4h or despite adequate fluid, ↑HR, systolic BP <100mmHg, ↑K⁺, ↑creatinine, acidosis.

Remember it is easier to treat fluid overload than acute kidney injury.

Table 12.4 *Classification of low urine output*[1]

	Volume in 1h	Volume in 24h
Normal urine output	>60ml (>1ml/kg)	>1600ml
Low urine output	<30ml (<0.5ml/kg)	<800ml
Oliguria	<17ml	<400ml
Anuria	<4ml	<100ml
Absolute anuria	None	None

[1] Volumes are defined for adult patients; in paediatrics values are based upon weight.

▶▶*Do not ignore patients with very low urine output, they will be amongst the sickest in the hospital.*

Think about *severe* acute kidney injury, shock; *most likely* hypovolaemia, hypotension, urinary retention, blocked catheter, prostatic hypertrophy; *other* rhabdomyolysis, chronic renal failure, renal vascular problems (eg thrombosis, emboli), urethral trauma.

Ask about abdominal pain, hesitancy, poor stream, fluid balance (oral and IV intake, vomiting, diarrhoea, stoma output, leaking wounds, fever/sweating), breathlessness, orthopnoea, postural dizziness; *PMH* kidney disease, solitary functioning kidney, prostate disease, ↑BP, heart disease, DM; *DH* nephrotoxic drugs (eg NSAIDs, gentamicin, ACEi, IV contrast).

Obs BP, HR, RR, fluid balance, CVP if possible.

Look for volume status (📖 p380), oedema, unrecorded leakage from wounds, stomas or surgical drains; palpable bladder, suprapubic pain, loin pain, enlarged prostate, evidence of infection or haemorrhage.

Investigations *urine* colour, dipstick, M,C+S; septic screen, if not responding to fluid challenges call for senior help and send urine for osmolality (📖 p591) and Na⁺; *blds* FBC, U+E, CK, osmolality; *bladder scan* if retention or a blocked catheter is suspected; *USS renal tract* will allow full assessment for structural causes, request a Doppler USS if renal artery stenosis/embolism is suspected.

Treatment insert a urinary catheter (📖 p546) and ask the nurses to keep an hourly fluid balance including any diarrhoea, vomiting and fluid loss from wounds. Consider asking for a catheter flush if already catheterised. Assess the patient and if in doubt treat as hypovolaemia with a fluid challenge (eg 500ml 0.9% saline over 10–15min, 📖 p381) and review in 1–2h. Beware post-obstructive diuresis if in retention/blocked catheter.

If urine output is still low despite treatment then get further senior advice. If a patient is volume depleted, it may need considerable fluid volumes to improve output, but assess frequently for volume overload. Always rule out urinary tract obstruction. Indiscriminate use of IV furosemide simply to improve output may make the fluid balance chart look better, but does nothing for your patient.

Table 12.5 *Common causes for low urine output*

	History	Examination	Investigations
Hypovolaemia (📖 p379)	Low fluid input, excess losses, post-op	Negative fluid balance, ↑HR, ↓JVP, ±↓BP (postural)	↑urea, concentrated urine, ↑ urine osmolality
Septic shock (📖 p480)	Malaise, symptoms of infection, acute illness	↑HR, ↑BP, ↑RR, exclude haemorrhage	May have ↓Hb, ↑↓WCC, ↑CRP, ±↑lactate
Acute kidney injury (📖 p372)	Severe illness, untreated low urine output	May be dehydrated or shocked	New onset ↑urea and creatinine, ↑CK if rhabdomyolysis
Chronic renal failure (📖 p373)	↑BP, lethargy, anorexia, previous kidney problems, DM	Pale, anaemic, oedema, bruising, peripheral neuropathy	Persistent ↑urea and creatinine, small kidneys on USS
Urinary retention (📖 p377)	Lower abdominal pain, previous prostate problems	Palpable bladder, often anuric, enlarged prostate	Full bladder on scan, relief on catheterisation

Hypovolaemia

This is by far the most common cause of low urine output in in-patients.
Symptoms, signs, investigations see Table 12.5.
Treatment increase fluid input; the rate of rehydration depends on the patient. If urine output is >0.5ml/kg/h simply increase the rate of current IV fluids. If <0.5ml/kg/h consider a fluid challenge (📖 p381) and prescribe some quick fluids to follow, eg 0.9% saline 1l/4h; review the patient in 1–2h.
Complications acute renal failure.

Fluid overload Prescribing of fluid volumes that exceed the ability of the kidneys to excrete may lead to iatrogenic fluid overload (eg failure to identify obstructive uropathy or cardiac failure as cause of low output).
Symptoms, signs, investigations (see 📖 p380).
Treatment (see 📖 p282 'Pulmonary oedema'). For mild overload reduce or stop IV fluids and review in a few hours; ask the nurses to record hourly obs and contact you if the patient's RR rises. If you are certain of overload, ensure no evidence of obstruction before trying 40mg furosemide IV. This will cause a diuresis in most patients, but potentially contribute towards acute renal failure if the patient was hypovolaemic. In certain settings (eg sepsis + cardiogenic shock) the patient may be intravascularly volume depleted, but symptomatically fluid overloaded – this requires senior assessment for HDU/ICU and inotropic support.
Complications pulmonary oedema.

Causes of low urine output covered elsewhere

Hypotension/shock	📖 p473	Cardiac failure	📖 p267

IV fluids[1]

Assessing volume status

HR, postural hypotension and low urine output (<0.5ml/kg/h) are sensitive signs of hypovolaemia while orthopnoea suggests overload.

Table 12.6 *Assessing volume status*

	History	Examination	Investigations
Mild-moderate fluid deficit (eg <1500ml in adult)	↓urine output, headache, thirst or poor oral intake, excessive fluid loss (eg diarrhoea, vomiting)	↑HR,[1] postural BP drop,[2] urine output <0.5ml/kg/h, dry mucous membranes, capillary refill >2s, ↓JVP	Dark urine, ↑urine osmolality; *blds:* ↑urea, ↑PCV/haematocrit, ↑albumin, ↑serum osmolality
Severe hypovolaemia *(as for mild plus ...)*	Drowsy, obtunded	Oliguria/anuria, ↓BP<100mmHg, sunken eyes, decreased skin turgor	↑creatinine
Fluid overload	Cardiac history, excess fluids, SOB, orthopnoea, cough, sputum (white/frothy), swelling	↑RR, ↓O₂ sats, ↑JVP, bilateral basal crackles, pitting oedema,[3] gallop rhythm (3rd heart sound)	Pulmonary oedema on CXR (📖 p582), abnormal ECG (📖 p572 – LVH, MI), ↑CVP

[1] Including upper range of normal, ie >90/min; remains slow if taking β-blockers or other rate limiting drugs (eg verapamil, diltiazem, digoxin).
[2] A drop of >20mmHg systolic/10mmHg diastolic is significant.
[3] Ankles if sitting, sacrum if in bed.

Fluid balance is calculated by measuring a patient's urine output and fluid input along with any losses from vomit, diarrhoea, or drains. The patient must be catheterised for accurate measurement.

Insensible losses are unrecordable fluid losses, eg sweating and breathing. 500–1000ml is usually lost each day, but this increases with pyrexia (from sweating), tachypnoea and burns; this loss will not be apparent from the fluid chart. Litres of fluid can be lost from burns and wound seepage which is missed unless the bandages are inspected.

Third-space fluids Also called 'fluid sequestration'; inflammation and injury causes capillary permeability to increase so that fluid and protein leak from the blood vessels (intravascular space) causing oedema. The patient is intravascularly hypovolaemic despite normal fluid balance and fluid should be replaced according to clinical signs, especially urine output. It is common in sepsis, pancreatitis and after major operations.

CVP lines Central venous pressure measurements are used primarily in ICU and HDU since they require a central line (📖 p534). By recording the pressure in the line at the level of the right atrium, an estimate of filling state is obtained. The normal range is 1–7mmHg (1–9cmH₂O); high pressure suggests fluid overload or heart failure while a low CVP suggests hypovolaemia. Trends are more important than absolute values; the CVP should rise with a fluid challenge; hypovolaemia has been corrected once this rise persists after the challenge has finished, or when there is no further rise in CVP with subsequent fluid challenges.

[1] NICE guidelines available at ⌖guidance.nice.org.uk/CG174

▶▶Resuscitation fluids

Rapid restoration of circulating volume is vital, particularly for those with evidence of severe hypovolaemia (Table 12.6). Give high-flow O_2, establish IV access and begin emergency management (📖 p472).

Fluid challenge This implies rapid delivery of a bolus of fluid with monitoring for effects to guide further fluid management. A bolus of 500ml crystalloid eg 0.9% saline IV (250ml if frail or heart problems, 10ml/kg in children) is infused over <15min. Reassess immediately: If evidence of hypovolaemia persists, consider further 250–500ml fluid boluses. Large volumes may eventually be needed, but seek senior help and involve ICU early.

Choice of fluid in resuscitation

Choice of synthetic resuscitation fluid has historically split into a debate between the use of crystalloids (aqueous solutions of mineral salts) and colloids (containing larger, insoluble molecules). Although colloids might theoretically exert an osmotic load keeping more fluid in the circulation, this effect may be overstated and must be set against the higher cost of colloids. Recent trial data have firmly come down in favour of the use of crystalloids, with evidence of increased rates of renal failure[1] and death[2] associated with colloid resuscitation. Evidence for choice of crystalloid is less robust, and both 0.9% saline and physiological salt solutions represent reasonable choices.

Of course, blood represents a highly physiological replacement fluid when used in haemorrhage, but is rarely a practical or necessary choice in other settings. Human albumin solutions should offer the same osmotic benefits as proposed for colloids, but in ICU study data any survival advantage appears small and limited to patients with severe sepsis.[3]

[1] Myburgh, J.A. et al. *NEJM* 2012 **367**:1901 available free at ⌂www.nejm.org/doi/full/10.1056/NEJMoa1209759
[2] Perner, A. et al. *NEJM* 2012 **367**:124 available free at ⌂www.nejm.org/doi/full/10.1056/NEJMoa1204242
[3] SAFE study investigators *NEJM* 2004 **350**:2247 available free at ⌂www.nejm.org/doi/full/10.1056/NEJMoa040232

Maintenance fluids

Prescribing 'routine' fluids is a common task for foundation doctors, and one your seniors are unlikely to take much interest in until you make a mistake. When asked to prescribe fluids, always consider *why* a patient is on fluids, *what* their electrolyte needs are (look at recent blood result), and *whether* further fluids should be given (is the patient able to drink?) If in any doubt, assess the patient for RR, JVP, and basal lung crepitations.

Maintenance requirements Typically adults require 25–30ml of water/kg/24h to cover their urine output and insensible losses (sweat, respiration, stool). This equals about 2–2.5l per day for a 70–80kg adult.[1] Several additional sources of fluid losses may occur in acutely ill patients:

- *Recordable* polyuria, NG aspirate, diarrhoea, vomiting, drains
- *Insensible* wound leakage, pyrexia, tachypnoea, burns
- *Third space* (📖 p380), eg pancreatitis, post-op.

As much as possible, intake should come through the GI tract – always maximise PO intake, and consider using NG fluids as an alternative to IV where inadequate PO intake persists ≥3d. Alternatively, for an elderly patient managing insufficient volumes PO and who has no need for an IV cannula, 1l 0.9% saline SC overnight (12h) may be all that is required. Always explore with seniors which patients need to remain NBM.

[1] Paediatric fluid requirements are on 📖 p383.

Estimating fluid requirements 24h requirements can best be estimated from review of an accurate fluid balance chart. This is especially useful in patients at risk of fluid overload. Three components need to be considered:
• Recorded losses over last 24h (from fluid chart)
• Estimate of insensible losses (usually 0.5–1.5l/24h)
• Estimate of fluid deficit (from history, examination, obs and fluid chart).
Where a fluid balance chart is not available, estimate needs as:
• Estimate of maintenance requirement from weight (25–30ml/kg/24h)
• Additional fluids if significant insensible losses are expected (0.5–1.5l/24h)
• Estimate of fluid deficit (from history, examination, obs).
Beware groups of patients who may need less fluids than estimated: elderly/frail, low BMI, heart problems, renal failure, partial oral intake.
Electrolyte and glucose requirements Estimation of electrolyte requirements should take into account current U+E, medications (especially diuretics and supplements) and fluid loss. Basic maintenance requirements are:
• ***Na$^+$, K$^+$, Cl$^-$*** 1mmol/kg/24h – eg typically 60–80mmol a day
• ***Glucose*** 50–100g/24h – 5% glucose contains 5g/100ml.
Table 12.7 shows the electrolyte content of some commonly used IV fluids. Due to potential to trigger dysrhythmias, the maximal safe rate of potassium administration outside of HDU/ICU is 10mmol/h.

Table 12.7 *Electrolyte constituents of common IV fluids*

	Na$^+$ (mmol/l)	K$^+$ (mmol/l)	Cl$^-$ (mmol/l)
5% glucose	0	0/20/40	0
Glucose saline[1]	30	0/20/40	30
0.9% saline[2]	154	0/20/40	154
Hartmann's	131	5	111
Packed red cells:			
Fresh	15	0.3	150
At expiry date	10	6.0	150

[1] 0.18% saline/4% glucose.
[2] 1l 0.9% saline/24h already exceeds daily Na$^+$ requirements. Large volume saline infusions result in hyperchloraemic metabolic acidosis and potential overload of renal sodium excretion capacity.

Prescribing Having decided the 24h fluid and electrolyte requirement, convert total needs into suitable 500–1000ml bags to run at appropriate rates. If there is any deficit the initial bags should be run more quickly to correct hypovolaemia. Where safe, prescribe the fluids so that they run out during the normal working day to reduce work for those on-call; if careful review is required before further fluid prescribing, this should be indicated on the chart.
A maintenance fluid regimen suitable for an otherwise well hospitalised patient who is NBM awaiting surgery is shown in Fig. 12.1. Although this may be appropriate for an adult with a healthy heart and kidneys, indiscriminate use of this regimen could lead to fluid overload.

Date	Route	Fluid	Additives	Vol	Rate	Signature
19.8.14	IV	5% glucose	40mmol KCl	1l	10h	ALJRivett
19.8.14	IV	0.9% saline	Nil	500ml	4h	ALJRivett
19.8.14	IV	5% glucose	20mmol KCl	1l	10h	ALJRivett

Fig. 12.1 Example of a maintenance fluids regimen.

Special cases

Post-op Patients may leave surgery with hypovolaemia due to blood loss and third space loss; they may require more fluids to make up this deficit. Despite lysis of cells during surgery causing a release of K^+, most post-operative patients who remain NBM will still require supplementary KCl in their post-operative fluid replacement after 24h.

Intestinal fluid losses Most intestinal fluids have a composition similar to 0.9% saline with 20mmol/l of KCl and should be replaced with this. For the exact composition of different intestinal fluids see section 9.2 of the **BNF**.

Heart problems Patients with previous heart disease are more prone to fluid overload and pulmonary oedema. Simple attention to fluid balance prevents problems in the majority of patients. If fluid overload develops the patient may require a ↓Na^+ diet, daily weights and fluid restriction (eg 1.5l/24h). There is no logic to the routine prescribing of furosemide alongside maintenance fluids.

Chronic liver failure Excess Na^+ may cause ascites. Restrict Na^+ by using 5% glucose; 1.5l/24h fluid restriction is sometimes required. If fluid resuscitation is required use salt-poor albumin (a blood product, see *BNF* section 9.2.2.2). Recheck U+E regularly to ensure not becoming hyponatraemic.

Acute renal failure Ensure adequate and timely administration of crystalloids to correct for any hypovolaemia. Avoid additional K^+ unless hypokalaemic. Further IV fluids should be determined by fluid balance ± CVP in HDU/ICU, along with regular repeat U+E.

Chronic renal failure A reduction in glomerular filtration rate (GFR) means that the kidney cannot excrete as much water, Na^+ or K^+. In mild renal failure excess fluids and Na^+ should be avoided, though acute deterioration in renal function is usually a sign of hypovolaemia. In severe renal failure restriction of Na^+, K^+ and fluid (eg 1.5l/24h) is required.

▶▶*If in doubt* Reassess and seek senior advice. Fluid prescribing is complex, the condition of your patient will change and there is no substitute for reassessing prior to prescribing the next bag of any fluid.

Children's maintenance fluids[1]

Milk volume babies >5d require 150ml/kg milk each day.
Maintenance calculate daily fluid (oral/IV) requirements from Table 12.8.

Table 12.8 *Maintenance fluids in children*

Weight	Fluids/kg/24h	Fluids/kg/h	Expected 24h volume
first 10kg	100ml/kg/24h	4ml/kg/h	0–1000ml
10–20kg	50ml/kg/24h	2ml/kg/h	1000–1500ml
above 20kg	20ml/kg/24h	1ml/kg/h	1500–3000ml

Example 23kg child: (10 × 100ml) + (10 × 50ml) + (3 × 20ml) = 1560ml/24h.

---

[1] Children are especially prone to iatrogenic electrolyte disturbances, especially hypo- and hypernatraemia, both of which can be fatal. Therefore, fluid choice requires specialist advice; 5% glucose + 0.45% saline is safe in most situations.

Potassium emergencies

Airway	Check airway is patent; consider manoeuvres/adjuncts
Breathing	If no respiratory effort – **CALL ARREST TEAM**
Circulation	If no palpable pulse – **CALL ARREST TEAM**

▶▶Call for **senior help** early if patient deteriorating.

Hypokalaemia

(K^+<2.5mmol/l or <3mmol/l with ECG changes)
- **ECG changes:** arrhythmias, prolonged PR interval, ST depression, small/inverted T waves, U waves (after T wave)
- **15l/min O_2** if SOB or sats <94%
- **Monitor** defibrillator's ECG leads, BP, pulse oximeter
- **Venous access**, take bloods for urgent repeat U+E, Mg^{2+}
- **Replace** K^+, 40mmol/l KCl in 1l 0.9% saline IV unless oliguric
  - do not replace K^+ faster than 10mmol/h outside of HDU/ICU
  - never give KCl STAT
- **ABG** to exclude severe alkalosis
- Call for senior help
- Reassess, starting with A, B, C ...

Hyperkalaemia

(K^+ ≥7mmol/l or >5.3mmol/l with ECG changes)
- **ECG changes:** arrhythmias, flat P waves, wide QRS, tall/tented T waves
- **15l/min O_2** in all patients
- **Monitor** defibrillator's ECG leads, BP, pulse oximeter
- **Venous access**, take bloods for urgent repeat U+E
- If ECG changes seen or K^+ ≥7mmol/l (arrhythmias, 🕮 p248):
  - 10ml of 10% calcium gluconate IV over 2min, repeat every 15min up to 50ml (five doses) until K^+ corrected
  - 10 units Actrapid® in 50ml of 50% glucose over 10min
  - salbutamol 5mg nebuliser
- **ABG** to exclude severe acidosis
- Consider Calcium Resonium® 15g PO or 30g PR
- Call for senior help
- Reassess, starting with A, B, C ...

Life-threatening causes

Hyperkalaemia	Hypokalaemia
• Renal failure	• Hypovolaemia
• Acidosis	• Alkalosis
• Tissue necrosis	

Electrolyte imbalance

▶▶Hypokalaemia (K^+<3.5mmol/l)

Worrying features ↓GCS, chest pain, palpitations, abnormal ECG.

Causes vomiting, diarrhoea, most diuretics, steroids and Cushing's, inadequate replacement in fluids, alkalosis, Conn's syndrome.

Symptoms weakness, cramps, palpitations, nausea, paraesthesia.

Signs muscle weakness, hypotonia, arrhythmias.

Investigations **blds** recheck U+E looking for coexisting electrolyte imbalances, in particular ↓Mg^{2+} *ABG* if alkalosis suspected *ECG* T wave flattening or inversion, U waves, ST depression, atrial arrhythmias.

Treatment if K^+ ≥2.5mmol/l with no ECG changes add 20–40mmol KCl to IV fluids or give Sando-K® 2 tablets/8h PO and monitor U+E; consider writing up Sando-K® only for 3–5d to prevent continuous unmonitored treatment. Replace any concurrent ↓Mg^{2+} (eg 8mmol $MgSO_4$ in 100ml 0.9% saline IV over 1h). If K^+ <2.5mmol/l or ECG changes see treatment plan, 📖 p384.

▶▶Hyperkalaemia (K^+ >5.3mmol/l)

Worrying features ↓GCS, chest pain, palpitations, abnormal ECG.

Causes haemolysed samples (likely if several hours taken to reach lab), renal failure, K^+-sparing diuretics (spironolactone, amiloride), ACEi, trauma, burns, excess K^+, large blood transfusions, Addison's disease.

Symptoms palpitations, dizziness, chest pain.

Signs assess haemodynamic stability, irregular pulse, stigmata of renal failure.

Investigations **blds** urgent repeat U+E; if K^+<7mmol/l with no new ECG changes or the sample is reported as haemolysed then await the repeat sample, otherwise follow the treatment plan (📖 p384); if on digoxin, check levels since digoxin toxicity will worsen hyperkalaemia; *ABG* for acidosis if acute renal failure *ECG* initially peaked T waves, later broad QRS and flat P waves, ultimately VF.

Treatment Ca^{2+} gluconate protects the heart against ↑K^+. Salbutamol and insulin move K^+ into cells to reduce plasma levels in the short term (1–2h) after which a rebound increase may occur. Furosemide (with IV fluids if necessary) or Calcium Resonium® (takes 24h, give with lactulose 30ml/6h PO) enhance K^+ excretion. If refractory or acidotic, dialysis may be necessary (📖 p373). Stop any causative or nephrotoxic medication.

Hyponatraemia (Na$^+$ <133mmol/l)

> *Worrying features* ↓GCS, irritable, seizures, ↑HR, ↓BP.

Ask about diarrhoea, vomiting, abdo pain, tiredness, urine frequency, quantity and colour, thirst, constipation, SOB, cough, chest pain, weakness, head trauma; *PMH* heart, liver or kidney problems; *DH* diuretics, opioids, antipsychotics, amiodarone, proton pump inhibitors, SSRIs, IV fluids.

Look for assess fluid balance and volume status (🕮 p380), basal creps, oedema (legs and sacrum), ascites, focal neurology, conscious level (if Na$^+$ <120mmol/l the patient may become irritable or confused, <110mmol/l there may be seizures or coma).

Investigations *blds* FBC, U+E, LFT, CRP, plasma osmolality; *urine* send paired sample for osmolality and Na$^+$; assess underlying cause as follows:

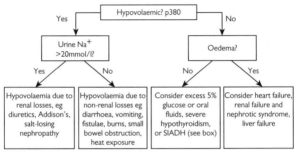

Fig. 12.2 Assessment of hyponatraemia.

Spurious ↓Na$^+$ (pseudohyponatraemia) can be caused by taking blood from an arm with IV fluids running, a lipaemic sample (labs should detect this) or osmotically active substances in the blood, eg in hyperglycaemia. Discuss with lab if unsure.

Syndrome of inappropriate ADH secretion (SIADH)

In this condition, inappropriate hypothalamic release of ADH leads to euvolaemic hyponatraemia. Beware of overcalling this diagnosis, which requires a careful workup:

- Concentrated urine despite dilute plasma (ie urine osmolality > plasma): generally plasma osmolality <275mosm/kg and urine osmolality >500mosm/kg
- No recent diuretics
- Clinical euvolaemia
- Urine sodium >20mmol/l
- Normal adrenal and thyroid function (check TSH and short Synacthen® test).

Causes include malignancy (lung, pancreas, lymphoma), lung infections, CNS infections or vascular events, drugs (eg SSRIs, tricyclics, carbamazepine, antipsychotics) or idiopathic. Management requires fluid restriction (initially 1l/24h) ± ADH antagonists (eg demeclocycline 300mg/12h PO).

Treatment Although acute hyponatraemia (<48h duration) can be rapidly corrected, chronic hyponatraemia (or where the timecourse is unclear) should be corrected slowly to prevent fluid overload or osmotic demyelination. Aim for a rise of no more than 10mmol/l/24h. Get senior help if seizures or coma (the rare situation where it may be necessary to raise Na^+ rapidly by ~5mmol/l using hypertonic saline) or if Na^+<120mmol/l. In all patients monitor fluid balance closely with catheter, regular obs and possibly CVP. Repeat U+E daily, or more frequently if neurological signs. Assess cause using Fig. 12.2 and treat accordingly.

- ***Hypovolaemic*** replace lost fluid with 0.9% saline according to degree of dehydration ($\square$ p382); severe hypovolaemia should be corrected ($\square$ p478) and takes precedence over hyponatraemia. Try to establish the cause of fluid loss and treat accordingly. Stop diuretics
- ***Normovolaemic or mild overload*** slow 0.9% saline IV eg 1l/8–10h, Na^+ levels should rise over a few days. If urine osmolality >500mOsmol/kg consider SIADH (see box)
- ***Oedematous*** urine Na^+ usually <10mmol/l, identify and treat the underlying cause (see relevant chapter).

> **Causes of hyponatraemia covered elsewhere**
>
> | Heart failure | $\square$ p267 | Renal failure | $\square$ p373 |
> |---|---|---|---|
> | Liver failure | $\square$ p313 | Nephrotic syndrome | $\square$ p376 |

Hypernatraemia (Na^+ >146mmol/l)

> *Worrying features* ↓GCS, ↑HR, ↓BP.

Causes fluid loss (diarrhoea, burns, fever, glycosuria eg DM, diabetes insipidus) or inadequate intake (impaired thirst response in elderly or hypothalamic disease); more rarely excess Na^+ (iatrogenic, Conn's syndrome).

Symptoms anorexia, nausea, weakness, hyperreflexia, confusion, ↓GCS.

Signs assess fluid balance, volume status ($\square$ p380), neurological deficit.

Investigations ***blds*** plasma osmolality (likely to be raised); ***urine*** osmolality (>400mOsmol/kg if fluid loss, <400mOsmol/kg if excess Na^+, normal range 350–1000mOsmol/kg); consider ***CT*** head or ***MRI*** if suspect central cause.

Treatment cells rapidly adapt to raised osmolality of extracellular fluid by retention and production of intracellular osmolytes. This prevents osmotic fluid losses from inside the cell, but if extracellular Na^+ concentration rapidly corrected, osmotic forces will now drive fluid into cells, causing lysis resulting in neurological damage and death. Hence aim for slow correction of Na^+ (10mmol/l/24h at the very most). Treatment is guided by volume status:

- ***Hypovolaemic*** give 0.9% saline 1l/6h (prevents sudden Na^+ shifts) until normovolaemic
- ***Normovolaemic*** encourage oral fluids or 5% glucose 1l/6h. Monitor fluid balance and plasma Na^+; consider a urinary catheter.

Hypocalcaemia (corrected Ca^{2+}<2.2mmol/l)

Although >99% calcium is stored in bones, and most of the remainder is intracellular, extracellular calcium is critical for neuromuscular and cardiac function. Albumin binds around 40% of extracellular calcium, so hypoalbuminaemia may give falsely low recordings of serum calcium; always check the 'corrected calcium'. Gut, renal, and bone calcium handling is critically regulated by vitamin D, which requires hydroxylation in functioning kidneys and liver to be active, and by PTH.

> *Worrying features* ↓GCS, chest pain, palpitations, ↓BP, abnormal ECG.

Causes vitamin D deficiency (elderly, Asians, Africans, chronic renal failure, intestinal malabsoprtion eg coeliac, Crohn's), hypoparathyroid, acute pancreatitis, alkalosis, ↓Mg^{2+}, alcoholism.

Symptoms spasm of hands and feet (carpopedal), twitching muscles, tingling around the mouth, fatigue, depression, dry skin, coarse hair.

Signs hyperreflexia, tetany, Trousseau's (spasm of hand from inflated BP cuff) and Chvostek's (unilateral twitching of face from tapping facial nerve 2cm anterior to auditory meatus), ↓BP, bradycardia, arrhythmias.

Investigations **blds** U+E, Ca^{2+}, PO_4^{3-}, Mg^{2+}, albumin, ALP, PTH, vitamin D **ECG** prolonged QT, ST abnormalities, arrhythmias.

Treatment treat arrhythmias according to 🕮 p248. If tetany is severe give 10ml 10% Ca^{2+} gluconate IV over 10min. Always assess for and correct coexistent ↓Mg^{2+}. If Ca^{2+} deficit is mild and the patient is asymptomatic, monitor. Prolonged ↓Ca^{2+} will need vitamin D replacement and Ca^{2+} supplements, eg Calcichew-D₃ Forte® one tablet/24h PO.

Complications arrhythmias, seizures, cataracts, bone fractures.

Primary hypoparathyroidism ↓PTH, despite ↓Ca^{2+}
• *Causes* iatrogenic (neck surgery, irradiation), autoimmune, metal overload
• *Investigations* ↓Ca^{2+}, ↓PTH, ↑PO_4^{3-}
• *Treatment* vitamin D, eg calciferol 1–2.5mg/24h PO.

Pseudohypoparathyroidism Genetic resistance to PTH, presents with ↓Ca^{2+} but high PTH and dysmorphic features (short stature, strabismus, short 4/5ᵗʰ metacarpals, low IQ, obesity);[1] treat as hypoparathyroid.

Rickets/osteomalacia Rickets is the childhood equivalent of osteomalacia, both characterised by vitamin D deficiency or defect in metabolism.
• *Features* ↓Ca^{2+}, ↓PO_4^{3-}, ↑ALP, decreased urine Ca^{2+}, crush fractures, spontaneous fractures (eg of ribs), rickets rosary (prominent costochondral junctions), long bone bowing and Looser's zones (pseudofractures, perpendicular to cortex, common in femoral/ humeral necks) on X-ray
• *Treatment* depends on cause, but usually simply by intake of adequate diet (egg yolk, milk, some fortified cereals); may require calciferol and Ca^{2+} supplements (eg Calcichew-D₃ Forte® one tablet/24h PO).

---

[1] Patients with the morphological appearance of pseudohypoparathyroidism but normal Ca^{2+} and PTH, are said to have *Pseudopseudohypoparathyroidism*. This is also the longest real word in the *Oxford English Dictionary*.

Hypercalcaemia (corrected Ca^{2+} >2.6mmol/l)

Worrying features ↓GCS, chest pain, palpitations, ↑HR, ↓BP, abnormal ECG.

Causes primary/tertiary hyperparathyroidism, malignancy (myeloma, bone metastases, PTH-related peptide secreting tumours), excess vitamin D supplements, sarcoidosis.
Symptoms **bones** (bone pain ±fractures), **stones** (renal), **moans** (depression), **groans** (abdo pain). Also vomiting, constipation, weakness, tiredness, thirst, polyuria, weight loss.
Signs hypertension, arrhythmias, dehydrated (shock if severe), cachexia, bony tenderness secondary to a local lesion – especially along spine.
Investigations **blds** FBC, U+E, Mg^{2+}, Ca^{2+}, PO_4^{3-}, ALP; send paired sample for PTH (may have to be on ice – discuss with lab); consider ESR, serum and urine electrophoresis; *ECG* short QT, arrhythmias; *CXR*; *bone scan*.
Treatment depends upon IV fluids to correct any volume deficit, then further fluid rehydration with coadministration of 40mg/12h PO or IV furosemide; consider catheterisation and CVP monitoring to assess fluid balance; monitor U+E, Ca^{2+}, and Mg^{2+} daily. IV bisphosphonates (eg pamidronate 30mg in 300ml 0.9% saline over 3h) are useful in refractory hypercalcaemia. Investigate and treat the cause.
Complications renal failure, arrhythmias, osteopenia, renal stones, peptic ulcers, pancreatitis.
Primary hyperparathyroidism ↑PTH from parathyroid tumour
• *Investigations* ↑PTH, ↑Ca^{2+}, ↑ALP, ↓PO_4^{3-}
• *Treatment* correct ↑Ca^{2+} then parathyroidectomy.
Secondary hyperparathyroidism ↑PTH caused by ↓Ca^{2+}; treat the underlying cause of ↓Ca^{2+} (📖 p388).
Tertiary hyperparathyroidism same presentation and treatment as primary, but caused by a parathyroid adenoma due to prolonged secondary hyperparathyroidism. Seen in end-stage renal failure.
Myeloma Plasma-cell malignancy secreting monoclonal immunoglobulins. Presentations include asymptomatic hypercalcaemia, renal failure, bleeding, infection or fracture.
• *Investigations* ↑ESR, ↑Ca^{2+}, normal ALP, often a degree of renal failure, monoclonal immunoglobulin band in urine or plasma (>30g/L, or >10% plasma cells on bone marrow biopsy else MGUS 📖 p396)
• *Treatment* correct ↑Ca^{2+} as above and with pamidronate IV; give adequate analgesia. Attempted cure requires bone marrow transplant. Lesions can be treated palliatively with radiotherapy or chemotherapy
• *Complications* infection, renal failure, haemorrhage.
Paget's disease Excess bone remodelling leads to structurally disorganised and weakened bone prone to fracture and deformity. Typically found in axial bones of elderly.
• *Features* ↑ALP, Ca^{2+} normal (but may be raised if immobile), lytic lesions and coarse trabeculations on X-ray
• *Treatment* analgesia, bisphosphonates, surgery for fractures and nerve entrapment
• *Complications* fractures, osteoarthritis, osteosarcoma (rare), cranial nerve compression (eg new deafness), high output heart failure.

Bone mets five cancers commonly metastasise to bone – these can be remembered as 'BLT with Kosher Pickle' • **B**reast • **L**ung • **T**hyroid • **K**idney • **P**rostate.

Haematology

Anaemia

Reduced red blood cell (RBC) mass, usually conveniently approximated as reduced haemoglobin concentration (eg ♂ <130g/L, ♀ <115g/L[1]). Causes easily divide into 3 basic mechanisms (reduced RBC production, increased RBC destruction, RBC loss) with clues found in abnormalities of RBC size and shape.

Worrying features Hb<80g/L, SOB, ↑HR, ↓BP, dizziness, fainting, lethargy, palpitations, chest pain, ↓GCS/restlessness.

Think about *most likely* haemorrhage, chronic blood loss (iron-deficiency anaemia), anaemia of chronic disease, renal failure **other** folate/B$_{12}$ deficiency (coeliac disease, Crohn's disease, partial gastrectomy, pernicious anaemia, elderly, alcoholism), haemoglobinopathy (📖 p397), haemolysis, alcoholic liver disease, malignancy/lymphoma/myeloma, myelofibrosis, hypothyroidism **dilutional** pregnancy, fluid resuscitation.

Ask about *any bleeding* (eg epistaxis, haematemesis, haemoptysis, haematuria, menorrhagia, melaena, PR bleeding); **evidence of hypoperfusion** dizziness, SOB (exertional/at rest), chest pain, palpitations; **clues to aetiology** weight loss, change in bowel habit, abdominal cramps, **PMH** or **FH** haemoglobinopathy; **DH** NSAIDs, trimethoprim, anticonvulsants, atypical antipsychotics; **SH** alcohol, vegetarianism, dietary fads.

Obs Resting tachycardia or postural BP drop suggest compromise.

Look for pallor (conjunctiva, nail beds, tongue), glossitis, mouth ulcers, hepatomegaly, splenomegaly, lymphadenopathy, jaundice; **CVS** bruits, signs of active bleeding, signs of heart failure; **PNS** peripheral neuropathy; **CNS** optic atrophy; **PR** melaena/blood.

Investigations *blds* FBC (with MCV – Table 13.1), blood film, iron, ferritin and TIBC, serum B$_{12}$ and folate,[2] reticulocyte count, direct antiglobulin test (see box), CRP, ESR, U+E, LFT, TFT, LDH, serum electrophoresis; **ECG** if CVS symptoms; **CXR** if suspicion of cancer and to help explain SOB; **other** urine Bence Jones protein, OGD, colonoscopy, bone marrow biopsy. See Table 13.2.

Treatment

Asymptomatic anaemia

- Look hard for a cause; exclude malignancy in patients >40yr
- Assess diet (B$_{12}$: meat, eggs, milk; folate: leafy greens, legumes; iron: meat, legumes, greens) and consider oral supplements (eg vegans).

Symptomatic anaemia or Hb <80g/L

Consider blood transfusion (📖 p398) and identify precipitating cause.

Direct antiglobulin test (Coombs test)

This test forms part of any haemolysis screen. Animal antibodies raised against human immunoglobulins cause RBC clumping in the presence of autoantibodies already bound to the RBC surface. The **indirect** antiglobulin test screens the serum of a potential transfusion recipient for antibodies against donor RBCs.

---

[1] Note since 2013 UK NHS laboratories report Hb in g/L, not g/dl.
[2] Always send *before* any transfusion, since transfusion may correct deficiencies.

Table 13.1 Mean cell volume (MCV) in different forms of anaemia

MCV <76fl	MCV 77–95fl	MCV >96fl
Iron deficiency	Pregnancy	B$_{12}$/folate deficiency
Thalassaemia	Haemorrhage	Alcohol
Haemoglobinopathies	Haemolysis	Liver disease
Sideroblastic anaemia	Renal failure	Thyroid disease
	Malignancy	Myelodysplasia
	Anaemia of chronic disease	Anti-folate drugs (eg methotrexate)
	Bone marrow failure	

Table 13.2 Laboratory findings in different forms of anaemia

	Iron	TIBC	Ferritin	MCV
Iron deficiency	↓	↑	↓	↓
Chronic disease	↓	↓	↔ or ↑	↔
Haemolysis	↑	↓	↑	↔

Abnormalities on the peripheral blood film
(OHCM9 📖 p322)

Acanthocytes	Irregularly shaped RBCs (liver disease)
Anisocytosis	RBCs of various sizes (megaloblastic anaemia/thalassaemia)
Blast cells	Nucleated precursor cells (myelofibrosis/leukaemia)
Echinocytes	Spiculated RBCs seen in renal failure
Howell–Jolly bodies	Nuclear remnants in RBCs (post-splenectomy)
Hypochromic	Pale RBCs (iron-deficiency anaemia)
Left shift	Immature white cells (infection or marrow infiltration)
Leukaemoid reaction	Reactive leucocytosis (infection/burns/haemolysis)
Poikilocytes	Variably shaped cells (iron or B$_{12}$ deficiency)
Reticulocytes	Immature RBCs (haemorrhage/haemolysis)
Right shift	Hypersegmented neutrophils (megaloblastic anaemia and liver disease)
Rouleaux	Clumping of RBCs (infection/inflammation)
Schistocytes	Fragmented RBCs (microangiopathic haemolytic anaemia)
Spherocytes	Spherical RBCs (autoimmune or hereditary)
Target cells	RBCs with central staining and outer pallor (liver disease/haemoglobinopathy)

Anaemia secondary to blood loss (📖 p478)

Symptoms chest pain, palpitations; may be history of peptic ulcer, recent surgery, trauma, epistaxis, haematemesis, melaena, or menorrhagia.

Signs ↑HR, ↓BP, postural BP drop, ↑RR, ↓GCS/restlessness, shock, pallor, sweating, cold, clammy; look at the wound site if post-op; PR: melaena. See Table 13.3.

Investigations **blds** initially may be normal; Hb, MCV, U+E (↑urea out of proportion to ↑creatinine in upper GI bleed), LFT, clotting, G+S/ X-match; once stable recheck Hb, reticulocytes; **OGD** if suspect upper GI source.

Acute treatment (📖 *p478*)
- Lay flat, elevate legs if hypotensive; give O₂
- IV access, take bloods, give rapid IV infusion (1l 0.9% saline STAT)
- If bleeding site is obvious, apply firm pressure and elevate
- Contact your senior – treat the cause (eg return to theatre if bleeding from operation site).

Table 13.3 *Acute blood loss*

▶▶**Measurement of haemoglobin does not accurately estimate the volume of blood loss in the first few hours after haemorrhage.**

Acute	Hb concentration may be normal initially, with red cells and plasma lost in equal proportions. With IV fluids or normal haemodilution a fall in Hb becomes evident
Intermediate	During IV fluid resuscitation Hb and clotting factors are diluted, unmasking loss of RBCs. Even in the absence of IV therapy the body retains salt and water in this circumstance, resulting in a natural haemodilution
Late	Homeostasis regulates the volume of fluid in the intravascular compartment and the Hb often rises as the 'clear' fluid (colloids/crystalloids) is eliminated. Without IV therapy Hb may remain low until erythropoiesis generates more RBCs

Anaemia of chronic disease (OHCM9 📖 p320)

Causes infection (eg TB, endocarditis), rheumatoid arthritis, malignancy, liver failure, most chronic diseases.

Symptoms fatigue, SOBOE, lethargy; may have very few symptoms/signs.

Investigations ↔ MCV, ↓TIBC/serum iron, ↔/↑ferritin.

Treatment treat the underlying disease; consider EPO in renal failure.

Haemolytic anaemia

Causes **acquired** autoimmune, microangiopathic,[1] mechanical heart valves, extracorporeal circuit, blood transfusion incompatibility, drugs, toxins, burns; **hereditary** haemoglobinopathy, G6PD deficiency, red cell membrane disorder (eg spherocytosis).

Signs mild jaundice, murmurs, lymphadenopathy, hepatosplenomegaly.

Investigations ↑bilirubin (unconjugated), reticulocyte count >85×10⁹/l (or >2%), ↑LDH, ↓haptoglobin, ↑urobilinogen.

Treatment depends upon the cause. Often steroids, immunosuppression ±splenectomy if autoimmune, treat precipitating cause if acquired.

[1] Microangiopathic haemolytic anaemia refers to destruction of red cells within capillaries. Schistocytes (fragmented red cells) are seen on a blood film. Causes include disseminated intravascular coagulation (DIC, 📖 p405), HELLP syndrome (📖 p505), thrombotic thrombocytopenic purpura (TTP), and haemolytic uraemic syndrome (HUS).

Iron-deficiency anaemia

Iron found in most diets containing adequate meat, legumes or greens.

Causes GI loss (gastroduodenal ulcer, oesophageal varices, IBD, malignancy), menorrhagia, poor diet, malabsorption syndromes, intestinal helminthiasis.

Symptoms abdominal pain, melaena or haematochezia, dysphagia, haemoptysis, haematemesis, diarrhoea; menorrhagia, epistaxis.

Signs pallor, koilonychia, glossitis, angular stomatitis; *PR* blood/melaena.

Investigations ***blds*** film (microcytic, hypochromic with anisocytosis and poikilocytosis), ↓serum iron, ↓ferritin, ↑TIBC; ***stool*** check for faecal occult blood; *OGD* ±*colonoscopy*; *CT* abdo if frail; *video capsule* endoscopy if suspect small bowel pathology.

Treatment iron supplements (ferrous sulphate 200mg/8h PO for 2wk, then 200mg/12h PO) – warn about side effects: change in bowel habit, black stools, nausea, epigastric pain. IV iron preparations available for those unable to tolerate or absorb oral iron. Transfuse if anaemia is severe enough to warrant (📖 p398), find and treat the cause.

> Treatment with oral iron raises the Hb by ~10g/L per week at best.

Folate/folic acid (vitamin B₉) deficiency

Folate found in spinach/green vegetables, nuts, liver, yeast. Body stores are small and depleted within weeks if dietary intake becomes inadequate.

Causes **malabsorption** alcohol, coeliac disease, Crohn's disease, tropical sprue; ↑**requirement** pregnancy, DM, lymphoma, malignancy; **drugs** anticonvulsants, trimethoprim, methotrexate.

Symptoms breathlessness, fatigue, headaches.

Signs glossitis, other features of anaemia.

Investigations ***blds*** B_{12}, folate, ↑MCV, look for malabsorption (📖 p308).

Treatment treat the cause; folic acid 5mg/24h PO for 4mth. For chronic haemolysis give long term, but exclude and treat any concurrent B_{12} deficiency as this may worsen B_{12} deficiency neuropathy.

> If planning pregnancy, folate should be taken 0.4mg/24h PO until 12/40 to reduce risk of foetal neural tube defects.

Vitamin B₁₂ deficiency

Vitamin B_{12} found in liver, kidney, fish, chicken, dairy products, eggs. Extensive total body stores and recycling from enterohepatic circulation means nutritional deficiency may take several years to manifest in the absence of other GI pathology: *suspect pathology if ↓B_{12}.*

Causes poor dietary intake, pernicious anaemia, malabsorption (as for folate deficiency), stomach/bowel resection, Crohn's disease.

Symptoms sensory neurological deficit, autoimmune disorders (eg vitiligo, infectious mononucleosis, Addison's disease), dementia.

Signs sore mouth (glossitis, angular cheilosis, mouth ulcers), neurological defects (peripheral neuropathy, optic atrophy), jaundice.

Investigations ***blds*** B_{12}, folate, ↑MCV, blood film, intrinsic factor/gastric parietal cell antibodies;[1] ↑methylmalonic acid (MMA).

Treatment dietary advice, hydroxocobalamin 1mg/72h IM for 2wk, then 1mg/3mth IM as maintenance dose.

---

[1] Gastric parietal cell antibodies sensitive (+ve in >90% with autoimmune gastritis, the end result of which is pernicious anaemia), but not specific (+ve in 5–10% of healthy individuals). Intrinsic factor antibodies are specific but less sensitive (+ve in 50–70%).

Leukaemia (OHCM9 📖 p346; see Table 13.4)

Table 13.4 *Epidemiology of common forms of leukaemia*

Type		Patient	Prognosis
Acute	Lymphoblastic (ALL)	2–4yr >60yr	Children 85% cure Elderly <20% cure
	Myeloid (AML)	Old>young, post-chemo	30% 5yr survival
Chronic	Lymphocytic (CLL)	>40yr, often male	60% 5yr survival
	Myeloid (CML)	Middle aged	90% 5yr survival

Symptoms recurrent/unusual infection, easy bruising, bleeding, joint pain, bone pain, malaise, weakness, abdo pain, weight loss, night sweats.
Signs pallor, petechiae, bruises, bleeding (check gums), lymphadenopathy, signs of infection, hepatosplenomegaly, focal neurology.
Investigations **blds** FBC (anaemia, ↑WCC, look at differential), blood film, U+E, LFT, ↑LDH, ↑urate, clotting; bone marrow **biopsy**.
Treatment **acute** antibiotics, blood and platelet transfusions; **chronic** chemoradiotherapy, bone marrow transplant or observation.
Complications infection, bleeding (DIC), hyperviscosity, cell lysis.

Lymphoma (OHCM9 📖 p354; see Table 13.5)

Table 13.5 *Basic epidemiology of lymphoma*

Type	Patient	Prognosis
Hodgkin's	Young adults or elderly, often male	60–90% 5yr survival
Non-Hodgkin's	Any age, especially the elderly	50% overall survival

Symptoms enlarged non-tender lumps, fever, night sweats, infection, itching, tiredness, weight loss, malaise, weakness, occasionally pain with alcohol.
Signs pale, lymphadenopathy, hepatosplenomegaly.
Investigations **blds** FBC, blood film, U+E, LFT, Ca^{2+}, LDH, urate; **CXR**, **CT/MRI** chest/abdo/pelvis; **biopsy** lymph node (Reed–Sternberg cell seen in Hodgkin's) and bone marrow.
Treatment chemoradiotherapy, steroids, bone marrow transplant.
Complications infection, bone marrow failure, SVC obstruction (📖 p283).

Paraproteinaemia Several diseases can cause an excess of a single (clonal) immunoglobulin including myeloma (📖 p389). Elderly patients may get a monoclonal gammopathy of undetermined significance (**MGUS**) distinguished from myeloma on the basis of paraprotein levels <30g/L, with <10% plasma cells on bone marrow biopsy and no evidence of end-organ damage. MGUS will progress to myeloma in <2% patients/year. In **Waldenström's macroglobulinameia**, ↑IgM from a lymphoplasmocytic lymphoma may lead to hyperviscosity.

Myeloproliferative disease (OHCM9 📖 p360)
Neoplastic diseases of myeloid progenitor cells with potential to transform to AML, including CML, as well as:
• Polycythaemia [rubra] vera (↑Hct; plethora, thrombosis)
• Essential thrombocytosis (↑platelets; thrombosis or bleeding)
• Myelofibrosis (marrow fibrosis; marrow failure, splenomegaly).

Pancytopenia – ↓Hb, ↓plts, and ↓WCC (OHCM9 📖 p358)
Marrow failure aplastic anaemia, malignancy, myelodysplasia, fibrosis.
Other hypersplenism, SLE, infection (eg TB, AIDS), B_{12}/folate deficiency.
Investigations **blds** FBC, blood film, B_{12}, folate; bone marrow *biopsy*.
Treatment Address underlying cause; blood and platelet transfusions.

Sickle-cell disease and trait[1] (OHCM9 📖 p334)

Point mutation in haemoglobin β-chain gene causes mutant Hb with tendency to polymerise under low oxygen tension. Resultant RBC deformities and increased endothelial adherence lead to haemolysis, vaso-occlusive crises and microinfarcts. With heterozygote frequencies as high as 30%, all patients with an African-Caribbean background must be screened by Hb electrophoresis before elective surgery.
Homozygote haemolytic anaemia, ↑reticulocytes, ↑bilirubin; history of sickle cell crises; hyposplenism.
Heterozygote (trait) normal Hb, usually healthy.
Complications vaso-occlusive crises with severe pain in long bones or acute abdomen; thromboses elsewhere may lead to splenic infarction, stroke, priapism, or myocardial and renal microinfarcts; sickle chest syndrome with chest pain, tachypnoea and pulmonary infiltrates is an emergency requiring ICU involvement; parvovirus B19 infection may lead to failure of erythropoiesis and aplastic anaemia.
Treatment supportive during crises, with opioid analgesia, vigorous IV hydration, warming, O_2 ± broad-spectrum antibiotics; exchange transfusion in severe crises; hydroxyurea may reduce frequency and severity of crises. Hyposplenism (due to splenic infarction) results in greater susceptibility to infection: penicillin prophylaxis, pneumococcal vaccination (5yrly) and meningococcal vaccination (single dose) should be offered, along with early identification and treatment of infections.

Thalassaemia[1] (OHCM9 📖 p336)

Genetic diseases of impaired production of different Hb chains with wide variety in severity and named after the defective globin chain. Common in Mediterranean, Arabian, and Asian populations. *β-thalassaemia major* (homozygote) and *α-thalassaemia* cause severe anaemia that requires transfusion (📖 p398). *β-thalassaemia minor* (heterozygote) causes a mild anaemia (>90g/L, MCV<75fl) that rarely requires treatment.
Treatment repeated transfusions with chelation therapy to combat iron overload; splenectomy reduces transfusion requirements.

Causes of lymphadenopathy

Infection local infection, EBV, CMV, hepatitis, HIV, TB, syphilis, toxoplasmosis, bartonella 'cat-scratch', fungal; **malignancy** lymphoma, leukaemia, metastases; **autoimmune** SLE, rheumatoid; **other** sarcoidosis, amyloidosis, drugs.

---

[1] For information on the NHS Sickle Cell and Thalassaemia antenatal and neonatal screening programmes, see ⊕**sct.screening.nhs.uk**

Transfusion of blood products

The understanding of blood groups and safe blood transfusion underpinned the huge advances in medicine and surgery of the 20th century. However, blood products carry risks which you must ensure do not outweigh benefits and consider alternatives before prescribing any transfusion.

When taking blood for blood bank samples it is essential to label the blood bottle at the bedside according to your hospital's transfusion protocols (usually involving **hand-labelling**) and check details against the patient's identification wristband. Errors here are disastrous, but still happen.[1]

Group and save (G+S) blood is analysed for ABO (Table 13.6) and Rh(D) grouping (see below) and for common red cell antibodies. Any further transfusion >72h after an initial transfusion will require a fresh G+S sample, since new antibodies may have formed.

Crossmatch (X-match) blood is analysed as for G+S, then fully screened for any antibodies against a compatible stored blood product.

Ordering blood products for elective use depend upon the type of surgery planned or the severity of deficit. Most hospitals issue guidance for juniors on pre-operative blood requests to prevent excess crossmatching resulting in waste. A G+S is sufficient for most procedures since a subsequent X-match can usually be done within 45min.

Ordering blood products for emergency use is a daily occurrence in most hospitals. In extreme emergencies blood can be issued without a full X-match (📖 p400), but this carries a greater risk of transfusion reactions. Ensure blood bottle and form are labelled fully and clearly, and indicate the quantity and type of blood product(s) needed as well as where they are needed. Speak to the haematology technician and arrange a porter to collect and deliver the blood products. ▶▶*If in doubt, ask.*

How many units to transfuse depends upon the clinical situation and following advice from a haematologist (where appropriate). In general, expect 1 unit to result in a Hb rise of approximately 10g/L in the absence of ongoing loss.

Checking blood products before they are given to a patient requires two people, both of whom must be familiar with local transfusion protocols;[2] this role will usually be taken by experienced nurses. Confirm and check the patient's name and DoB against their wristband and the compatibility label on the blood product. Next check the name, DoB, hospital number and blood product number, blood group and expiry date on each bag and the form; initial against each unit on the prescription once checked.

Table 13.6 *ABO blood groups*

Blood group	Serum antibodies	UK frequency	Comment
O	Anti-A, Anti-B	44%	Universal donor
A	Anti-B	45%	
B	Anti-A	8%	
AB	None	3%	Universal recipient

[1] For those who find transfusion protocols overly burdensome, the UK transfusion incident reports available at 🖰**www.shotuk.org** make sobering reading.

[2] See 🖰**transfusionguidelines.org.uk** for UK national transfusion guidelines.

Packed red cells

Indication	Symptomatic/severe anaemia or severe haemorrhage
Immunology	Needs ABO and Rh(D) compatibility between donor and recipient
Volume	220–320ml
Donor	Each unit from one donor
Shelf life	35d at 4°C; must be used within 4h once removed from fridge
Cost	~£130 per unit

Whole blood is seldom used and all blood is now leucocyte-depleted.

Platelets

Indication	Symptomatic/severe thrombocytopenia, platelet dysfunction
Immunology	Rh(D) compatibility more important than ABO, but not crucial[1]
Volume	~300ml (adult dose is 300ml; one unit, ~300 x 10^9 platelets)
Donor	Usually pooled from four donors
Shelf life	5d at room temperature – must be kept agitated
Cost	~£210 per unit

For invasive procedures (eg LP or liver biopsy) transfuse to achieve a *documented* platelet count >50 x 10^9/l. Since transfused platelets have a short half-life, which may be further reduced in pathological thrombocytopenia, time the transfusion as close to the procedure as possible.

Fresh frozen plasma (FFP)

Indication	Replacement of coagulation factor deficiency (if no safe single factor concentrate available), multiple coagulation deficiencies (associated with severe bleeding), disseminated intravascular coagulation (DIC), massive blood transfusion
Immunology	Rh(D) compatibility more important than ABO, but not crucial[1]
Volume	~250ml; adult dose is 10–15ml/kg (usually three to four units)
Donor	Each unit from one donor
Shelf life	1–2yr at –30°C; must be used within 4h once thawed
Cost	~£30 per unit (~£120 per adult dose)

Cryoprecipitate (cryo)

Indication	Contains fibrinogen, von Willebrand's factor and factors VIII, XIII; used in DIC and massive transfusion
Immunology	Rh(D) compatibility more important than ABO, but not crucial[1]
Volume	250ml (adult dose 500ml; two units)
Donor	Each (250ml) unit from five donors
Shelf life	1–2yr at –30°C; must be used within 4h once thawed
Cost	~£165 per unit (~£330 per adult dose)

>50% adults will be chronically infected with Cytomegalovirus (CMV). New CMV infection in immunocompromised individuals (eg organ or bone marrow transplant, dialysis, HIV) can be fatal, hence products from CMV –ve donors should specifically be requested for immunosuppressed patients who are known to be CMV –ve.

[1] Because of the presence of serum antibodies, compatibility is reversed for non-red cell blood products so AB becomes the universal donor and O the universal recipient. Rh(D) status is unaffected: Rh(D) –ve recipients should receive Rh(D) –ve blood products if possible.

Red cell transfusion

Indications To correct symptomatic or severe anaemia; to replace blood loss in haemorrhage. Trigger factors for transfusion are described in the 'When to transfuse' section. Generally a unit of packed cells raises the Hb by 10g/L in an adult.

Contraindications **absolute** Patient refusal (eg Jehovah's Witness); **relative** Pernicious anaemia/macrocytic anaemia, CRF/fluid overload.

Prescribing Blood should be prescribed on the fluid part of the drug chart (some hospitals may have dedicated transfusion charts). If the patient is hypovolaemic from haemorrhage then each unit of blood should be infused quickly (STAT-30min), though for more elective transfusions each unit can be administered at 3–4h. In elective transfusions it may be necessary to give furosemide 20–40mg STAT PO/IV with alternate units (starting with the second unit) to prevent fluid overload in patients with LV dysfunction. See Figs 13.1 and 13.2.

In acute haemorrhage it may be necessary to obtain blood quickly. Table 13.7 illustrates options available in this situation:

Table 13.7 *Options for crossmatching of packed red cells*

O-negative	Universal donor. Often stored in the ED, theatres or blood bank. Does not first require a specimen from patient.
Group-specific	ABO and Rh(D) status specific. Takes ~15min
Full crossmatch	ABO, Rh(D) status and antibody tested. Takes ~45min

Transfused blood must be given through a dedicated giving set with an in-line filter. A standard IV cannula of any size may be used; for rapid infusion, larger-bore cannulas, eg 16G (grey) are needed. Blood should not be left unrefrigerated for more than 4h and cannot be returned to blood bank if it has been unrefrigerated for >30min.

Monitoring of the patient should be undertaken regularly during transfusion, paying close attention to HR, BP, RR and temp. A small rise in temp and HR are common. See 🔲 p402 for transfusion reactions. Close monitoring requirements may strain nursing staffing levels and affect safety, hence only urgent transfusions should be performed out of hours.

Date	Route	Fluid	Additives	Vol	Rate	Signature
01/09/14	IV	Red cells	Nil	1 unit	4h	JFRivett
01/09/14	IV	Red cells	20mg furosemide	1 unit	4h	JFRivett

Fig. 13.1 Example of an elective transfusion.

Date	Route	Fluid	Additives	Vol	Rate	Signature
01/09/14	IV	Red cells	Nil	1 unit	STAT	HL Dixon
01/09/14	IV	Red cells	Nil	1 unit	STAT	HL Dixon
01/09/14	IV	Red cells	Nil	1 unit	30min	HL Dixon

Fig. 13.2 Example of an emergency transfusion.

When to transfuse

While consumption of blood products has remained pretty constant over the last few years, the size of the donor pool has shrunk, making blood and blood products more scarce. Up-to-date information on blood stocks in the UK can be viewed on the National Blood Service website.[1]

Why not transfuse? Besides the fact that blood products are expensive and have limited availability, they carry significant risks (see Table 13.8).

Transfusion triggers Hb values of 80g/L are often considered a trigger to thinking about transfusion. However, many patients are asymptomatic at these values and have sufficient haemoglobin to provide tissue oxygenation. In an otherwise fit patient (eg a young man who has undergone repair of an open femoral fracture), transfusion is often not required for an Hb 80g/L, though a frail arteriopath may suffer with SOB or anginal symptoms at an Hb of 90g/L and may benefit from slow transfusion of 2 units. Interestingly, more conservative transfusion strategies have proven to be safe, and possibly advantageous, in acute GI bleed[2] and ICU studies.[3]

If in doubt speak to your senior after assessing the patient for signs or symptoms relating to anaemia ±hypovolaemia (□ p380).

Always ensure the cause for the anaemia is known, or appropriate investigations including serum B_{12}/folate/iron studies have been sent. This is easy enough to forget in the heat of the moment, but measurements made post-transfusion will include a contribution from the donor and lead to missed deficiencies.

Table 13.8 *Complications of blood and blood product transfusion*

Immunological	Non-immunological
Anaphylaxis	Transmission of infection:
Urticaria	• Bacteria (staph/strep)
Alloimmunisation	• Viruses (HIV, HCV, CMV etc)
Incompatibility	• Parasites (malaria etc)
Haemolytic transfusion reactions	• Prion (vCJD)
Non-haemolytic transfusion reactions	Fluid overload/heart failure
Transfusion-associated lung injury	Iron overload (repeated transfusions)

▶▶Massive blood transfusion

Replacement of one or more circulating volumes (usually >10units) within a 24h period, or >50% circulating volume in 3h.

Consider that platelets, clotting factors and fibrinogen will have been lost/diluted and that these should also be transfused, as well as electrolytes and minerals. Speak to a haematologist who will advise appropriately.

Activate all hospitals should have a massive blood transfusion protocol, which you can activate by calling the haematology lab. They will issue blood products and advise upon administration and further testing as appropriate.

Ensure that steps are being taken to prevent further blood loss and that senior members of the team have considered a transfusion ceiling if appropriate.

[1] Available at ⏚**www.blood.co.uk**. More detailed guidelines issued by the British Committee for Standards in Haematology make interesting reading for the enthusiast, available at ⏚**www.bcshguidelines.com**

[2] Villanueva, C. *et al. NEJM* 2013 **368**:11 available free at ⏚**www.nejm.org/doi/full/10.1056/NEJMoa1211801**

[3] Hébert, P.C. *et al. NEJM* 1999 **340**:409 available free at ⏚**www.nejm.org/doi/full/10.1056/NEJM199902113400601**

Transfusion reactions
- These are potentially fatal, so must be managed urgently
- ABO incompatibility is the most serious complication; reactions are seen within minutes of starting the transfusion
- Low-grade pyrexia is common during a transfusion, though a rapid rise in temp at the start is worrying.

Signs ↑temp, ↑HR, ↓BP, cyanosis, dyspnoea, pain, rigors, urticaria, signs of heart failure.

Investigations **blds** FBC, U+E, bilirubin, LDH, blood film, direct anti-globulin test, clotting, repeat G+S (check blood group), antibody screen, blood cultures (if pyrexia persists); **urine** free haemoglobin; **CXR** if signs of heart failure.

Treatment
- As outlined in Table 13.9
- Inform senior and haematologist early
- Re-check labelling on blood products and return bags to laboratory.

Table 13.9 ▶▶*Acute transfusion reactions (OHCM9 📖 p343)*

Features	Management
≥2 of: • Temp >40°C • Chest/abdo pain • ↑HR/↓BP • Agitation • Flushing	Likely **haemolytic transfusion reaction** (ABO incompatibility – potentially life-threatening) Stop transfusion. **Call senior help**. 15l/min O₂, 1l 0.9% saline STAT (via new giving set), hydrocortisone 200mg STAT IV, chlorphenamine 10mg STAT IV. Monitor BP, urine output. Check ECG, U+E (↑K+), clotting/fibrinogen
• Temp <40°C • Shivering	Likely **non-haemolytic transfusion reaction** Slow transfusion. Give paracetamol 1g/6h PO Monitor obs (HR, BP, temp) Call senior help if no improvement or worsening
• ↑HR/↓BP • Bronchospasm • Cyanosis • Oedema	Likely **anaphylaxis** (📖 p470) Stop transfusion. **Call senior help**. 15l/min O₂, adrenaline (epinephrine) 0.5mg (1:1000) IM, 1l 0.9% saline STAT (via new giving set), hydrocortisone 200mg STAT IV, chlorphenamine 10mg STAT IV
• Urticaria • ±↑temp <40°C • ±↑itch	Likely **allergic reaction** Observe closely to exclude anaphylaxis Slow transfusion. **Inform senior**. Monitor obs (HR, BP, temp) Hydrocortisone 200mg STAT IV, chlorphenamine 10mg STAT IV
• Fluid overload	Slow transfusion. 15l/min O₂ and sit upright Consider furosemide 40mg STAT IV. Catheterise. See 📖 p282 **Call senior help** if no improvement or worsening

Following a blood transfusion

It takes ~6–12h after a transfusion for the concentration of the RBCs to settle; FBC measurement before this is likely to give an inaccurate value.

The Jehovah's Witness and blood products

Healthcare professionals must not be frightened to talk to any patient about sensitive matters if it may affect their care, and patients who are Jehovah's Witnesses are no different. You might feel uncomfortable talking to a Jehovah's Witness about what they regard as acceptable practice, but they will welcome the fact you are open and addressing an issue which is an important part of their religion. You are also likely to learn a great deal about their religion and about the person inside. Most Jehovah's Witnesses carry an advanced directive stating their requests with regards to blood products.

Acceptable treatments includes non-blood volume expanders (saline, Hartmann's, glucose, gelatins (Gelofusine®), starches (Voluven®), dextrans), agents which control haemorrhage (recombinant factor VIIa (NovoSeven®), tranexamic acid) and agents which stimulate red cell production (recombinant erythropoietin; check preparation is free from human albumin), IV iron.

Unacceptable treatments are those which involve the transfusion of donor whole blood, packed red cells, white cells, fresh frozen plasma and platelets. Pre-operative autologous (self-donated) blood is also not usually acceptable.

Treatments which individuals may consider include blood salvage (intra-operative and post-operative), haemodilution, haemodialysis and cardiac bypass (pumps must be primed with non-blood fluids). Some fractions of plasma or cellular components may be considered acceptable by some individuals (cryoprecipitate, albumin, immunoglobulins, clotting factors, and haemoglobin-based O_2 carriers). Transplants including solid organ (heart, liver) as well as bone and tissue may also be accepted.

For further information the Hospital Liaison Committee for Jehovah's Witnesses, has several centres all over the country run by Jehovah's Witnesses. Hospital switchboard will have contact details of your local representatives though there is also a 24h contact service for urgent advice for patients and Healthcare professionals (0208 906 2211); non-urgent enquiries can be sent via email to his@wtbts.org.uk.

Paediatric patients, consent and Jehovah's Witnesss[1]

Children aged 16 or 17 can consent to any treatment. Parental agreement is not legally required, although in practice discussion should involve parents. Children under the age of 16 may still consent to treatment, including transfusion, if they have sufficient maturity, understanding and intelligence to enable them to understand what is being proposed (see Gillick competence, 📖 p28).

The law on *refusal* of treatment is more complex. Children under the age of 18 have no automatic right to refuse recommended treatment; parental agreement will over-ride any such a refusal. On rare occasions, parents may refuse life-saving treatment on behalf of a minor. In an immediately life-threatening situation where further delay may cause harm, treatment such as blood products may be given in the child's best interests, but the team should always involve consultant paediatricians and hospital ethicists where practical. If the requirement is less immediate then the consultant will be able to seek further legal advice, which might involve approaching the High Court for a specific Issue Order under Section 8 of The Children's Act 1989.

[1] For an excellent review see Woolley, S. *Arch Dis Child*. 2005 **90**:715 available free online at ⏎www.ncbi.nlm.nih.gov/pmc/articles/PMC1720472

Clotting emergencies

↑PT/INR (OHAM3 📖 p582)

Most likely over-anticoagulation with warfarin (see Table 13.10), consider DIC (see 📖 p405), and acute liver failure (see 📖 p313).

For other causes of ↑PT/INR see 📖 p567.

Table 13.10 *Management of raised PT/INR*

Patient not bleeding	Patient bleeding
INR 5–8	**Medical emergency**
• Withhold warfarin until INR <5 • Identify cause of ↑INR	• Seek senior help urgently • Discuss with haematologist • Vitamin K 5mg STAT IV
INR 8–12	• Consider factors II, VII, IX and X
• Withhold warfarin until INR <5 • Vitamin K 2mg STAT PO/IV • Daily INR – consider admission • Identify cause of ↑INR	• Beriplex®/Octaplex® • or FFP 15ml/kg STAT • Withhold warfarin until INR <5 • Identify cause of ↑INR
INR >12	
• Withhold warfarin until INR <5 • Vitamin K 5mg STAT PO/IV • Admit for daily INR • Identify cause of ↑INR	

↑APTT (OHAM3 📖 p582)

Most likely over-anticoagulation with heparin (📖 p407), consider DIC (see 📖 p405).

For other causes of ↑APTT see 📖 p567.

Bleeding

▶▶Disseminated intravascular coagulation (OHAM3 📖 p596)
Pathological activation of the clotting cascade results in formation of microvascular thrombi and multiorgan failure. Consumption of fibrinogen, platelets, and clotting factors results in haemorrhagic complications.

Signs bleeding + petechiae with signs of underlying precipitant (see box)

Investigations blds ↓platelets, ↑PT/INR, ↑APTT, ↓fibrinogen, ↑↑D-dimer.

General treatment request urgent senior help and discuss with haematologist. Treat underlying cause (most commonly sepsis), supportive measures for BP, acidosis, hypoxaemia, and maintain normothermia. Blood transfusion to compensate for anaemia (may exacerbate coagulopathy).

Correction of coagulopathy give FFP (15ml/kg, ie 3–4 units) if PT or APTT >1.5 × control. Platelets, cryoprecipitate (rich in fibrinogen) or factor concentrates may be advised by haematologist.

Complications massive haemorrhage, end-organ failure, death (DIC is an independent predictor of mortality in trauma or sepsis).

Common precipitants of DIC	
• Septicaemia (Gram –ve > Gram +ve)	• Obstetric emergencies
• Disseminated malignancy	• Liver failure
• Incompatible blood transfusion reactions	• Severe trauma/burns.

Thrombocytopenia
Often an incidental finding, but patients may present with bleeding (gums, epistaxis) or easy bruising. Spontaneous bleeding tends not to occur until platelet counts <20×10⁹/l, but if surgery or an invasive procedure is planned then aim for counts >50×10⁹/l. Reduced production (eg aplastic anaemia, leukaemia), increased consumption (eg immune thrombocytopenic purpura (ITP), haemolytic-uraemic syndrome), and drug-induced (eg amiodarone, carbamazepine) forms are all recognised. Treatment includes identification and reversal of cause, with guidance by a haematologist. Avoid IM injections. Consider heparin-induced thrombocytopenia (HIT) if occurs 4–14d after commencing heparin (📖 p406).

Bleeding disorders (OHCM9 📖 p338)
Haemophilia A factor VIII deficiency; X-linked recessive, but 30% of cases have no FH due to new mutation. **Presents** with bleeding in childhood, usually haemarthrosis. **Investigations** ↑APTT and ↓factor VIII. **Treatment** avoid NSAIDs and IM injections. Seek senior help early, and ensure team speaks to haematologist on-call if patient is bleeding.

Haemophilia B (Christmas disease) factor IX deficiency; X-linked recessive. Clinically treat in the same fashion as haemophilia A.

von Willebrand disease mild but common (1/1000) autosomal dominantly inherited coagulopathy associated with deficiency of von Willebrand factor (vWF). **Presents** with mucocutaneous bleeding and menorrhagia. **Investigations** ↑APTT; PT and platelets normal; specialist specific assays. **Treatment** is not usually required. Discuss with haematologist on-call if problematic bleeding.

Anticoagulation

Anticoagulant drugs are used to prevent thrombotic events in those at risk of thrombosis or to prevent clot propagation after a thrombotic event has occurred. Recent years have seen a number of new agents become available. Generally parenteral routes are preferred in the acute setting, with oral dosing used for those who require longer term therapy.[1]

Table 13.11 *Anticoagulant treatment options*

		Uses				Notes
		VTE[1]	TP[2]	ACS	CVA[3]	
Heparin (unfractionated)	IV	✓	✓	✓	✓	Also used in arterial thrombus; risk of HIT (see box); reverse by stopping ± with protamine
Heparin (low molecular weight: LMWH)	SC	✓	✓	✓	✓	Lower risk of HIT (see box); preferred option in pregnancy; monitor anti-Factor Xa levels only in those at risk of bleeding; partial reversal with protamine
Fondaparinux	SC		✓[4]	✓		Preferred option in ACS; monitoring not required; no specific reversal agent – discuss with haematology
Warfarin	PO	✓			✓	In use since 1954; see 🛇 p407
Dabigatran	PO		✓[5]		✓[6]	Routine monitoring not required; no specific reversal agent – discuss with haematology
Apixaban	PO		✓[5]		✓[6]	
Rivaroxaban	PO		✓[5]		✓[6]	

[1] VTE: Venous thromboembolism (PE/DVT treatment and prevention of recurrence).
[2] TP: Thromboprophylaxis – see below.
[3] CVA: Prevention of stroke and systemic embolism in eg AF, mechanical heart valves.
[4] Licensed for TP in medical patients and subset of surgical patients (GI + hip/leg orthopaedics).
[5] Licensed for TP only in hip/knee orthopaedic surgical patients.
[6] Licensed in atrial fibrillation in absence of mitral valve disease or replacement and with ≥1 risk factor: eg previous CVA/TIA/PE/DVT, diabetes, CCF, HTN, age ≥75 years.

All anticoagulants should be avoided in patients with active bleeding or at high risk of bleeding. Seek specialist advice in patients with renal failure, liver failure and haemophilia.

Unfractionated heparin

This has a rapid onset of action, a short half-life (0.5–2.5h, but longer in hypothermia) and is reversible with protamine (1mg protamine over 10min IV neutralises ~100 units unfractionated heparin within 15min). This makes it the best, if cumbersome option for situations where effective but rapidly reversible anticoagulation is desired (eg patients with metallic valves awaiting surgery or at risk of bleeding). Administration is by bolus followed by a continuous infusion set at a rate determined according to 6h measurements of the APTT – check your local policy.

Heparin-induced thrombocytopenia (HIT)[1]

The development of procoagulant antibodies in those receiving heparin may lead to thrombocytopenia with thrombosis. Perform a baseline FBC and consider HIT in those with ↓plt >30% and/or new thrombosis within 4-14d of starting heparin. Discuss any suspected cases with haematology.

[1] British Committee for Standards in Haematology guidelines available free at 🖰**onlinelibrary. wiley.com/doi/10.1111/bjh.12059/full**

[1] Exceptions to this include those with active cancer and a DVT or PE, in whom longer term therapy with LMWH is more effective than warfarin.

Thromboprophylaxis[1]

In medical patients Consider if mobility significantly reduced for ≥3 days, or ongoing reduced mobility **and** 1 or more risk factors of: age >60yr,[2] active cancer, dehydration, obese, PMH or FH of DVT/PE, known thrombophilia, on COCP/HRT, significant active medical comorbidity.

In surgical/trauma patients Consider if 1 or more of above risk factors, or if 1 or more of: significantly reduced mobility, total anaesthetic time >90min, pelvic/lower limb surgery lasting >60min, significantly reduced mobility, acute inflammatory or intra-abdominal condition.

Bleeding risk Balance benefits of thromboprophylaxis against bleeding risk, including any active bleeding, acquired or inherited bleeding disorders, concurrent use of anticoagulants (eg warfarin), LP/epidural/spinal anaesthesia within the previous 4h or within the next 12h, acute stroke, thrombocytopenia, uncontrolled hypertension (≥230/120 mmHg).

Treatment In addition to good hydration and early mobilisation, where benefits outweigh bleeding risk, offer pharmacological therapy. In most instances this will be with LMWH (eg enoxaparin 40mg/24h SC or 20mg/24h if eGFR <30ml/min). Alternatives include fondaparinux (inhibits activated factor Xa), rivaroxaban or apixaban (direct activated Xa inhibitors) and dabigatran (thrombin inhibitor) – see Table 13.11. Compression stockings offer less effective prophylaxis for those in whom pharmacological therapy is contraindicated, but should be avoided in those with vascular disease or stroke.

Warfarin antagonises the vitamin K-dependent synthesis of factors II, VII, IX, and X. Warfarin slows clot formation, as measured by the INR.

Counselling advise patients of the risks and benefits of therapy and discuss the need for compliance with INR monitoring. Discuss the large number of drug interactions and the need to inform doctors of warfarin therapy before starting any new medication (see Table 13.12).

Loading should always be initiated according to local guidelines, with close monitoring of INR and dose adjustment. Warfarin may be prothrombotic over the first 36–48h, as levels of regulatory proteins C and S fall faster than clotting factors; hence, with the exception of very slow loading regimens (<5mg/day), continue LMWH for at least 72h after starting warfarin and until INR therapeutic.

Target INR will generally be in the range 2–3. In those with prosthetic heart valves, or previous thromboembolism whilst on warfarin, higher targets (range 3–4) may be required, despite increased bleeding risk.

Treatment duration is lifelong for most indications (or until risks>benefits). In DVT/PE, treatment should be reviewed at 3mth, and early cessation considered where a clear, temporary provocative factor can be identified.

Stopping warfarin for a procedure may require no additional cover (low-risk indications eg AF) or cover with heparin (LMWH or unfractionated according to local policy). Metallic mitral valves carry a much higher risk of thrombus formation than valves in the higher pressure aortic position.

Discharging patients requires suitable anticoagulation service follow-up to be in place, with current dosing documented (eg UK 'yellow book').

Over-anticoagulation with warfarin see 📖 p404

Table 13.12 *Drugs interacting with warfarin – consult Appendix 1 of BNF*

Drugs which ↑INR	Alcohol, amiodarone, cimetidine, simvastatin, NSAIDs
Drugs which ↓INR	Carbamazepine, phenytoin, rifampicin, oestrogens

[1] NICE guidelines available at 🖰 guidance.nice.org.uk/CG92
[2] Age >35yr if pregnant or up to 6 weeks post-partum.

Skin and eyes

Rash emergency

▶▶Call for **senior help** early if patient unwell or deteriorating.
- **15l/min O₂** if short of breath, O₂ sats <94% or unwell
- **Monitor** pulse oximeter, BP, defibrillator ECG leads if unwell
- Obtain a full set of **observations** including temp, BP, and RR
- Take **history** if possible/check notes/ask ward staff
- **Examine patient:** skin examination and condensed CVS, RS, abdo
- Establish likely causes and rule out **serious causes**
- Look for the findings listed in Table 14.1 which may aid diagnosis.

Table 14.1 *Features of serious causes of rash*

Finding	Life-threatening diagnoses to consider
Shock (↑HR, ↓BP)	Meningococcal septicaemia ⊞ p413
	Allergic reaction/anaphylaxis ⊞ p470
	Necrotising fasciitis ⊞ p413
Wheeze/SOB	Allergic reaction/anaphylaxis ⊞ p470
Purpura	Meningococcal septicaemia ⊞ p413
Post-operative	Necrotising fasciitis ⊞ p413
	Allergic reaction/anaphylaxis ⊞ p470
Following drug administration	Allergic reaction/anaphylaxis ⊞ p470
	Erythema multiforme major ⊞ p418
Mouth involvement	Allergic reaction/anaphylaxis ⊞ p470
	Erythema multiforme major ⊞ p418
	Meningococcal septicaemia ⊞ p413

Rash

Worrying features RR >30, sats <92%, wheeze, systolic <100mmHg, confusion, tachy/bradycardia, rapidly changing or non-blanching rash.

Think about *life-threatening* meningococcal septicaemia, necrotising fasciitis, toxic epidermal necrolysis, Stevens–Johnson syndrome, urticaria (anaphylaxis), staphylococcal scalded skin syndrome; **other acute** cellulitis, viral exanthem (eg chickenpox, measles), shingles, fungal infections, erythema nodosum, erythema multiforme, Henoch–Schönlein purpura, ecchymosis; **chronic** psoriasis, dermatitis (eg atopic, contact), vasculitis, erythema ab igne, bullous disease.

Ask about speed of onset, distribution of rash, associated symptoms, exacerbating and relieving factors, family history; **PMH** previous skin disease, joint/GI disease, immunosuppression, weight loss; **DH** allergies, vaccinations, antibiotics, previous drugs to treat skin disease; **SH** occupation, exposure to irritants, pets, exposure to others with illness/skin disease.

Obs temp, RR, BP, HR, O₂ sats.

Look at hands and nails for pitting, Janeway lesions or Osler's nodes, splinter haemorrhages, and then examine affected area and rest of skin. Try to form a description of the lesions based upon size, shape, colour, palpability, blisters and associated features (📖 p138). Also examine the scalp and mouth. Other examination as dictated by history.

Investigations **blds** if suspect infection or systemic disease; FBC, CRP, ESR, U+E; blood cultures. Further specialist investigations are listed in Table 14.2.

Table 14.2 *Investigating cutaneous infections*

Test	Use	Example
Blister fluid	Viral culture	Herpes simplex
Blood test	Autoantibodies	Systemic lupus erythematosus
	Serology	Streptococcal cellulitis
Nail clippings	Fungal culture	Onychomycosis
Patch testing	Allergy testing	Nickel allergy
Skin biopsy	Culture	Mycobacteria/fungi
	Histology	Pemphigus
	Immunohistochemistry	Cutaneous lymphoma
Skin scrapings	Fungal culture	Tinea
	Microscopy	Scabies
Skin swab	Bacterial culture	Impetigo
Wood's light	Fungal fluorescence	Scalp ringworm

Treatment depends upon cause; see following topics.

Bacterial infections causing a rash

Impetigo
Superficial epidermal infection typically seen around the faces of children.
Symptoms weeping, spreading erythema, highly contagious
Signs erythema with yellow crust and serous discharge; occasionally blisters.
Investigations **skin swabs** show *Staphylococcus aureus* in >90% of cases, but group A streptococci (*S. pyogenes*) can sometimes be found.
Treatment of localised disease can be achieved with topical fusidic acid (Fucidin®)/8h for 1wk. More extensive impetigo may require oral antibiotics, eg flucloxacillin 500mg/6h PO (for staphylococci) and phenoxymethylpenicillin 500mg/6h PO (for streptococci). Ensure close contacts are examined and treated if necessary; encourage good hand hygiene and avoidance of sharing towels.

Erysipelas
Epidermal streptococcal infection with involvement of cutaneous lymphatics; results in tense, well-demarcated erythema and lymphadenopathy; typically seen on face or legs. *Treatment* as for cellulitis.

Cellulitis
Non-necrotising infection of the dermis.
Symptoms hot, sometimes tender area of erythema, usually on leg or face; may be spreading; history of trauma to skin (insect bite, cannula site). May be systemic effects: fever, anorexia, N+V, diarrhoea.
Signs blanching warm spreading erythema (outline area with marker to observe response to treatment), ±mild oedema, break in the skin, serous discharge, lymphadenopathy in draining nodes, ↑temp, ↑HR, ↑RR.
Investigations **blds** ↑WCC and NØ, ↑CRP/ESR; blood cultures if pyrexial; D-dimer likely to be raised in infection so not useful in differentiating cellulitis from DVT; **skin swabs** not usually helpful, but check multisite **MRSA swab** results; **USS** to exclude DVT (depending on Wells' score 📖 p450) or ruptured Baker's cyst.
Treatment – check local guidelines; likely organisms include *S. aureus* (may be MRSA) or group A streptococci:
- If patient is systemically well and has no other significant comorbidities, oral antibiotics (flucloxacillin 1g/6h PO; if MRSA suspected or proven doxycycline 200mg STAT then 100mg/24h PO)
- If signs of systemic upset (↑temp, ↑HR, ↑RR) or coexisting disease (DM, IHD, PVD) admit for short-course IV antibiotics (flucloxacillin 1g/6h IV; if MRSA suspected or proven vancomycin 1g/12h IV)
- If profoundly unwell, request senior help immediately and consider ▶▶necrotising fasciitis (📖 p413)
- Painful or restricted eye movement, proptosis or visual disturbance all suggest ▶▶orbital cellulitis, an ophthalmology emergency.

Erythematous cannula sites

Cannulae should be resited every 72h to prevent local infection. If a cannula site is red and inflamed or pus is present, take a skin swab for C+S, remove cannula, and clean and dress the site. Give flucloxacillin 1g/6h PO or clarithromycin 500mg/12h PO (if penicillin allergic) for 5d.

▶▶Necrotising fasciitis (OHAM3 📖 p473)

Symptoms rapidly spreading painful erythema with features of systemic sepsis, fever, sweating, N+V, diarrhoea, anorexia, ↓GCS; may occur at break in skin or operation site but often no apparent skin trauma.

Signs rapidly spreading blanching erythema (outline area with marker to observe rate of spreading), blisters, ±oedema, lymphadenopathy in draining nodes, sometimes crepitus over tissues, ↑temp, ↑HR, ↑RR, ↓BP.

Investigations **blds** ↑WCC and NØ, ↑CRP/ESR; **blood cultures and skin swabs/tissue aspiration** may identify infective organism(s) but do not withhold treatment to do these tests if patient is systemically unwell; **X-ray** may reveal gas in subcutaneous tissues of affected area.

Treatment – ▶▶this is a surgical emergency.

- Seek senior help **immediately** (the moment you suspect, *not* once you have watched the fasciitis evolve and confirm your suspicions)
- Surgical debridement is the most important measure, **consult senior surgeon without delay**
- Likely to need a combination of IV benzylpenicillin, gentamicin, clindamycin, and metronidazole – seek urgent microbiology advice.

Pathogens may be a mixture of aerobic and anaerobic organisms seen following abdominal surgery or in diabetics (type 1), a group A streptococcus (type 2) or clostridia (type 3 – gas gangrene).

Outcome depends upon speed of identification and initiation of treatment, as well as comorbidity and the site affected. Extensive tissue loss from surgery and necrosis is common; overall mortality is ~25%.

▶▶Meningococcal septicaemia (OHCM9 📖 p832)

Symptoms include fever, joint and muscle ache, non-blanching (purpuric) rash, N+V, diarrhoea, anorexia, malaise; meningitis frequently occurs, reflected by headache, neck stiffness and photophobia.

Signs ↑temp, ↑HR, ↑RR, cap refill >2s, ↓BP, non-blanching petechial or purpuric rash; **meningism/photophobia if meningitis also present** (📖 p360).

Investigations **blds** ↑WCC and NØ, ↑CRP/ESR, meningococcal PCR, deranged clotting if severe sepsis (DIC); **blood cultures** do not withhold antibiotics before taking these if patient is systemically unwell.

Treatment – ▶▶this is a medical emergency

- **A**irway, **B**reathing (give O₂), **C**irculation (obtain IV access)
- Seek help immediately – contact your seniors as soon as you suspect
- If patient is in shock (systolic BP <100), involve ICU team urgently
- 0.9% saline 1l STAT IV and goal-directed fluid resuscitation (📖 p481)
- Ceftriaxone 4g STAT IV if septicaemia is suspected
- Inform public health consultant once patient is stable.

Pathogen Neisseria meningitides, a Gram-negative diplococcus; since the introduction of a vaccine for serogroup C, serogroup B accounts for the majority of infections seen in Europe and North America.

Outcome depends upon speed of identification and initiation of treatment. Mortality for meningococcal septicaemia is about 10% in the developed world. Complications in survivors include neurological deficits (eg cognitive impairment, deafness), limb amputation, renal failure and adrenal failure (Waterhouse–Friderichsen syndrome).

Viral infections causing a rash

Chickenpox (varicella zoster virus – VZV) (OHCM9 📖 p400)

Symptoms begin with fever and malaise 14–21d after exposure to VZV. The typical rash then develops: Flat lesions initially, evolving to itchy scabs. Older children and adults are at risk for the development of pneumonitis or encephalitis, manifesting as breathlessness or altered mental function.

Signs ↑temp, ↑HR, and presence of evolving rash; macules, papules, vesicles, pustules, scabs, in centripetal distribution (spreading out from the trunk). ↑RR and ↓O_2 sats suggest respiratory involvement. Altered personality, ↓GCS, or ataxia suggests CNS involvement.

Investigations not usually undertaken but **vesicular fluid** can be examined under electron microscopy or sent for viral **PCR**; **serology** viral antibody titres can be monitored but this is seldom necessary; **CXR** may show diffuse consolidation in varicella pneumonitis; **CT brain** to exclude other causes of neurology in presumed varicella encephalitis.

Treatment for simple cutaneous disease is symptomatic with antipyretics and topical antihistamines. Antiviral therapy is usually given to patients >16yr (aciclovir 800mg/5h PO). In the immunocompromised or those with rare complications (pneumonitis, encephalitis) use aciclovir 10mg/kg/8h IV. Consider ICU admission for respiratory support in pneumonitis.

Pregnancy Primary VZV infection during the 1st 20wk of pregnancy is associated with 1–2% risk of foetal anomalies and spontaneous abortion; infection within 5 days of delivery is also associated with a risk of neonatal VZV infection. Women without a clear history of chickenpox should have viral specific IgG titres checked and if negative, should be offered VZV vaccination before becoming pregnant. The vaccine cannot be used in pregnancy, when primary infection may require zoster immune globulin (ZIG) to prevent the onset of disease, and oral aciclovir if the disease develops – discuss with microbiology.

> **Chickenpox** very rarely occurs in the same individual twice. **Shingles** only occurs in patients who have had chickenpox previously; the virus lies dormant in the dorsal root/cranial nerve ganglia. **Non-immune individuals** can catch chickenpox from patients who have either chickenpox or shingles; the infectious period runs from 48h prior to onset of the rash until all lesions crust over.

Shingles (herpes zoster)

Symptoms initially focal pain, followed by classical blistering rash in a dermatomal distribution (will not cross the midline), ±malaise.

Signs observations often normal; erythematous papules, evolving into vesicles with pustules which crust over after ~7d. Typical occurs in a thoracic or lumbar dermatome.

Investigations not usually undertaken but **vesicular fluid** can be examined under electron microscopy or sent for viral **PCR**.

Treatment antiviral therapy limits post-herpetic neuralgia if started within 72h (aciclovir 800mg/5h PO); parenteral antivirals should be used in immunocompromised (aciclovir 10mg/kg/8h IV). Treat pain with simple analgesia (paracetamol, NSAIDs) and amitriptyline 25mg/24h PO.

- **Herpes zoster ophthalmicus**: Involvement of the ophthalmic branch of the trigeminal nerve (CN Va); may lead to sight threatening keratitis; apply 3% aciclovir ointment to eye/5h and **seek ophthalmic opinion**
- **Ramsay–Hunt syndrome** (OHCM9 📖 p505): facial pain, vesicles in external auditory canal and ipsilateral facial palsy; complete recovery in <50%.

Measles (Rubeola)

Symptoms prodrome of fever, coryza and cough; rash spreading from face and neck to trunk and limbs.

Signs ↑temp, ↑HR, conjunctivitis, pathognomonic grey 'Koplik' spots on buccal mucosa seen ~2d prior to appearance of maculopapular rash.

Investigations none required routinely; respiratory swab **PCR** in critically ill.

Treatment supportive care; vitamin A supplements if malnourished; complications include pneumonitis, pneumonia, encephalitis; subacute sclerosing panencephalitis is a degenerative CNS disease appearing ~10yr after infection.

Rubella (German measles)

Symptoms rash with fever and coryza; adults may experience arthralgia.

Signs discrete macular rash spreading from face to trunk and limbs; features of concurrent illness/infection (↑temp, ↑HR, etc); tender lymphadenopathy.

Investigations none routine; *blds* ↑viral specific IgM during infection.

Treatment supportive care; primary infection during 1st trimester of pregnancy carries ~90% foetal anomalies (eg deafness, cataracts).

Viral exanthema (the viral rash)

Symptoms rash associated with prodromal symptoms of viral illness (fever, myalgia, arthralgia, headache); may or may not be itchy.

Signs widespread maculopapular rash; features of concurrent illness/infection (↑temp, ↑HR, pharyngitis, etc). Rash associated with numerous viruses (echovirus, parvovirus, EBV, measles) so not diagnostic.

Investigations none required routinely; discuss with virology if unwell.

Treatment simple analgesia and topical antihistamines; resolves over ~7d.

Fifth disease ('slapped cheek' fever)

Symptoms non-itchy rash on cheeks, which feel burning hot; later spreads to trunk and limbs; headache; otherwise well; usually in children.

Signs dense erythematous rash on cheeks, and reticulate erythema (net-like rash) on proximal limbs; caused by parvovirus B19.

Investigations none required routinely.

Treatment rash will subside over 7–10d; treat concurrent symptoms.

Herpes simplex virus (cold sore/genital herpes)

Symptoms small painful blisters usually around mouth or in genital area.

Signs vesicles or pustules around mouth (usually HSV1) or in genital area (usually HSV2). Often resolve, but then return months or years later.

Investigations not usually undertaken but **vesicular fluid** can be examined under electron microscopy or sent for viral **PCR**.

Treatment consists of aciclovir 200mg/5h PO for primary HSV infections and painful genital infections. Treat facial and genital 'cold sores' with aciclovir 5% to affected area/4h topically.

Molluscum contagiosum (water blisters)

Symptoms small, non-itchy spots, occurring on trunk and limbs in childhood (skin contact) and around groin in early adulthood (sexual transmission); highly contagious.

Signs small translucent vesicles (1–3mm), which look fluid-filled, but are actually solid, often with the central depression (punctum). Caused by a poxvirus, and usually resolve spontaneously after 6–12mth.

Investigations none routine; screen for other STDs in adults (📖 p465).

Treatment cryotherapy can be used in older children and adults.

Fungal infections causing a rash

Dermatophytes are pathogenic fungi capable of causing a range of diseases.

Tinea corporis ('ringworm'): mildly itchy, asymmetrical rash which spreads with a slightly raised, scaly edge, often leaving a clear centre.

Tinea faciei superficial, itchy infection of face.

Tinea cruris is essentially ringworm in the groin, though this lesion is often red and more plaque-like with a well demarked border.

Tinea pedis also known as 'athlete's foot', is usually found in the webspaces of the toes, resulting in itchy skin which is fissured and macerated. If found elsewhere on the foot it is often more diffuse and scaly, but just as itchy. Pustules are not uncommon in more aggressive disease.

Treatment of small focal areas of tinea can be achieved with topical antifungal creams (terbinafine, clotrimazole, miconazole, etc); more widespread infections require oral therapy (terbinafine, itraconazole).

Candida albicans

Candida is a yeast, and thrives in warm moist areas, in children's nappies (nappy rash), in body folds (intertrigo), and also in interdigital webspaces, mimicking tinea pedis. The rash is erythematous with a ragged, peeling edge which may contains small pustules. The mouth and genital tract can also be affected and present with small white plaques/white discharge.

Treatment consists of removing predisposing factors (ensure skin remains clean and dry) and topical antifungal creams (as for tinea); use drops (eg nystatin) or pessaries (eg clotrimazole) for oral and genital tract infections respectively; resistant infections may require oral therapy (eg fluconazole).

Infestations causing a rash

Scabies is an intensely itchy rash, often worse at night, caused by the scabies mite, *Sarcoptes scabiei*. Commoner in children and with social overcrowding. The rash is papular and usually in the interdigital webspaces of the hands and feet, around the ankles, wrists, axillae and umbilicus. Linear skin burrows are pathognomonic but not always present. The diagnosis can be confirmed by microscopic examination of skin scrapings, looking for mites or their eggs. Highly contagious.

Treatment with a scabicide (malathion or permethrin) is only successful if the whole body is treated, if all close contacts are treated and if bedding and clothing are washed. Itching may last up to 4wk after treatment.

Lice are blood-sucking parasites. **Head lice** (Pediculosis capitis) are commonest in children, spread by direct contact and can result in scalp excoriation. The presence of eggs ('nits') in the hair confirms the diagnosis. **Body lice** (Pediculosis corporis) are associated with poverty and not often seen in the developed world; excoriations on the skin are often the only sign. **Pubic lice** (Phthiriasis pubis or 'crabs') are transmitted by sexual contact and largely affect the coarse hairs of the pubic region, but can infest leg and body hair, as well as eyelashes and eyebrows.

Treatment is with malathion or permethrin, but resistance is common and close contacts should also be treated; clothing and bedding should be thoroughly washed.

Chronic inflammatory rashes (OHCS8 📖 p596)

Dermatitis (eczema)[1] found in ~10% of the population in various forms:
- **Atopic** onset usually in childhood; associated with asthma and allergies
- **Contact** inflammatory response to skin irritant; may blister
- **Venous stasis** seen in lower limbs of older patients; hyperpigmented
- **Seborrhoeic** itchy scaling of scalp associated with reaction to skin fungi.

Symptoms include itchy, dry skin, or patches of infected skin.

Signs erythematous patches with excoriations from itching; in atopic eczema these typically affect the flexures of the elbow, knees and around the neck; vesicles and serous weeping may be a feature. Superimposed bacterial or viral infections are common. Affected skin may develop chronic lichenification and hyperpigmentation.

Treatment is multifactorial and depends on underlying cause. Attempt identification and avoidance of known irritants. In atopic eczema, triple therapy with topical steroids (📖 p178), topical emollients and bath oil and soap substitutes form the mainstay; step 4 treatments such as UVB/PUVA, ciclosporin and azathioprine may be prescribed by a dermatologist (Fig. 14.1). Treat bacterial superinfection promptly eg flucloxacillin 500mg/6h PO.

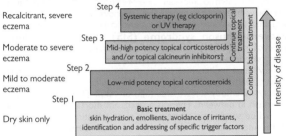

Fig. 14.1 Step-wise management of atopic eczema. † Calcineurin inhibitors include pimecrolimus (Elidel®) and tacrolimus (Protopic®).

Psoriasis[2] inflammation of the dermis, with epidermal hyperproliferation. Occurs in ~2% of the population, with peak incidences in the early 20s then again in the 50s. Exacerbations can be precipitated by infections, drugs (eg lithium, β-blockers), UV light, alcohol and stress.

Symptoms itchy, dry patches of skin which can bleed when scratched.

Signs of **chronic plaque psoriasis** are pink/red scaly plaques, especially on the extensor surfaces of elbows and knees, lower back and scalp; nail pitting is common; **pustular psoriasis** affects palms and soles; **guttate psoriasis** occurs suddenly, often 2–3wk after a streptococcal throat infection, causing numerous small pink papules on the trunk; **flexural psoriasis** tends to occur in later life, and forms in the groins, natal cleft and submammary area

Treatment is symptom-led and largely topical; emollients, mild to moderate topical steroids, vitamin D analogues, retinoids and purified coal tar are common topical treatments. Use of UVB/PUVA, anti-TNF therapy, methotrexate and ciclosporin may be considered by a dermatologist.

---

[1] NICE childhood eczema guidelines available at ⌁guidance.nice.org.uk/CG57
[2] NICE psoriasis guidelines available at ⌁guidance.nice.org.uk/CG153

Other causes of rash

Urticaria also known as 'hives' or 'nettle rash' is characterised by the formation of intensely pruritic papules or plaques ('weal') which are pale initially but become erythematous with a surrounding rim of pale skin or erythema ('flare'). Common in response to certain topical chemicals (eg nettle sting) but also in response to systemic drugs (sometimes part of anaphylaxis) or antigens (during a blood transfusion). Can also occur as part of the rare hereditary angioedema syndrome, due to deficiency in plasma C1 esterase inhibitor (OHCS8 ☐ p603).

Erythema nodosum is characterised by tender, erythematous nodules, typically on the shins. Commoner associations include: infections (tuberculosis, streptococcal, *Mycoplasma pneumoniae* and EBV), sarcoidosis, inflammatory bowel disease, autoimmune disorders, pregnancy and drugs (sulfonamides and the oral contraceptive pill) (OHCS8 ☐ p588).

Erythema multiforme is a hypersensitivity rash and has two subtypes. *Erythema multiforme minor* produces 'target' lesions, with a red centre, a clear circular area, and an outer red ring. *Erythema multiforme major* is a similar rash with involvement of one or more mucous membranes (classically the mouth). Often no precipitant is identified (~50%) but associations are recognised with several infections (eg HSV, adenovirus, *Mycoplasma pneumonia*) and drugs (eg sulfonamides, NSAIDs, penicillins) (OHCS8 ☐ p588).

Stevens-Johnson syndrome (SJS) and toxic epidermal necrolysis (TEN) represent different extents of severe, life-threatening skin inflammation (considered by some to be an extreme form of erythema multiforme) that is usually drug induced. Widespread blisters, with sloughing, erythematous macules and mucosal erosions affect <10% body surface area (SJS) or >30% (TEN) with an overlap diagnosis in between. There is a significant mortality and senior help should be sought immediately, with close attention to skin care, fluid replacement and prevention of superinfection (OHCS8 ☐ p609).

Pemphigus and pemphigoid are rare primary blistering diseases. Pemphigus causes superficial blisters and often involves the mucous membranes of the mouth; the blisters are delicate and burst easily, so areas of raw skin are often more noticeable than blisters. Pemphigoid causes tense blisters in older patients, and seldom affects the mouth. Both forms are autoimmune and require dermatology assessment (OHCS8 ☐ p602).

Pyoderma gangrenosum presents with nodules or pustules which often ulcerate, leaving a blackened ulcer with a purulent surface. Associated with inflammatory bowel disease, primary biliary cirrhosis, and rheumatoid arthritis amongst others, the exact cause remains unclear. Needs urgent dermatology assessment (OHCS8 ☐ p588).

Henoch–Schönlein purpura is self-limiting small vessel vasculitis typically seen following a simple upper respiratory tract infection in childhood. Petechiae and purpura develop on the legs and buttocks and may be associated with abdominal pain, arthralgia and oedema (OHCS8 ☐ p197).

Granuloma annulare is a common, benign inflammatory disorder of unclear aetiology, characterised by clusters of papules appearing on the hands, feet or trunk which later merge into a ring. Associations include T1DM, but most cases appear in otherwise healthy individuals (OHCS8 ☐ p586).

Table 14.3 *Common skin manifestations in systemic disease*

Diabetes mellitus (📖 p328)	Candidiasis, necrobiosis lipoidica (non-itchy yellow maculopapular lesions on the shins), folliculitis (infected hair follicles), skin infections
Coeliac disease (📖 p308)	Dermatitis herpetiformis (itchy papules and vesicles on knees, elbows, back and buttocks)
IBD (📖 p309)	Erythema nodosum, pyoderma gangrenosum
Rheumatoid arthritis (📖 p454)	Rheumatoid nodules (firm nodules either loose or attached to deep structures over extensor surfaces, classically the elbows), vasculitis, pyoderma gangrenosum
SLE (📖 p457)	Facial butterfly rash, photosensitivity, red scaly rashes, diffuse alopecia (hair loss)
Hyperthyroidism (📖 p326)	Pre-tibial myxoedema (non-pitting plaques and nodules, classically on the shins), clubbing, alopecia
Hypothyroidism (📖 p334)	Sparse coarse hair, dry skin, asteatotic eczema (pruritic, dry, cracked skin)
Neoplasia	Acanthosis nigricans (velvety, brown pigmented plaques, often around the neck), dermatomyositis, ichthyosis (scaly skin), pruritus
Drug eruptions (OHCS8 📖 p609)	Maculopapular rash (±fever and eosinophilia); urticaria; erythema multiforme, Stevens-Johnson syndrome
Vasculitis	Palpable purpuric rash typically on shins; wide range of other pathologies including telangiectasia, urticaria, ulcers (see 📖 p593 for autoantibodies in diagnosis)
HIV (📖 p490)	Infections (oropharyngeal candida, facial/genital molluscum contagiosum, herpes simplex, varicella zoster – 📖 p414); seborrhoeic dermatitis or psoriasis (📖 p417); Kaposi sarcoma (enlarging purple patches or plaques seen on feet, arms, legs or oral mucosa)

Skin lumps

Worrying features weight loss, night sweats, hard irregular lump, ↑size.

Think about *serious* skin cancer, sarcoma, lymphoma, TB; ***common*** lipoma, sebaceous cyst, abscess, boil, carbuncle, ganglion, fibroma, lymph node, naevi, skin tags, keratocanthoma, keloid scarring.

Ask about location, speed and duration of onset, change with time, pain, other lumps, trauma, bites, infections, skin changes, systemic symptoms (eg weight loss, vomiting, fever); ***PMH*** previous lumps, cancer, radiotherapy; ***SH*** foreign travel, sun exposure, occupation; ***FH*** skin cancer.

Look for site, size, shape, consistency (hard, firm, soft, fluctuant), tenderness, temperature, surface, association with skin (moves with skin – intradermal, skin moves over it – subcutaneous), overlying skin (colour, punctum, ulcerated), edges, mobility/tethering, pulsatility, transillumination, relationship to nearby structures, lymphadenopathy, splenomegaly.

Investigations *blds* consider FBC, U+E, LFT, CRP, ESR; *imaging* CXR, USS, CT/MRI; *biopsy* FNA, punch biopsy, excision biopsy.

Lipoma
Common, benign tumour of mature fat cells.
Symptoms single or multiple, non-painful, can cause pressure effects, common on the trunk and neck, never found on palms/soles of feet.
Signs smooth, well-defined, soft, subcutaneous, mobile, no skin changes.
Management can be surgically excised if causing distress.

Epidermoid cyst (sebaceous cyst)
Proliferation of epidermal cells within dermis.
Symptoms single or multiple, painful if infected, common on the trunk, neck and face, almost never found on palms/soles of feet.
Signs firm, well-defined, intradermal, mobile; overlying punctum is common; may discharge white/cheesy material; can become inflamed.
Management consider flucloxacillin 500mg/6h PO if inflamed/tender, may also require incision and drainage; surgical excision once non-inflamed.

Ganglion cyst
Cystic lesion of joint or synovial sheath of tendon.
Symptoms single, non-painful; 80% occur at wrist.
Signs smooth, well-defined, subcutaneous, transilluminable.
Management conservative; can be aspirated or excised, but ~40% recur.

Fibroma
Benign tumour of connective tissue; can occur in any organ.
Symptoms and signs vary according to tissue affected, usually slow growing with no overlying skin changes.
Management biopsy/imaging if any doubt; excision often possible.

Sarcoma
Rare, but devastating malignant tumour of connective tissue.
Symptoms single, painful, progressive enlargement, weight loss.
Signs firm/hard, tethered, regional lymphadenopathy.
Management combination of surgery, radiotherapy and chemotherapy.

Melanocytic naevi (moles)

Benign proliferation of melanocytes.

Worrying signs ↑size, change in pigmentation, irregular outline, bleeding, itching, inflammation (may suggest transformation to melanoma, 📖 p422).

Symptoms and signs most common are acquired naevi that develop during childhood as small, flat pigmented areas and may progress to pale, raised, fleshy naevi with age; congenital melanocytic naevi are larger, present from birth and carry a higher risk of transformation to melanoma.

Management refer to specialist if worrying signs are present.

Lymphadenopathy

Worrying signs non-tender, >3wk, >1cm, hard, irregular surface, tethering, weight loss, night sweats, fatigue, absence of infection.

Causes **isolated** local/regional infection; **multiple** see 📖 p397.

Symptoms lump usually in the neck, axilla or groin.

Signs firm, subcutaneous; usually mobile, well-defined, smooth surface.

Management enlarged lymph nodes can often be treated by 'watchful waiting' however, biopsy or image if worrying signs are present.

Abscess

Accumulation of pus within cavity due to infection or foreign body.

Symptoms typically single, painful, onset over days, may be febrile/unwell.

Signs fluctuant, well-defined, under the skin; tender, inflamed (red, hot); may spontaneously discharge; common on neck, axilla, groin, perineum.

Management incision and drainage ±antibiotics eg flucloxacillin 1g/6h PO.

Boil (furuncle)

Abscess forming in inflamed hair follicle, typically with *S. aureus* infection.

Symptoms single, painful, common on neck, axilla, groin, perineum.

Signs red, tender, hot, central punctum, may discharge pus.

Management often discharges spontaneously, otherwise treat as abscess; multiple furuncles may coalesce into a *carbuncle* which requires drainage and extended antibiotic therapy.

Warts

Benign proliferation of epidermis associated with infection with human papillomavirus (HPV); can occur in various sites.

Common warts are papular lesions with a rough surface with black dots within them, often on the hands and feet. Spread is by direct contact.

Plantar warts (veruccas) are usually flat or inward growing with black dots ('heads'). Often painful if over pressure areas.

Plane warts are small, flesh-coloured, flat-topped lesions usually on the face or backs of the hands without black dots.

Anogenital warts are transmitted sexually and associated with different HPV subtypes from non-genital warts; subtypes 16 and 18 are strongly associated with cervical carcinoma, so ensure recent cervical smear in any ♀ with genital warts (or in ♀ partner, of any affected individual).

Treating warts is often difficult. Topical keratolytic agents (such as salicylic acid or trichloracetic acid) is usually first-line treatment, and cryotherapy (freezing) is undertaken by many general practitioners as well as in dermatology clinics. Non-genital warts often resolve spontaneously over ~2–3yr.

Actinic keratosis

Scaly lesions seen on sun-exposed skin of fair skinned individuals. Can progress to skin cancer; can be surgically removed or topically treated.

Skin cancers

Basal-cell carcinoma (BCC)

Commonest form of skin cancer, accounting for ~75% of diagnoses.
Risk factors exposure to UV light (sunlight and sunbeds), PMH or FH of BCC, exposure to arsenic.
Appearance slow growing sore on sun-exposed skin; most are **nodular** (waxy appearance, rolled pearly edges and central ulceration—'rodent ulcer' typically found on face); other variants include **superficial** (flat, red, scaly patches – found on trunk) and **pigmented**.
Investigation biopsy and histology if large, followed by surgical excision; usually fully excised initially if small and sent for histological analysis.
Treatment excision (including Mohs' surgery), topical chemotherapy, radiotherapy, cryosurgery.
Prognosis BCC rarely metastasise but can cause local tissue destruction (eg ear, lip) and very infrequently cause death.

> *Mohs' surgery* involves surgical removal of the obvious tumour and a thin layer of tissue from the site. This layer is frozen and stained then examined under a microscope. If there are tumour cells present, a further (deeper) layer of tissue is removed, and the process is repeated until the layer is tumour-free. This procedure minimises the need for large skin excisions and gives the best cosmetic outcome.

Squamous-cell carcinomas (SCC)

These account for approximately 20% of cutaneous malignancies.
Risk factors exposure to UV light (sunlight and sunbeds) or to industrial carcinogens (eg arsenic, tar), chronic ulcer inflammation, immunosuppression, premalignant conditions (eg Bowen's disease, actinic keratosis).
Appearance variable; typically fleshy plaque or papule arising on sun-exposed skin (~70% on head and neck), often with bleeding, scaling or ulceration; other forms include **Marjolin ulcer** (new area of induration at edge of leg ulcer); **keratoacanthoma** is a rapidly growing nodule with central ulceration that usually spontaneously regresses and is considered by most as a variant of SCC.
Investigation usually none, may be biopsied.
Treatment surgical excision or radiotherapy; topical chemotherapy, photodynamic therapy and immunomodulators used if unsuitable for surgery.
Prognosis if localised disease, excision gives 95% cure rate but SCC can metastasise rapidly via local lymph nodes with poor outcome.

Malignant melanoma

Accounts for ~4% of all skin cancers, but majority of skin cancer deaths.
Risk factors pale-skin, sun exposure, sunburn, multiple/congenital naevi.
Symptoms/signs A new, or changing mole, as assessed by ABCDE criteria:[1] **A**symmetry, **B**order irregularity, **C**olour variation, **D**iameter increasing or >6mm, **E**volving over time.
Management surgical excision, ±lymph node removal, ±chemotherapy.
Prognosis depends upon completeness of excision, lymph node involvement, presence of ulceration and tumour thickness; these are combined to give a stage (stage I: 5yr survival 85-99%; stage IV: 10%).

1 Abbasi, N.R. et al. *JAMA* 2004 **292**:2771 available free at jama.ama-assn.org

Breast lumps

> *Worrying features* >50yr, fixed, hard, enlarging lesion with skin tethering, breast eczema, new nipple inversion or bloody nipple discharge; **PMH** or **FH** breast cancer.

Think about *serious* breast cancer; **common** fibroadenoma, fibroadenosis, abscess, isolated cyst, seroma, trauma (fat necrosis).
Ask about onset, duration, change with menstrual cycle, pain, trauma, skin changes, nipple changes, nipple discharge; **PMH** previous lumps, breast cancer, breastfeeding, pregnancy; **DH** OCP, HRT; **FH** breast cancer.
Look for see ⬜ p141 for breast examination
Management breast lumps require a triple assessment of **clinical examination**, **imaging** (mammography ±USS) and **histology** (FNA or core biopsy); these should be offered via a '1-stop' breast clinic.

Fibroadenoma
Symptoms and signs young women (<40yr) with highly mobile, non-tender, well-defined, and small lump (breast mouse), otherwise well.
Management refer to breast surgeon; usually not excised unless >40yr, suspicious USS appearance or >4cm.

Fibroadenosis (fibrocystic change)
Symptoms and signs 35–50yr, single or multiple, painful and tender lumps, size and pain vary with menstrual cycle.
Management refer to breast surgeon; often assessed with USS and aspiration, but may require mammography and excision.

Abscess
Risk factors breastfeeding, DM, smoking, steroids, trauma.
Symptoms and signs single, red, hot, tender lump, fluctuant, may discharge pus from the nipple, fever.
Management refer to surgeon for incision and drainage with antibiotics.

Breast seromas
Collections of serous fluid; common after breast surgery.
Symptoms and signs may discharge fluid, non-tender, fluctuant.
Management refer to surgeon for percutaneous drainage.

Breast cancer[1]
Most common non-skin cancer in UK; women aged 50–70yr are offered 3yrly screening mammography; overall 5yr survival is 80%.
Risk factors age, family history, oestrogen exposure (early menarche, late menopause, nulliparity, obesity), previous breast cancer.
Symptoms finding on screening (mammography), breast lump, nipple inversion or bloody discharge, skin changes, weight loss, bone pain.
Signs palpable, non-tender mass (often hard, poorly defined), skin dimpling, peau d'orange (prominent pores), nipple eczema (Paget's), lymphadenopathy.
Investigations **mammography ±USS** (for women <35yr with dense breasts); **biopsy/FNA** for histological evidence of cancer; **staging** may require LFT, Ca^{2+}, USS liver ±axilla, CT, bone scan.
Treatment varies with tumour stage, tumour markers, grade and the patient's wishes. Options will include combinations of surgery, chemotherapy, radiotherapy, hormonal modulation, and monoclonal antibodies.
Complications metastases (bones, lung, liver, brain), recurrence, lymphoedema, seroma, cosmetic appearance, psychological.

[1] NICE guidelines available at ⊸guidance.nice.org.uk/CG80 and ⊸guidance.nice.org.uk/CG81

Leg ulcers

Loss of epithelial integrity with failure to heal.

Think about venous insufficiency, peripheral vascular disease, neuropathic (eg DM), pressure ulcers, trauma, infection, pyoderma gangrenosum (📖 p418), vasculitides, skin cancer, steroids.

Ask about onset, duration, pain, trauma, claudication; **PMH** peripheral vascular disease, ↑BP, CVA, MI, angina, varicose veins, DVT, DM; **DH** steroids; **SH** smoking, alcohol.

Look for number, site, size, base, edge, depth, shape, colour, oedema, eczema, vascular disease (peripheral pulses, hair loss, cold), neuropathy (sensation), infection (discharge, lymphadenopathy).

Investigations **blds** FBC, CRP, fasting glucose (if not known DM; HbA$_{1c}$ if known DM); consider ESR, complement, RhF, ANA, ANCA; **ankle brachial pressure index** (ABPI, 📖 p448) ±duplex **USS** or **CT angiogram** if ABPI abnormal; **wound swab** (±X-ray if osteomyelitis suspected); **biopsy** atypical areas.

Table 14.4 *Clinical assessment of leg ulcers*

	Venous (~80%)	Arterial (~10%)	Neuropathic (~10%)
History	Obesity, immobility, varicose veins, DVT	Intermittent claudication, HTN, DM, IHD, smoker	Numbness, DM, family history
Leg	Pigmented, varicose veins, swollen, hot	Shiny, hairless, cold	Joint destruction
Site	Medial aspect of legs	Lateral malleolus, toes, dorsum of foot	Heel, metatarsal head, pressure points
Size	Can be very large	Usually small	Usually small
Base	Usually superficial with sloughy exudate	Deep with a dark, dry base, few signs of healing	Can be very deep (extend to bone)
Edge	Irregular, areas of repeated healing and exacerbation	Well defined, often circular	Surrounded by thickened skin
Sensation	Painful	Painful	Relatively painless

Management Ensure good nutrition and treat the cause, where possible. Healing often takes weeks to months and is commonly managed by community nurses, with ulcer clinic visits where appropriate:

- **Venous** provided ABPI is >0.8 apply compression bandaging (eg 4-layer 'Charing Cross') with absorbable dressings to dry out the slough. Emollients and steroid creams also help; may need debridement/grafting
- **Arterial** avoid compression bandages; address vascular risk factors and refer to a vascular surgeon for consideration for bypass or angioplasty
- **Neuropathic** careful footcare to avoid repeated injury, often needs surgical debridement and antibiotics; osteomyelitis is common; assess for and treat coexistent vascular disease; specialist diabetic foot team if DM
- **Infection** ulcers usually have bacteria present; infection or cellulitis should be suspected if there is pus, excessive pain, surrounding erythema or pyrexia. Swab the ulcer and treat as for cellulitis (📖 p412).

No improvement consider other diagnoses (including TB and cancer) or dermatitis from therapeutic agents. Ensure swabs sent; discuss with dermatology and consider biopsy. May need curettage or skin grafting.

Acute red eye emergency

▶▶Call for **senior help or speak to on-call ophthalmologist** urgently if patient has new onset ↓visual acuity (VA) in affected eye.

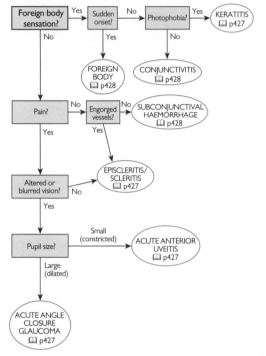

Fig. 14.2 Determining the likely cause of the acute red eye.

►►Keratitis (OHCS8 📖 p432)

Corneal inflammation with white slough on cornea; may ulcerate.

Symptoms eye irritation/foreign body sensation often on background of chronic gritty/irritated eyes or in contact lens wearers. If ulceration occurs, pain, photophobia, and altered visual acuity may develop.

Signs mild localised redness, often only in one sector of the cornea (unlike conjunctivitis which is usually bilateral and diffuse with a discharge); normal visual acuity unless ulceration. Fluorescein with a blue light may show corneal ulceration with corneal haze.

Management if ulceration present or suspected, refer urgently for ophthalmologist to consider infectious or autoimmune causes and for definitive care. This is likely to include corneal swabs/scrapes and antibiotic eyedrops under close supervision.

►►Episcleritis and scleritis (OHCS8 📖 p432)

Inflammation of white outer coating; often underlying autoimmune disorder.

Symptoms mild eye ache and tenderness; pain, photophobia and altered visual acuity are uncommon in episcleritis, but may feature in **scleritis**.

Signs mild localised redness (often involving just one sector, but occasionally diffuse); normal visual acuity; otherwise normal examination in episcleritis. In **scleritis** the globe may be tender to touch and there may be ↓visual acuity.

Management urgent ophthalmology review to consider **scleritis**.

Likely ophthalmic management topical steroids or non-steroidal agents for episcleritis, potentially oral immunosuppressants for **scleritis**.

►►Acute anterior uveitis (iritis) (OHCS8 📖 p430)

Inflammation of pigmented parts of eye; associated with systemic disease (eg IBD, arthropathies, sarcoid); pain on pupillary constriction.

Symptoms blurred vision, photophobia, and pain if severe.

Signs red eye, ↓visual acuity, cornea usually clear, pupil may be irregular and small, ±hypopyon (pus in the anterior chamber).

Management refer urgently to ophthalmologist.

Likely ophthalmic management intensive topical steroids, dilating agents.

►►Acute angle closure glaucoma (OHCS8 📖 p430)

↑Intraocular pressure due to blockage of anterior chamber drainage.

Symptoms aching eye pain (usually unilateral and severe), often associated with N+V; blurred vision and haloes around lights are common.

Signs red eye, ↓visual acuity, hazy cornea (if severe); pupil often mid-dilated, can be unreactive to light and oval shaped (rugby ball-like); globe tender and firm to touch. ↑intraocular pressure; usually >40 mmHg.

Management emergency referral to ophthalmologist; antiemetics and IV opioids may be needed for symptoms but should not delay referral.

Likely ophthalmic management constrict the pupil (miosis) with pilocarpine drops, and reduce aqueous formation with acetazolamide PO/IV. Mannitol IV is also sometimes used to reduce intraocular pressure. Definitive care achieved with peripheral iridectomy to allow constant drainage of aqueous even when pupil dilated.

Superficial foreign body (FB) and corneal abrasions

Symptoms sudden onset discomfort/foreign body sensation; lacrimation and redness; occurs, eg whilst hammering or chiselling without eye protection or following minor trauma to the eye. A contact lens may sometimes have been 'lost' and cause FB sensation.

Signs red, watering eye; FB may be visible. Always evert both top and bottom lids to check for FBs here as well; visual acuity is usually normal. Fluorescein with a blue light may show corneal ulceration/abrasion(s).

Treatment may need to anaesthetise the eye with topical local anaesthetic (proxymetacaine, tetracaine, or oxybuprocaine) to allow examination and treatment. Gently pick up FB with cotton bud, or irrigate lavishly with sterile 0.9% saline. Re-examine eye afterwards to ensure all FBs have gone. Protect the eye with an eye shield until local anaesthetic has worn off and give chloramphenicol eye drops 0.5% 4h topical or ointment 1% 6h topical for 3d. **If unable to remove FB or evidence of corneal abrasion speak to senior, or on-call ophthalmologist**.

Conjunctivitis

Symptoms eye discharge, ±FB sensation, itch, concurrent cold, hayfever.

Signs red eye, discharge, normal visual acuity, clear cornea.

Treatment can be highly contagious so care should be taken with handwashing. **Bacterial** topical antibiotics (eg chloramphenicol drops 0.5%) to both eyes every 2h whilst awake for 2d, then 6h for 1wk; **viral** may need topical antibiotics to prevent secondary infections, but usually self-limiting; **allergic** identify allergen if possible and encourage avoidance; topical antihistamine, (eg azelastine), or mast-cell inhibitors (cromoglicate) may offer relief; artificial tears (eg Viscotears®) may help if dry eyes are a problem.

Table 14.5 *Determining the cause of a conjunctivitis*

	Bacterial	**Viral**	**Allergic**
Discharge	Sticky, pus-like	Watery	Watery
Itch	+/–	+/–	++++
Recurrent	+/–	+/–	Often seasonal
Contagious	Yes	Yes	No
Uni- or bilateral	One, then both	One, then both	Both
Other symptoms	Often none	Common cold	Hay fever

Subconjunctival haemorrhage

Symptoms often an incidental finding by the patient and usually benign; can sometimes initially cause mild FB sensation. Pain, photophobia, or altered vision should suggest an alternative diagnosis.

Signs diffuse area of bright red blood under the conjunctiva, very different to inflamed blood vessels seen in other forms of red eye; normal VA.

Treatment check BP, and if recurrent check FBC and clotting; may need eye protection (eg tape at night) if swollen and unable to close readily; discuss with ophthalmologist only if recurrent or severe.

Sudden visual loss

Worrying features **severe deficit, additional neurology, scalp pain.**

Think about retinal vein occlusion, retinal artery occlusion, giant-cell arteritis, retinal detachment, arteriosclerotic ischaemic optic neuropathy, vitreous haemorrhage; angle closure glaucoma.

Ask about loss of vision; often painless.

Look for ↓visual acuity or no vision in affected eye, pupil unresponsive to light (suggests optic nerve disorder); abnormal retina on fundoscopy. Check for other neurological signs, for scalp pain/tenderness and ECG for AF.

Management immediate referral to on-call ophthalmologist.

▶▶**Giant-cell (temporal) arteritis** (📖 p361); ↓visual acuity in affected eye, typically with temporal headache/pain, may be retinal splinter haemorrhages or disc oedema.

▶▶**Retinal artery occlusion** (OHCS8 📖 p435)
Symptoms sudden, painless and severe loss of vision.
Signs relative afferent pupillary defect; pale retina with 'cherry spot' macula.
Risk factors for vascular disease (DM, smoker, ↑lipids, IHD).
Treatment if seen within 1h of onset, you may attempt to dislodge the embolus by pressing hard on the globe, then suddenly releasing; most damage will be irreversible.

▶▶**Retinal vein occlusion** (OHCS8 📖 p435)
Symptoms sudden, painless and severe loss of vision; may be segmental.
Signs relative afferent pupillary defect; engorged, red retina in affected area.
Risk factors include age, chronic glaucoma, HTN, polycythaemia.
Treatment supportive; laser photocoagulation may reduce macular oedema.

▶▶**Vitreous haemorrhage** (OHCS8 📖 p434)
Symptoms sudden painless loss of vision; floaters.
Signs relative afferent pupillary defect; loss of red reflex; unable to see retina.
Risk factors DM (proliferative retinopathy), bleeding disorder, trauma.
Treatment should resolve spontaneously; prevent further episodes by laser photocoagulation of proliferative vessels; vitrectomy if persistent.

Optic neuritis may be associated with a sub-acute, painless, unilateral loss of vision, often with associated loss of colour discrimination (best assessed by asking the patient to identify the colour of a red Neurotip™). Fundoscopy may reveal a swollen, bulging optic disc. *Causes* include demyelinating disease (this may be a first presentation of MS). *Treatment* is supportive, with resolution occurring over a few weeks.

Gradual visual loss

Think about refractive error, cataracts, macular degeneration, chronic glaucoma, diabetic retinopathy, optic atrophy, drug toxicity, optic neuroma; inherited disease.

Ask about painless loss of vision, symptoms of underlying disease.

Look for ↓visual acuity or no vision in affected eye, pupil unresponsive to light or relative afferent pupillary defect (suggest optic nerve disorder), abnormal cornea, lens, retina, or optic disc on fundoscopy.

Management needs full ophthalmic assessment. If in-patient try and arrange for review in eye clinic prior to discharge, or refer back to GP.

Cataracts (OHCS8 📖 p442)
Causes DM, steroids, trauma, eye surgery; congenital.
Symptoms blurred vision (bilateral), poor distance judgement (unilateral).
Signs ↓visual acuity, cataract visible in lens; retina and red reflex visible unless cataract is dense.
Treatment cataract surgery is performed on a single eye at a time if the cataract(s) are interfering with lifestyle (eg reading or driving). They are usually done as a day-case procedure under local anaesthetic; the lens is removed (phaecoemulsion) and an artificial lens implanted.

Age-related macular degeneration (OHCS8 📖 p438)
Causes age related, smoking.
Symptoms deterioration of central vision.
Signs ↓visual acuity, but normal visual fields; normal disc, but macula often pigmented or bleeding upon fundoscopy.
Treatment is aimed at reducing further visual loss; 'wet' (neovascular) forms can be treated with anti-angiogenic monoclonal antibodies (eg ranibizumab) or laser photocoagulation.

Chronic (open angle) glaucoma results in peripheral visual field loss in those with ↑intraocular pressure (IOP). *Signs* include cupping and atrophy of the optic disc. *Treatment* aims to ↓IOP by ↓aqueous formation (topical β-blockers eg timolol, or carbonic anhydrase inhibitors eg dorzolamide) or ↑reabsorption (prostaglandin drops, eg latanoprost); surgery involves trabeculectomy (allows aqueous drainage into subconjunctiva).

Registration of visual impairment

A consultant ophthalmologist can apply on behalf of a patient to register as blind or partially sighted; this is a voluntary not a statutory process. Registration entitles the individual to some tax allowances, benefits, and some concessions for public transport and other public facilities. Generally acuity <3/60 (after correction) qualifies as 'blind', whilst corrected vision <6/60 qualifies as 'partially sighted'; restriction of visual fields or loss of central vision may also qualify.

The Royal National Institute of Blind People advise on benefit entitlements, aids for the house and independent living, and for guide dogs:

Royal National Institute of Blind People
105 Judd Street, London, WC1H 9NE
0303 123 9999 ☞www.rnib.org.uk

Other visual disturbances

▶▶Photophobia

Causes **neurological** meningitis, subarachnoid haemorrhage, migraine, encephalitis, hangover; **ophthalmic** glaucoma, scleritis, keratitis and corneal injury, iritis, cataracts.

Symptoms bright light causes discomfort or exacerbates pain (especially painful having fundoscopy performed).

Signs dislike of light; intolerant of fundoscopy. Check for signs of meningism (📖 p360) and for focal neurology; perform full eye examination.

Treatment treat for likely cause(s); seek senior help urgently.

Diplopia – double vision

Causes extra-ocular muscle palsy, cranial nerve palsy, myasthenia gravis, orbital fracture, multiple sclerosis.

Symptoms double vision which is corrected by closing one eye or at extremes of gaze is called binocular diplopia; monocular diplopia is rarer and is not corrected by closing one eye, being caused by a structural abnormality within the eye.

Signs double vision usually relieved by occluding vision in one eye (the outer image will disappear when the affected eye is covered), loss of conjugate gaze, ↓ROM of eye when testing all movements in turn, fatigability of muscles, other evidence of associated disease (MS, CVA, etc).

Treatment discuss with senior; refer to neurologist/ophthalmologist.

Tunnel vision

Causes glaucoma, severe cataracts, alcohol consumption, retinitis pigmentosa, migraine.

Symptoms loss of peripheral vision with preservation of central vision, as though looking through a tunnel.

Signs check for visual field defect, ↓visual acuity, cataracts, or abnormal retina; check BP and blood glucose.

Treatment treat the cause.

Haloes around lights

Causes glaucoma, cataracts, post-corrective surgery, idiopathic.

Symptoms haloes and glare from lights, often more obvious at night.

Signs look for ↓visual acuity, cataracts.

Treatment treat the cause.

Floaters and flashing lights

Causes retinal detachment, vitreous detachment, migraine, idiopathic (non-sinister).

Symptoms dark flecks or webs which drift about in the line of vision; flashing lights, usually in the periphery of vision even when eye closed.

Signs often very few signs if non-sinister cause; ↓visual acuity, visual field, or abnormal fundoscopy may feature in retinal or vitreous detachment.

Treatment often not necessary. If lots of new floaters have appeared quickly or there are associated flashing lights, haloes or newly impaired visual acuity refer urgently to ophthalmologist.

Emergency department

Trauma

Worrying features shock, tachypnoea, ↓GCS, significant mechanism. [1]

Think about *emergency* severe trauma (📖 p232); ***common*** head injury, neck injury, concealed bleeding, fractures, dislocations, sprains, strains, bruises, incisional wounds, lacerations, abrasions, foreign bodies.
Ask about location at time of injury, activity prior to injury, cause/mechanism/direction of injury, ability to walk/move immediately after and now, exacerbating/relieving actions, pain, associated symptoms, time of last meal; *PMH* all medical problems, clotting abnormalities, kidney problems, GI problems, surgery, admissions, psychiatric problems; *DH* tetanus status, allergies; *SH* occupation, dominant hand, normal mobility, help at home.

Important questions to help assess RTAs

Collision speed (both vehicles combined)? Wearing seatbelt? Airbags deployed? Position in car (driver/passenger side, front/back)? Injuries/fatalities of other vehicle occupants? Patient trapped in car? What stopped the car? Was the car written off?

Obs HR, BP, RR, GCS, blood glucose, temp.
Look for (see 📖 pp146–152 for specific joint examinations); resting position, bruising, swelling, deformity, skin changes, active range of movement, tenderness (bony vs. soft tissue), passive range of movement, stability of joint, ability to use joint eg walking, always check:
• Joints directly above and below the site of injury
• Distal sensation/circulation (pulse, capillary refill) of affected limbs.
Investigations *X-ray* if fracture/dislocation is possible or to exclude a radio-opaque foreign body (eg some glass, metal).

Consequences of trauma covered elsewhere			
Wounds	📖 p436	Neck injury	📖 p440
Head injury	📖 p438	Epistaxis	📖 p460

Treatment Analgesia (📖 p86) should be given prior to examination and investigation to allow time for the drugs to act.
The following injuries need senior review or referral:
• Wounds with involvement of deep structures, eg tendons
• Wounds in cosmetically sensitive areas, eg face
• Wounds in functionally sensitive areas, eg hands, genitals
• Wounds with loss of skin tissue
• Displaced fractures
• Unstable fractures
• Open fractures
• Fractures with skin tenting or associated dislocation
• Dislocation of major joints (ie hip, knee, ankle, shoulder, elbow)
• Injuries with neurovascular compromise.

[1] eg fall from >1m or 5 stairs; axial load to head – eg diving; high-speed motor vehicle collision; rollover motor accident; ejection from a motor vehicle; accident involving motorised recreational vehicles; bicycle collision.

Soft tissue injuries (sprains, strains)

A sprain is minor damage to a ligament while a strain is caused by minor damage to a muscle. Both are managed the same way:

- **Rest** initially, but weight-bear or exercise as soon as symptoms allow
- **Ice** to reduce swelling over the first 48h; keep the ice away from the skin (eg use a tea towel) and apply for 10–15min at a time
- **Elevation** reduces both swelling and pain.

Prescribe adequate analgesia (eg paracetamol 1g/6h PO and ibuprofen 400mg/6h PO) and give reassurance. Compression is not routinely recommended as it can delay regaining full mobility.

Natural history symptoms often worsen over 24–48h then start to improve; they may take up to 6wk to resolve completely. Most heal completely, otherwise physiotherapy strengthening exercises can help.

Dislocations

- Provide adequate analgesia
- Document deficits in distal circulation and sensation and at-risk nerves
- X-ray before and after reduction (except ankle dislocation which should be reduced urgently, with senior supervision)
- Recheck and document any deficits in distal circulation and sensation and at-risk nerves. Appropriately immobilise/strap.
- Discharge with analgesia and orthopaedic follow-up if necessary.

Natural history symptoms improve dramatically with reduction though some discomfort may be present for days/weeks. Further dislocation is common and may need physiotherapy or surgical treatment.

Fractures

Types **hairline** very small fracture, no bony displacement; **simple** 2 bone sections; **comminuted** ≥3 bone sections; **open/compound** break in skin overlying a fracture.

You should suspect a fracture if there is a history of high forces, bony tenderness, swelling or reduced range of movement (ROM).

Treatment

- **Analgesia only** eg single rib or coccyx fractures, these do not need imaging unless a complication is suspected (eg pneumothorax)
- **Immobilisation** (eg backslab, sling) analgesia, fracture clinic follow-up for fractures that do not need an urgent orthopaedic review
- **Orthopaedic referral** if unstable, compound (open) or neurovascular compromise.

Natural history pain worst after the injury with little improvement by day 3–5. Simple fractures should heal over 6wk with minimal complications; serious fractures may reduce range of movement permanently.

▶▶*Open/compound fractures* resuscitate (🕮 p472). Seek immediate senior help, especially if distal sensation/circulation impaired or coexisting dislocation. Give analgesia (eg IV morphine), take a digital/polaroid photo, cover the wound with iodine/saline-soaked swabs, start IV antibiotics (eg co-amoxiclav 1.2g/8h IV), review tetanus status, X-ray; refer urgently to orthopaedics.

Wounds

Ask about mechanism of injury, paying particular attention to bites (animal or human), foreign bodies (eg metal/broken glass), contamination with soil or manure and when the wound occurred. Always ask about and document tetanus status.

Look for record the site, size (measure) and type of the wound (see Table 15.1), check distal sensation, pulse/cap refill and movement, look and feel inside the wound (usually with local anaesthetic) to assess depth, presence of foreign bodies and involvement of deep structures (eg tendons).

Table 15.1 *Types of wound*

Puncture	Deep wound with a small skin defect, eg cat bite, nail
Incisional wound	Wound caused by sharp objects, eg knife/broken glass, often have straight edges and can be deep
Laceration	Wound following blunt trauma, eg banging head on pavement, edges are often ragged and bruised
Abrasion	Graze
Full thickness	Wound that fully penetrates the skin (epidermis and dermis) so that subcutaneous fat is visible
Superficial	Wound that does not fully penetrate the skin

Cleaning all wounds should be thoroughly cleaned with sterile water or 0.9% saline. Abrasions may need to be scrubbed and deeper wounds may need cleaning with high-pressure 0.9% saline (use a syringe and green needle hub with the needle broken off). Cleaning can be done after local anaesthetic infiltration.

Important rules
- X-ray all wounds involving broken glass or metal foreign bodies
- Wounds should not be closed if:
  - older than 12h (unless facial)
  - very dirty or infected
  - foreign bodies present
  - bites
- Refer wounds that involve tendons or joints (to orthopaedics), arteries (to vascular surgeons) or nerves (to orthopaedics or plastics).

Primary closure is closing the wound in ED; several options are available:
- **Glue** for faces, children and small wounds (<2cm) if the edges are not gaping. The glue should just hold the edges together, not enter the wound. Be very careful not to get the glue in the eye
- **Steristrips ™** for small wounds, especially pretibial or facial lacerations
- **Sutures** (📖 p560) for wounds which are large, deep or over joints. Simple, interrupted stitches of non-absorbable suture are used for the vast majority. A layered closure with absorbable sutures may be required if the wound is especially deep; seek senior help.

Delayed primary closure the wound is left open for 3–5d then reviewed and closed if no infection is evident.

Secondary closure allowing the wound to heal without intervention.

Tetanus status should be documented for all wounds. Ensure adequate prevention (eg wound irrigation) and remember that patients over 50yr and immigrants may have received no previous tetanus vaccinations.

Table 15.2 *Tetanus prophylaxis*

Immunisation status	Clean wound	Tetanus-prone wound[1]
Full course (5 injections) **or** booster <10yr ago	No prophylaxis needed	HATI[2] only if contaminated with manure
Partial course **and** booster ≥10yr ago	Tetanus booster	Tetanus booster and HATI[2]
Not immunised or unknown	Start tetanus course	Start tetanus course and give HATI[2]

[1] Tetanus-prone wounds:
* Heavy contamination especially with soil or manure (remember gardeners)
* Infection or wounds >6h old
* Puncture wounds (eg cat bites, nails)
* Devitalised tissue.

[2] Human anti-tetanus immunoglobulin.

Antibiotics (check local guidelines) eg flucloxacillin 1g/6h PO for 5d for puncture wounds, and wounds involving bones (eg crushed fingertips). Co-amoxiclav 625mg/8h PO for 5d for heavily contaminated wounds (consider leaving these wounds open). Antibiotics are no substitute for thorough wound irrigation/washout.

Animal/human bites treat with eg co-amoxiclav 625mg/8h PO for 5d.

Assaults the notes you make may be used in a legal case many years from now so think carefully about what you write. For example:
* Distinguish facts from hearsay; make it clear where information came from, eg 'Patient alleges assaulted with an iron bar'
* Document injuries accurately including location, size (measure) and type of wound (see Table 15.1); use simple line diagrams. Do not interpret what potentially caused the wound.
* Write your notes imagining them being read out in public by someone wishing to make you appear stupid.

Osteoporosis (OHGP3 p516)

The ED is a common place of presentation for elderly fallers; often there may be no significant injury sustained, but the patient may not be so fortunate next time. The 1yr mortality after a fractured neck of femur is 30%, so never miss an opportunity to think about prevention of falls (p443) and osteoporosis. Risk factors include early menopause, ↑age, ♀ sex, ↓BMI (especially previous eating disorder), family history, steroid usage, alcohol excess and malabsorption disorders.

Management in all: smoking cessation, regular weight-bearing exercise, falls reduction measures (p443), Ca^{2+} and vitamin D supplements (eg Adcal-D₃® 2 tabs/24h PO). Further treatment with a bisphosphonate (eg alendronic acid 70mg/weekly PO) or strontium ranelate (2nd line) should be based upon estimated 10yr fracture risk. The WHO have developed the FRAX tool for this purpose, available online at www.shef.ac.uk/FRAX Although bone mineral density can be formally assessed by DEXA scanning, the FRAX tool does not absolutely require this value. FRAX results are linked to guidance developed by the UK National Osteoporosis Guidance Group (NOGG) on whether to initiate treatment, give lifestyle advice, or request DEXA.

Head injury

> *Worrying features* ↓GCS, vomiting, seizures, basal skull fracture, amnesia.

Think about *emergency* unconscious, ↑ICP, extradural haematoma, subdural haematoma; ***common*** concussion.

Ask about mechanism of injury, time of injury, loss of consciousness, seizures, memory (before, during and after), blood/fluid from nose or ears, vomiting, weakness/tingling/numbness in limbs, time of last meal, dizziness, visual changes, headache; *PMH* clotting abnormalities, all previous medical, surgical or psychiatric problems; *DH* anticoagulants, tetanus status; *SH* occupation, normal mobility, help at home.

Obs GCS, HR, BP, RR, glucose.

Look for GCS (📖 p340), orientation, CSF leaking from ears (otorrhoea) or nose (rhinorrhoea), Battle's sign (bruising over the mastoid processes, a late sign), blood behind eardrum (haemotympanum), 'panda' eyes, (bruising around the eyes), focal neurology (eg weakness or numbness); if head injury caused by fall think about what precipitated the fall (?dysrhythmia, hypoglycaemia, postural hypotension; see 📖 p443).

Investigations *CT* if indicated (Fig. 15.1).

Treatment – involve a senior when dealing with any head injury
▶▶*Unconscious* bleep an anaesthetist immediately and see 📖 p338.
CT head according to the CT criteria (Fig. 15.1) ± admission.
Criteria for admission:
• New, clinically significant abnormalities on imaging
• Not returned to GCS 15 after imaging, regardless of the imaging results
• Criteria for CT scanning fulfilled, but scan not done, either because CT not available or because patient not sufficiently co-operative/ stable to allow scanning
• Continuing worrying signs (eg persistent vomiting, severe headaches)
• Other sources of concern (eg drug or alcohol intoxication, other injuries, shock, suspected non-accidental injury, meningism, cerebrospinal fluid leak).

Subdural haematoma
Venous bleed into the skull; can be acute (↓GCS and ↑ICP, usually post-trauma) or chronic (fluctuating conscious level over days in eg elderly, alcoholics, patients on anticoagulation).
Management CT diagnosis; drained by craniotomy or burr hole.

Extradural haematoma
Arterial bleed into skull often from middle meningeal artery after trauma.
Symptoms/signs initially well but ↓GCS over 4–8h as blood collects.
Management CT diagnosis; drained by craniotomy or burr hole.

Post-concussion syndrome
Patients may have concussion symptoms for months after a head injury, eg headaches, dizziness, tiredness, depression, memory problems.

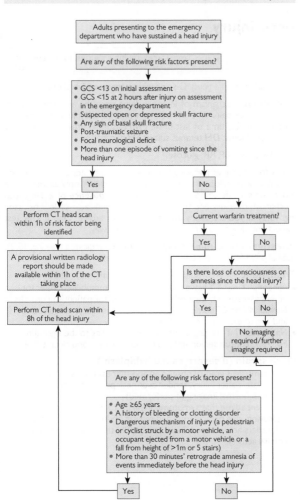

Fig. 15.1 NICE head injury guidance; Selection of adults for CT scanning of head. National Clinical Guideline Centre (2014) Head Injury: Triage, assessment, investigation and early management of head injury in children, young people and adults. Clinical Guideline 176 (Partial update of NICE CG56). Copyright © NCGC. Reproduced by permission.
NICE guidance available at ⌐guidance.nice.org.uk/CG176

Neck injury

Worrying features ↓GCS, large forces, multiple injuries, focal neurology.

Think about *emergency* C-spine injury; ***common*** whiplash.

Ask about mechanism of injury, walking since the accident, comfort sitting up, neck pain, time of neck pain onset, head injury, weakness or tingling of limbs, time of last meal; ***PMH*** asthma, previous medical or surgical problems; ***DH*** tetanus status; ***SH*** occupation.

Obs GCS, HR, BP, RR, glucose.

Look for midline vs. paravertebral neck tenderness, steps, deformity, look for limb weakness, loss of sensation, other injuries; ►► only examine neck movements if safe to do so. This requires the ***absence*** of a dangerous mechanism of injury and the ***presence*** of an indicator of low risk (see Fig. 15.2). If you are in any doubt, seek senior advice. Only if safe, test the patient's ability to turn their neck 45° each way.

Investigations ***C-spine X-ray or CT neck*** if indicated (see Fig. 15.2); see 📖 p594 for interpretation of C-spine X-ray.

Treatment – ►►consult a senior when dealing with neck injuries
- *Abnormal X-rays/CT* leave the patient's neck immobilised, refer for urgent assessment, treat other injuries, monitor patient's neuro obs
- *Normal X-rays/CT* do not exclude ligamentous injury; consult senior and aim to examine neck and clear it clinically
- *No X-rays/CT* if imaging is not required according to the algorithm in Fig. 15.2, consult senior and aim to examine neck and clear it clinically.

Neck sprain (if severe called 'whiplash')
- *Symptoms/signs* gradual onset pain and stiffness not usually present immediately after injury; tender over neck paravertebral >midline
- *Diagnosis* normal imaging (if performed)
- *Treatment* advise that symptoms are likely to worsen before improving, give paracetamol and regular NSAIDs, heat/ice may help, soft collars are not used, initial rest (≤48h) then gradual return to normal activity.

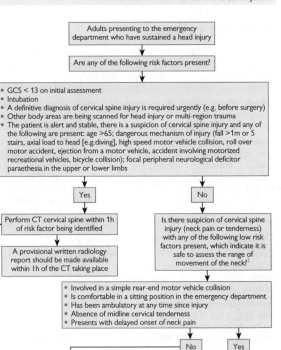

Fig. 15.2 NICE neck injury guidance; Selection of adults and children (age 10+) for imaging of the cervical spine. National Clinical Guideline Centre (2014) Head Injury: Triage, assessment, investigation and early management of head injury in children, young people and adults. Clinical Guideline 176 (Partial update of NICE CG56). Copyright © NCGC. Reproduced by permission. NICE guidance available at ⌂guidance.nice.org.uk/CG176

---

[1] i.e. in the absence of at least one of these indicators of 'low risk', the cervical spine should be considered potentially unstable and it is not safe to move the neck – proceed to three-view imaging within 1h.

Children under 10 years

Separate guidelines exist for use in children – see ⌂guidance.nice.org.uk/CG176

Falls and collapse

> *Worrying features* ↑↓HR, ↓BP, chest pain, palpitations, head injury, loss of consciousness, recurrent vomiting, incomplete recovery, focal neurology, long time spent on hard surface, hypothermia.

Think about *serious* MI, dysrhythmias, shock, sepsis, CVA, seizure, hypoglycaemia, hypoxia, PE; ***common*** postural hypotension, mechanical fall (see box), syncope (vasovagal, situational, cardiac; Table 15.3), ataxia.

Ask about symptoms and activity before falling (aura, dizziness, chest pain, palpitations), speed of onset, visual changes, loss of consciousness (can you remember: falling, being on the floor, getting up?), incontinence, recovery, head injury, other injuries, mechanism of injury, length of time spent immobile; ***PMH*** previous falls (and investigations), heart problems, DM, Parkinsonism; ***DH*** anticoagulants, antihypertensives, antiepileptics, hypoglycaemics, diuretics, nitrates; ***SH*** usual mobility and aids, ability to eat and drink independently, alcohol.

Obs temp, HR, lying and standing BP, glucose, GCS, sats, RR.

Look for pulse volume, HR and regularity, carotid bruit, volume status (📖 p380), heart murmurs (aortic stenosis), focal neurology, ability to stand, ability to walk, bruising, lacerations or haematomas on the head or body, movement of all limbs, sites of tenderness.

Investigations consider ***ECG*** dysrhythmia or MI (± cardiac monitor); ***blds*** FBC, U+E, CRP, cardiac markers (repeat at 12h); investigate for injuries as appropriate: ***CT*** if focal neurology, persistent ↓GCS or post-head injury (📖 p438); ***X-ray*** if clinical suspicion of a fracture.

Table 15.3 *Common causes of syncope*

	History	Examination	Investigations
Vasovagal syncope (📖 p260)	Onset in seconds, precipitated by fear, stress, pain or standing	±Postural drop, otherwise normal	Normal
Cardiac syncope (📖 p250–261)	Sudden onset and recovery, chest pain, palpitations, SOB	Fast, slow, irregular or absent pulse	Dysrhythmia or MI on ECG, pauses on 24h Holter monitor, ±↑cardiac markers
Neurological (📖 p340)	Rapid onset, headache, ↓GCS, weakness, altered sensation	Focal neurology, persistent ↓GCS, ataxia	CVA or intracranial haemorrhage on CT; check glucose
Seizure (📖 p346)	±Aura, poor recall, limb movements, tongue biting, post-ictal confusion/drowsiness, incontinence	Drowsy, injuries, ±Todd's paresis	Initial investigations often normal, check glucose

Treatment 15l/min O$_2$ and lie flat initially. Exclude serious conditions (HR, ECG, BP, glucose) and establish IV access. Treat according to diagnosis.

Some precipitants of falls to consider			
Seizures	📖 p346	Hypoglycaemia	📖 p323
Focal neurology	📖 p353	Sepsis	📖 p483
GCS + confusion	📖 p340	Chest pain	📖 p241
Head injuries	📖 p438	Tachyarrhythmias	📖 p250
Postural drop	📖 p474	Bradyarrhythmias	📖 p258
Vertigo	📖 p363	Hypoxia	📖 p271
		Ataxia	📖 p363

Situational syncope

Similar to vasovagal syncope (📖 p260), but brought on by a specific action:
Micturition middle-aged/elderly men; advise to sit down to urinate.
Carotid sensitivity can be brought on by shaving.
Cough brought on by coughing fits.

The elderly, recurrent falls and the 'mechanical' label[1]

We all trip over things from time to time, but it's a pretty rare occurrence, so think again before you ascribe the lazy label of 'mechanical' fall to the elderly lady lying on the trolley in front of you. Age, dementia, and other processes of nature may well be irreversible, but the challenge is to identify and deal with the *reversible*, before the next fall leads to a fractured femur and inexorable decline. Consider delirium (📖 p341), peripheral neuropathy (📖 p355), untreated Parkinsonism (📖 p349), poorly controlled arthritis (📖 p454), cerebellar disease/ataxia (📖 p363). ↓Vitamin D is common in the elderly and leads to ↓muscle tone and bone frailty – check plasma levels and consider oral supplementation (eg Adcal-D₃® 2 tabs/24h PO). Is there a history of alcohol excess? Are diuretics and urge incontinence forcing the patient to rush for a bathroom (📖 p377)? Does the patient have and correctly use appropriate walking aids (sticks, frames) and is the home environment safe (liaise with OT)? Has poor vision been assessed and corrected as much as possible (bi/varifocal lenses are associated with ↑falls risk)?

Even if you are still unable to identify anything reversible, always assess for osteoporosis and consider treatment (📖 p437).

---

1. NICE guidelines available at ⌨guidance.nice.org.uk/CG161

Acutely painful limb emergency

Airway	Check airway is patent; consider manoeuvres/adjuncts
Breathing	If no respiratory effort – **CALL ARREST TEAM**
Circulation	If no palpable pulse – **CALL ARREST TEAM**

▶▶Call for **senior help** early if patient deteriorating.
- **Sit patient up**, unless pain will not allow
- **15l/min O₂** if ischaemia suspected
- **Monitor** O₂ sats, HR, BP, temp:
  - is the patient shocked or febrile?
- Brief **history**/check notes/ask ward staff:
  - arterial/cardiac problems or DM
  - recent trauma/surgery
- **Examine** patient: condensed RS, CVS and abdo exam
- **Examine all limbs**: vascular, neuro and joint exams:
  - is the pain localised to a joint or specific area?
  - check distal sensation, pulses and cap refill (ischaemia?)
- **Venous access**, take bloods:
  - FBC, ESR, U+E, CRP, ±cardiac markers, ±sickle-cell, D-dimer, clotting, G+S
- Check pulses with **Doppler** if available
- **ECG** to exclude acute MI, AF
- **ABG** if systemically unwell
- Analgesia, eg IV morphine titrated to pain
- **Consider** serious causes and treat if present:
  - **acute ischaemia** 15l/min O₂, analgesia, heparin, (vascular) surgeons
  - **compartment syndrome** 15l/min O₂, remove plaster, orthopaedics, consider fasciotomy
  - **septic arthritis** 15l/min O₂, joint aspiration, orthopaedics
  - **necrotising fasciitis** 15l/min O₂, fluids, IV antibiotics, surgeons
  - **gangrene** 15l/min O₂, fluids, IV antibiotics, surgeons
- Call for **senior help**
- **Reassess**, starting with A, B, C …

Life- and limb-threatening causes

Acute ischaemia	🕮 p446	Septic arthritis	🕮 p455
Compartment syndrome	🕮 p447	Necrotising fasciitis	🕮 p413
Myocardial infarction (arm)	🕮 p244	Gangrene	🕮 p447
Spinal cord compression	🕮 p357	Sickle-cell crisis	🕮 p397

Acute limb pain

Worrying features sudden onset, severe pain, ↓sensation, ↓power, absent distal pulses, cold to touch; shock, pyrexia, recent surgery/trauma.

Think about *serious* acute ischaemia, septic arthritis, compartment syndrome, gangrene, necrotising fasciitis; ***common*** muscular, joint or bone pain, DVT, cellulitis, thrombophlebitis, sciatica; ***other*** osteomyelitis, Baker's cyst, vasculitides, myositis, peripheral neuropathy. See Table 15.4.

Ask about location, trauma, speed of onset, change on moving and raising, back pain, chest pain, SOB; *PMH* recent surgery, previous limb pain, DM, MI, CVA, DVT, PE; *DH* anticoagulants; *SH* exercise tolerance.

Obs temp, BP, HR, O₂ sats, RR.

Look for *vascular assessment* colour, mottling, hot/cold, cap refill, pulses (compare both sides); *neurological assessment* power, sensation, reflexes; *orthopaedic assessment* evidence of trauma, swelling (distal, joint, calf), range of movement (active and passive), muscle, joint or bone tenderness (see 🕮 p146–152 for specific joint examinations); *respiratory assessment* if SOB or suspect DVT.

Investigations most limb pain can be diagnosed from clinical examination; consider the following investigations: *blds* FBC, U+E, ESR, CRP, D-dimer, venous lactate, blood cultures; *Doppler* for pulses (?ischaemia); *ECG* for AF; *X-rays* for joint disease or bone fractures; *ABG* if hypoxic and suspicion of PE/DVT.

Management ensure adequate analgesia (🕮 p86). Try to determine what structure is causing the pain (eg skin, muscle, joint, bone); if there is no obvious structure consider arterial problems, infection or DVT.

Superficial thrombophlebitis
Inflammation and thrombosis of a vein, which can progress to DVT.

Symptoms gradual onset of tenderness over a vein.

Signs red, tender area with hard palpable vein/varicosity.

Risk factors IV cannula, varicose veins, IVDU, DVT risk factors (🕮 p450).

Investigations no specific investigations but have a low threshold for blood and Doppler studies to exclude underlying DVT.

Treatment resite/remove IV cannula, elevation, exercise, compression, NSAIDs (eg ibuprofen 200–400mg/6h PO); if DVT suspicion, start LMWH.

Complications Post-phlebitic pain; if thrombophlebitis recurs or affects other sites (migratory) suspect malignancy or vasculitis.

Muscle pain
Causes trauma, strains, fibromyalgia, infection, rhabdomyolysis, drugs (statins, ACEi, steroids), inflammation (polymyalgia rheumatica, polymyositis, dermatomyositis, SLE), metabolic (↓Ca²⁺, ↓K⁺, ↓Na⁺, alkalosis), endocrine (hypo/hyperthyroid, Cushing's), referred joint pain.

Investigations often none; FBC, U+E, Ca²⁺, CK, ESR, CRP, X-ray.

Treatment simple analgesia including NSAIDs, rest for first 24h then gradually exercise the joint, ice packs, and elevation. Consider physiotherapy referral if persists.

Table 15.4 *Common causes of limb pain*

	History	Examination	Investigations
Acute ischaemia	Rapid onset, distal >proximal, painful (worse with legs raised)	Pulseless, cap refill >2s, pale, cold, weak, reduced sensation	Doppler pulse ↓ or absent; obstruction on angiography
Infection (eg cellulitis)	Gradual onset, feels unwell, history of trauma or bite	Pyrexia; red, tender, warm, swollen	↑WCC, ↑CRP, ↑ESR, often ↑D-dimer
DVT	Gradual onset, painful (improved with legs raised)	Red, swollen, hot, tender leg	↑D-dimer; thrombosis on Doppler USS
Compartment syndrome	Recent trauma or surgery ±POP	Severe pain on passive movement	Increased compartment pressure
Joint	Trauma, pain on movement, unable to bear load	Tender over joint, joint effusion, pain on movement (active = passive)	Abnormal X-ray (eg arthritic changes); abnormal synovial fluid
Muscle	Trauma, pain on movement	Tender ±swelling on muscle/tendon insertion, pain on movement (active >passive)	Normal X-rays, may have a ↑CK
Bone	Trauma, pain on movement and at rest	Bony tenderness with swelling and reduced range of movement	Abnormal X-ray

Cause of limb pain covered elsewhere			
Ulcers	📖 p424	Swelling	📖 p441
Back pain/sciatica	📖 p356	Joint pain	📖 p452
Cellulitis	📖 p412	Rashes	📖 p411–419
Chronic limb pain	📖 p448	Necrotising fasciitis	📖 p413
DVT	📖 p450	Trauma	📖 p434

▶▶Acute limb ischaemia

This is an *emergency*; ischaemia is irreversible after 6h.

Worrying signs ↓sensation; purple, non-blanching mottling.

Causes emboli, thrombosis, dissecting aneurysm, trauma.

Risk factors arterial graft, peripheral vascular disease, previous thrombo-emboli, AF, prosthetic heart valves, recent MI, dehydration, malignancy.

Symptoms unilateral painful, tingling, weak limb, worse on raising limb.

Signs absent pulses, slow cap refill (compare with opposite limb), cold and pale (can be red if limb below heart), reduced power and sensation.

Investigations a hand-held Doppler probe will show a reduced or absent pulse; angiography may demonstrate an obstruction.

Treatment this needs urgent surgery – call a senior surgeon who will consider embolectomy, intra-arterial thrombolysis, bypass or amputation. Give 15l/min O_2 and analgesia (eg morphine); IV access with IV fluids if dehydrated; may require heparinisation (📖 p406) pre- or post-op.

Complications amputation, gangrene, ↑K^+, renal failure, sepsis.

▶▶Gas (wet) gangrene

This is an ***emergency***; *Clostridium* infection causing necrosis and sepsis.
Symptoms unwell with painful extremities or wound.
Signs pyrexia, shock, tender brown/black area with blistering and oedema, muscle necrosis, crepitus (from gas in tissue).
Risk factors ischaemia, DM, malignancy, surgery/trauma.
Investigations **blds** FBC, U+E, LFT, CRP, CK, blood cultures, clotting; **ABG** acidosis; **Gram stain** of pus or necrotic tissue; **X-ray** may show gas (dark patches in soft tissues).
Treatment call a senior surgeon who will consider urgent debridement. Give 15l/min O$_2$, fluids and broad-spectrum antibiotics (eg benzylpenicillin 2.4g/4h IV, clindamycin 600mg/6h IV, and metronidazole 500mg/8h IV).
Complications amputation, sepsis, death.

Dry gangrene

Ischaemic muscle necrosis without infection.
Signs well-defined, painless, shrivelled brown/black area.
Treatment debridement or amputation may help prevent infection; alternatively conservative management awaiting autoamputation.
Complications wet gangrene.

▶▶Compartment syndrome

This is an ***emergency***; call a senior surgeon if suspected.
Symptoms excessive pain following an injury or fracture, distal tingling, numbness or weakness.
Signs pain at rest, worse on passive stretching of a muscle, reduced sensation (loss of two point discrimination), redness, swelling, slow cap refill; absent pulse and pallor are late signs.
Risk factors long bone fractures and plaster casts, significant injury, crush injury, vascular injury, anticoagulants, burns.
Investigations clinical diagnosis; **blds** FBC, U+E, CK, clotting; it is possible to measure compartment pressure by inserting a manometer through the skin (eg Wick catheter), pressures >30mmHg indicate need for urgent fasciotomy, although some surgeons advocate avoiding intervention if compartment pressure is ±20mmHg of diastolic pressure.
Treatment 15l/min O$_2$; elevate limb (lie the patient flat); ensure adequate analgesia; IV fluids if dehydrated (monitor urine output); remove plaster cast if present; discuss with surgeons regarding urgent fasciotomy.
Complications rhabdomyolysis, ↑K$^+$, neurological damage, amputation.

Osteomyelitis

Risk factors DM, immunocompromise, open fractures, prostheses.
Symptoms fever, bone pain, malaise (or fever without focus).
Signs bony tenderness, warm, red, swollen.
Investigations **blds** ↑WCC, ↑ESR, ↑CRP, blood cultures; **imaging** X-ray (insensitive since there are rarely changes in the first 10d), USS (may show periosteal lifting), MRI (gold standard); **bone biopsy** where indicated.
Culture try to obtain a sample for microbiology prior to starting antibiotics (by swabs, USS-guided aspiration or bone biopsy in theatre).
Treatment high-dose antibiotics (discuss with microbiology) for at least 6wk; often requires central access; surgical drainage of abscess if present.
Complications septic arthritis, fracture, amputation, seeding to other sites.

Chronic limb pain

Peripheral arterial disease (PAD)

Chronic limb ischaemia causes intermittent claudication/critical ischaemia.

- *Intermittent claudication* cramp in calf, thigh or buttock on walking a fixed distance, worse uphill, relieved by stopping or rest
- *Critical ischaemia* pain in limb at night, relieved by hanging legs out of bed; arterial ulcers, dry gangrene.

Signs **early** cool, hairless, pulseless limbs; **late** pain and pallor on elevation.
Investigations **blds** FBC, U+E, lipids, ESR; *ECG*; *ABPI* (ankle brachial pressure index, see box); *imaging* CT or Doppler arteriography.
Treatment address vascular risk factors (exercise, stop smoking, treat DM, ↑BP and ↑cholesterol); aspirin 75mg/24h PO, avoid β-blockers; refer to vascular team for consideration of angioplasty or bypass graft.
Complications acute ischaemia, gangrene, rest pain, ulcers.

Ankle brachial pressure index (ABPI)

With the patient lying flat, a Doppler probe is used to record the systolic BP (ie lowest pressure at which the pulse is occluded) in each arm (cuff around upper arm, probe over brachial artery) and twice in each leg (cuff around calf, probe over posterior tibial and dorsalis pedis). The result is expressed as a ratio of the highest ankle pressure for each leg, to the highest brachial pressure.

Example: left ankle posterior tibial pressure of 126, dorsalis pedis pressure of 124, brachial pressures of 138 and 142; ABPI = 126/142 = 0.89

Normal	0.8–1.3	Moderate PVD	0.5–0.8
Severe PVD	<0.5	Calcification	>1.3

Lumbar spinal stenosis

Symptoms cramp in thigh or leg on walking, worse on walking downhill or standing, associated back pain. See Table 15.5.
Signs pain on straight leg raise/back extension, often no neuro symptoms.
Investigations lumbar spine X-ray and MRI spine.
Treatment exercise, NSAIDs, steroid injections, spinal decompression.
Complications cord compression, cauda equina syndrome (📖 p357).

Table 15.5 *Nerve entrapment syndromes*

Syndrome	Symptom
Carpal tunnel syndrome (median)	Aching of wrist and forearm, tingling of thumb, index, middle, ±ring finger
Ulnar entrapment (wrist or elbow)	Tingling of ring and little fingers, ±forearm
Radial tunnel syndrome or posterior interosseous syndrome	Weak extension of fingers and thumb
Meralgia paraesthetica	Tingling lateral thigh
Common peroneal compression	Weak dorsiflexion of foot

Chronic limb pain covered elsewhere

Osteoarthritis	📖 p454	Gout	📖 p455
Peripheral neuropathy	📖 p355	Sciatica/radiculopathy	📖 p357
Limb ulcers	📖 p424	Analgesia in chronic pain	📖 p86

Limb swelling

Worrying features weight loss, night sweats, pain, hard irregular lump, vomiting, SOB and chest pain.

Think about causes depend upon site (Table 15.6).

Table 15.6 *Clinical assessment of limb swelling*

Pitting	**Bilateral:** congestive cardiac failure, nephrotic syndrome, renal failure, ↓albumin, early lymphoedema, venous insufficiency, trauma, SVC/IVC obstruction (arms/legs)
	Unilateral: cellulitis[1], deep vein thrombosis, early lymphoedema, venous insufficiency, trauma
Non-pitting	**Bilateral:** chronic congestive cardiac failure, lymphoedema, chronic venous insufficiency, trauma, compartment syndrome
	Unilateral: lymphoedema, chronic venous insufficiency, trauma, compartment syndrome

[1] The diagnosis of bilateral cellulitis is a rare one, and more usually represents a misdiagnosis (eg elderly with CCF, venous insufficiency and venous stasis eczema).

Ask about *swelling* location, onset, duration, redness, warmth, pain (severity, radiation), associated rash, history of trauma, insect bites/stings; *systemic symptoms* nausea and vomiting, pyrexia, sweating, weight loss; *PMH* recent operations, fractures or immobility, cancer (±radiotherapy), DM, IBD, IHD, polycythaemia, thrombocytosis, thyroid disease; *DH* COCP/HRT, steroids, amlodipine, drug allergies; *SH* recent long distance travel, alcohol, smoking.

Obs temp, HR, BP, RR, sats, urine output, blood glucose.

Look for *swollen limb*: site, size, shape, colour, tenderness and temperature of swelling, evidence of trauma, skin breaks between toes (for leg cellulitis), nail condition, tortuous veins; *systemic* evidence of malignancy (eg cachexia, abdominal/rectal mass, clubbing, lymphadenopathy); evidence of chronic liver disease (p313, eg ascites, jaundice, spider naevi); surgical scars (eg previous mastectomy/axillary clearance), evidence of cardiac failure (p282, bibasilar creps, wheeze); in ♀: gravid uterus, consider *PV* tenderness, palpable masses.

Investigations target according to likely causes (see following sections).

Lymphoedema (OHGP3 p1039)
Accumulation of interstitial fluid due to abnormal lymphatic drainage; may be congenital, or secondary to surgery, radiotherapy, malignancy or filariasis.
Symptoms limb swelling, reduced mobility, recurrent infections.
Signs acute lymphoedema may be pitting, but as it becomes more chronic the tissues become woody and pitting is less likely. Chronic oedema from congestive cardiac failure can also become woody and non-pitting.
Risk factors female sex, malignancy, breast cancer surgery (especially axillary node clearance), radiotherapy, family history, obesity.
Treatment **medical** elevation of the limb, compression bandages, massage of the limb in a proximal direction (to aid fluid return), exercise, weight loss, antibiotics if 2° skin infection present; no evidence for use of diuretics; **surgical** excisional techniques available, but radical.
Complications cellulitis, ulcers, psychological problems, pain.

Deep vein thrombosis[1,2] (OHCM9 📖 p580)

Symptoms unilateral swelling and/or pain.

Signs warm, red, tender, swollen limb (eg leg >3cm compared to other calf measured 10cm below tibial tuberosity), pitting oedema.

Risk factors age >60yr, obesity, recent surgery/immobility/long distance travel, oestrogen (pregnancy, HRT, OCP), PMH or FH PE/DVT, malignancy, thrombophilia, medical comorbidity (eg CCF, IBD, active inflammation).

Investigations **blds** FBC, U+E, D-dimer (see box). Assess the DVT probability (risk score Table 15.7 ±D-dimer) to determine the need for further investigation with Doppler ultrasonography.[3] If suspected PE (📖 p278), perform **ECG** and consider **ABG**.

Treatment Commence parenteral anticoagulation (eg enoxaparin 1.5mg/kg/24h SC) if USS +ve or delayed >4h. If confirmed DVT, start oral anticoagulation (📖 p407).

Complications PE, post-thrombotic syndrome (chronic pain and swelling).

Pre-test probability in DVT

Symptoms and signs of DVT are non-specific; likewise, the much over-ordered D-dimer blood test is a non-specific marker of thrombosis. The application of clinical scoring systems, which combine established risk factors with reliable clinical findings, allow the identification of low-risk patients, in whom a negative D-dimer has a robust negative predictive value. In higher risk patients, Doppler ultrasonography is justified, regardless of the D-dimer assay result.

The Wells score has proven to be clinically reliable and is widely used in modified '2 level' form.[4] The following measures score 1 point each if present:

- Active cancer (treatment ongoing or in past 6mth, or palliative)
- Leg paralysed or in plaster
- Recent bed rest >3d or major surgery within 12wk
- Previous documented DVT
- Visible collateral superficial veins (non-varicose)
- Pitting oedema
- Tenderness along veins
- Whole leg swollen
- >3cm calf swelling (cf other calf).

Subtract 2 points if there is another diagnosis that is as or more likely (eg cellulitis).

Table 15.7 *The 2 level DVT Wells score*

Score	Risk of DVT	Management[5]
≤1	Unlikely (5.5%)	D-dimer test, if +ve USS, if –ve unlikely to be DVT
≥2	Likely (28%)	Arrange USS; LMWH if delay in USS >4h

Where risk score ≥2 but USS -ve, perform D-dimer test: if +ve, repeat USS in 6–8d.

[4] Wells, P.S. *et al. NEJM* 2003 **349**:1227 (available free at 🖰NEJM.org); a good overview of the use of clinical scoring alongside further tests is Scarvelis, D. *et al. CMAJ* 2006 **175**:1087 available free at 🖰www.ncbi.nlm.nih.gov/sites/ppmc/articles/PMC1609160

[5] Most hospitals will also have their own guidelines which you should consult, particularly regarding logistics of arranging USS through ambulatory pathways.

Venous insufficiency

Symptoms bursting/throbbing leg pain, relieved by elevating legs, worse on standing; previous DVT or thrombophlebitis.

Signs pain ↓ by lifting legs, red discolouration, swelling, varicose veins.

Investigations Duplex ultrasound, D-dimer if DVT suspected.

Treatment compression bandages (if ABPI >0.8), varicose vein surgery.

Complications varicose veins, thrombophlebitis, ulcers, cellulitis.

[1] See also thromboprophylaxis, 📖 p406; NICE guidelines at 🖰guidance.nice.org.uk/CG92

[2] NICE DVT/PE guidelines at 🖰guidance.nice.org.uk/CG144

[3] Most radiology departments will only scan the leg veins above the knee, since below knee DVTs carry a much lower risk of PE; there is a low risk (1–2%) of clot extension into more proximal veins—for this reason, in those with a high pre-test probability, a positive D-dimer and a negative Doppler USS, consider repeat Doppler USS at 1–2wk.

Post-cannula swelling

Tissuing is where an IV cannula has not been inserted correctly and is sited only partially in the vein or outside the vein altogether, meaning that fluid or drugs cannot be infused/injected.

Treatment remove cannula and re-site if required, elevate the affected limb and give simple analgesia for pain.

If no improvement consider possibility of infection of cannula site (□ p412); assess swelling for collection – if in doubt request USS – if present, start IV ABx (eg co-amoxiclav 1.2g/8h IV) and discuss drainage with surgeons.

Baker's cyst

Symptoms pain and swelling behind the knee, may radiate to calf; similar to symptoms of DVT, common in osteoarthritis.

Signs fluctuant swelling in the popliteal fossa; can also have calf swelling.

Investigations distinguishable from DVT by **USS**.

Treatment conservative (NSAIDs, ice packs).

Angioedema

Episodic subcutaneous and submucosal oedema, 2° to ↑vascular permeability occurring in hereditary, idiopathic, drug-induced and antigen-driven forms.

Symptoms colicky abdominal pain, shortness of breath (laryngeal oedema), dysphagia, watery diarrhoea, pruritus (in antigen-driven cases).

Signs well demarcated swelling (eg hands/feet/face), dyspnoea ±stridor (if largyngeal/tongue swelling leads to airway compromise), urticaria.

Investigations diagnosis made clinically; **blds** ↑tryptase (from mast cell degranulation) if reaction was anaphylactic, ↓complement levels help confirm diagnosis (see 'Anaphylaxis' □ p470).

Treatment assess airway – if any concerns ▶▶request immediate senior help since IM adrenaline (0.5ml (0.5mg) 1:1000 adrenaline STAT) and urgent intubation may be required; nebulised salbutamol (5mg NEB STAT) or nebulised adrenaline (5ml (5mg) of 1:1000 adrenaline) may also help; give antihistamines (eg chlorphenamine 10mg IV STAT) and steroids (eg hydrocortisone 200mg IV STAT). Identify and stop any likely precipitant (eg new ACEi) and avoid in future; request C1 esterase inhibitor assays and consider referral to an immunologist if severe/frequent episodes and precipitating cause not clear (androgens, tranexamic acid and FFP are all used to prevent attacks in hereditary angioedema).

Limb swelling covered elsewhere			
Cellulitis	□ p412	Renal failure	□ p373
Compartment syndrome	□ p447	Nephrotic syndrome	□ p376
Heart failure	□ p282	Cirrhosis	□ p316
Pre-eclampsia	□ p504	Anaphylaxis	□ p470
SVC obstruction	□ p283		

Joint pain

> *Worrying features* fever, weight loss, severe pain, rashes.

Think about *emergency* septic arthritis; ***polyarthritis*** rheumatoid, osteoarthritis, ankylosing spondylitis, psoriatic arthritis, connective tissue disease (eg SLE), reactive arthropathy, rheumatic fever, polymyalgia rheumatica, IBD; ***monoarthritis*** septic arthritis, trauma, crystal arthropathy (gout, pseudo-gout), monoarthritic presentation of polyarticular disease, leukaemia, endocarditis, sickle-cell, haemophilia.

Ask about *description of pain* site, relieving/exacerbating actions, duration, other joint involvement; *inflammatory symptoms* morning stiffness, pain that improves with exercise but not rest, alternating buttock pain, nocturnal pain during 2nd half of night only; *systemic* fever, night sweats, weight loss, nausea, rashes, altered bowel habit, mouth ulcers, dysuria, visual disturbance, dry eyes or mouth, trauma; *PMH* joint pain, gout, haemophilia, sickle-cell, trauma, IBD, heart problems; *DH* steroids, anticoagulants, thiazide diuretics; *FH* joint disease, IBD; *SH* occupation, mobility, help at home, change in lifestyle due to symptoms. **Obs** temp, HR, BP.

Look for see 📖 p146–152 for specific joint examinations; always check the joint above and below; *look* resting position/deformity, swelling, rashes, erythema; *feel* warmth, tenderness, nodules; *move* reduced range of movement (passive and active), crepitus; *systemic* finger clubbing, psoriasis (check nails and scalp), enthesitis (tenderness at tendon insertions eg Achilles), muscle tenderness, back flexion, sacroiliitis (pain on pelvic squeeze), gait, ulcers, lymphadenopathy, hepatomegaly, splenomegaly.

Investigations *blds* FBC, U+E, CK, CRP, ESR, RhF, ANA; also consider: sickle-cell, urate, anti-dsDNA, complement titres, antiphospholipid antibodies; *urine* dipstick ±send for casts; *imaging* X-ray affected joints; *joint aspiration* (M,C+S, crystals).

Classification of rheumatological disease

Systemic rheumatic disease
Inflammatory diseases affecting joints, with multiple extra-articular manifestations; autoantibodies aid classification but role in pathogenesis unclear. Examples include rheumatoid arthritis, SLE, myositis, scleroderma, mixed connective tissue disease.

Spondylarthropathies (seronegative arthopathies)
Group of chronic disorders with inflammation of the sacroiliac joint (sacroiliitis), vertebrae (spondylitis). All are associated with HLA-B27; serum rheumatoid factor is usually negative (hence 'seronegative'). Includes ankylosing spondylitis, psoriatic arthritis, reactive arthritis and enteropathic arthopathies.

Vasculitis
Inflammatory destruction of blood vessels; may be 2° to other inflammatory or infectious conditions; 1° forms include giant-cell arteritis, Churg–Strauss syndrome, Behçet's disease, polyarteritis nodosa, Wegener's granulomatosis.

Crystalline arthropathy
Crystal deposition in joints seen in gout and pseudogout; usually mono/oligoarticular.

Infectious arthritis
Joint infection, seen in septic arthritis; often occurs in already damaged joint. Also seen in disseminated gonococcal infection.

Table 15.8 *Common causes of joint pain*

	History	Examination	Investigations
Rheumatoid arthritis	Symmetrical; typically hands and wrists; malaise	Inflamed, swollen joints, early deformity	↑ESR, +ve RhF, erosive changes
Osteoarthritis	Chronic onset; typically in hands, hips and knees	Non-inflamed, ↓ROM	Normal blds; joint space narrowing, osteophytes
Septic arthritis	Fever, single joint, rapid onset	Tender, swollen, hot, red, unable to move	↑WCC/CRP/ ESR, +ve culture
Gout	Acute onset, severe single joint pain	Red, tender, swollen, tophi	Urate crystals on joint aspirate
Pseudo-gout	Gradual onset, single joint pain	Red, tender, swollen	CPP crystals on joint aspirate
Polymyalgia rheumatica	Elderly, symmetrical shoulder/pelvic pain	Muscle tenderness, pain on movement	↑↑ESR, ↑ALP
Ankylosing spondylitis	Back pain, stiffness, young male	↓Back flexion and chest expansion	↑ESR, −ve RhF, HLA-B27 +ve
Reactive arthritis	Lower limb pain, dysuria, eye pain	Inflamed joints, conjunctivitis, keratoderma blennorrhagica	↑ESR, −ve RhF, X-ray normal; throat/genital swabs for eg chlamydia
Psoriatic arthritis	Psoriasis, variable joint involvement	Psoriasis, nail changes, dactylitis	↑ESR, −ve RhF, erosive changes
SLE	Fever, malaise, weight loss, rash, lethargy	Malar rash, ulcers	ANA, dsDNA +ve, ↓Hb, ↓WCC, ↑ESR/CRP
Rheumatic fever	Sore throat, migratory joint pain, rash, fever	Murmur, chorea, nodules	↑ESR/CRP, ASOT +ve
IBD	Migratory arthritis, abdo pain, diarrhoea, PR bleeding	Abdo tenderness, erythema nodosum	Distinctive colonoscopy
Leukaemia	Weight loss, bruising, weakness	Petechiae, bruises, lymphadenopathy	↑↑WCC, ↓Hb
Sickle-cell	Dactylitis in children, septic arthritis all ages	Swollen, hot, tender monoarthritis	Sickle-cell positive, ↓Hb
Haemophilia	Sudden onset, single joint in children	Haemarthrosis, tender, swollen	↑APTT, ↓factor VIII or IX

Causes of joint pain covered elsewhere			
Trauma	📖 p434	Leukaemia	📖 p396
Osteomyelitis	📖 p447	IBD	📖 p309
Sickle cell	📖 p397	Haemophilia	📖 p405

Rheumatoid arthritis[1]

Chronic inflammatory disease causing symmetrical peripheral arthritis and systemic manifestations; associated with considerable morbidity and mortality.
Common joints PIP, MCP and MTP joints, wrist, elbow, knee, ankle.
Risk factors female sex (but worse prognosis in males), family history.
Symptoms morning stiffness, malaise, fatigue, mild fever, weight loss.
Signs swelling, redness, hand deformity (Swan neck or Boutonnière deformities and ulnar deviation of fingers; Z-deformity of thumb), nodules (elbows).
Investigations **blds** ↓Hb, normal MCV, ↑ESR, Rh factor +ve (80%), ANA +ve (30%); ***X-ray*** erosions, cysts, osteopenia, narrow joint space, deformity.
Treatment analgesia, NSAIDs, exercise, physiotherapy, corticosteroids, disease-modifying anti-rheumatic drugs (DMARDs) eg sulfasalazine, methotrexate, azathioprine, ciclosporin should be started at diagnosis ideally in combination, biological therapies (anti-TNFα eg infliximab), surgery (reconstructive, synovectomy, joint replacement, fusion).
Flare ups analgesia, splinting, corticosteroids (oral or intra-articular).
Complications joint destruction, septic arthritis, antiphospholipid syndrome.
Systemic manifestations MI, pericardial or pleural effusions, pulmonary fibrosis, Sjögren syndrome (dry eyes and mouth), episcleritis, nerve entrapment (🕮 p448), vasculitis, Felty syndrome (splenomegaly + neutropenia).

American College of Rheumatology diagnostic classification

≥4 of the following for ≥6wk supports a diagnosis of rheumatoid arthritis
- Morning stiffness >1h
- Symmetric arthritis
- Rheumatoid nodules
- +ve rheumatoid factor
- Arthritis of ≥3 left or right PIP, MCP, wrist, elbow, knee, ankle, and MTP joints
- Arthritis of ≥1 of PIP, MCP, wrist joints
- Typical radiographic changes

Osteoarthritis[2]

Common joints knees, hips, spine, DIP and PIP joints.
Risk factors age, female sex, previous trauma, obesity.
Symptoms pain worse with activity, stiffness on resting.
Signs initially none; effusion, deformity, reduced range of movement.
Investigations **blds** normal; ***X-ray*** loss of joint space, subchondral sclerosis, bone cysts and osteophyte formation.
Treatment exercise (especially strengthening of muscles near affected joints), weight loss, walking aids, analgesia (🕮 p86, eg paracetamol, NSAIDs (topical before PO), COX-2 inhibitors), steroid/local anaesthetic joint injections; joint replacement if refractory to medical therapy.
Complications disability, immobility, chronic pain, joint destruction.

Polymyalgia rheumatica

Symmetrical myalgia affecting muscles of neck, shoulder, hips or thighs.
Risk factors >50yr, female sex, giant-cell (temporal) arteritis.
Symptoms bilateral morning pain and stiffness in proximal muscles lasting >1h, weight loss, fatigue, malaise, depression, mild fever.
Signs muscle tenderness, normal power; ↓range of movement (from pain).
Investigations **blds** ↑↑ESR (typically >50mm/h), ↑CRP, ↑ALT, ↑ALP, ↓Hb, normal MCV, normal CK; temporal artery biopsy if suspect giant cell arteritis (🕮 p361).
Treatment prednisolone 20mg/24h PO, gradually reduced (over months).

[1] NICE guidance available at 🕮 **guidance.nice.org.uk/CG79**
[2] NICE guidance available at 🕮 **guidance.nice.org.uk/CG59**

▶▶Septic arthritis
Common joints single knee or hip.

Risk factors joint disease, prosthetic joint, immunosuppression, ↑age, DM, trauma.

Symptoms acute onset painful joint, swelling, fever.

Signs swollen, hot, tender, red, painful joint, often held slightly flexed, ↓range of movement.

Investigations **blds** ↑WCC, CRP and ESR, +ve blood culture; *joint aspiration* ↑WCC, organisms on Gram stain, +ve culture; *X-ray* as baseline.

Organisms staphylococci, *Streptococcus pyogenes*; Gram −ve bacilli or fungi in elderly or debilitated; TB.

Treatment analgesia, urgent orthopaedic referral, high-dose IV antibiotics for ≥6wk (eg co-amoxiclav 1.2g/8h IV) after diagnostic joint aspiration; may need repeated aspiration/surgical washout.

Complications joint destruction, 2° osteoarthritis, septicaemia.

Gout (urate crystal arthropathy)
Common joints monoarticular in 90%: eg great toe MTP, ankle, knee.

Risk factors ↑age, male sex, thiazide diuretics, red meat, alcohol.

Symptoms acute onset painful joint, ±fever; ↓range of movement.

Signs swollen, hot, tender, red, painful joint; *chronic* tophi (white/yellow or skin coloured nodules of urate) over Achilles, elbow, knee or ear.

Investigations exclude septic arthritis; **blds** ↑WCC/ESR/CRP; *joint aspiration* −ve birefringent needle-shaped crystals; *X-ray* normal.

Treatment **acute attack** rest, high fluid intake, reduce thiazide diuretics, alcohol and red meat, NSAIDs (eg diclofenac 50mg/8h PO) or steroids (eg prednisolone 40mg/24h PO for 3d, then tapered over 3wk); avoid colchicine (causes diarrhoea); *recurrent attacks* allopurinol (100mg/24h PO) reduces urate levels; do not start during acute attacks.

Pseudo-gout (calcium pyrophosphate crystal arthropathy)
Common joints mono/oligoarticular: knee, wrist, hips.

Risk factors age, family history, trauma, haemochromatosis.

Symptoms and signs are similar to gout, though less intense.

Investigations exclude septic arthritis; **blds** ↑WCC/ESR/CRP; *joint aspiration* weak +ve birefringent rhomboid-shaped crystals; *X-ray* calcification.

Treatment rest; NSAIDs (eg diclofenac 50mg/8h PO); intra-articular or oral steroids (eg prednisolone 40mg/24h PO for 3d, then tapered over 3 weeks); no effective prophylactic treatment.

Ankylosing spondylitis
Common joints sacroiliac, spine.

Risk factors male sex, HLA-B27.

Symptoms back pain worst at night, morning stiffness >1h, heel pain.

Signs fixed spinal kyphosis, restricted chest expansion, heel tenderness (enthesitis), pain on loading sacroiliac joints; uveitis.

Investigations **blds** ↑WCC/ESR/CRP, −ve RhF, HLA-B27 (92%); *X-ray* spinal and sacroiliac erosions, squared vertebrae, syndesmophytes (ossified edges of vertebral discs), fusion of spine (bamboo spine).

Treatment exercise; NSAIDs, sulfasalazine, biological therapies (anti-TNFα eg infliximab); spinal surgery.

Complications spinal fusion, aortic regurgitation, pulmonary fibrosis, restricted ventilation.

Reactive arthritis[1]

Arthritis developing 2–4wk after genitourinary or gastrointestinal infection.
Common joints asymmetrical affects large joints eg knee, ankle, hips.
Organisms triggers include *Chlamydia, Campylobacter, Shigella* and *Salmonella.*
Risk factors HLA-B27.
Symptoms recent diarrhoea or genitourinary infection; regardless of trigger, initial symptoms are often dysuria and urethral discharge; acute asymmetrical oligoarthritis with malaise, fatigue ±fever; heel pain, gritty eyes.
Signs bilateral conjunctivitis, swollen joints, tender tendon insertion points (enthesitis), genital ulceration, nail thickening; vesicles, pustules or plaques on genitals, palms or soles of feet (keratoderma blennorrhagica).
Investigations **blds** ↑WCC/ESR/CRP, –ve RhF and –ve ANA; **X-ray** initially normal; consider stool/throat/genital swabs for causative organism.
Treatment NSAIDs, rest, intra-articular or oral steroids; sulfasalazine or methotrexate if severe; 1% chloramphenicol ointment/6h for eyes; doxycycline 100mg PO/12h for 3mth if caused by *Chlamydia.*
Complications recurrent/chronic arthritis, ankylosing spondylitis (5%).

Enteropathic arthopathies

These rheumatological diseases are seen in the context of bowel inflammation, such as IBD, or after a gastrointestinal infection. All share an association with HLA-B27 and highlight a fascinating but poorly understood gut–joint immunological axis. Sacroiliitis, spondylitis, and asymmetrical hip or knee inflammation are accompanied by enthesitis (inflammation of points of insertion of tendons/ligaments into bone). Treatment of any underlying condition improves the arthritis.

Psoriatic arthritis (see also 📖 p417)

Common joints five distinct patterns of disease:
- Asymmetrical oligoarthritis (often fingers/toes + flexor tendons)
- Symmetrical polyarthritis (may resemble rheumatoid but involves DIP)
- Spondylitis ±sacroiliitis (may resemble ankylosing spondylitis)
- Asymmetric DIP arthropathy with nail changes
- Arthritis mutilans (widespread destruction of joints of hands).

Risk factors psoriasis (joint symptoms may present first), family history.
Symptoms vary with pattern; skin changes (of any form of psoriasis).
Signs nail ridging, pitting and lifting (onycholysis); psoriasis (check scalp, perineum, umbilicus); enthesitis, dactylitis (swollen fingers).
Investigations **blds** ↑WCC/ESR/CRP, –ve RhF and ANA; **X-ray** mild erosive changes especially in hands; osteopenia less extensive than rheumatoid.
Treatment rest, splinting; treat skin lesions (📖 p417); NSAIDs, intra-articular or oral steroids, methotrexate, ciclosporin; biological therapies (anti-TNFα eg infliximab); reconstructive surgery.
Complications joint destruction, immobility, antiphospholipid syndrome.

---

[1] The term 'Reiter's syndrome' is to be avoided, in light of the involvement of Hans Reiter (1881–1969) in the Nazi party, eugenics and 'research' in concentration camps.

Systemic lupus erythematosus (SLE)

Chronic, relapsing-remitting, multi-organ inflammatory disease; joint pain represents one of the commonest initial presentations of SLE.

Common joints symmetrical or asymmetrical; PIP, MCP, wrists, knees.

Risk factors ♀ (90%); African or South East Asian ethnicity.

Symptoms **systemic** malaise, fever, weight loss **musculoskeletal** joint or muscle pain **skin** photosensitive malar or discoid rash, oral ulcers **renal** oedema, haematuria **neurological** seizures, psychosis **lung** pleuritic chest pain, dyspnoea **cardiac** exertional chest pain or pain on sitting forwards (pericarditis) **GI** abdo pain, diarrhoea **haematological** pallor, frequent infections, recurrent miscarriage.

Signs arthritis (swelling, tender), malar/discoid rash, oral ulcers, altered mental state, pericardial or pleuritic rubs, peritonitis.

Investigations **blds** ↓Hb/WCC/plts, ↓C4±C3, ↑ESR, ANA +ve (95%, but non specific), dsDNA +ve (70%, highly specific, reflects disease activity), anti-Sm +ve (40%, most specific), U+E; **urine** blood, protein, casts; **X-ray** non-erosive arthritis, pleural effusions; **echo** valve vegetations, pericardial effusion.

Treatment NSAIDs, hydroxychloroquine ± oral steroids (for flares) in mild disease; methotrexate, azathioprine, mycophenolate in more severe disease; limited evidence for biological therapies (eg belimumab, rituximab).

Complications IHD, stroke, antiphospholipid syndrome (10%).

Drug induced certain drugs can cause a lupus-like syndrome that resolves promptly upon drug withdrawal; these include isoniazid, methyldopa, hydralazine and diltiazem.

American College of Rheumatology diagnostic classification

The presence of ≥4 of the following supports a diagnosis of SLE:

- **A**rthralgia
- **R**enal disease
- **A**NA +ve
- **S**erositis (pleuritic or pericardial)
- **H**aematological abnormalities (↓Hb/WCC/plts)
- **P**hotosensitivity
- **O**ral ulcers
- **I**mmunological tests (eg anti-dsDNA, anti-Sm)
- **N**europsychiatric symptoms (seizures, psychosis)
- **M**alar rash
- **D**iscoid rash

Can be remembered by the mnemonic 'A RASH POINts MD'.

Antiphospholipid syndrome (APS)

Antibodies to membrane phospholipids (formerly confusingly referred to as 'lupus anticoagulant') are found in severe inflammatory diseases as well as in normal individuals. APS is the association of antiphospholipid antibodies with arterial or venous thromboembolism, or recurrent or late-term miscarriage.

Rheumatic fever

This migratory polyarthritis occurring 2–6wk after a streptococcal infection was previously a common cause of childhood mortality and structural heart disease, but is now rare in the developed world.

Diagnosis requires 2 major or 1 major and 2 minor 'Jones' criteria:

- *Major* Carditis (new murmur, valve lesions, CCF); migratory large joint polyarthritis; Aschoff bodies (firm, painless nodules on wrist, elbow or knee); erythema marginatum (pink rings on trunk or limbs); Sydenham's chorea (face or arms)
- *Minor* Prolonged PR interval (if carditis not counted); arthralgia (if polyarthritis not counted); ↑WCC/CRP/ESR; fever, previous rheumatic fever.

Treatment penicillin, NSAIDs ±steroids (see *Children's BNF*).

Neck lumps

Worrying features >45yr, weight loss, night sweats, hard irregular lump.

Think about *serious* malignancy (primary, metastases, lymphoma); **common** many of the lumps on 🕮 p420; see Table 15.9 for lumps found only in the neck.

Table 15.9 *Location and causes of neck lumps*

Location	Causes
Midline	Goitre, thyroid isthmus mass, dermoid cyst, thyroglossal cyst
Anterior triangle	Lymph node, thyroid mass, salivary gland mass, branchial cyst, carotid artery aneurysm
Posterior triangle	Lymph node, cervical rib, pharyngeal pouch

Ask about location, onset, duration, change with time, pain, other lumps, trauma, bites, infections, skin changes, systemic symptoms (eg weight loss, vomiting, fever), sore throat, cough, hoarse voice; **PMH** previous lumps, cancer, radiotherapy, thyroid problems; **SH** foreign travel, smoking, alcohol intake; **FH** thyroid disease, cancer.

Look for assess as for other lumps (🕮 p420) along with the following: movement on swallowing, movement on tongue protrusion, dentition, mouth ulcers, lumps inside the mouth, lumps in the tongue, appearance of the tonsils (?asymmetry), ear examination, facial nerve palsies.

Investigation *blds* consider FBC, U+E, LFT, TFT, CRP, ESR; *imaging* CXR, USS, CT/MRI; *biopsy* fine needle aspiration (FNA) especially for thyroid or salivary gland lumps, USS-guided biopsy, excision biopsy.

Management a neck lump should always be taken seriously and referred to ENT unless it is clearly a reactive lymph node.

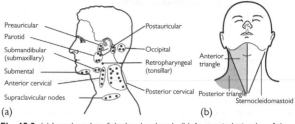

Fig. 15.3 (a) Lymph nodes of the head and neck. (b) Anatomical triangles of the neck.

Thyroid lump/goitre

Symptoms and signs midline or anterior triangle mass, moves with swallowing but not with protruding tongue, may be hypo/eu/hyperthyroid.

Management send TFT, arrange USS and refer to ENT for fine needle aspiration; increasing risk of malignancy with increasing age.

Salivary gland lump

Causes stone, gland inflammation (eg mumps), malignancy.

Symptoms and signs lump in sublingual, submandibular, or parotid gland.

Management refer discrete lumps to ENT for fine needle aspiration; increasing risk of malignancy with increasing age; suspect mumps if diffuse uni- or bilateral parotid enlargement with fever (supportive management).

Thyroglossal cyst

Embryological remnant from the descent of the thyroid gland.

Symptoms and signs young patient (<40yr) with single lump by the hyoid which moves with swallowing and protruding tongue, may be inflamed.

Management confirm presence of functioning thyroid gland, since may be the only thyroid tissue; refer to ENT for removal (Sistrunk procedure).

Dermoid cyst

A benign, cystic teratoma which may contain fat or hair.

Symptoms and signs single subcutaneous lump, found in the midline of the neck or next to the eye in young patients (<20yr).

Management refer to ENT for complete removal, can recur.

Branchial cyst

Incomplete closure of an embryological branchial arch, resulting in a cyst.

Symptoms and signs slowly enlarging smooth mass, typically presenting in 2nd or 3rd decade; most arise from 2nd branchial arch, appearing at the anterior border of sternocleidomastoid; may be tender, or enlarge after URTI.

Management refer to ENT for surgical excision, may recur.

Pharyngeal pouch (Zenker diverticulum)

Symptoms and signs elderly patient with upper oesophageal dysphagia; regurgitation of undigested food; halitosis; mass rarely palpable.

Management confirmed by contrast swallow, treated by surgical myotomy.

Cervical rib

Congenital abnormality, with an extra rib arising from C7.

Symptoms and signs hard mass in posterior triangle; usually unilateral; may have Raynaud's, distal muscle weakness or pain. Adson's sign is loss of radial pulse on elevation of arm on affected side.

Management may require physiotherapy or excision if causing problems.

ENT

> *Worrying features* unilateral hearing loss, mastoid pain, unilateral tonsillar enlargement, hoarse voice >3wk, stridor, dysphagia, systemic symptoms, night sweats.

Earache and deafness (OHGP3 📖 p942)

Think about serious acute mastoiditis; ***common acute*** URTI, foreign body otitis media, otitis externa, tonsillar pathology; *serious chronic* cholesteatoma, acoustic neuroma; ***common chronic*** glue ear, chronic suppurative otitis media (CSOM), earwax, presbyacusis (age-related deafness).

Ask about onset, duration, discharge, itching, hearing loss, speech problems, runny nose, sore throat, trauma, malaise.

Look for pyrexia, appearance of eardrum (?perforated), effusion, colour of canal, discharge, tonsils, lymphadenopathy, dental abscess, mastoid/sinus pain.

Management most earache simply requires analgesia, consider:
- **Otitis media** red, bulging drum ± effusion; pus/bloody discharge if drum perforated; analgesia, antibiotics if <2yr old, moderate to severe pain, or T>39°C (eg amoxicillin at dose appropriate for age; check children's *BNF*)
- **Otitis externa** itching, tender, discharge ± pus; clean canal and keep dry (may need aural toilet by ENT), give gentamicin + steroid ear drops
- **Ear wax** olive oil (drops into ear/6h for 5d) prior to syringing with warm water (ensure drum not perforated)
- **Glue ear** persistent middle ear effusion with deafness usually lasts 3–6mth; a 2–6wk course of amoxicillin may help. ENT referral for grommets is only required if persistent and falling behind at school
- **CSOM** central perforation of drum, treat as for otitis externa
- **Cholesteatoma** squamous epithelium proliferating within middle ear; unilateral deafness with chronic, painless discharge; requires ENT referral
- **Acoustic neuroma** unilateral deafness ±tinnitus or vertigo; requires ENT referral
- **Presbyacusis** bilateral hearing loss with age, consider hearing aid.

Epistaxis (nosebleeds)

Ask about onset, duration, previous episodes, trauma, ↑BP, NSAID/anticoagulation therapy, bleeding tendency, cirrhosis, alcohol.

Look for postural BP change, shock; evidence of trauma/fracture.

Investigations if persistent/recurrent: BP; FBC, clotting, LFT.

Management resuscitate if needed (📖 p472); try to stop bleeding:
- Tilt head down, apply pressure to the soft fleshy part of the nose for 15min
- Pack with nasal tampons leaving the attached ribbon visible to aid removal after 48h (irrigate with saline first); if further bleeding refer to ENT for cautery.

In severe, persistent bleeding, continue resuscitation and refer urgently to ENT.

Sore throats (OHGP2 📖 p932)

Think about serious peritonsillar or retropharyngeal abscess, leukaemia/ neutropenia; ***common*** viral URTI, tonsillitis, glandular fever.

Ask about duration, coryzal symptoms, odynophagia, otalgia, night sweats, drug history.

Look for pyrexia, enlarged tonsils ± pus, red throat, lymphadenopathy; fever, odynophagia, neck stiffness ± dyspnoea suggest possible abscess.

Management urgent FBC if possibility of neutropenia (eg chemotherapy, azathioprine); urgent ENT referral for drainage and IV antibiotics if abscess suspected; otherwise reassure, gargle with soluble aspirin, regular analgesia (paracetamol and ibuprofen) ± over-the-counter medications (eg Difflam® see *BNF*). Consider antibiotics (eg phenoxymethylpencillin 500mg/6h PO) if persistent or pus seen over tonsils.

Persistent consider alternative diagnosis including EBV serology; consider tonsillectomy in those with ≥5 disabling sore throats/year for 2yr.

Groin lumps

> *Worrying features* testicular mass, painful lump, tenderness, vomiting, constipation.

Think about *serious* testicular cancer, testicular torsion, strangulated hernia; **common** lymph node, inguinal hernia, femoral hernia, hydrocele, varicocele, spermatocele, epididymitis/orchitis, ectopic testis, urogenital prolapse, saphena varix, groin abscess. See Fig. 15.4.

Ask about location, onset, duration, change with time, pain, reducibility, other lumps, trauma, skin changes, coughing, lifting, nausea, vomiting, constipation, weight loss, urinary incontinence; **PMH** previous lumps, cancer; ♀: previous pregnancies, type of delivery; **SH** foreign travel, IVDU, recent intercourse, condom usage; **FH** cancer.

Look for see 📖 p156 for female genital examination, 📖 p155 for male.

Management most lumps can be identified from history and examination; painful lumps need immediate referral to surgeons to exclude testicular torsion or strangulated hernias. Testicular lumps need urgent (2wk) referral.

Inguinal hernia
Risk factors ♂, increasing age, chronic cough, constipation, heavy lifting, previous abdominal surgery, ascites, obesity.
Symptoms often asymptomatic apart from lump.
Signs examine with the patient lying, then repeat standing up: scars, external genitalia, tenderness, reducibility (by patient and yourself), cough impulse, check other side; only 'indirect' hernias extend into the scrotum.
Management **conservative** weight loss, truss, high-fibre diet, stop smoking, treat lung disease; **surgery** day surgery, either open or laparoscopic.
Complications irreducible hernia, strangulation.

Femoral hernia
As for inguinal hernia but more common in women and greater risk of irreducibility and strangulation; surgical repair at earliest opportunity.

▶▶Strangulated hernia
An irreducible hernia where the blood supply has been compromised.
Symptoms irreducible, painful lump near a hernial orifice (usually inguinal or femoral); may have nausea, vomiting, absolute constipation, abdo pain.
Signs tender, red lump ±abdominal distension, ±peritonism.
Investigations **blds** FBC, U+E, glucose, amylase, CRP, G+S; **AXR** (exclude bowel obstruction); **erect CXR** (exclude bowel perforation).
Management request urgent senior review; NBM, analgesia (eg morphine 5mg IV PRN (titrate to pain) with cyclizine 50mg/8h IV), IV access and fluids (📖 p381); book emergency theatre.

Saphena varix
Dilated proximal long saphenous vein due to incompetent valves.
Symptoms and signs single, soft, compressible, bluish lump below the inguinal ligament, disappears on lying, cough impulse present.
Management high saphenous vein ligation.

Groin abscess

Common in IVDU after injection in groin with dirty needles; manage as for skin abscess (📖 p421), but consider DVT, endocarditis, HIV and atypical infections.

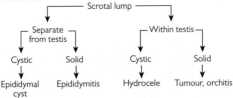

Fig. 15.4 Differential diagnosis of a scrotal lump.

▶▶Testicular torsion

This is an emergency – if you suspect torsion, get a senior review immediately as testicular tissue will become necrotic in hours.

Symptoms lower abdominal pain, swollen/painful testis, nausea, vomiting.

Signs ↑HR, high riding/horizontal-lying testis, thickened spermatic cord (early sign), −ve Prehn's sign (elevating testis does not relieve pain: if +ve more suggestive of epididymitis), absent cremasteric reflex.

Differential diagnosis epididymo-orchitis, hydrocele, testicular tumour.

Management request urgent senior review; diagnosis may be confirmed on Doppler USS but this should not delay emergency surgical exploration; NBM, analgesia (eg morphine 5mg IV PRN (titrate to pain) with cyclizine 50mg/8h IV), IV access and fluids (📖 p381); book emergency theatre.

Complications testicular necrosis, infertility, contralateral torsion if not fixed.

Hydrocele

Fluid in the tunica vaginalis surrounding the testis.

Symptoms and signs enlarged 'testicle', soft, non-tender, smooth, well-defined, transilluminable.

Investigations can be secondary to a testicular tumour, **USS** if in doubt.

Management conservative if asymptomatic; surgical intervention involves eversion and suturing of the tunica vaginalis; aspiration ± sclerosant is an alternative in patients unsuitable for surgery, but associated with recurrence.

Spermatocele (epididymal cyst)

Benign cystic accumulation of sperm within the head of the epididymis.

Symptoms and signs soft, small, well-defined, spherical, transilluminable, separate (superior) to the testis; painless, but may be uncomfortable.

Management transscrotal excision, only if symptomatic.

Varicocele

Varicose veins within the spermatic cord, associated with subfertility.

Symptoms and signs soft, tubular lumps like a 'bag of worms' above the testicle, resolves on lying, cough impulse present; may be uncomfortable.

Management usually none; surgical ligation can improve fertility.

Ectopic testis

Embryological failure of testis to descend through inguinal canal.

Symptoms and signs usually diagnosed in childhood; smooth, well-defined, spherical mass between inguinal ring and scrotum, empty scrotal sac on the same side.

Management surgical orchidopexy to reduce cancer risk.

Epididymitis/orchitis

Infection of epididymis/testis after UTI or STI; may mimic testicular torsion.

Causes Chlamydia species, *N. gonorrhoea*, *E. coli*, viral eg mumps.

Symptoms and signs acute testicular swelling and pain, tender, enlarged testis ±urethral discharge, fever.

Management exclude testicular torsion (📖 p463) and assess for STI (📖 p465) and UTI (urine dipstick/M,C+S); most infections will respond to doxycycline 100mg/12h PO and analgesia.

Testicular cancer

Symptoms painless lump felt within testicle, difference in size of testicles.

Signs hard, non-transilluminable, irregular surface to testicle, may have a 2° hydrocele.

Investigations **blds** FBC, LFT, α-FP, β-hCG, LDH; *imaging* scrotal USS, CXR and CT for staging; *biopsy*.

Management surgical removal with radiotherapy and/or chemotherapy.

Prognosis 98% 5yr survival.

Urogenital prolapse

Risk factors multiple childbirth, vaginal deliveries, large babies, heavy lifting, age, chronic cough, constipation, obesity.

Symptoms vaginal lump, dragging sensation, urinary frequency/urgency, urinary incontinence, constipation, intercourse problems.

Signs **PV** exclude masses, prolapse may be seen on asking patient to 'bear down' during speculum examination.

Treatment weight loss, stop smoking, treat constipation, pelvic floor exercises; *interventional* ring pessaries;[1] *surgery* hysterectomy, pelvic floor repair.

Table 15.10 *Types of urogenital prolapse*

Uterine prolapse	**First degree**	cervix remains within vagina
	Second degree	cervix visible at introitus
	Third degree	procidentia; uterus protruding from vagina
Vault prolapse	Prolapse of the vaginal wall after hysterectomy; may contain small intestine or omentum	
Urethrocele	Urethra bulges onto the lower anterior vaginal wall	
Cystocele	Bladder wall bulges on the anterior vaginal wall	
Rectocele	Rectal wall bulges into the middle posterior vaginal wall	
Enterocele	Intestinal loops herniate into the upper posterior vaginal wall	

[1] Review every 6mth to replace, check for bleeding/ulceration and symptoms. Prescribe topical oestrogen to reduce the risk of ulceration.

Sexually transmitted infections (STIs)

Until recently known as venereal disease (after Venus, the Roman goddess of love) patients may present to the emergency department or their GP complaining of symptoms of an STI. These patients should always be given information about and encouraged to attend the local sexual health clinic, ideally with any current partner. Since coinfection with multiple STIs is common, these clinics offer comprehensive screening, sexual health advice and contact tracing where necessary. Some common infections include:

- **Gonorrhoea** (*Neisseria gonorrhoeae*) Symptoms usually appear 1–14d after exposure and include yellow/green discharge with dysuria in both sexes. Diagnosis involves Gram staining and culture of high vaginal or urethral swabs, and PCR. Usually sensitive to cephalosporins, as increasingly resistant to fluoroquinolones (ciprofloxacin, levofloxacin).
- **Chlamydia** (*Chlamydia trachomatis* serovars D-K) Symptoms usually appear 1–3wk after exposure and include watery/white discharge ± dysuria in both sexes. Infection can often go unnoticed (especially in women). Diagnosis involves antigen detection or PCR, using live cells acquired from endocervical (♀) or urethral (♂) swabs using a special swab and transport medium. Usually sensitive to tetracyclines or macrolides.
- **Lymphogranuloma venerum** (*Chlamydia trachomatis* serovars L1–3) Increasingly common amongst homosexual men in Europe. Primary infection is marked by the appearance of a painless ulcer at the inoculation site after 3–12d; secondary disease appears after up to 6mth, with tender unilateral lymphadenopathy, or proctitis in anal inoculation. Diagnosis is either serological or with PCR. Usually sensitive to tetracyclines or macrolides.
- **Syphilis** (*Treponema pallidum*) Symptoms can take up to 3mth to appear. Primary disease causes a painless genital ulcer. Secondary disease causes perianal plaques, a non-itchy rash and flu-like symptoms. Diagnosis is serological, usually using a combination of a nontreponemal screening test (eg VDRL), with confirmation using a treponemal specific test (eg FTA-ABS). Treatment is with IM benzylpenicillin.
- **Genital herpes** (herpes simplex virus, usually type 2) Symptoms usually appear 2–7d after exposure, causing itching, tingling or small fluid-filled vesicles in genital area. Diagnosis is clinical, supported by PCR where necessary. Episodes can be treated with antivirals (eg aciclovir), but this does not 'cure' the disease (see also 🕮 p415).
- **Genital warts** (human papillomavirus, especially types 6, 11) Small fleshy tags or larger cauliflower-shaped lesions. Diagnosis is clinical, supported by PCR testing where necessary. Always ensure a recent cervical smear in affected women. Treatment is with topical keratolytic or cryotherapy. Likely to recur (see also 🕮 p421).
- **Pubic lice** (*Pthirus pubis*) Symptoms take 1–14d after exposure and include pruritus in hairy infected areas in both sexes. Diagnosis is by light microscopy. Treatment is with parasiticidal topical preparation which should be repeated at 7d to kill lice emerging from surviving eggs (see also 🕮 p416).

Burns emergency

Airway	If airway involved – **CALL ANAESTHETIST**
Breathing	If no respiratory effort – **CALL ARREST TEAM**
Circulation	If no palpable pulse – **CALL ARREST TEAM**

▶▶Call for **senior help** early if patient deteriorating or >10% burns.

Airway/C-spine

- **Apply** collar, sandbags, and tape if C-spine injury is possible
- **Look** for burns to the face and neck, singed eyebrows, facial hair or nasal hairs, soot around the nostrils or in the sputum, facial swelling
- **Listen** for snoring noises, stridor, hoarse voice
- **Intubation** if inhalation injury suspected to prevent airway obstruction.

Breathing

- **15l/min O_2** if SOB or sats <94%
- **Count** RR; rapid breathing suggests inhalation injury
- **Monitor** O_2 sats and RR
- **Escharotomy** if circumferential chest burns are restricting breathing.

Circulation

- **Venous access**, send bloods for
  - FBC, U+E, glucose, clotting, G+S
  - carboxyhaemoglobin (COHb) – try the blood gas machine
- **Give** 0.9% saline 1l STAT
- **Give** morphine IV (eg 10mg titrated to pain) and cyclizine 50mg IV
- **Monitor** HR with defibrillator ECG leads and BP for signs of shock.

Disability

- **Assess GCS** and check glucose
- **Look/feel** for pupil reflexes, limb tone and plantar reflexes.

Exposure

- **Measure** the extent of 2nd-/3rd-degree burn, see Fig. 15.5
- **Cover the burn** with cling film as analgesia, avoid creams
- Check **temp**.

Further resuscitation

- Obtain **history** and **examine** the patient
- **Calculate** fluid requirements and adjust rate accordingly (see 'Burns fluid resuscitation')
- **Catheterise** to monitor urine output
- **CXR** for trauma and as a baseline (signs of inhalation injury after 24h)
- **ABG** if respiratory distress
- **Monitor** circulation of all limbs with burns
- Call for **senior** help
- **Reassess**, starting with A, B, C …

Serious complications

• Hypovolaemia	📖 p472	• Coexisting trauma	📖 p434
• Carbon monoxide poisoning	📖 p469	• Limb ischaemia	📖 p446
• Inhalation injury	📖 p469	• Restriction of breathing	📖 p270

Measuring the burn

Burn sizes are expressed as a percentage of the skin surface covered by 2nd- or 3rd-degree burns. 1st-degree burns (erythema only) are not counted. The Lund and Browder chart[1] in Fig. 15.5 works for children and adults:

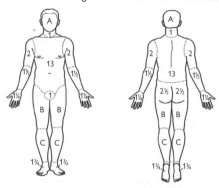

Relative percentage of body surface area affected by growth						
Area	<1yr	1yr	5yrs	10yrs	15yrs	Adult
A (½ of head)	9½	8½	6½	5½	4½	3½
B (½ of one thigh)	2¾	3¼	4	4¼	4½	4¾
C (½ of one leg)	2½	2½	2¾	3	3¼	3½

Fig. 15.5 Lund and Browder chart. [1]

The palm (not including fingers) of a patient's hand is about 0.75–1% of their body surface area and this can be used for smaller burns. Alternatively the 'rule of nines' can be used for adults:

Head	Each arm	Each leg	Trunk front	Trunk back	Perineum
9%	9%	18%	18%	18%	1%

Burns fluid resuscitation

The burn size is used to calculate fluid requirement for resuscitation using the following formula:

- $(4 \times$ weight (kg)) $\times$ percentage of burn = volume over 24h (ml)

Give half over the first 8h after injury (ie over 6h if presented at 2h):

- (Volume over 24h (ml) $\div$ 2) $\div$ 8 = rate per hour (ml)

The other half is given over 16h:

- (Volume over 24h (ml) $\div$ 2) $\div$ 16 = rate per hour (ml)

So for a 70kg man with 30% burns the rate is 525ml/h for the first 8h then 263ml/h for the next 16h. This is only a guide, monitor the volume status and urine output to maintain volume (📖 p380).

[1] Reproduced from Lund, C.C., Browder, N.C. *Surg Gynaecol Obstet* 1944 **79:**352.

Burns

> *Worrying features* HR >100, systolic BP <100mmHg, RR >30, O_2 sats <92%, signs of inhalation injury, full thickness or circumferential burn, fires indoors, explosions, >10% skin involvement.

Think about *life/limb threatening* see 🕮 p466; **most likely** cutaneous burns, chemical/electrical burn, carbon monoxide poisoning, non-accidental injury, associated injuries (fractures, wounds, eye/ear trauma).

Ask about mechanism of burn, time of burn, explosions, smoke, cause of fire, place where fire occurred, duration of exposure, immediate treatment, falls/jumping out of windows, trauma, breathing difficulty, pain; **PMH** cardiac or respiratory problems, previous burns/trauma; **DH** allergies, tetanus status; **SH** smoking (COHb result), housing (do they have somewhere to go?)

Obs temp, RR, BP, HR, O_2 sats.

Look for soot around nostrils/mouth, facial burns, swelling, singed facial hair, nostril hair or eyebrows, stridor, hoarse voice, degree of burn (see Table 15.11), colour, sensation, blistering, extent of burn, location of burn, circumferential burns, other trauma.

Depth of burn is assessed by the appearance, blanching, sensation and bleeding when pricked with a needle; it can be difficult to assess especially as different depths may be close together so that a patient may report pain in an area of full thickness burn. Always get a senior's opinion.

Investigations *blds* COHb if fire occurred inside; *consider* ABG, CXR.

Table 15.11 *Classifying burn severity*

Depth	Superficial	Partial dermal	Deep dermal	Full thickness
Degree	1st	2nd		3rd
Colour	Red	Pink, blisters	Bright red, mottled	White, brown, black, leathery
Blanching	Yes	Yes	No	No
Sensation	Yes	Yes	Yes	No
Bleeding	Yes	Yes	Slow	No

Treatment

Major burns (>10% skin surface) resuscitate as per protocol (🕮 p467).
Minor burns cool with running cold water for 10–20min as soon as possible after the injury. Offer analgesia (🕮 p86) and cover the burn with cling film until management has been determined. The following should be referred to plastics for assessment:
• All burns to the face, hand, or genitalia unless small and superficial
• All deep dermal/full thickness burns larger than a postage stamp.
Ask for their advice on dressings (often minimal as some dressings alter the appearance of the burn).
Other burns should be cleaned with water and dressed.

Dressings

If referring straight to plastic surgery cover the burn in cling film. Otherwise aim to keep the burn covered with a sterile and non-adherent dressing:

- **Silver sulfadiazine cream** (eg Flamazine®) silver has antibiotic effects to reduce the risk of infection; it should be pasted on 3–5mm thick
- **Paraffin impregnated gauze** (eg Jelonet®) this is a non-adherent dressing; it can be applied over silver sulfadiazine cream
- **Sterile gauze** and crepe bandages can be used on top of Jelonet®
- **Polythene bag/glove** this can be placed over a burn to the hand treated with silver sulfadiazine cream
- **Paraffin wax/Vaseline®** can be applied often for areas difficult to dress
- The burn should be reviewed and redressed in 2–3d.

> #### Tetanus
> Burns can cause inoculation with tetanus; manage in the same way as wounds (🕮 p437).

▶▶Inhalation injury

Inhalation of smoke can cause delayed obstruction of the airway.

Symptoms breathlessness, hoarse voice, dysphagia, confusion.

Signs singed facial hair or eyebrows, soot around the nostrils or palate, facial/neck burns, stridor, drooling, swelling near the airways, wheeze.

Investigations ↓PEFR; **blds** ↑COHb (see 'Carbon monoxide poisoning'); **ABG** acidosis, hypoxia, hypercapnia; **ECG** exclude dysrhythmia/ischaemia; **CXR** ARDS after 24h.

Management symptoms or signs of inhalation injury should prompt early intubation, high-flow humidified O_2, salbutamol.

Complications pulmonary oedema, ARDS, upper airway obstruction.

▶▶Carbon monoxide poisoning

This must be considered in all patients involved in fire-related injuries.

Symptoms headache, vomiting, malaise, lethargy, dysrhythmias.

Signs often none, O_2 sats will be falsely high, cherry-red lips (rare).

Results COHb available on some gas analysers – seek advice. >30% is considered serious; very heavy smokers may have a COHb of up to 15%; **ABG** may show metabolic acidosis; **ECG** to exclude dysrhythmia/ischaemia.

Management 15l/min O_2 by tight fitting mask and reservoir for >24h (use humidified O_2); consider mannitol, ventilation, hyperbaric O_2.

Complications cerebral oedema, pulmonary oedema, MI, dysrhythmia.

▶▶Chemical burns

These can be severe, especially if alkalis are involved. They should be washed in running water for at least 20min; larger burns may need fluid replacement as for thermal burns (🕮 p467). Toxbase (🕮 p493) will give advice on the treatment of specific chemical burns.

▶▶Electrical burns

These can cause dysrhythmias, cardiac damage and severe muscle damage resulting in renal failure or compartment syndrome. **ECG** in all patients; **blds** FBC, U+E, ↑CK; **urine** dipstick if severe or high voltage (>1000V) for blood (actually detecting myoglobinuria).

Anaphylaxis in adults (OHCM9 📖 p806)

Airway	If airway involved – **CALL ANAESTHETIST**
Breathing	If no respiratory effort – **CALL ARREST TEAM**
Circulation	If no palpable pulse – **CALL ARREST TEAM**

▶▶Call for **senior help** early if anaphylaxis suspected.
- **Sit patient up** unless hypotensive, then lay flat with legs elevated
- **15l/min O₂** in all patients
- **Monitor** pulse oximeter, BP, defibrillator ECG leads if unwell
- Request full set of **observations**
- Take brief **history** if possible/check **drug chart**/ask ward staff
- **Examine patient**: look for early signs of anaphylaxis (see box)
- Establish **likely cause** and stop further exposure (eg IV antibiotics)
- **Adrenaline**, 1:1000 solution, 0.5ml (0.5mg) **intramuscular**:
  - **repeat after** 5min if no improvement
- Large-bore **venous access**, take bloods if time permits:
  - FBC, U+E, mast cell tryptase (see 'Investigations')
- IV infusion of **1l 0.9% saline** STAT
- Consider nebulised β-agonist for **bronchospasm**:
  - salbutamol 5mg, or
  - adrenaline 1:1000 solution, 5ml (5mg)
- Re-assess
- Consider **adjuncts** to treatment:
  - antihistamine, eg chlorphenamine 10mg slow IV
  - hydrocortisone 200mg slow IV
- Ensure **senior help** has been requested.

Intramuscular adrenaline should be given if the diagnosis of anaphylaxis is likely but **not if the symptoms are mild** or the patient is well.

Early signs of anaphylaxis

• Urticaria	• Flushing
• Bronchospasm/stridor	• Abdominal pain
• Vomiting and/or diarrhoea	• Sense of impending doom.

▶▶Anaphylaxis

Worrying signs BP <90mmHg systolic, ↓O$_2$ sats, chest tightness, stridor.

Common precipitants	
Drugs	Penicillins, anaesthetic drugs, contrast media, blood products
Environmental	Latex, stings, eggs, fish, strawberries, nuts

Symptoms chest tightness, wheeze, breathlessness, itching, swelling, anxiety/fear/agitation, GI disturbance (vomiting, abdominal pain, diarrohea).

Signs see box; later hypotension, tachycardia, tongue/periorbital swelling, wheeze, cyanosis. Treat all patients with physical signs.

Investigations ▶▶if you suspect anaphylactic shock commence treatment

(see 📖 p470): seconds count. Subsequently check for serum mast cell tryptase to confirm global mast cell degranulation (send three samples of clotted blood: one during the reaction once adrenaline has been given, one 1h post-reaction, and one 6–24h post-reaction).

Follow-up by immunologist; consider adrenaline for self-injection (eg EpiPen®).

Adrenaline (epinephrine) preparations	
1:1000	Preparation – 1ml ampoule. Give 0.5ml (0.5mg) IM 1mg in 1ml
1:10,000	Preparation – 10ml syringe in cardiac arrest drugs, or 10ml ampoule 1mg in 10ml

Intramuscular adrenaline should be given if the diagnosis of anaphylaxis is likely but **not if the symptoms are mild** or the patient is well.

Hypotension emergency

Airway	If airway involved – **CALL ANAESTHETIST**
Breathing	If no respiratory effort – **CALL ARREST TEAM**
Circulation	If no palpable pulse – **CALL ARREST TEAM**

▶▶Call for **senior help** early if patient deteriorating

Systolic <100mmHg:
- Lay patient flat and **elevate the legs** if dizzy
- **15l/min O₂** if SOB or sats <94%
- **Monitor** pulse oximeter, BP, defibrillator ECG leads if unwell
- Request full set of **observations** and **ECG**
- Take brief **history** if possible/check **notes**/ask ward staff
- **Examine patient**: condensed RS, CVS, abdo and neuro exam
- Establish **likely cause of shock**
- Large-bore **venous access**, take bloods:
  - FBC, U+E, CRP, D-dimer, cardiac markers, blood cultures
- IV infusion of **1l 0.9% saline** STAT
- **Treat** most likely cause, see following sections
- **Arterial blood gas**, but don't leave the patient alone
- Consider requesting urgent **CXR**, portable if too unwell
- Call for **senior help**
- **Reassess**, starting with A, B, C …

Life-threatening causes

- Hypovolaemic/haemorrhagic shock (📖 p478)
- Septic shock (📖 p480)
- Cardiogenic shock (tamponade/tension pneumothorax/heart failure) (📖 p479)
- Anaphylactic shock (📖 p470)
- Neurogenic shock (spinal shock) (📖 p481).

Hypotension (systolic <100mmHG)

Worrying features ↓GCS, ↑↓HR, stridor, ↓O₂ sats, bleeding, chest pain, dizziness, ↓urine output, renal failure, severe back pain, non-blanching rash.

Think about *life-threatening* shock (hypovolaemic/haemorrhagic, septic, cardiogenic, anaphylactic, neurogenic), dysrhythmia (brady- or tachyarrhythmia); *other* postural hypotension, vasovagal episode, Addison's disease/adrenal insufficiency, drugs (β-blockers, ACEi, Ca²⁺ channel blockers, diuretics, nitrates).

Ask about *assess severity* shortness of breath, ↓GCS, feeling faint/ dizzy on standing, what is timecourse, and what BP does patient usually run (inspect recent obs charts); *consider cause* palpitations, chest pain, blood loss (haematemesis, melaena, PV bleeding), trauma, abdominal/back/loin pain, diarrhoea, vomiting, polyuria, fever, sweats, cough, urinary symptoms, itch/urticaria, spinal trauma or anaesthetic, weight loss, skin darkening; *PMH* AAA, gastroduodenal ulcers, pregnancy, diabetes insipidus and DM, infections (urinary, chest, cardiac, blood), immunocompromise, angina, MI, previous DVT/PE, Addison's disease, postural hypotension; *DH* cardiac medications (β-blockers, ACEi, Ca²⁺ channel blockers, diuretics, nitrates), blood transfusions, antibiotics, anticoagulants, recent anaesthetics, steroids (?withdrawal), allergies (?anaphylaxis); *FH* PE/DVT, Addison's/autoimmune disease; *SH* smoking, alcohol, recreational drug abuse.

Obs HR, BP, postural BP, RR, sats, temp, GCS, fluid balance.

Look for volume status (📖 p380), pulse rate/rhythm/volume, evidence of diarrhoea or vomiting, source of bleeding (limbs, chest, abdomen, back, mouth, PR, PV), palpable abdominal aortic aneurysm, abdominal guarding or tenderness, warm peripheries or fever, flushed appearance, sweating, urticaria, dyspnoea, focal signs in the chest (consolidation, tension pneumothorax, or pulmonary oedema), calf swelling or tenderness, wasting of small muscles of the hands or ↑skin pigmentation.

Investigations *serial BP* repeat BP manually to confirm diagnosis and check bilateral BP; *ECG* dysrhythmia, evidence of LVH/strain/MI; *blds* FBC, U+E, glucose, G+S (X-match if haemorrhage), CRP; consider D-dimer, cardiac markers, clotting, blood cultures, mast cell tryptase; *urine* dipstick and M,C+S, consider catheter; *CXR* consolidation, mediastinal widening; do not request if you suspect tension pneumothorax – perform immediate needle decompression (📖 p279); *pelvic X-ray* in trauma; *CT chest* may be necessary if aortic dissection suspected. Consider also central venous pressure monitoring via a central line, continuous arterial pressure can be monitored via an arterial line; *urgent echo* LV function, aortic root dilation/dissection, pericardial fluid (tamponade effect), massive PE, aortic/mitral valve prolapse.

Treatment ▶▶Call for senior help early Secure airway; O₂ (15l/min), lie as flat as tolerated ±elevate legs; monitor BP; IV access (secure appropriately large-bore cannula in antecubital fossa). If active bleeding give IV colloid and consider urgent blood transfusion (O-negative, type specific, or full X-match, 📖 p400). Otherwise give fluid challenge (📖 p381) at rate appropriate for degree of compromise and comorbidities (eg 1l 0.9% saline STAT if young, septic and ↓GCS; 250ml 0.9% saline 30min if elderly, CCF and alert). Try to establish and treat the likely cause.

Postural (orthostatic) hypotension

Drop in BP of >20/10mmHg measured >1min after standing from lying position; can occur when sitting from a lying position in severe disease.

Causes **volume depletion** dehydration, bleeding; **iatrogenic** antihypertensives, diuretics, nitrates, antidepressants; **autonomic neuropathy** DM, Guillain–Barré, syphilis, Parkinson's disease, ageing.

Symptoms dizziness ± loss of consciousness when standing.

Signs ↓systolic BP >20mmHg or ↓diastolic >10mmHg upon standing; ↑HR (in most instances; absence of tachycardia suggests autonomic aetiology).

Investigations lying/standing BP usually diagnostic. Other investigations as appropriate to investigate cause of syncope/collapse (📖 p442).

Acute treatment ensure patient safety. Review medications and identify likely precipitants; can these be stopped or changed for a drug without this side effect? Optimise control of DM. Identify and treat precipitating disease.

Chronic treatment advise simple lifestyle changes such as elevating the head of the bed, getting out of bed/chairs slowly and holding onto something as standing. In autonomic neuropathy, consider graduated stockings for lower legs, increasing salt and fluid intake, and mineralocorticoids (eg fludrocortisone 100–200micrograms/24h PO).

Complications falls and subsequent bone and soft tissue injuries including intracranial bleeding and fractured neck of femur.

Assessing the hypotensive in-patient

When on-call, you will frequently be asked to assess patients with low BP. Key factors to help identify the acutely unwell include a sudden ↓BP (inspect recent obs charts), other abnormal obs (↑temp, ↑RR, ↓urine output, ↓GCS, ↑HR – but beware those on a β-blocker). Early warning scores (📖 p224) can be helpful in this regard: Patients with worrying obs require urgent IV fluids and further assessment (?current diagnosis, ?sepsis, ?shock – 📖 p473), whilst the fit 30-year-old in the bed opposite, who feels quite well with his BP of 90/50mmHg, may safely be left to sleep.

▶▶Leaking abdominal aortic aneurysm (AAA) (OHCM9 📖 p656)

Most AAAs are asymptomatic, enlarging gradually until their dramatic presentation with sudden rupture and an associated dismal mortality. In the UK, the NHS AAA screening programme offers all men USS screening at 65yr, allowing elective repair where necessary.

If you suspect a ruptured/leaking AAA:

• Fast-bleep for senior help and vascular surgeon immediately
• Order urgent O −ve blood and urgent X-match 8 units.

Symptoms severe constant or colicky abdominal pain radiating to the back, collapse or feeling faint.

Risk factors ↑age, male, ↑BP, smoking, IHD, ↑cholesterol, known AAA.

Signs expansile abdominal mass (pushes hands apart, not just pulsating) – examination will **not** cause rupture; ↑HR, ±↓BP, ↑RR, pale, sweating, cool extremities, distension, tenderness, ↓peripheral pulses in legs.

Investigations none if unstable; urgent **CT** aids diagnosis and management.

Management emergency O₂ (15l/min); **resuscitate** large-bore IV access for bloods and STAT colloid/blood (keep systolic BP 90–100mmHg, do not raise above this as ↑risk of leak from AAA); prepare to transfer to theatre or interventional radiology suite; observations every 15min. Those unfit for intervention require palliative care (📖 p91).

Shock

Classification of shock

Shock has many definitions, but is essentially a problem at the cellular level and results from inadequate tissue perfusion. There are several causes, and the key to treating shock successfully is establishing the precipitating factor(s) quickly, based upon cutaneous signs and a very brief history. See Tables 15.12–15.14.

- *Hypovolaemic* shock (📖 p478) is caused by a reduced circulating volume, often secondary to haemorrhage. The patient is usually pale, cool to touch, has moist skin and is tachycardic
- *Septic* shock (📖 p480) is mediated by a loss in vascular tone due to pathogenic toxins and endogenous inflammatory mediators. The circulatory volume is likely to be normal, but loss of peripheral vascular resistance results in ↓BP and inadequate tissue perfusion. The patient is usually warm, flushed, vasodilated and tachycardic
- *Cardiogenic* shock (📖 p479) results from pump failure (heart failure) or inadequate filling of the pump (eg massive PE). This can occur as part of a chronic picture or acutely following a massive MI. The patient is pale and clammy, feels cool to touch and usually tachycardic, though a profound bradycardia may itself result in cardiogenic shock. ↑JVP and peripheral oedema if right ventricular failure, basal lung crepitations if left ventricular failure – both if biventricular failure
- *Anaphylactic* shock (📖 p470), like septic shock, results from loss of vascular tone, mediated by histamine release, amongst other endogenous factors. Like septic shock, the patient is often flushed and peripherally warm, with a rapid weak pulse, wheeze, stridor, urticaria and oedema
- *Spinal* shock (📖 p481) also results from loss of vascular tone, but mediated by trauma of the cord or following spinal anaesthesia. Loss of sympathetic innervation of the vascular beds or the heart can produce a drop in BP and a reduced cardiac output. Patients have mixed cutaneous clinical signs, but the most striking feature will be the neurological deficit.

Treat all hypotensive patients, especially if HR >100. A BP of 100mmHg systolic may be critically low if the patient is normally hypertensive (eg elderly); use HR and other clinical markers as a guide. Always consider giving a fluid challenge (📖 p381) early, particularly if you remain unclear on the type of shock you are faced with. In the absence of florid evidence of failure, you are unlikely to push any adult into gross cardiac failure with eg 500ml 0.9% saline IV STAT, which should help with circulatory support whilst you assess and plan further. See Table 15.15.

Complications whatever the cause of shock, prolonged hypotension will result in hypoperfusion of vital organs and subsequent disruption to physiology, which may be irreversible (eg brain – ↓GCS/coma, kidneys – ARF/ATN, liver – ischaemic hepatitis, heart – myocardial ischaemia/MI).

Table 15.12 *Clinical markers in shock*

	Hypovolaemia	Sepsis	Cardiogenic	Anaphylaxis	Spinal
HR	↑	↑	↑/↓	↑	↑/↓
BP	↔/↓	↓	↓	↔/↓	↓
JVP	↓	↓	↑	↓	↓
Peripheries	Cool	Warm	Cool	Cool/warm	Warm

Table 15.13 *Main causes of shock*

Hypovolaemic	• External blood loss (eg scalp laceration)
	• Internal blood loss (eg ruptured AAA/pelvic fracture)
	• Severe dehydration
	• inadequate fluid intake (eg starvation)
	• excessive fluid loss (eg diarrhoea, polyuria)
	• 3rd-space loss (eg pancreatitis)
Septic	• Septicaemia
	• blood-borne infection, ?source
Cardiogenic	• Pump failure/ineffective pump
	• severe LV dysfunction
	• outflow tract obstruction (eg aortic dissection)
	• dysrhythmia (tachy- or bradyarrhythmia)
	• Inadequate pump filling
	• pulmonary embolism
	• cardiac tamponade
	• tension pneumothorax (or large simple)
Anaphylactic	• Systemic inflammatory response/vasodilatation
Spinal	• Loss of sympathetic (vascular) tone ± ↓cardiac output
	• dilatation of arterioles/venous pooling
	• loss of sympathetic drive of the heart (T1–T4)

Table 15.14 *Causes of lactic acidosis – metabolic acidosis with ↑lactate*

Tissue hypoxaemia	**Non-hypoxaemic tissues**
Inadequate perfusion	Sepsis
Severe anaemia	Renal and hepatic failure
Severe hypoxia	Uncontrolled DM
Catecholamine excess	Acute pancreatitis
Severe exercise	Paracetamol overdose
Drug-induced	**Rare hereditary causes**
Metformin	Glucose-6-phosphatase deficiency
Methanol	Fructose-1,6-diphosphatase deficiency
Ethanol	
Aspirin (salicylates)	
Salbutamol	

Table 15.15 *Estimated blood loss – classification of haemorrhagic shock*

Based on an otherwise healthy 70kg adult man

	Class I	Class II	Class III	Class IV
Blood loss (ml)	<750	750–1500	1500–2000	>2000
Blood loss (% blood volume)	<15%	15–30%	30–40%	>40%
HR	↔/↑	↑	↑↑	↑↑
BP	↔	↔	↓	↓↓

The key message is that ↓BP is a relatively late sign in bleeding and requires prompt management to stop the source of bleeding and give adequate fluid resuscitation. Seek urgent senior help..

▶▶**Hypovolaemic shock** (OHAM3 📖 p315)

Common causes	
Haemorrhage	Trauma (external/internal bleeding), ruptured AAA, GI bleed
Salt + water loss	Diarrhoea, vomiting, burns, polyuria (DI and DM)
'3rd-space' loss	Acute pancreatitis, ascites

Worrying signs BP <90mmHg, ↓GCS/restlessness, oliguria, mottled skin, unresponsive to fluid challenge, ongoing bleeding ▶▶**call senior help.**

Symptoms dizziness on standing (±lying), SOB, ± chest pain; **symptoms of underlying disease** trauma to limb/chest/abdomen/pelvis, pain (eg chest/back/abdomen), melaena/haematemesis, diarrhoea, urinary frequency, epigastric pain radiating to back, abdominal swelling/bloating.

Signs BP <100mmHg systolic, ↑HR, weak/thready pulse, postural hypotension, cool peripheries/cap refill >2s, ↓JVP, ↓GCS/restlessness, oliguria, mottled skin in severe hypotension.

Signs of underlying disease obvious source of bleeding: external (wound/GI bleed) or internal (haemothorax, ascites/tense abdomen, pelvic instability, swollen thighs); burns, palpable AAA (📖 p474), tender epigastrium, Grey-Turner's sign/Cullen's sign (📖 p296), melaena on PR.

Investigations **blds** FBC (↓Hb; may be normal early in acute blood loss), U+E (↑urea in GI bleed, ↓K⁺ in diarrhoea/vomiting), LFT, amylase, clotting, osmolality, X-match (consider O-ve and type-specific blood whilst awaiting match); **ABG** acidosis in haemorrhage, DKA and pancreatitis, alkalosis in vomiting; **ECG** ischaemia; **CXR** haemothorax; **pelvic X-ray** pelvic fracture; **abdo USS/CT** AAA (though if ruptured AAA may need theatre before imaging) or free intra-abdominal fluid; **urine** Na⁺ and osmolality in diabetes insipidus **stool** M,C+S (ova, cysts and parasites, C. diff. toxin).

Acute treatment of severe haemorrhage call senior help; lay flat and elevate legs; O₂ (15l/min); IV access (2 large-bore cannulae in antecubital fossa, take blood for FBC, clotting, urgent X-match); 1l 0.9% saline STAT; attempt to stop bleeding by compression if appropriate, further 1l 0.9% saline STAT if no ↑BP or ↓HR; consider urgent blood transfusion (O-negative, type specific, or full X-match, 📖 p400); identify likely cause of haemorrhage and commence appropriate management. Seek early involvement of surgeons/ICU. 'Permissive hypotension' is employed in the early phase of resuscitation in haemorrhagic shock so do not push systolic BP >100mmHg.

Acute treatment of non-haemorrhage hypovolaemia call senior help; lay flat and elevate legs; O₂ (15l/min); IV access (secure appropriately large-bore cannula in antecubital fossa); 1l 0.9% saline STAT; further 1l 0.9% saline STAT if no ↑BP or ↓HR; identify likely cause of hypovolaemia and commence appropriate treatment; pancreatitis (📖 p296), severe diarrhoea (📖 p306), vomiting (📖 p304), burns (📖 p466), fever and sweating (📖 p482), ascites (📖 p316). Seek early involvement of ICU.

Further treatment once appropriate management initiated, recheck observations, including glucose, repeat U+E and FBC (±ABG); catheterise and monitor urine output; reassess frequently, starting with A, B, C.

▶▶Cardiogenic shock (OHAM3 📖 p314)

Common causes

Pump failure	LV dysfunction (post-ACS), aortic dissection, dysrhythmia
Inadequate filling	Pulmonary embolism, pneumothorax, cardiac tamponade

Worrying signs BP <90mmHg, ↓GCS/restlessness, oliguria, mottled skin, chest pain, hypoxaemia ▶▶**call senior help.**

Symptoms dizziness on standing (±lying), SOB, ±chest pain **symptoms of underlying disease** chest pain ±pleuritic, ±radiating to back/left arm/jaw, breathlessness, orthopnoea, palpitations.

Signs BP <100mmHg systolic (check both arms), ↑/↓ HR, weak pulse, cool peripheries, ↑JVP, ↓GCS, oliguria, mottled skin in severe hypotension.

Signs of underlying disease ↓O_2 sats, signs of pneumothorax (↓expansion, ↑percussion note, ↓breath sounds on affected side, tracheal deviation), pulmonary oedema, pitting oedema, stigmata of hyperlipidaemia, Beck's triad in cardiac tamponade (↓BP, ↑JVP, faint heart sounds).

Investigations ▶▶if you suspect cardiogenic shock identify most likely cause and treat prior to undertaking investigations; seconds count. Most useful investigation will be immediate **ECG** ischaemia, dysrhythmia, small complexes; **CXR** pneumothorax, cardiomegaly, fluid overload; **ABG** hypoxaemia; **blds** FBC, U+E, glucose, clotting, X-match; **other imaging** as appropriate, including **echocardiogram** (cardiologist on-call or ED senior) for dissection, massive PE, cardiac tamponade, LVF.

Acute treatment 15l/min O_2. Further management depends on pathology:

Causes of cardiogenic shock covered elsewhere

Bradyarrhythmia	📖 p258	Aortic dissection	📖 p247
Tachyarrhythmia	📖 p250	Pulmonary embolism	📖 p278
Heart failure	📖 p282	Pneumothorax	📖 p279

▶▶Cardiac tamponade (OHAM3 📖 p156)

Collection of fluid (usually blood) in pericardium, compressing ventricles and reducing ability of heart to fill.

Causes trauma, pericarditis, post-MI, dissecting aortic aneurysm.

Signs tachycardia, hypotension, Beck's triad (↓BP, ↑JVP, faint heart sounds).

Investigations **CXR** cardiomegaly, pulmonary oedema; **ECG** small complexes, tachycardia, ischaemia; **echo** pericardial fluid, poor stroke volume.

Acute treatment 15l/min O_2, IV access, needle pericardiocentesis.

▶▶Emergency needle pericardiocentesis (OHAM3 📖 p158)
Get senior help

- Monitor heart rhythm on ECG monitor; have IV fluids running and defibrillator close
- Clean skin on chest/upper abdomen with antiseptic
- Connect 18G cannula to 20ml syringe via a 3-way tap
- Advance needle to the left of xiphisternum, aiming for tip of left scapula
- Withdraw syringe as advancing, watching for ectopics on ECG
- Ectopics imply needle in myocardium, withdraw a little into the pericardial space
- Aspirating 20–40ml can improve BP, but fluid likely to reaccumulate
- Patient needs definitive cardiothoracic input urgently.

▶▶**Septic shock** (OHAM3 📖 p376)

Common sources of infection resulting in septicaemia	
Chest Pneumonia	Intra-abdominal Perforation; biliary tract
Skin/soft tissues Cellulitis; gangrene	Urinary tract UTI; pyelonephritis
Heart Endocarditis	Post-op Wound infection; bowel leak

Worrying signs BP <90mmHg, ↓GCS/restlessness, DIC, oliguria, mottled skin, petechial rash, unresponsive to fluid challenge ▶▶**call senior help.**

Symptoms dizziness on standing (±lying), SOB, ±chest pain **symptoms of underlying disease** sweats, shivers, nausea and vomiting, breathlessness, cough, dysuria, urinary frequency, abdominal pain, wound/skin pain, headache, confusion.

Signs fever, BP <100mmHg systolic, tachycardia ± bounding pulse, warm peripheries, ↓JVP, ↓GCS, oliguria, mottled skin in severe hypotension.

Signs of underlying disease cellulitis, non-blanching petechial rash (meningococcal septicaemia), chest crepitations (pneumonia), abdominal/loin/suprapubic tenderness (intra-abdominal infection).

Investigations **blds** FBC (↑WCC ±↓Hb), U+E, LFT, ↑CRP/ESR, glucose, clotting/fibrinogen, procalcitonin;[1] **bld cultures** try to take at least 2 sets from different sites, plus additional cultures from any central lines; **ABG** acidosis, ↓BE, ↑lactate; **ECG** ischaemia; **urine dipstick** blood, protein, nitrites, leucocytes; send for M,C+S; **erect CXR** consolidation, free air under diaphragm; **culture** skin/wound swabs, sputum; **echo** valvular lesion/vegetation (if suspect endocarditis; transoesophageal more sensitive than transthoracic; **other imaging** as appropriate.

Acute treatment call senior help; lay flat and elevate legs; O₂ (15l/min); IV access (secure appropriately large bore cannula in antecubital fossa); 1l 0.9% saline STAT; give IV antibiotics appropriate to likely source of infection (see 📖 p179); repeat 1l 0.9% saline bolus STAT if no ↑BP or ↓HR. Consider central line to monitor CVP and arterial line for serial ABGs and invasive BP monitoring. Seek early involvement of ICU as may need inotropic/ventilatory support. **Goal-directed therapy** in sepsis aims to restore tissue perfusion and O₂ delivery and ensure early administration of antibiotics; this greatly improve outcomes (see 📖 p481).

Further treatment continue broad-spectrum antibiotic therapy until advised of alternative, more targeted therapy by microbiologist. Aggressive fluid therapy may be required to ensure adequate tissue perfusion. Monitor for the development of DIC which can result in necrosis and gangrene, as well as profound bleeding (📖 p405).

▶▶**Toxic shock** is a specific form of septic shock, caused by the production of a toxin by Gram-positive bacteria (typically *Staphylococcus aureus*).

Risk factors ♀ (in association with the use of tampons).

Signs and symptoms fever (T >38.9°C), ↓BP (<90mmHg systolic), diffuse macular rash ±desquamation, vomiting, diarrhoea, ↓GCS.

Treatment is the same: fluid resuscitation, broad-spectrum antibiotics initially, **remove source of infection/pus**, support impaired organ function. ICU admission is often required.

---

[1] Procalcitonin levels rise in bacterial sepsis; normal levels in setting of raised inflammatory markers suggest non-septic cause of inflammation and may help reduce inappropriate antibiotic use.

SIRS, sepsis, and survival

Some useful definitions in sepsis include:
SIRS (**S**ystemic **I**nflammatory **R**esponse **S**yndrome): present if ≥2 of:
- HR>90
- RR >20 or PaCO$_2$ <4.3 kPa
- Temp <36 or >38.3°C
- WCC <4 or >12 x 10^9/l

Sepsis: SIRS + known or suspected infection.
Severe sepsis: sepsis + signs of hypoperfusion or organ failure including ↓urine output, elevated urea or creatinine, abnormal LFTs, coagulation disturbance, hypoxia or ARDS, or a raised serum lactate.
Septic shock: hypotension persists despite adequate fluid challenge, or requires use of vasopressors or inotropes.
Septic shock is common, serious, and survivable. This simple maxim has driven intensivists to seek better ways of managing sepsis. One vital realisation was the importance of early intervention, which may often be delivered by non-intensivists and junior doctors. A key study by Rivers[1] in 2001 showed a clear survival benefit in patients with sepsis who were randomised to receive initial care according to a standardised approach referred to as 'Early Goal Directed Therapy' (EGDT).
Since 2002, the 'Surviving Sepsis' campaign has represented an international attempt to improve diagnosis, survival and management in sepsis, through education, audit and research, and provides an excellent range of resources (⬚www.survivingsepsis.org). Key steps in sepsis management include:
- Early measurement of serum lactate: if ≥4mmol/l commence EGDT
- Collection of blood cultures prior to antibiotic administration
- Administration of broad-spectrum antibiotics within 3h of admission with sepsis, or within 1h of recognition of severe sepsis
- Aggressive early fluid therapy (30ml/kg crystalloid as boluses until lactate <4mmol/l, systolic BP ≥90mmHg and MAP ≥65mmHg).

Other key steps include ongoing fluid resuscitation to keep CVP 8–12mmHg, the appropriate use of vasopressors to maintain MAP ≥65mmHg, mechanical ventilation and good glycaemic control, all of which the ICU team will be only too happy to undertake after you have helped to save the patient's life with the simple measures listed.

[1] Rivers, E. *et al.* NEJM 2001 **345**:1368 available free at ⬚www.nejm.org/doi/full/10.1056/NEJMoa010307

▶▶**Spinal (neurogenic) shock**

Common causes

Trauma	Traumatic transection of spinal cord at any level
Iatrogenic	Spinal anaesthesia

Symptoms usually motor/sensory dysfunction below level of lesion; bowel and bladder dysfunction.
Signs ↓BP, warm peripheries; may not be able to mount tachycardia if lesion above T1–T4 (origin of sympathetic supply to the heart), focal neurology ±up-going plantar relaxes, loss of anal tone.
Investigations imaging of spinal cord as appropriate.
When to treat BP <100mmHg systolic, symptomatic of ↓BP, organ failure.
Acute treatment call senior help; lay flat and elevate legs (providing spinal injury not suspected); O$_2$ (15l/min); 1l 0.9% saline STAT; catheterise. If trauma involve spinal/orthopaedic surgeons. If iatrogenic, (eg epidural) stop epidural and consult anaesthetist. Seek early involvement of ICU.

Pyrexia

> *Worrying features* ↑HR, ↓BP, ↓GCS, ≥40°C, purpuric rash, +ve blood cultures.

Think about *serious* septic shock (🕮 p480); *most likely* **infection** including UTI, pyelonephritis, cellulitis, septic joint, wound infection, URTI, pneumonia, gastroenteritis, endocarditis, abscesses, meningitis; **iatrogenic** transfusion reaction, infected line, drug reaction, neuroleptic malignant syndrome; *other* PE/DVT, inflammatory conditions and malignancy.

Ask about *urinary* frequency, dysuria, pyuria; *respiratory* cough, sputum production and colour, haemoptysis, breathlessness, chest pain, sore throat/ear, coryza, contact and immunisation to TB; *joints/ skin* arthropathy, rash, erythema, breaks to skin; *neurological* headache, photophobia, neck stiffness; *systemic* appetite, weight loss, night sweats; *PMH* immunosuppression (DM, lymphoma/leukaemia, HIV, transplant, cystic fibrosis), underlying lung disease, TB, recurrent UTI, prosthetic heart valve or valvular lesion; *DH* immunosuppression (including steroids), blood transfusions, new drugs commenced (eg antipsychotic), allergies; *SH* any contacts with similar symptoms, exposure to TB, smoking, recreational drug use (IVDU, ecstasy).

Obs temp (?swinging), HR, BP, RR, sats, blood glucose, urine output.

Look for pulse rate/rhythm/volume, cap refill, warm peripheries, sweating, flushing, tachypnoea, tremor, splinter haemorrhages, break in skin, needle tracks in arms/feet/groin, focal skin/wound infection, bronchial breathing/crackles/reduced air entry, heart murmur, suprapubic/loin tenderness, red catheter/line sites, joint swelling.

Investigations septic screen (🕮 p483); *urine dipstick* and M,C+S (🕮 p590); *blds* FBC, ↑NØ (bacterial), ↑LØ (viral), ↑EØ (drugs/parasites/ allergy), blood film (may suggest haematological malignancy/malaria), U+E, LFT, inflammatory markers (CRP, ESR), cultures (🕮 p515); consider: D-dimer if DVT/PE suspected (🕮 p450) and procalcitonin (🕮 p480); *sputum* C+S, if active TB suspected request urgent 'smear' microscopy for acid-fast bacilli (AFB); *stool culture*, *skin swabs*; *ABG* respiratory failure or metabolic acidosis (🕮 p584); *CXR* pneumonia/effusion; *echo* if you suspect bacterial endocarditis; transoesophageal is more sensitive than transthoracic;[1] *LP* if meningitis suspected (after CT head).

Treatment assess the severity of illness, have a low threshold for treatment as septic shock (🕮 p480). If signs of infection, consider broad-spectrum antibiotics (🕮 p179) until culture results known. Repeat septic screen if new rise in temp >38°C even if already commenced on antibiotics.

Symptom management paracetamol (1g/6h PO) ±ibuprofen (400mg/6h PO) for pyrexia; an electric fan may also produce symptomatic relief. Give adequate analgesia (🕮 p86) and ensure adequate hydration (consider IV fluids if nauseated or NBM); supplementary O₂ if sats <94%.

Request early *senior review* if in doubt of diagnosis or patient unwell.

---

[1] This may be true, but the cardiologists may take a good deal of persuading.

The septic screen

In many patients the likely source of a fever will be obvious, and investigations and management can be tailored specifically towards that; in others it is less clear, and a more widespread approach is required.

History a thorough history can sometimes shed new light on the potential cause or highlight the potential for immunocompromise.

Examination of all the patient's systems and a top to toe examination of the skin and joints may reveal a source of infection. All line sites should be inspected and changed if old or inflamed – send the tips of removed lines to microbiology for culturing.

Investigations see box.

Septic screen

- FBC (repeat every 2d)
- Inflammatory markers, ESR, CRP (repeat every 2–4d)
- Urine culture (separate samples from any nephrostomies/urostomies)
- Sputum culture, if indicated
- Blood cultures (3 sets at 6–8h intervals from different veins; additional sets from any central lines)
- Microbiology swabs of wounds/pressure areas/cannula or central line sites
- CXR if productive cough or abnormal clinical signs present.

If infectious source still not identified, consider:
- Procalcitonin (will be negative if non-infective cause, ☐ p480)
- Stopping all antibiotics (if stable) and repeating all cultures after 48h
- Echocardiogram if new murmur or new stigmata of bacterial endocarditis
- Check sickle-cell status
- Blood film for parasites (if malaria is suspected)
- Lumbar puncture if CNS infection suspected or needs excluding (CT first).

Pyrexia of unknown origin (PUO) (OHCM9 ☐ p388)

Classically defined as a recurrent fever (T >38.3°C), persisting for >3wk, without obvious cause despite >1wk of in-patient investigations. Causes include infection (30%), malignancy (30%), non-infectious inflammatory disease (eg connective tissue disease, vasculitis; 20%), and drug reactions. Always repeat a detailed history and examination, clearly summarise all investigations and results so far and discuss with an infectious disease physician. Despite your best efforts, in ~10% of cases a cause is never found.

Iatrogenic causes of pyrexia

- Transfusion reactions (☐ p402)
- Infected lines:
  - cannula, central lines, arterial lines, urinary catheters, long-lines, etc.
- Drug-induced (most due to hypersensitivity reactions):
  - antibiotics (eg erythromycin, nitrofurantoin, isoniazid, penicillins)
  - cardiovascular medications (eg atropine, hydralazine, nifedipine)
  - malignant hyperthermia (eg anaesthetic agents)
  - neuroleptic malignant syndrome (eg antipsychotic drugs)
  - miscellaneous (eg aspirin, allopurinol, phenytoin, opioid withdrawal).
- Post-operative:
  - atelectasis (often 24h post-op).

Urinary tract infection, including pyelonephritis (OHCM9 📖 p292)

Worrying signs ↓BP/shock (📖 p480), temp >40°C, new renal impairment. Elderly patients can be afebrile or hypothermic but heavily bacteraemic.

Symptoms **cystitis** urinary frequency, dysuria, urgency, pyuria, haematuria, suprapubic pain; **pyelonephritis** fever, rigors, vomiting, loin pain.

Risk factors ♀, sexual intercourse, catheterisation, DM, immunosuppression, pregnancy, structural abnormalities of urinary tract, stones, elderly.

Signs warm peripheries, vasodilation, tachycardia, suprapubic/loin pain.

Investigations **Urine dipstick** (see box and 📖 p590) C+S if clinical suspicion of UTI and in all pyrexial/vomiting children; *blds* FBC (↑WCC, ↑NØ), U+E (↑urea, ↑creatinine if ↓urinary tract obstruction p377), ↑inflammatory markers, ↑glucose (?DM); **bld cultures** if ↑temp or systemically unwell.

Acute treatment (UTI) if ↓BP/shock treat as septic shock (📖 p480); otherwise paracetamol (for fever) and consider empirical antibiotic therapy (eg trimethoprim 200mg/12h PO, or co-amoxiclav 1.2g/8h IV if septic) whilst awaiting sensitivities; ↑oral fluid intake. Treat for 3d (simple infection in ♀) or 7d (if structural urinary tract abnormality, immunosuppressed or ♂).

Acute treatment (pyelonephritis) if ↓BP/shock treat as septic shock (📖 p480); admit for IV antibiotics if septic, pregnant, frail elderly, immunosuppressed or structurally abnormal urinary tract. Give paracetamol and start empirical antibiotic therapy (eg co-amoxiclav 625mg/8h PO or 1.2g/8h IV) whilst awaiting sensitivities; ↑oral fluid intake. Treat for 7–10d.

Further investigation consider renal USS ±referral to urology if: failure to respond to treatment, recurrent UTIs (especially in ♂), pyelonephritis (after 1st episode in ♂, 2nd episode in ♀), *Proteus* species isolated or microscopic haematuria persisting after resolution of symptoms.

Simple measures to prevent urinary tract infections

- Drink >2l fluid day
- Voiding at 2–3h intervals
- Double voiding
- Voiding before bedtime and after sexual intercourse
- Wipe front to back after micturition (♀).

Recurrent urinary tract infections

- Avoidance of constipation (prevents outflow obstruction)
- Drinking cranberry juice[1]
- Antibiotic prophylaxis (eg trimethoprim)
- Avoidance of irritants in bathwater (bubble bath etc).

[1] Kontiokari, T. et al. *BMJ* 2001 **332**:1571 available free at 🖰www.bmj.com

Just how useful is a urine dipstick?

A MSU culture demonstrating a urinary pathogen at >10⁵ CFU/ml is the gold standard test in suspected UTI. Dipsticks allow 'near patient' testing for various markers that may allow for a modest improvement in clinical diagnosis:

- **Nitrites** many uropathogens reduce nitrate to nitrite; +ve in ~30% confirmed UTIs, but highly specific. False −ves occur with organisms that do not reduce nitrate or polyuria
- **Leucocyte esterase** a marker for pyuria; will be positive in ~80–90% confirmed UTIs; false-positives occur with contamination from eg vagina
- **Blood** +ve in ~70–80% confirmed UTIs; false +ves occur with contamination from eg menstrual bleeding, renal stones
- **Protein** reflect organisms and cells in urine; +ve in ~50% confirmed UTIs.

Study data from UK primary care[2] show that where clinical suspicion of a UTI exists, the presence of nitrites, leucocytes or blood can support a diagnosis, but that evaluation of protein provides no additional information. Combining test results increases sensitivity, but decreases specificity. Even when all tests are −ve, 24% of symptomatic women will have a UTI confirmed by MSU culture. *If UTI suspected, send an MSU.*

[2] Little, P. et al. *Health Technol Assess* 2009 **13**(19) available free at 🖰www.journalslibrary.nihr.ac.uk/hta/volume-13/issue-19

Endocarditis (OHAM3 ▢ p96)

Symptoms fatigue, anorexia, weight loss, fever, night sweats, dyspnoea.

Risk factors prosthetic valve, valvular lesion (aortic >mitral), congenital cardiac defect, pacemaker/central line, mural thrombus (post-MI), recurrent bacteraemia (IV drug users, severe dental disease), atrial myxoma.

Signs fever (90%), new murmur (85%), neurological deficit (40%), splinter haemorrhages, Janeway lesions, Osler's nodes, Roth spots, conjunctival haemorrhage, tachycardia, warm peripheries, CCF, evidence of IVDU.

Investigations for diagnostic criteria see below; **blds** FBC (↑WCC, ↑NØ, ↓Hb), U+E, LFT, ↑ESR/CRP; **bld cultures** take 3 sets (prior to commencing ABx) from different sites at intervals of >1h; **ECG** non-specific changes, new AV block if aortic valve disease; **CXR** pulmonary oedema, septic pulmonary emboli if tricuspid disease; **echo** valvular lesion/vegetation (sensitivity 90% for transoesophageal; 60% for transthoracic); **V/Q scan** if pulmonary emboli suspected; **urine dipstick** blood ± protein.

Acute treatment try to obtain at least 3 sets of blood cultures prior to commencing antibiotics even if patient unwell. Empirical treatment should include a penicillin (benzylpenicillin or flucloxacillin) and gentamicin, ±vancomycin if ?MRSA. Give O₂ as needed, paracetamol and other supportive measures (anti-emetics, IV fluids if dehydrated, diuretics if CCF).

Further treatment give antibiotic therapy for at least 4–6wk, targeted according to microbiology advice. Valve replacement may be indicated in refractory CCF, aortic root abscess (lengthening PR interval, RBBB), failure of prosthetic valve, persistent sepsis despite antibiotics.

Complications valve destruction, cardiac failure, AV block, intracardiac abscess, embolism (to brain, limbs, lungs), septicaemia, death.

Duke criteria for infective endocarditis (IE)[1]

Definite IE – 2 major, or 1 major and 3 minor, or 5 minor criteria
Possible IE – findings fall short of 'definite' but not 'rejected'
Rejected IE – firm alternative diagnosis or resolution within <4d of therapy.

Major criteria
● Blood cultures:
  • +ve for *typical* organism on ≥2 separate occasions[2]
  • +ve for organism *consistent* with IE on 2 occasions >12h apart
  • +ve for organism *consistent* with IE on 3/3 or 3+/4 cultures taken >1h apart
● Evidence of endocardial involvement defined as +ve echocardiogram.[3]

Minor criteria
● Predisposing heart condition or drug use
● Fever >38°C
● Vascular phenomena (septic emboli, Janeway lesion, intracranial or conjunctival haemorrhage)
● Immunologic phenomena (glomerulonephritis, Osler's nodes, Roth spots, +ve rheumatoid factor)
● Microbiological evidence (+ve blood cultures failing to meet major criteria)
● Echocardiographic findings (consistent with IE but not meeting major criteria).

[1] Durack, D.T. et al. *Am J Med* 1994 **96**:200 (subscription required).
[2] *Streptococcus viridans, Streptococcus bovis*, HACEK group (*Haemophilus* sp, *Actinobacillus actinomycetemcomitans, Cardiobacterium hominis, Eikenella corrodens, Kingella* sp). *S. aureus* or *Enterococci* in absence of 1° focus.
[3] Evidence of an intra-cardiac vegetation or abscess, new valvular regurgitation, or dehiscence of prosthetic valve.

Neutropenia

Neutrophil counts $<1 \times 10^9/l$ increase susceptibility to infection. Severe neutropenia ($<0.5 \times 10^9/l$) necessitates urgent assessment for infection.

Causes of neutropenia typically seen following marrow suppression from chemotherapy (usually 7–10d later) for an underlying malignancy. Other causes of neutropenia present less often to hospital, but include several rare congenital syndromes, infections (viral, brucellosis, TB), a large number of drugs (eg amiodarone, penicillins, cephalosporins, carbimazole, propylthiouracil, ACEi, antipsychotics, anticonvulsants, sulphonylureas), hypersplenism (eg Felty syndrome) or anti-neutrophil antibodies and marrow failure secondary to either infiltration or B_{12}/folate deficiency.

▶▶*Febrile neutropenia* requires prompt medical action – see box and Table 15.16.

Non-febrile neutropenic patients without any signs of infection, are still immunocompromised; question if hospital is appropriate as they may be safer at home. If admission is necessary, ensure a clean side-room is used and the patient should have reverse barrier nursing to prevent staff introducing infection. Check for a cause of neutropenia and look at FBC to exclude a significant pancytopenia. Discuss prophylactic antibiotics with haematology and microbiology. Remove unnecessary IV cannulae, central lines or urinary catheters; if left in, change IV cannulae every 48h.

▶▶Febrile neutropenia (OHAM3 📖 p690)

Definitions	• Neutropenia: NØ$<0.5 \times 10^9/l$ (or $<1.0 \times 10^9/l$ and predicted to ↓) • Pyrexia: >38.3°C at any point or >38°C sustained >1h • beware the possibility of normo/hypothermia in the very sick, or those on steroids or NSAIDs
Source of infection	• Often not clear clinically; consider: mouth/teeth/gums, sinuses, URTI/LRTI, diarrhoea, Hickman/central line, urine, skin, perianal. • Microbiological diagnosis made in only about 40% of cases
Investigations	• Monitor FBC and differential, ±clotting, U+E, LFT, glucose • Culture blood (peripheral and from central lines), urine, sputum • Swab central line ports and skin folds • Consider stool and CSF cultures; CMV and aspergillus PCR • CXR • Repetitive clinical examination to identify source of infection
Treatment	• Resuscitate (O_2, IV fluids; if in septic shock, see 📖 p480) • Commence antibiotics early (see Table 15.16) • Early involvement of haematology and microbiology • Consider antifungal prophylaxis

Table 15.16 *Empirical antibiotic therapy for febrile neutropenia*

Early discussion with microbiology is advised (check your local policy guidelines)	
1st line	Tazocin® 4.5g/8h IV + gentamicin 5mg/kg/24h IV
2nd line	Add in vancomycin 1g/12h IV if known or suspected MRSA
3rd line	Consider adding in amphotericin if fever not settling

Further therapy, including the use of recombinant granulocyte-colony stimulating factor (G-CSF) will be advised by haematology: low risk patients who remain apyrexial at 48h may be switched to oral therapy and antibiotics stopped as the neutrophil count recovers.

Notifiable diseases

Notification of a number of diseases (see box) is mandatory under the Health Protection (Notification) Regulations 2010 and the Public Health (Control of Disease) Act 1984. The statutory requirement for notification of certain infectious diseases was introduced over 100 years ago to help identify and stem outbreaks and epidemics of certain infectious diseases (initially cholera, diphtheria, smallpox, and typhoid). This remains the primary purpose of the legislation today. If a patient has been diagnosed with a notifiable disease, or is strongly suspected of having a notifiable disease, a notification certificate should be completed and sent to the 'Proper Officer' of the local authority (or discussed by telephone if the case is urgent). Seek advice from microbiology if you have any concerns. Ensure you know the patient's address, home circumstances, any foreign travel and their clinical history before referring the case.

UK Notifiable diseases

- Anthrax
- Botulism
- Brucellosis
- Cholera
- Diarrhoea (infectious, bloody)
- Diphtheria
- Encephalitis (acute)
- Food poisoning
- Haemolytic uraemic syndrome
- Invasive group A streptococcal disease
- Legionnaires' disease
- Leprosy
- Malaria
- Measles
- Meningitis: all types
- Meningococcal septicaemia
- Mumps
- Paratyphoid fever
- Plague
- Poliomyelitis (acute)
- Rabies
- Rubella
- SARS
- Scarlet fever
- Smallpox
- Tetanus
- Tuberculosis
- Typhoid fever
- Typhus fever
- Viral haemorrhagic fever
- Viral hepatitis: all types
- Whooping cough
- Yellow fever.

Disease surveillance is carried out nationally by the Health Protection Agency (HPA) who publish a very interesting and informative weekly report of the numbers and location of the various notifiable diseases. These reports, and further information on notification can be found at: ⁿwww.hpa.org.uk/infections/topics_az/noids/menu.htm

HIV is not a notifiable disease, but it is often voluntarily reported to the HPA, typically by a senior clinician or laboratory scientist.

Infections covered elsewhere			
Pneumonia	📖 p276	Meningitis/Encephalitis	📖 p360
Cellulitis	📖 p412	Tonsilitis	📖 p461
Gastroenteritis	📖 p307	Cholecystitis	📖 p295
Endometritis	📖 p507	Sexually transmitted	📖 p465

Recurrent/unusual infections

Patients reattending with recurrent infections may be identified by their GP. In hospital, isolation of an unusual pathogen will usually trigger further investigation, and a microbiologist will often suggest further investigations, as well as treatment.

Opportunistic infections are commonly seen in HIV (📖 p490) and other immunocompromised states (see Table 15.17, p489). Identification of an unusual pathogen does not infer immunocompromise, it merely makes it more likely. Equally, immunocompromised patients will also develop 'standard' infections with 'standard' pathogens.

Causes of immunocompromise are diverse and diagnosis requires meticulous history taking, examination and investigation (mostly blood-based), from which microbiology and infectious disease physicians will be able to offer advice. DM, ↑age, steroids (📖 p177) and immunosuppressants can cause a relative increase in susceptibility to infections, though less so than neutropenia.

Malaria (OHCM9 📖 p394)

A common cause of fever in the tropics, malaria is the most deadly vector-borne disease in the world, found in Central/South Americas, sub-Saharan Africa, India, Southeast Asia and parts of the Middle East. Consider malaria in any traveller who presents with fever or unexplained illness within 1mth of travel to these endemic areas, regardless of prophylaxis.

Plasmodium *falciparum, vivax, ovale* and *malariae* all cause human malaria.

Transmission is through the bite of an infected female *Anopheles* mosquito, which typically occurs at night. The use of bed nets, mosquito repellents, long-sleeved clothing, and prophylaxis all reduce (but do not eliminate) the risk of infection.

Presentation is with fever, typically a few weeks after infection, though incubation periods vary according to the species of *Plasmodium*, as well as the patient's previous exposure. The classic cyclical fever, peaking every 2–3d is rare. Other symptoms include headache, vomiting, fatigue, and arthralgia/myalgia.

Severe forms of malaria include cerebral (↓GCS), severe anaemia, renal and respiratory failure. All are more common with *P. falciparum*.

Diagnosis requires identification of parasites on ≥3 thick and thin blood films drawn 12–24h apart. Thick films are more sensitive and allow quantification of parasitaemia, whilst thin films aid identification of species. Many labs will offer rapid and sensitive tests based upon immunohistochemical identification of parasite antigens, or PCR.

Treatment depends upon species. *P. falciparum* is typically resistant to chloroquine (which is used for other species); alternatives include artesumate, mefloquine and Malarone®; discuss with infectious diseases.

Prophylaxis should be encouraged in all travellers to endemic areas. Choices include chloroquine, proguanil, doxycycline, mefloquine and Malarone®. Further advice is available in the *BNF* section 5.4.1.

Table 15.17 *Opportunistic pathogens in the immunocompromised* (OHCM9 📖 p477)

Candidiasis	Ubiquitous fungus, typically causing white oral plaques (thrush), though can form in skin folds, genitalia and oesophagus; in severe cases causes septicaemia. Treated locally with nystatin or systemically with fluconazole or amphotericin B
CMV retinitis	Most common in HIV+ patients. Reduction in visual acuity, ±blindness. 'Mozzarella pizza' appearance on fundoscopy. Treated with ganciclovir or foscarnet
Cryptococcus neoformans	Encapsulated yeast, causing eye infections, but most commonly meningitis, often without neck stiffness. India ink stains help identify organism; confirm on culture. Amphotericin B (±flucytosine) followed by fluconazole is used to control, though cure in HIV+ patients is rare
Herpes simplex virus (types 1 or 2)	Cold sores/genital lesions. More serious CNS infections (meningitis/encephalitis) require high-dose IV aciclovir
Pneumocystis jiroveci (formerly carinii)	The most common opportunistic infection seen in HIV+ patients, this unicellular fungus typically causes a severe pneumonia. Also seen in patients with leukaemia and following bone marrow transplantation. Suspect in any immunocompromised patient with fever, dyspnoea, and non-productive cough. CXR typically shows diffuse bilateral infiltrates, but may be normal. Diagnose based upon culture of induced sputum or bronchoalveolar lavage samples. Treat with co-trimoxazole (trimethoprim + sulfamethoxazole). HIV patients with CD4+ counts <200 should receive this as prophylaxis or secondary prophylaxis following PCP
Tuberculosis (TB)	This is the commonest of the mycobacteria which present clinically. Frank pulmonary TB in the immunocompromised may result from primary infection or reactivation of a primary infection many years prior. Treatment should be aggressive with quadruple therapy (📖 p491). Compliance is crucial and should be emphasised. Always consider MDR-TB
Mycobacterium avium intracellulare	M. avium and M. intracellulare are 2 ubiquitous nontuberculous species of mycobacterium that cause disseminated infection in HIV+ patients with CD4+ counts <50; pulmonary infection is also seen in those with chronic lung disease. Prolonged combination antituberculous therapy is required
Tinea corporis	Fungal skin infections are common in the healthy, but more so in the immunocompromised. Treat with topical agents (nystatin, clotrimazole, terbinafine) unless more invasive disease (📖 p416)
Toxoplasma gondii	Protozoal infection, associated with eating undercooked meat or food contaminated with cat faeces. Usually subclinical, unless HIV+ patient, where causes chorioretinitis, meningitis/ encephalitis or intracerebral abscesses. Treat with sulfadiazine and pyrimethamine. Secondary prophylaxis required
Varicella-zoster virus	Can cause severe cutaneous manifestations (chickenpox and shingles, 📖 p414), pneumonitis or encephalitis in immunocompromised. Requires high-dose IV aciclovir or foscarnet. Urgent ophthalmology input if ophthalmic shingles

HIV/AIDS[1]

Probably arising from primates in Africa, and first described in 1981, the HIV epidemic spread rapidly and silently around the globe in the absence of understanding or testing. 1% of the adult population are now infected, with 3 million new infections and 2 million deaths a year.

Transmission blood-borne; mother to child (during birth or breastfeeding), sexual intercourse, IV drug users, needle-stick injuries, blood products.

Stages of infection

- *Acute seroconversion* 2–6wk after infection; 50% will develop symptoms: sore throat, fever, malaise, maculopapular rash, lymphadenopathy
- *Asymptomatic* a symptom-free period lasting 8–10yr; may have persistent generalised lymphadenopathy
- *Symptomatic* as the immune system fails and the virus mutates, the patient becomes more susceptible to common pathogens (eg colds, gastroenteritis); constitutional symptoms include weight loss and fatigue
- *AIDS* diagnosis with an AIDS-defining illness (see box).

Symptoms often asymptomatic (+ve HIV test); may present with Kaposi's sarcoma or opportunistic infection(s) (see box): cough, shortness of breath, weight loss, lethargy, recurrent fever, confusion, headaches, diarrhoea, abdominal pain, dysphagia.

Signs rashes (Kaposi's sarcoma is a red/purple, slightly raised papule or plaque often on the head, neck, trunk or mucous membranes); wasting, generalised lymphadenopathy, oral/genital candidiasis.

Counselling always obtain consent prior to any HIV test and discuss how the result will be communicated; length counselling is rarely required.[1] Never give a result to a 3rd party.

Investigations **HIV antibody** tests used for diagnosis: can take up to 3mth to give a positive result after infection; **HIV PCR** used to monitor treatment; more sensitive than the antibody tests and give a viral load to quantify infection; **CD4 count** used to monitor and plan treatment.

Label all bodily fluid samples as 'high risk' if HIV is suspected.

Treatment with a combination of drugs (HAART: Highly Active Anti-Retroviral Therapy) should be led by a GUM or infectious disease specialist, and guided by the CD4 count. Treatment is usually initiated with 2 nucleoside reverse-transcriptase inhibitors (NRTI) + 1 non-nucleoside reverse transcriptase inhibitor (NNRTI). 2 NRTIs + 1 protease inhibitor (PI) is a 2nd-line therapy. Multiple new classes of drug are coming to market. Co-trimoxazole and isoniazid are used as prophylaxis against *Pneumocystis jirovecii* and TB. Ensure appropriate vaccinations given,[1] but caution with live vaccines (eg BCG, MMR, yellow fever).

Post-exposure prophylaxis (PEP) healthcare workers exposed to potential infection, or individuals attending the emergency department after a high-risk exposure, may be offered PEP, pending serological testing; seek local guidance.

Prognosis untreated mortality >90% with progression to AIDS in 8–10yr; appropriate treatment, where available, dramatically improves survival.

Common AIDS-defining conditions

Kaposi's sarcoma	Progressive multifocal leucoencephalopathy
Pneumocystis jirovecii pneumonia (PCP)	Recurrent non-typhi salmonella septicaemia
CMV retinitis	Cerebral toxoplasmosis
Chronic mucocutaneous herpes	Cryptococcal meningitis
Mycobacterium avium intracellulare	Non-Hodgkin's lymphoma
Miliary or extrapulmonary TB	Primary cerebral lymphoma
Oesophageal candidiasis	HIV-associated wasting
Chronic cryptosporidial diarrhoea	HIV-associated dementia

[1] Range of useful British HIV association guidelines (including on testing) available at ⁂www.bhiva.org/Guidelines.aspx

Tuberculosis (TB)[1,2]

Responsible for 2 million annual global deaths, and latently infecting 3 billion people, TB was in decline in the UK through most of the 20th century. Rates began to increase in the 1990s, mostly in London and major cities.

Transmission by air droplets generated by a person with infectious stage TB.

Risk factors immunocompromise (eg HIV+ve), social deprivation, migrants from, or travel to, high prevalence countries (eg South-East Asia, Africa).

Outcomes of exposure
- *Immune destruction* of inhaled bacilli by a competent immune system
- *Primary TB* infection may be asymptomatic, or cause cough, fever, etc
- *Latent TB* after primary infection most patients become asymptomatic with the mycobacteria dormant within a tubercle; CXR may show apical fibrosis
- *Active TB* disease in a specific organ (see Table 15.18) or throughout the body (miliary); usually reactivation of latent TB (eg due to immunocompromise) or a rarely continuation of primary TB.

Table 15.18 *Sites of active TB*

Pulmonary	Commonest (80%): cough, fever, breathlessness, weight loss
Meningeal	Sub-acute meningitic symptoms: fever, headache, ↓GCS
Genitourinary	Frequency, dysuria, loin pain, haematuria; ♂epididymitis; ♀PID, infertility
Bone	Back pain, stiffness; paraspinal abscess or cord compression
Skin	Jelly-like nodules/ulcers on face and extremities (lupus vulgaris)
GI	Affects any part of GI tract—typically ileocaecal; weight loss, abdo pain
Miliary	Haematological spread to multiple tissues: liver, spleen, lungs, marrow

Symptoms and signs see Table 15.18; systemic features include fever, night sweats, weight loss, anorexia, lethargy, erythema nodosum.

Isolation if you suspect TB and patient requires admission to hospital, isolate patient in −ve pressure side room until 3 sputum samples have been urgently tested for mycobacteria. All visitors/staff must wear face masks; if the patient is moved through the hospital they should wear a mask. If mycobacteria are identifiable on initial urgent sputum smears, these so-called 'smear +ve' patients must remain isolated; retest after 2wk of treatment: they should no longer be infectious.

Investigations **CXR** consolidation (often apical), cavitation, fibrosis, calcification, hilar lymphadenopathy, pleural effusion; **sputum** 3 early morning cultures for Ziehl–Nielsen (ZN) stain for acid-fast bacilli (AFB), takes 3–12wk; sputum may be induced with nebulised saline; bronchoscopy with lavage and biopsy may be necessary in those with high index of suspicion; **Mantoux** tuberculin skin test based upon hypersensitivity response to intradermal mycobacterial antigens: may be false −ve if immunocompromised, whilst result may be +ve in latent infection or after BCG vaccine; **interferon-G release assays** eg T-SPOT® TB: sensitive and specific; do not reliably differentiate active and latent infection; **HIV** consent all patients with TB for testing; **drug sensitivity testing** previously performed in culture over several weeks, now based upon rapid genetic testing.

Treatment **initial phase (2mth)** standard therapy involves rifampicin, isoniazid, pyrazinamide and ethambutol; **continuation phase (4mth)** rifampicin and isoniazid are continued for fully sensitive isolates. Resistant organisms will require alternative regimens; side effects are common eg hepatitis (all antibiotics), neuropathy (isoniazid), visual changes (ethambutol). Full compliance is essential: Directly Observed Therapy (DOT) is recommended where risk of poor compliance.

Drug resistance multi-drug resistant TB (MDR-TB) is resistant to isoniazid and rifampicin; consult with infectious disease specialists early.

Contact tracing all individuals who have shared an enclosed space with someone with active TB should have further testing guided by risk and previous vaccination.[2]

Vaccination BCG (Bacillus Calmette–Guérin) is a live vaccine that decreases the risk of developing TB by between 50 and 70%; it used to be given in the UK to everyone at 13yr but is now given at birth to at-risk groups only.

[1] See ⌂www.who.int/tb for useful information and educational resources.

[2] NICE guidelines available at ⌂guidance.nice.org.uk/CG117

Overdose emergency

Airway	Check airway is patent; consider manoeuvres/adjuncts
Breathing	If no respiratory effort – **CALL ARREST TEAM**
Circulation	If no palpable pulse – **CALL ARREST TEAM**
Disability	If GCS ≤8 – **CALL ANAESTHETIST**

Drug overdoses are often deliberate but can happen accidentally at home or in a hospital. The emergency management is the same.

▶▶Call for **senior help** early if patient unwell or deteriorating.

- **Lie patient down** ask a colleague to observe for vomiting and be ready to turn them onto their side
- **Assess respiration** RR, O_2 sats, O_2 requirement, consider blood gas:
  - call anaesthetist if poor respiratory effort, it will only get worse
- **Assess CVS** HR, BP, consider fluid resuscitation (🕮 p381)
- **Venous access**, take bloods:
  - FBC, U+E, LFT, salicylate, paracetamol, glucose, PT/APTT
- **Monitor** pulse oximeter, BP cuff, defibrillator ECG leads if unwell
- Take brief **history** to establish the medication(s), quantity and timing
- **Consult the Toxbase/Poisons service** (🕮 p493) for info on the specific overdose
- Consider **gastric lavage** if <1h since overdose
- **Examine patient** condensed CVS, resp, abdo and neuro exam
- Repeat set of **observations** and **ECG**
- **Consider**:
  - urine toxicology
  - urinary catheter
  - ABG
- **Follow management plan from Toxbase/Poisons service (🕮 p493)**
- If patient deteriorating:
  - call for senior help
  - **reassess** starting with A, B, C …

Life-threatening causes

• Paracetamol	🕮 p495
• Other overdoses	Check Toxbase/Poisons service (🕮 p493)

Overdose and deliberate self-harm[1]

> *Worrying features* violent method, intention to die, ongoing wish to die, previous attempts, preparation, concealment.

Think about *emergency* psychosis, acute suicidal intent; ***common*** depression, grief, stressful situations, relationship breakdown.

Ask about *medical* medications taken, dose, number of tablets, time-frame, ingestion of alcohol, symptoms (vomiting, tinnitus, dizziness, abdo pain), mechanism of injuries; ***psychiatric*** events leading to overdose, expected outcome, intent (eg call for help, to kill themselves), suicide note, extent of planning/preparation (eg spontaneous), circumstances of seeking help, expectation of being found, current intent (eg still suicidal), alcohol intoxication prior to events, recent stresses (relationships, work, money, family, legal); ***PMH*** previous suicide attempts and methods, psychiatric care, chronic illness; risk factors for paracetamol toxicity (if paracetamol overdose, 📖 p495); ***DH*** regular medications, alternative medicines (eg St John's wort), tetanus status, allergies, alcohol intake, substance abuse; ***SH*** who do they live with? Who is at home? Relationships, family, friends, employment.

Obs temp, HR, BP, RR, GCS, glucose.

Look for[1] *medical* orientation, conscious level, pupil size, reflexes, tone, tremor, sweating, agitated, abdo tenderness, sweating, nutritional state; ***psychiatric*** (mental state examination once medically stable and not intoxicated, see 📖 p160) neglect, scars on wrist/forearms, eye contact, withdrawn, abnormal posture or movements, anxiety, paranoia, flat affect, speech form and content, thought form and content including delusions, perception including hallucinations, concentration, memory, insight into actions. See Table 15.19.

Investigations[2] paracetamol and salicylate levels in all overdoses (ideally 4h post-overdose); consider **blds** glucose, FBC, U+E, LFT, PT/APTT **ECG**; **ABG**.

Management[2]

Severe overdose stabilise the patient according to 📖 p492 and get senior help early.

Severe trauma call the trauma team and see 📖 p232.

Paracetamol see 📖 p495.

Other trauma see 📖 p434.

Risk assessment (📖 p494) this determines the psychiatric management of the patient. Once medical problems are resolved the patient must be discussed with the on-call liaison psychiatrist. They will recommend further in-patient psychiatric assessment or discharge home with appropriate psychiatric follow-up.

Acutely suicidal patients must not leave the hospital without psychiatric assessment. If necessary they can be restrained or sedated (📖 p364) under the Mental Health Act (1983); always seek senior advice and help.

---

[1] NICE guidelines available at ⌐guidance.nice.org.uk/CG16
[2] Guidance on specific overdoses can be obtained from the UK National Poisons Information Service at ⌐www.toxbase.org (all UK NHS emergency departments should have a login).

Table 15.19 *Features of common overdoses*

	Symptoms and signs	Investigations
Salicylates (aspirin)	Vomiting, ↑RR, tinnitus, vertigo, sweating	Respiratory alkalosis then metabolic acidosis; ↑↓glucose, ↑salicylate levels
Tricyclic antidepressants (TCAs)	Dilated pupils, blurred vision, seizures, ↓GCS, dysrhythmia, tachycardia	Acidosis, prolonged PR, QRS and QTc heart block, ventricular dysrhythmias
Digoxin	Nausea, confusion, hallucinations, yellow haloes around lights, anorexia	Dysrhythmias, ST depression ('reverse tick' shaped, 🕮 p259); effects more severe if ↓K+
Opioids	Pinpoint pupils, ↓RR, ↓GCS	Respiratory acidosis, opioids on urine toxicology
Benzodiazepines, barbiturates, alcohol	↓GCS, ↓BP, ↓tone, ↓reflexes	Respiratory acidosis (mixed acidosis if excess alcohol); blood and urine toxicology
Ecstasy, amphetamines, cocaine	Thirst, confusion, agitation, tremor, dilated pupils ↑HR, ↑BP, ↑temp	Urine toxicology; ECG abnormalities (dysrhythmia, ischaemia)

Assessing risk after suicide attempts

This is a difficult judgement that requires experience; making the wrong decision could result in a preventable death. All cases should be discussed with the on-call psychiatrist. The mnemonic 'SAD PERSONS' was originally developed to teach medical students to assess suicide risk; this has been modified into a validated scoring system for use in the emergency department setting (Table 15.20).[1] It is by no means foolproof; trust your instinct and ask for help if you are in any doubt

Table 15.20 *Modified 'SAD PERSONS' score*

Sex: Male	Score +1
Age <19yr or >45yr	Score +1
Depressed or hopeless	Score +2
Previous suicide attempts or psychiatric care	Score +1
Excessive alcohol or drug use	Score +1
Rational thinking loss: psychotic or organic illness	Score +2
Separated, widowed or divorced	Score +1
Organised or serious attempt at suicide	Score +2
No social support	Score +1
Stated future intent (determined to repeat or ambivalent)	Score +2

Interpreting the score

Score <6	May be safe to discharge, depending upon circumstances
Score 6–8	Probably requires psychiatric assessment
Score >8	Likely to need admission and urgent psychiatric assessment

Other important risk factors include stressful life-events, unemployment or retirement, identifying with others who have committed suicide, chronic illness (medical or psychiatric) and availability of lethal weapons or drugs (eg farmers or vets).

[1] Hockberger et al. J Emerg Med. 1988 **6**:99 (subscription required).

Paracetamol overdose

Paracetamol is the most widely used analgesic in the UK and the world. It is contained in a large number of preparations available over the counter, leading to the potential for both accidental and deliberate overdose. In the UK, paracetamol is the commonest drug overdose, and the commonest cause of acute liver failure, but only rarely leads to death (approximately 130 deaths and 15–20 liver transplants a year).

Symptoms and signs occur in 3 phases; initially patients may have no specific symptoms, or mild nausea and vomiting; after 24h, RUQ pain ±evidence of liver failure (↑PT ↑ALT ↑AST); after 3–5d recovery may begin, or fulminant hepatic failure will develop with coagulopathy, ↓blood glucose, encephalopathy and acute kidney injury (hepatorenal syndrome).

Investigations Paracetamol and salicylate levels 4h after overdose or as soon as possible if >4h; less reliable in staggered overdose (tablets taken over >1h) – begin acetylcysteine regardless; LFT (↑ALT), U+E, clotting, blood glucose; **ABG** (pH<7.3 despite adequate fluid resuscitation predicts mortality).

Treatment activated charcoal PO given within 1h if ingestion of >150mg/kg. Acetylcysteine helps replace the substrates necessary to eliminate the toxic products formed when normal hepatic metabolism of paracetamol is overwhelmed, and should be given to all those with a staggered overdose or a blood paracetamol level above the treatment threshold on the nomogram in Fig. 15.6.

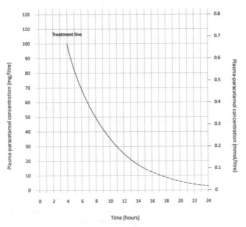

Fig. 15.6 Paracetamol overdose treatment nomogram. Reproduced from *Drug Safety Update* September 2012, vol 6, issue 2: A1 © MHRA.

In adults three doses of acetylcysteine are given:
- 150mg/kg IV infusion in 200ml 5% glucose or 0.9% saline over 1h
- 50mg/kg IV infusion in 500ml 5% glucose or 0.9% saline over 4h
- 100mg/kg IV infusion in 1000ml 5% glucose or 0.9% saline over 16h.

Start treatment within 8h of ingestion – do not wait for level if patient presents close to or after this time. Discontinue treatment if the plasma concentration is later reported as below the treatment line and patient is asymptomatic with normal LFTs, creatinine and PT. Discuss patients with acidosis, encephalopathy, worsening renal function or PT prolongation with hepatologist on call (or at nearest liver centre if not available locally)

Side effects Flushing, rash, pruritus, urticaria, nausea and vomiting are all relatively common during treatment. More severe anaphylactoid reactions (↓BP, ↑HR, bronchospasm) should be managed as per 🕮 p470 with infusion slowed or stopped.

Vaginal bleeding

Worrying features ↑HR, ↓BP, weight loss, anaemia, abdominal pain, +ve pregnancy test.

Think about *emergency* massive bleed, ectopic pregnancy, miscarriage; ***common*** menstruation, dysfunctional uterine bleeding, trauma, ectropion, contraceptive-related, infection, cervical or endometrial polyps, malignancy (cervix, uterus, ovaries), foreign body, miscarriage, fibroids, pelvic inflammatory disease; ***rare*** clotting abnormalities, hypothyroid. See box and Table 15.20.

Causes of vaginal bleeding

Menorrhagia	Dysfunctional uterine bleeding, fibroids, endometriosis, polyps, pelvic inflammatory disease, endometrial cancer, IUCD/foreign body, clotting disorder, hypothyroid
Postcoital	Ectropion, polyps, infection, cancer (cervix, uterus), trauma
Intermenstrual	Polyps, ectropion, infection, IUCD/foreign body, pregnancy, hormonal contraception, cancer (cervix, uterus)
Postmenopausal	▶▶Endometrial cancer until proven otherwise, other cancer (cervix, ovarian), atrophic vaginitis, infection, polyps

Ask about possibility of pregnancy, timing of bleeding (between periods, during periods, after intercourse), duration of bleeding, amount of bleeding (pads, tampons, clots, flooding), menstrual pain, effect on lifestyle, other vaginal discharge, weight loss, abdo pain, trauma, dyspareunia (pain during intercourse), lumps; ***PMH*** anaemia, clotting problems, thyroid problems; ***DH*** contraceptive pills or injections, IUCD, anticoagulants, aspirin; ***SH*** sexual activity; ***O+GH*** usual cycle and bleeding, pregnancies, miscarriages, terminations, last smear test and result, STIs, date of last menstrual period (LMP).

Obs HR, BP, postural BP, RR, temp, pregnancy test.

Look for abdo tenderness/guarding, pelvic masses, inguinal lymphadenopathy, exclude PR bleeding; ***internal examination*** (📖 p156) vulval lesions, size of uterus, uterine masses, adnexal tenderness or masses, presence of blood/discharge; ***speculum exam*** (📖 p157) ulceration, ectropion, bleeding, lumps, prolapse, triple swab if infection is suspected.

Investigations ***pregnancy test*** by urinary β-hCG is absolutely essential; consider ***blds*** serum β-hCG, FBC, CRP, clotting, U+E, LFT, TFT; ***USS*** pelvis (trans-vaginal). May need diagnostic laparoscopy or hysteroscopy.

Treatment

- *Signs of shock* call for senior help; resuscitate as for other causes of blood loss (📖 p478)
- *Positive pregnancy* test and abdominal tenderness: assume an ectopic pregnancy (📖 p498); secure two sites of good IV access (grey or bigger), X-match 4 units and contact a gynaecologist immediately
- *Postmenopausal bleeding* refer urgently to rule out cancer
- *Otherwise* consider likely diagnoses and rule out serious conditions. See Table 15.20.

Table 15.20 *Common causes of vaginal bleeding*

	History	Examination	Investigations
Ectopic	Abdo pain; LMP >4wk, PV bleeding	Abdo tenderness ± peritonism, shock	+ve β-hCG; ↓Hb; empty uterus may be seen on USS
Miscarriage	PV bleeding, crampy pain	Open/closed os, products of conception	β-hCG +ve, ±foetus or empty uterus on USS
Dysfunctional uterine bleeding	Menorrhagia	Normal	Normal
Fibroids	Menorrhagia	Bulky uterus	Visible on USS
Endometrial cancer	Postmenopausal bleeding, abdo pain	Usually normal; inguinal lymphadenopathy	Thickened endometrium on USS; mass on hysteroscopy
Pelvic inflammatory disease	Abdominal pain, vaginal discharge, dyspareunia	Abdominal tenderness, foul-smelling discharge	+ve cultures
Infection	Vaginal discharge, itching, foul odour	Erythema, swelling, discharge	+ve cultures
Ectropion/erosion	Intermenstrual or postcoital bleeding; use of OCP or pregnant	Red ring or flare around external os	Normal
Polyps	Intermenstrual or postcoital bleeding	Polyp may be visible on speculum examination	Polyp on hysteroscopy
Cervical cancer	Postcoital bleeding, dyspareunia, discharge	Mass, ulcer or bleeding cervix	Colposcopy and biopsy
Ovarian cancer	Lower abdo pain, weight loss, ±bleeding	Adnexal mass, abdominal distension	↑CA-125; mass on USS or CT
Hypothyroid	Constipation, cold intolerance, tiredness, menorrhagia	Dry skin, goitre, bradycardia, slow relaxing reflexes	↓T₄, ↑TSH
Clotting abnormality	Family history, bleeding, bruising, joint swelling	Bruises, joint swelling or deformity	Abnormal clotting or bleeding time

Causes of vaginal bleeding covered elsewhere			
Pelvic inflammatory disease	📖 p500	Miscarriage	📖 p503
Clotting abnormalities	📖 p405	Hypothyroid	📖 p334

Infection (cervicitis, vaginitis)

Infection with candida or STIs (📖 p465); similar symptoms can be caused by a lack of oestrogen (atrophic vaginitis), allergy or foreign body.

Symptoms itching, vaginal discharge, dysuria, superficial dyspareunia, abnormal odour, small amounts of bleeding.

Signs vaginal or cervical erythema, swelling, exudates, discharge.

Investigation high vaginal, endocervical and chlamydial swabs.

Treatment treat the cause eg antibiotics, antifungals, oestrogens.

▶▶**Ectopic pregnancy**[1] (OHCS8 📖 p262)

A gynaecological emergency, usually presenting at 6–9wk gestation. Consider this in every woman of child-bearing age presenting with collapse, acute abdominal pain ±PV bleeding.

Symptoms abdominal pain, shoulder tip/back pain, PV bleeding, recent amenorrhoea, dizziness; *ruptured ectopic* collapse, shock, peritonism.

Risk factors ↑maternal age, previous ectopic, tubal surgery, previous STIs/PID, IUCD, assisted conception techniques, smoking.

Signs **abdo** unilateral iliac fossa pain (75%) ±mass (50%); if rupture guarding; ↑HR ±↓BP; **PV** bleeding (50%), extreme cervical pain.

Investigations **blds** β-hCG (serum and urine), FBC, G+S/X-match; transvaginal **USS** foetal sac/pole in the adnexae, free fluid.

Differentials miscarriage, appendicitis, pelvic infection, ovarian cyst.

Management IV access (14–16G), IV fluids and urgent referral to gynae; **medical** methotrexate increasingly used for small (<3.5cm) early ectopics in stable patients **surgical** laparoscopic/open salpingectomy/salpingostomy or oophorectomy; send sample for histology.

Dysfunctional uterine bleeding

Menorrhagia without any detectable abnormality.

Symptoms heavy bleeding during periods only, interfering with daily activities, otherwise well.

Signs normal systemic and gynaecological exam.

Investigations **blds** may have mild iron deficiency anaemia, otherwise normal.

Management tranexamic acid 1g/6h PO or mefenamic acid 500mg/8h PO (both started on the first day of periods and whilst flow is heavy), cyclical progesterone, combined OCP, Mirena® coil; in severe cases endometrial ablation/resection or hysterectomy may be considered.

Cervical ectropion/erosion

Temporary extension of the uterine epithelium through the cervical os into the vagina in response to oestrogen eg combined OCP or pregnancy.

Symptoms often asymptomatic; intermenstrual bleeding, postcoital bleeding, menorrhagia.

Signs red flare or ring around the external os on speculum examination.

Investigations none required but must have usual smear test screens.

Treatment usually none, change of contraceptive, cautery/cryosurgery.

Cervical and endometrial polyps

Uterine growths that may pass through the external os into the vagina.

Symptoms often asymptomatic, menorrhagia, intermenstrual, postcoital or postmenopausal bleeding.

Signs may be visible on speculum examination.

Investigations **hysteroscopy** endometrial polyps may be seen; if removed they should be sent for histology, but 99% are benign.

Treatment surgical removal with cautery of the base with silver nitrate via speculum or hysteroscopy.

---

[1] NICE guidelines available at ⤷**guidance.nice.org.uk/CG154**

Fibroids (uterine leiomyoma)

Benign tumours of the uterine smooth muscle.

Symptoms may be asymptomatic, menorrhagia, prolonged periods, pelvic pain, urinary frequency or incontinence, infertility, abdominal mass.

Signs palpable mass on abdominal or vaginal examination, bulky uterus.

Investigations **blds** may have anaemia; visible on pelvic **USS**.

Treatment symptoms improve after menopause so treatment is often conservative; *medical* GnRH agonists (eg goserelin, leuprorelin) cause a temporary menopause to shrink the tumour; *radiology* uterine artery ablation; *surgery* myomectomy, hysterectomy.

Endometrial (uterine) cancer

This is common and presents early, so all postmenopausal or irregular perimenopausal bleeding must be referred to gynaecologists.

Risk factors age, overweight, high fat diet, polycystic ovaries, late menopause, no pregnancies, family history, tamoxifen; OCP is protective.

Symptoms postmenopausal or intermenstrual bleeding, menorrhagia, watery vaginal discharge, lower abdo pain, dyspareunia.

Signs usually normal unless advanced.

Investigations transvaginal **USS** to assess endometrial thickness; *biopsy* via aspiration sampling; *hysteroscopy* ± dilation and curettage (D+C).

Treatment total abdominal hysterectomy and bilateral salpingo-oophrectomy ±radiotherapy or palliative treatment with radiotherapy.

Prognosis overall 5yr survival 80%.

Cervical cancer

Risk factors human papillomavirus, early first intercourse, multiple partners, smoking, others STIs, lack of screening.

Vaccination against HPV types 16 and 18 is routinely offered to all 12yr-old girls in UK (Cevarix®); predicted to lead to ↓70% cervical cancer incidence.

Screening all women aged 25–64yr are offered screening by cervical smear (3yrly from 25–49yr; 5yrly from 50–64).

Symptoms asymptomatic (abnormal smear tests); postcoital, intermenstrual or postmenopausal bleeding, dyspareunia, vaginal discharge.

Signs ulceration, mass or bleeding on cervix.

Investigations **colposcopy** ± biopsy; *CT/MRI*.

Treatment **low stage (1a)** hysterectomy and radiotherapy; **high stage (>1b)** chemotherapy and radiotherapy.

Prognosis overall 5yr survival 65%.

Ovarian cancer[1]

Risk factors family history, age, early menarche, late menopause, no pregnancies, infertility, overweight; OCP is protective.

Symptoms lower abdo pain (similar to ovarian torsion 🕮 p500), weight loss, bloating, irregular periods, postmenopausal bleeding, urinary frequency, constipation, pain on intercourse.

Signs adnexal mass, abdominal distension/mass, ascites, leg oedema, DVT.

Investigations **blds** ↑CA-125, α-FP, β-hCG; **USS** or **CT** abdomen/pelvis.

Treatment surgical removal of all visible tissues (uterus, ovaries, omentum) and chemotherapy.

Prognosis usually poor due to late presentation; overall 5yr survival 30%.

[1] NICE guidelines available at **guidance.nice.org.uk/CG122**

Gynaecological causes of pain

▶▶Consider ectopic pregnancy in every woman of child-bearing age presenting with collapse, acute abdominal pain and PV bleeding (📖 p498).

Pelvic inflammatory disease (PID)

Infection and inflammation of the upper genital tract commonly with STIs (📖 p465) eg *Chlamydia trachomatis* or *Neisseria gonorrhoeae*.

Symptoms lower abdominal pain (90%), vaginal discharge (75%, may be foul-smelling), intermenstrual/postcoital bleeding (40%), pyrexia (30%), dysuria, dyspareunia, nausea, vomiting, infertility, general malaise.

Signs **abdomen** tenderness; **PV** adnexal tenderness, cervical excitation.

Risk factors young age at first intercourse, multiple sexual partners, no barrier contraception, smoking.

Differential diagnosis appendicitis, endometriosis, ovarian cysts, ectopic pregnancy, other STIs, HIV, urinary tract infection.

Investigations **MSU**; **genital swabs** (high vaginal, endocervical, Chlamydia) for M,C+S; **blds** FBC, CRP, cultures; **USS** (to exclude ovarian cyst).

Management IV access for fluids, analgesia; remove IUCD; antibiotics (eg ceftriaxone 250mg IM STAT, then metronidazole 400mg/12h PO and doxycycline 100mg/12h PO for 14d); refer to GUM for contact tracing.

Complications untreated may lead to chronic pelvic pain and infertility; tubo-ovarian abscess, septicaemia, 2° infertility, ectopic pregnancy.

Ovarian cyst/torsion

Torsion most commonly occurs with fibromas and dermoid cysts.

Symptoms severe, sudden onset lower abdominal pain, iliac fossa pain radiating to the flank, nausea, vomiting, fever.

Signs **abdomen** tenderness; **PV** adnexal tenderness.

Risk factors developmental abnormalities, early pregnancy, women undergoing hormonal stimulation for IVF.

Differential diagnosis appendicitis, diverticulitis, ectopic pregnancy, urinary tract infection.

Investigations **urine** dipstick ±MSU; urine and serum β-hCG (to exclude pregnancy/ectopic); **USS**.

Management IV access for fluids, analgesia; laparoscopy if not settling.

Complications infection, peritonitis, adhesions, infertility (rare).

Endometriosis

Endometrial tissue found outside the endometrial cavity that bleeds with the menstrual period; called adenomyosis if in the uterine muscle wall.

Symptoms often asymptomatic; painful periods, pelvic pain before/with periods or constantly (adhesions), deep dyspareunia, infertility, rectal pain.

Signs generalised pelvic tenderness, fixed (retroverted) uterus, palpable nodule on uterosacral ligaments; large uterus in adenomyosis.

Investigations **laparoscopy** (though it is a common incidental finding).

Management **medical** preventing cyclical hormone changes can shrink ectopic tissue: continuous combined OCP; GnRH agonists (eg goserelin, leuprorelin); **surgery** laparoscopic laser ablation of ectopic tissue and division of adhesions, bilateral salpingo-oopherectomy ±hysterectomy.

Contraception

Contraception (OHGP3 📖 p748)

Ideally, this should be discussed with both partners; options include:
- *Barrier methods* condoms, caps, diaphragm, femidoms, sponges; condoms reduce transmission of STIs (no other contraceptives have this effect)
- *IUCD* local progesterone-releasing (Mirena®) or copper-containing plastic device; **side effects** bleeding, pain, pelvic infection, ectopic pregnancies, expulsion
- *Oral contraceptive pill* either oestrogen and progesterone (combined, COC) or progesterone only (POP); **side effects** acne, bleeding, breast tenderness, bloating, weight gain, mood changes, nausea, DVT/PE
- *Hormones by other routes* eg implants (3yr) and injections (3mth)
- *Sterilisation* for couples who have completed families; NB male sterilisation is 10 times more effective than female sterilisation.

Effectiveness is usually quoted as the percentage of *typical users* who would avoid pregnancy if having regular unprotected intercourse for 1 year. Male sterilisation >99.9%, female sterilisation 99.7%, Mirena® 99.9%, COC 99.7%, POP 99.5%, Depo 99.5%, Implants 99.9%, IUCD 99%, barrier methods 85–98%, coitus interruptus 70%.

Pill checks (OHGP3 📖 p752)

Women on the COC or POP need reviews every 3–6mth:
Problems headaches, weight gain, bloating, breakthrough bleeding, depression, acne, breast tenderness, hypertension (check BP).
Education stop smoking, DVT risks (reattend immediately if painful ±swollen leg), missed pill rules (see box).

> ### Advice for missed pills
>
> **COC** if <12h since missed dose, take the pill immediately then at the usual time; no extra precautions. If >12h take next pill at normal time; alternative contraception for next 7d, start another pack without a break if due to finish pack within 7d.
>
> **POP** if >3h since missed dose, take pill immediately and then take the next dose at the normal time; alternative contraception for 7d.
>
> If patient develops vomiting or diarrhoea whilst on either pill, advise her to use barrier contraception until 7d after resolution of symptoms.

Emergency contraception (OHGP3 📖 p748)

Discuss timings, LMP, risk of PE/migraine, future contraception, STI testing.
Levonorgestrel available over the counter as a single 1500microgram tablet within 72h then barrier contraception until next period.
Copper IUCD inserted within 5d; more effective but infection is a risk so needs STI screen (📖 p465) and consider prophylactic antibiotics.

Menopause and HRT (OHGP3 📖 p708)

HRT helps alleviate menopausal symptoms, including hot flushes and vaginal atrophy. Much attention has focused on the ↑risk of PE/DVT, stroke, breast, ovarian and endometrial cancers associated with HRT usage. In general, HRT should only be prescribed after a discussion of these risks with the patient, and then at the lowest effective dose for the shortest necessary period of time, with regular review. The risks of HRT are summarised in section 6.4.1 of the *BNF*.

Early pregnancy (1ˢᵗ trimester)

Diagnosing pregnancy

Symptoms missed period, urinary frequency, nausea, vomiting, malaise, nipple tingling/itching, breast enlargement.

Signs enlarged uterus, cervix looks bluish (venous engorgement).

Investigations **Urine** β-hCG usually positive from the first day of the missed period; **Serum** β-hCG only measure if urine β-hCG is +ve; useful for assessing 1ˢᵗ trimester complications (should increase by >66% every 2d) **USS** transvaginal yolk sac should be detectable within the endometrium from about 5/40 gestation.

Management give the news sensitively, consider who is present (eg relatives), offer congratulations if appropriate; start folic acid 0.4mg/24h PO (more if on anticonvulsants); ask GP to refer to antenatal clinic.

Health promotion exercise, no smoking or alcohol, no vitamin supplements (vitamin A is teratogenic), avoid unpasteurised cheese, shellfish and raw eggs (listeria), and cat faeces (toxoplasmosis).

When to give Anti-D in rhesus (D) −ve women

<20/40: Anti-D 250units IM (deltoid) within 72h of the following situations:

- Ectopic pregnancy
- Spontaneous miscarriage <12/40 with instrumentation eg EPRC
- Spontaneous miscarriage >12/40
- Threatened miscarriage >12/40 if bleeding persists this is repeated every 6wk until delivery
- Surgical or medical terminations <20/40
- Amniocentesis/chorionic villus sampling (CVS)
- Abdominal trauma.

>20/40: Anti-D 500units IM (deltoid) within 72h of the following situations:

- Routinely at 28/40 and 34/40 gestation
- Antepartum haemorrhage
- External cephalic version (ECV) attempts
- Abdominal trauma
- Delivery of rhesus-positive baby (none if baby rhesus-negative).

Table 15.21 *Selected NICE obstetric guidelines*

Topic	Web reference
Routine antenatal care	⁂guidance.nice.org.uk/CG62
Hypertension in pregnancy	⁂guidance.nice.org.uk/CG107
Diabetes in pregnancy	⁂guidance.nice.org.uk/CG63
Multiple pregnancy	⁂guidance.nice.org.uk/CG129
Mental health	⁂guidance.nice.org.uk/CG45
Intrapartum care	⁂guidance.nice.org.uk/CG55
Caesarian section	⁂guidance.nice.org.uk/CG132
Postnatal care	⁂guidance.nice.org.uk/CG37
Ectopic pregnancy and miscarriage in early pregnancy	⁂guidance.nice.org.uk/CG154

Miscarriage (Table 15.22)

Loss of pregnancy <24/40 gestation.

Differentials ectopic pregnancy (📖 p498), ectropion, infection, polyp.

Symptoms vaginal bleeding (may see products of conception), crampy lower abdominal pain, nausea, vomiting, dizziness.

Table 15.22 *Types of miscarriage*

Miscarriage	PV findings	USS findings
Threatened	Bleeding, closed os	Intrauterine pregnancy with heart beat
Inevitable	Bleeding, open os	Intrauterine pregnancy with heart beat
Missed	None/bleeding	Intrauterine pregnancy, no heart beat
Incomplete	Bleeding, open os	Retained products of conception
Complete	Bleeding settling	Empty uterus

Signs may be shocked (↑HR, ↓BP); abdominal tenderness suggests ectopic; *PV* check size of uterus, exclude adnexal tenderness; *speculum* open/closed cervical os, clots, products of conception.

Investigations **blds** FBC, G+S, β-hCG **urine** β-hCG **USS** transvaginal.

Management if there is marked abdo/cervical tenderness exclude an ectopic (📖 p498) by USS and serial serum β-hCG. If shocked insert a grey cannula, fluid resuscitate (📖 p472) and remove products of conception from the os (can cause vasovagal); ergometrine 0.5mg IM is given for severe bleeding. Offer all patients analgesia (📖 p86).

- *Threatened* no treatment has demonstrated any benefit; bed rest is often suggested but does not affect outcome; 25–50% will abort
- *Inevitable/incomplete* the products of conception usually pass without intervention or with mifepristone; surgical removal by ERPC may be considered for pain, bleeding or large quantities of tissue in the uterus
- *Missed* evacuation of products of conception medically eg mifepristone or surgically by EPRC.

ERPC Evacuation of Retained Products of Conception is performed under spinal or general anaesthetic; send evacuated material for karyotyping and histology.

Counselling Offer those affected a chance to ask questions and provide written material for them to take away. Up to 40% of pregnancies end in miscarriage and of these 80% are due to a foetal abnormality eg chromosomal; it should be stressed that miscarriage is almost never due to the actions of the mother.

Recurrence ≥2 unexplained consecutive miscarriages should prompt investigation eg parental karyotypes, karyotype of the products of conception, maternal antiphospholipid antibodies, maternal pelvic USS.

Termination of pregnancy (TOP)

Patients are referred by GPs or family planning centres. Future contraception should be discussed.

Methods **medical** (<9wk) mifepristone 600mg PO, then 1mg gemeprost PV 36–48h later; **surgical** dilatation and evacuation or vacuum aspiration.

Complications haemorrhage, infection, retained products of conception, uterine perforation, feelings of guilt, depression.

Later pregnancy (2ⁿᵈ/3ʳᵈ trimester)

Table 15.23 *Normal ranges in later pregnancy*

Parameter	Range	Parameter	Range
Haematocrit	No change	Albumin	25–40g/l
Haemoglobin	95–150g/L	Urea	1.6–6mmol/l
WCC	5–16 x 10⁹/l	Creatinine	35–75μmol/l
Platelets	150–400 x 10⁹/l	PaO₂	11.0–14.0kPa
ESR	44–114mm/h	PaCO₂	3.6–4.2kPa
Fibrinogen	3000–6200mg/L	HCO₃	18–23mmol/l

Hypertension in pregnancy[1] (BP >140/90mmHg)

Hypertension occurs in up to 20% of pregnancies; 90% will be associated with known chronic hypertension, but some women will develop newly ↑BP, typically after 20/40 gestation (pregnancy-induced or gestational).

Pre-eclampsia is hypertension with development of proteinuria (>0.3g/24h) and may develop from ≥20/40 gestation until 6wk post-partum.

Risk factors **for pre-eclampsia** <18yr or >35yr, first pregnancy, BMI >30, chronic ↑BP, DM, SLE, thrombophilia, PMH or FH pre-eclampsia.

Symptoms usually asymptomatic, headache, vomiting, visual disturbance.

Signs evaluate for signs of 2° causes of ↑BP (📖 p263) or end-organ damage (📖 p265); *pre-eclampsia:* RUQ tenderness, oedema, papilloedema, hyperreflexia, clonus.

Investigations **urine** M,C+S, 24h collection for protein (essential if dipstick ≥2+ protein); **blds** in chronic hypertension ensure secondary causes of hypertension excluded (📖 p263) and recent screening for baseline evidence of end-organ damage (📖 p265); if suspect pre-eclampsia: FBC (plts <100×10⁹/l suggests pre-eclampsia, ITP or HELLP), U+E, ↑urate (sensitive but not specific for renal damage), LFT, clotting (for DIC, 📖 p405), G+S. See Table 15.23.

Assess the foetus USS (foetus growth, size, presentation, liquor volume, foetal movements), umbilical artery Doppler, CTG.

Management **hypertension** stop any existing treatment with ACEi, ARB or chlorothiazide and refer to antenatal medical clinic for monitoring ± antihypertensive therapy; options include labetalol or Ca²⁺-channel antagonists; if suspect *pre-eclampsia* admit ±treat with IV hydralazine or labetalol and MgSO₄; consider expediting delivery.

▶▶Eclampsia

New onset tonic-clonic seizures or unexplained coma during pregnancy or postpartum; usually develops on background of pre-eclampsia.

Signs and symptoms headache, hyperreflexia, clonus, oedema, seizures

Management ▶▶*Obstetric crash call* move into left lateral position, protect airway, 15l/min O₂, IV access (FBC, U+E, LFT, clotting, G+S), check BP, check glucose; MgSO₄ 4g over 20min IV, then maintenance dose of 2g/h IV; if diastolic >110mmHg give hydralazine or labetalol IV (📖 p266). Once stabilised, establish close foetal monitoring and consider **urgent delivery.**

After delivery treat BP >160/110mmHg (📖 p266), strict fluid balance, monitor FBC, U+E, LFT, observe for ≥5d.

---

[1] NICE guidelines available at ⌁guidance.nice.org.uk/CG107

▶▶HELLP (Haemolysis, Elevated liver enzymes, Low Platelets)

Develops in 10% of cases of severe pre-eclampsia.
Symptoms upper abdominal pain, headache, malaise, vomiting.
Signs RUQ tenderness, oedema, ↑BP.
Results ↓Hb, ↑bilirubin, ↑ALT, ↓plts, proteinuria.
Management resuscitate, FFP/plts/blood transfusion, urgent delivery.
Complications DIC, haemorrhage (brain, liver), eclampsia.

Gestational diabetes mellitus (see also ▢ p328)

Any degree of glucose intolerance first detected during pregnancy.
Screening although some advocate universal screening, current NICE guidance[1,2] is to offer a 2h 75g oral glucose tolerance test (OGTT) at booking to women with: previous gestational DM or baby >4.5kg, BMI >30, 1st-degree relative with DM, South Asian, black Caribbean or Middle Eastern ethnicity.
Symptoms often asymptomatic, glucose on urine dipstick.
Signs large for dates, polyhydramnios.
Investigations **blds** plasma glucose ≥7.8mmol/l after OGTT (▢ p328); self-monitoring of capillary blood glucose; regular **USS** to assess foetal growth.
Treatment diet changes and exercise will achieve good glycaemic control in 80%; start insulin or oral hypoglycaemics after 1–2wk if this fails; stop treatment after birth and repeat OGTT at 6wk.
Complications congenital abnormalities, stillbirth, pre-eclampsia, polyhydramnios, large baby, traumatic delivery; **neonate** birth injury (eg shoulder dystocia, brachial plexus trauma), respiratory distress syndrome, polycythaemia, hypoglycaemia, jaundice.

▶▶Antepartum haemorrhage

Vaginal bleeding after 24/40 gestation.
Causes placenta praevia, placental abruption; gynae causes see ▢ p486.
Severe bleeding call senior help; lay flat and elevate legs; O₂ (15l/min); secure 2 large bore IV cannulae (take blood for FBC, clotting, G+S), 1l 0.9% saline STAT; urgent blood (O-negative, type specific, or full X-match, ▢ p400); consider urgent delivery.
Mild bleeding admit, IV access (FBC, clotting, G+S), monitor HR and BP, **PV** only if placental site known; **USS**; consider anti-D (▢ p502).

Anaemia in pregnancy

Screening checked FBC at 12, 28 and 36wk, treat if Hb <110g/L.
Treatment ferrous sulphate 200mg/24h PO and folic acid 0.4mg/24h PO.

Breech presentation

Should be noted from antenatal examination and scans. External cephalic version can be attempted at 37/40 gestation (Rhesus –ve mothers will need anti-D ▢ p502). Elective Caesarean section is often performed.

Gestation >41/40

The risk of stillbirth increases after 42/40 gestation. If the baby has not been delivered by 41/40 then the mother should be seen in antenatal clinic to discuss induction methods. Induction methods include:
- Prostaglandin vaginal gel to 'ripen' the cervix
- Artificial rupture of membranes (AROM, amniotomy)
- Oxytocin infusion.

---

[1] NICE antenatal care guidelines available at ⌁guidance.nice.org.uk/CG62
[2] NICE diabetes in pregnancy guidelines available at ⌁guidance.nice.org.uk/CG63

Delivery[1]

See 📖 p554 for the procedure for normal vaginal delivery.

Prematurity

Birth <37/40 gestation can have serious effects on the baby's survival and risk of disability, especially <32/40. Key components of management of a woman in preterm labour include early and close liaison with obstetrics and paediatrics, maternal steroids (beclometasone 12mg/12h IM) if 24–34/40, consideration of tocolytics, consideration of transfer to a hospital with neonatal intensive care.

Premature rupture of membranes (PROM)

Rupture of membranes prior to onset of labour. Beyond 37/40 gestation, delivery should occur within 24h to reduce the risk of maternal/foetal infection; consider use of IV oxytocin or vaginal prostaglandin gel to induce labour. If <37/40 gestation, admit for IV antibiotics, close monitoring and specialist consideration of the use of steroids, and induction of labour.

Foetal monitoring

- *Doppler probe* listen for decelerations at the end of a contraction
- *CTG* (see box)
- *Foetal blood* sampling (through a dilated cervix from the foetal scalp) to check for acidosis, representing hypoxia (normal pH >7.25).

▶▶Foetal distress (worrying CTG, abnormal foetal blood sample) may indicate need for urgent delivery.

Reading the cardiotocograph (CTG)

CTGs measure foetal HR and uterine tone (contractions). They are usually printed with a scale of 1cm/min. There are four features to note:
- **Baseline** foetal HR (should be 110–160bpm)
- **Variability** (spikes and dips, should be ≥5bpm)
- **Acceleration** (transient increase in HR of >15bpm for >15s)
- **Decelerations** (transient decrease in HR of >15bpm for >15s).

There are three types of deceleration:
- **Early** occur with contractions; the lowest HR is when uterine tone is highest; these are physiological, reflecting compression of the foetal head
- **Late** occur after the contraction; the lowest foetal HR is 20–30s after the maximal uterine tone; these are abnormal
- **Variable** the relation to uterine tone and the degree of deceleration vary between contractions; these are abnormal.

▶▶Worrying features baseline outside of normal, reduced variability, early decelerations of >40bpm, late decelerations, persistent variable decelerations, prolonged decelerations.

Difficult deliveries

Failure to progress if the baby is not coming out get senior help and consider: maternal position, maternal technique, episiotomy, instrumental delivery (forceps/ventouse), emergency LSCS.
Shoulder dystocia 'HELPERR': call **H**elp, **E**pisiotomy, hyperextend the mother's **L**egs onto the abdomen, suprapubic **P**ressure, **E**nter (turn the shoulder with fingers), **R**emove the posterior arm, **R**oll onto all fours.

[1] NICE intrapartum care guidelines available at ⌁guidance.nice.org.uk/CG55

After delivery (post-partum)[1]

▶▶Post-partum haemorrhage

Loss of >500ml blood during the first 24h after delivery. May be primary – loss of > 500ml blood during the first 24h after delivery, or secondary – excessive bleeding >24h and <12wk postnatally.

Causes failure of uterine contraction, tears, retained placenta, clotting disorders.

Severe bleeding call senior help; lay flat and elevate legs; O_2 (15l/min); secure 2 large-bore IV cannulae (take blood for FBC, clotting, G+S), 1l 0.9% saline STAT; urgent blood (O-negative, type specific, or full X-match, 🔲 p400); compress the uterus bimanually, give Syntocinon® 10 units/h in 500ml 0.9% saline, deliver/check placenta, remove any retained placental tissue and repair tears; may need evacuation under anaesthetic or emergency hysterectomy.

Mild bleeding IV access (FBC, clotting, G+S), 0.9% saline, monitor HR and BP, vaginal examination.

Pyrexia

Causes endometritis, wound infection, mastitis, UTI, URTI, DVT.

Ask about mode of delivery, premature ruptured membranes, pyrexia in labour, pain, cough/SOB, PV bleeding/discharge, dysuria, breast pain.

Look for abdo/loin tenderness; **PV** uterine/adnexal tenderness, lochia (period-like discharge), breast tenderness, leg swelling.

Investigations **urine** M,C+S; **blds** FBC, CRP, G+S, bld cultures; **culture** high vaginal swab, sputum, wound swab.

Management according to the cause:

- *Wound infection* of tear or episiotomy: antibiotics (eg flucloxacillin 500mg/6h PO and metronidazole 400mg/8h PO)
- *Endometritis* tender uterus, offensive lochia (vaginal discharge): antibiotics (eg co-amoxiclav 625mg/8h PO; 1.2g/8h IV if signs of sepsis)
- *Mastitis* tender, red breast: encourage to continue breastfeeding (to prevent milk stagnation), NSAIDs (eg ibuprofen 400mg/6h PO), antibiotics (eg flucloxacillin 500mg/6h PO).

Breast problems (see 🔲 p173 for prescribing in breastfeeding)

Cracked nipples nipple shields or emollient cream.

Breast abscess refer to surgical team for incision and drainage.

Post-natal psychiatric problems[2]

With the exertion and trauma of labour, dramatic hormone changes and the immediate demands of motherhood, it is perhaps unsurprising that 85% of women experience mood disturbance during the post-partum period. For most, this goes no further than transient and mild *Postpartum 'Baby blues'* 1–10d after delivery, with rapidly fluctuating mood and irritability. 10% may experience *Postnatal depression*, typically 6–16wk after delivery; this resembles depression in any other adult (🔲 p367) and may necessitate antidepressants (eg SSRIs given for a minimum of 6mth), counselling or psychiatric referral. *Puerperal psychosis* affects 0.2% of women, typically presenting 3–7d after delivery with acute psychosis (🔲 p365); this is a ▶▶*psychiatric emergency* necessitating urgent referral and involvement of social services.

[1] NICE postnatal care guidelines available at ⌁guidance.nice.org.uk/CG37

[2] NICE obstetric mental health guidelines available at ⌁guidance.nice.org.uk/CG45

Procedures

Practical procedures

In experienced hands procedures seem easy and highly rewarding, but it takes practice. Learning new procedures can make you feel frustrated, embarrassed, and guilty about inflicting pain. When you are learning a new procedure, especially if it is your first time, ask one of your seniors to take you through it and supervise you. Try to get as much practical experience as you can so that you can work more independently and eventually teach others.

Before starting always introduce yourself and obtain informed consent (verbal or written, 📖 p29) before carrying out the procedure. Explain in clear, simple language what the procedure involves, how it will feel, and why it is necessary and ask if they have any questions. Mentally prepare yourself by thinking through each step of the procedure.

The procedure as you perform the procedure take your time, plan ahead, and be confident in your actions. Make sure you and the patient are as comfortable as possible and in the right position. Ask for an assistant – useful if you have forgotten anything.

If things go well at the end of the procedure always clean up and always dispose of your own sharps. Check the patient is alert, comfortable, and well.

If things go wrong ask for help early. Stay calm and reassure the patient while you wait for help to arrive. See 📖 p30 if there is a serious problem.

Writing in the notes write your name, date, and time of the procedure. Document that you obtained informed consent, why the procedure was undertaken, if there were any problems during it, who supervised and/or assisted you, and what your management plan is, eg sending CSF sample for M,C+S. You should also document the details of any equipment used, such as putting the reference sticker from a urinary catheter wrapping in the notes. Always write that the patient is comfortable afterwards, assuming this is true.

Learning and assessment You will start to learn practical procedures as a medical student. Increasingly, skills labs and simulated manikins are used for formal teaching, prior to your first supervised efforts on patients. Repetition and feedback will help shape your skills, along with reflection on your efforts: think about what you did well, what you could do differently and how you would teach someone else doing the procedure. By the end of F1, you will need to be signed off as competent for the core 15 procedures listed in Table 1.2 (📖 p9) and maintain and improve these skills through F2. You can record your progress using the table on 📖 p512. F1/F2 DOPS forms now receive much less emphasis, and are meant to provide feedback simply on the way you interact with a patient whilst performing the skill.

Things to remember to put on a procedures trolley

- Gloves ± sterile
- Needles (various sizes)
- 0.9% saline
- Antiseptic solution
- Syringes
- Local anaesthetic
- Plenty of swabs – you can never have too many
- Dressings and tape
- Specimen pots/bottles
- Kidney dishes/galipots
- Sharps bin.

Laboratories

There are six main laboratories associated with a hospital:
- Biochemistry
- Haematology and blood bank
- Microbiology
- Histopathology (including cytology)
- Immunology
- Genetics (only available in certain larger hospitals).

Biochemistry this department deals with the processing of blood samples for salt and mineral levels, eg U+E, LFT and hormone levels such as cortisol, TFT etc. It also deals with monitoring drug levels, eg sodium valproate and ABG samples if there is not a blood gas machine in the clinical areas. In general 'gel' bottles are used for biochemistry samples but check with your lab if you are unsure or taking blood for an unusual test (see 📖 p517).

Haematology this lab processes samples for FBC, ESR, clotting studies, G+S and crossmatching. It also examines blood films if there is clinical suspicion of haematological disease, eg haemolytic anaemia, leukaemia or malaria.

Microbiology this specialty is concerned with identifying bacteria, viruses, fungi and parasites in samples of various bodily fluids from patients. It examines specimens under the microscope to look for cells, cultures them in an incubator to try and grow pathogens and if any bugs grow, it investigates which antibiotics can be used to kill them or prevent their growth. It deals with specimens such as blood, urine, faeces, CSF, and swabs taken from any site on the body. Microbiologists also use advanced molecular biology techniques to identify organisms that are difficult to culture, as well as assay antibiotic levels and are a useful source of advice when prescribing antibiotics for complex cases after discussion with your team's seniors. They usually produce the hospital antibiotic guideline policy in combination with the pharmacists.

Histopathology this specialty deals with tissue samples, eg biopsies and specimens removed during operations or post-mortems. Pathologists examine these samples both macro- and microscopically to determine the nature of the tissue and the underlying disease process. They use different slicing and staining techniques to examine specimens under the microscope to determine the disease process or progression.

Immunology performs tests to assess the immune system for underactivity (immunosuppression) or overactivity (autoimmune disease); many of these involve measuring antibody levels eg ANA. Samples for antibody analysis usually go in the plain tubes (📖 p517).

Genetics this lab has two subdivisions:
- Cytogenetics that look for chromosomal abnormalities eg assessing an amniocentesis sample for trisomy 21 (Down's)
- Molecular genetics that look for mutations in DNA, eg cystic fibrosis.

The blood tube used for these tests varies between centres; the sample quality (fresh, free-flowing) is especially important for cytogenetics.

Achievement of Core Foundation Skills

This page is for you to record your personal progress towards achieving independence in all 15 of the key practical procedures identified by the GMC as required by the end of F1. During F2 you should maintain and build on these skills. Links to relevant pages in this book are shown.

Skill	Key dates and progress	
	First attempted	Signed off
Venepuncture 📖 p514		
IV cannulation 📖 p518		
Giving IV medication and fluids 📖 p526		
ABG 📖 p522		
Blood culture 📖 p515		
IV fluid prescribing and infusion 📖 p380		
Blood transfusion 📖 p398		
Local anaesthetic injection 📖 p558		
SC injection 📖 p524		
IM injection 📖 p524		
Perform and interpret an ECG 📖 p528		
Perform and interpret peak flow 📖 p130		
Urethral catheterisation (♀) 📖 p546		
Urethral catheterisation (♂) 📖 p546		
Airway care and adjuncts 📖 p230		

Taking blood (venepuncture)

| **Consent** verbal | **Level** F1 | **Difficulty** 1/5 |

Indications diagnosis, monitoring physiological state, therapeutic drug monitoring.

Contraindications *absolute* competent patient refusal, ipsilateral AV fistula.

Site usually antecubital fossa but can use any vein (eg hands, arms, feet, and groin (femoral stab 📖 p516)); never use a limb with an AV fistula (dialysis) or an IV infusion.

Equipment non-sterile gloves, tourniquet, antiseptic swab, vacutainer hub and needle, gauze, tape, sharps bin, blood bottles (see 📖 p517).
Checks patient comfortable, vein exposed, accessible and not pulsing, cotton wool to hand, no IV fluids going into the limb of selected vein.
Patient position upper limb sit the patient upright, with arm extended and below the heart; ***lower limb*** lay patient flat on their back.

Procedure wash hands and wear non-sterile gloves. Assess both arms and select an appropriate vein. Tighten the tourniquet proximally and palpate along the course of the vein to assess its direction and depth. Swab the skin and allow it to dry; and hold the vein steady with your non-dominant hand. Warn the patient and advance the needle into the vein at 20° to the skin; feel for the slight 'give' as you enter the vein and hold your position as you insert the blood bottle into the hub. Once the bottles are filled, unclip the tourniquet and gently cover the puncture site with cotton wool. Withdraw the needle, then apply pressure to the cotton wool. Press (or ask the patient to press) on the cotton wool for 2min (longer if bleeding) then tape it in place. Dispose of the needle and hub into the sharps bin. Fill the blood tubes at the patient's bedside, label them, and complete the accompanying request forms.

Confirmation blood flows freely into the bottle.

Complications pain, bleeding, haematoma, failure, infection.

Safety steady the patient's arm on a pillow to reduce movement and risk of needle-stick injury, dispose of needles into a sharps bin immediately, do not resheath them.

Alternatives
- Blood samples can be taken from cannulae when they are first inserted.
- Central venous lines can be used to sample blood. You will need 2 syringes and a 3rd with a suitable solution to flush the line (always check whether the line needs to be left with heparinised saline in it or just flushed with saline); wear sterile gloves, clean the port thoroughly with alcohol wipes, withdraw 5ml of blood in the first syringe and dispose of it; next withdraw the blood for your sample in the 2nd syringe, before flushing the line with the solution drawn up in 3rd syringe.
- Needle and syringes can be used for smaller veins which may collapse from the suction from vacutainers. For these veins use a small needle (eg blue, 23G) or 'butterfly' (Fig. 16.1; 📖 p521) but beware of haemolysis causing artificially ↑K^+ and ↑LDH.

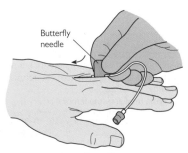

Fig. 16.1 Taking blood using a butterfly needle.

- If you are unable to obtain blood from the upper limb look at the veins in the leg/foot; if you still cannot find veins ask your senior to try before considering a femoral stab.

Hints and tips

- In patients with poor veins spend a long time finding a suitable vein rather than stabbing blindly
- In children use topical local anaesthetic, see 📖 p521
- In adults choose veins by palpation with the tourniquet on rather than their appearance; a bouncy vein is usually easy to take blood from
- Tie the tourniquet tightly and ask the patient to clench their fist repeatedly with their arm below their heart; tap the vein to make it more prominent
- It is best to use a green (21G) vacutainer needle for U+E samples to prevent haemolysis and spuriously ↑K^+; if using a needle and syringe, aspirate blood slowly and gently. Only use blue (23G) needles for very fine veins
- Pull the skin and vein taut to prevent movement away from the needle, especially in older patients
- Going through the skin is the most painful bit, once under the skin you can take several attempts to manoeuvre the needle into the vein
- If you can only obtain a small sample consider using paediatric tubes; see the minimum blood requirements on 📖 p517
- If you decide to use a needle and syringe, never force blood into blood tubes; the results are spectacular, messy, and embarrassing. Consider pulling the top off.

Procedure for taking blood cultures

Indicated by a repeated/persistent temp >37.5°C or one-off ≥38.3°C when a causative organism or source is not already known.

In suspected bacterial endocarditis take 3 sets (6 bottles) from 3 separate veins.

Procedure as for normal blood-taking with needle and syringe except:
- Wear sterile gloves (strict aseptic technique for central lines)
- A set of blood cultures is two bottles (one aerobic and one anaerobic)
- After using the chlorhexidine swab do not touch the vein again
- Once the blood has been obtained replace the used needle with a fresh one
- Flip off the culture bottle lids, swab the top with a clean chlorhexidine wipe, insert the needle and fill each bottle with 5–10ml.

Femoral stab

| **Consent** verbal | **Level** F1 | **Difficulty** 2/5 |

Indications taking blood when alternative sites are not possible.
Contraindications *absolute* competent patient refusal; *relative* local infection, coagulopathy.
Site either side of groin medial to the femoral artery (Fig. 16.2).

Equipment non-sterile gloves, antiseptic swab, 10–20ml syringe, 21G green needle, gauze, tape, sharps bin, appropriate blood bottles (see p517).
Checks patient comfortable, groin exposed, cotton wool to hand.
Patient position patient flat on their back with groin exposed.

Procedure wash hands and wear non-sterile gloves. Feel for the femoral pulse and choose the side where it is most prominent. Swab the skin thoroughly then place your fingers over the artery; warn the patient and insert the needle vertically 1cm medial to your fingers. Pull back on the syringe as you advance and stop moving as soon as you get flashback. Fill the syringe then withdraw. Exert pressure over the area with cotton wool for at least 2min and dress it with a plaster once bleeding has subsided. Fill the blood tubes and label them at the patient's bedside, dispose of the needle and syringe in a sharps bin and complete the accompanying request forms.

Confirmation blood flows freely into the syringe.
Complications pain, bleeding, haematoma, infection, failure; bright red, pulsatile flashback suggests you hit the artery; continue to aspirate the required amount of blood as arterial blood can be used for all routine tests, but press firmly for ≥5min after withdrawing the needle to ensure haemostasis.
Hints and tips to remember the anatomy of the femoral region, work in a lateral to medial direction and think 'NAVY':

- **N**erve (femoral nerve, most lateral)
- **A**rtery (femoral artery)
- **V**ein (femoral vein)
- **Y**-fronts (vital undergarment, best removed prior to procedure).

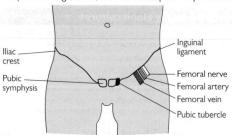

Iliac crest

Pubic symphysis

Inguinal ligament

Femoral nerve
Femoral artery
Femoral vein
Pubic tubercle

Fig. 16.2 Anatomy of the femoral region.

Blood tubes

The colours and contents of the various blood bottles vary between suppliers and hospitals. Use Table 16.1 as a guide to which bottle is used for each test and to make sure the sample is suitable. Fill in the colour of blood bottles and specific blood tests used in your hospital. We have left space at the bottom for other blood tubes.

Table 16.1 *Blood tubes*

Colour	Contents	Tests	Special instructions
	EDTA	FBC, reticulocytes, HbA$_{1C}$, sickle screen, Hb electrophoresis, malaria screen	1ml minimum but aim to fill; gently mix to prevent clotting
	EDTA	ESR	Always fill to the line and gently mix to prevent clotting
	EDTA	Blood transfusion (G+S, crossmatch)	4ml minimum; always handwrite ≥3 forms of patient identification
	Sodium citrate	D-dimer, APTT, PT/INR, thrombophilia screen, fibrinogen	Always fill to the line and gently mix to prevent clotting
	Glucose separating gel	U+E, LFT, amylase, TFT, CRP, Cl$^-$, Mg^{2+}, Ca^{2+}, PO$_4^{3-}$, HCO$_3^-$, urate, LDH, total protein, digoxin, paracetamol and salicylate, lithium, other drug levels, tumour markers, β-hCG, protein electrophoresis, cardiac markers	1.5ml minimum but aim to fill; try to use a green vacutainer needle to prevent haemolysis and inaccurate K$^+$ result
	Plain	Some endocrine tests, drug levels, serology	1.5ml minimum but aim to fill
	Fluoride oxalate	*Blood* glucose, lactate, alcohol; *CSF* glucose, protein, oligoclonal bands	*Blood* fill to the line, mix gently; *CSF* 6 drops; mix gently
	Heparin	Some endocrine tests	Mix gently, may need to be transported on ice

IV cannulation

| **Consent** verbal | **Level** F1 | **Difficulty** 2/5 |

Indications unwell patients, shock, IV fluids/drugs, blood product transfusions, other routes of drug administration not tolerated.

Contraindications *absolute* competent patient refusal, ipsilateral AV fistula.

Site the forearm and back of the hand on the non-dominant arm are usually more convenient sites for the patient, but any vein can be used (eg hands, arms, feet, legs), antecubital fossa in an emergency, never use a limb with an AV fistula (dialysis).

Equipment tourniquet, non-sterile gloves, antiseptic swab, cannulas (appropriate size, see Table 16.2), cannula dressing, 5ml syringe with saline flush, cotton wool, blood collection tubes and adaptor if blood sample required, sharps bin.
Checks patient comfortable, skin is clean and free of infection, vein exposed, accessible and not pulsing, cotton wool ± syringe to hand.
Patient position upper limb sit the patient upright, with arm extended and below the heart; **lower limb** lie patient flat on their back.

Procedure wash hands and wear non-sterile gloves. Assess both arms and select an appropriate vein. Tighten the tourniquet proximally and palpate along the course of the vein to assess its direction and depth. Local anaesthetic can be given intradermally or topically prior to this procedure. Swab the skin with 2% chlorhexidine, allow it to dry then hold the vein steady with your non-dominant hand. Warn the patient and advance the cannula through the skin at 20° with the bevel facing upwards and proximally. Look for flashback, then advance the cannula and needle a little further before withdrawing the metal needle whilst firmly advancing the plastic cannula. Dispose of your sharp as soon as possible at the bed-side. Press with your thumb over the tip of the cannula in the vein.
- **Taking blood** if blood leaks out try lifting the arm, if still leaking remove the tourniquet. Attach the adaptor and each blood tube in turn, then remove the tourniquet
- **Not taking blood** remove the tourniquet.

Place the cap on the end of the cannula, secure with the adhesive dressing and flush with 2–5ml 0.9% saline through the side port. Date the dressing and document date and time of insertion in the notes. Dispose of the needle into a sharps bin.

Confirmation flashback seen, saline flush requires minimal pressure and does not form a proximal subcutaneous 'bleb' or cause pain.

Complications *early* haematoma, tissuing (fluid/drugs enter subcutaneous tissues), local damage, air embolism; *late* thrombophlebitis, cellulitis.

Safety never reinsert the metal needle into the plastic cannula once you have fully removed it as this increases the risk of needle-stick injuries and bits of the plastic cannula may shear off and embolise, steady the patient's arm on a pillow to reduce movement and the risk of needle-stick injury, dispose of needles into a sharps bin immediately.

Alternatives central venous cannulation (📖 p534), alternative route of drug administration (PO/IM/SC/PR).

Hints and tips
• See comments under 'Taking blood'
• Start distally in a limb and work your way proximally if you fail to cannulate initially
• Veins are easier to cannulate at the junction of two veins
• Try to avoid cannulae over a joint as these are uncomfortable and more likely to tissue
• If you go through the wall of the vein, withdraw a small distance until flashback recurs and try to advance the plastic cannula
• In confused patients and children, always cover the cannula with a crêpe bandage and tape the IV line to their skin to minimise auto-extraction and further cannulation practice.

Table 16.2 *Intravenous cannulae*

Colour	Size	Flow rate (ml/min)	Use
Blue	22G	31	Small fragile veins
Pink	20G	55	IV drugs and fluids ±blood
Green	18G	90	Blood, fluids, drugs
White	17G	135	Blood, fluids, drugs
Grey	16G	170	Rapid blood, fluids, drugs
Orange	14G	265	Rapid blood, fluids, drugs

Cannula care
• Inspect cannula daily, looking for inflammation and replace it every 72h
• If asked to replace it, check cannula is still necessary
• If blocked, try flushing the line gently with 0.9% saline and check the giving set isn't kinked
• Remove the cannula if the surrounding skin becomes red, swollen or tender as a result of cannula insertion.

Taking blood in children

Never use a needle and syringe, *never* use a snapped off broken needle.
Consent verbal from parent ±child   **Level** F1   **Difficulty** 3–5/5

Indications diagnosis, monitoring physiological state, drug monitoring.
Contraindications *relative* parental refusal, preserving veins.
Planning before you take the blood get all the equipment ready, think about the amount of blood and which bottles you need, work out where the child, parent and staff will go, think about distraction and topical anaesthesia (eg EMLA).
Choosing a vein the appearance of the vein is more important than the feel in very young children (they can be too small to palpate); common sites include hands, feet and forearms. Antecubital fossa and saphenous veins should only be used if there is no chance of a long line being inserted.

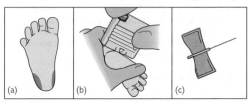

(a)   (b)   (c)

Fig. 16.3 (a) Safe area for heel prick. (b) Use of a Tenderfoot® for heel prick. (c) A cut-off butterfly.

Heel prick

• **Age range** babies <10d; though works on fingers at all ages if desperate
• **Samples** <1ml of blood, ie 2 bottles, not K⁺, clotting or blood cultures
• **Analgesia** pacifier dipped in 20% glucose, swaddling
• **Staff** can be performed alone in babies.
• **Advantages** easy, usually quick, does not use up a site for cannulation
• **Disadvantages** small quantities, can take a long time, messy.

Procedure grip the heel tightly between index finger and thumb. Choose a site on the outside of the heel (Fig. 16.3a) and wipe with an antiseptic swab then apply a small amount of Vaseline®. Hold the lancet (Fig. 16.3b) firmly against the skin and squeeze the heel as you release the lancet. Catch the blood as it drips out; you may need to gently squeeze the foot. Apply cotton wool.

Keeping it 'fun' it is essential to make the experience as pleasant as possible – not least of all to make it easier the next time. Use a special treatment room, involve the play therapist, keep their parents with them, smile, offer distraction, and, most importantly, give out stickers.

Winged needle/cut-off butterfly (Fig. 16.3c)

- **Age range** <1yr (but works at any age)
- **Samples** not blood cultures
- **Analgesia** pacifier dipped in 20% glucose, swaddling, Ametop®/EMLA®
- **Staff** two extra – one to hold the child, one to act as tourniquet.
- **Advantages** relatively easy to hit the vein, can get large quantities
- **Disadvantages** very messy, can clot if flowing slowly.

Procedure locate suitable vein (between the knuckles can be surprisingly good if no others are visible). Ask a colleague to act as a tourniquet. Stretch the skin to fix the vein; a baby's fist fits well between the thumb and index finger if their wrist is flexed. Insert the needle slowly until blood drips out of the needle; catch sufficient blood then remove the needle and apply cotton wool.

Butterfly

- **Age range** >1yr
- **Samples** not blood cultures
- **Analgesia** Ametop®/EMLA®, cold spray, distraction (play therapist)
- **Staff** two extra – one to hold the child, one as tourniquet and distraction.
- **Advantages** clean, can get large quantities
- **Disadvantages** hard to hold butterfly whilst drawing on syringe.

Procedure locate suitable vein. Ask a colleague to act as a tourniquet. Stretch the skin to fix the vein; insert the needle slowly until there is flashback. Hold the butterfly in place whilst gently filling the syringe until there is sufficient blood; remove the butterfly and apply cotton wool.

Cannula

- **Age range** any
- **Samples** any including blood cultures
- **Analgesia** pacifier dipped in 20% glucose, swaddling, Ametop®/EMLA®, cold spray (ethyl chloride), distraction (play therapist)
- **Staff** two extra – one to hold the child, one as tourniquet and distraction
- **Advantages** sterile, easy to obtain large samples, clean
- **Disadvantages** makes future cannulation harder, can be difficult.

Procedure locate suitable vein. Ask a colleague to act as a tourniquet. Stretch the skin to fix the vein. Hold cannula between thumb and middle finger with bevel facing up. Gently insert the cannula until you see flashback then use your index finger to gently advance the plastic cannula into the vein. Secure the cannula in place with a couple of steristrips™ then completely remove the needle (into a sharps bin at the bedside) and collect blood from the cannula by allowing it to drip into the tubes. Remove the tourniquet and secure the cannula further with an adhesive dressing. Attach the extender to the cannula and flush with 2ml 0.9% saline. Wrap the surrounding area and the extender tube in gauze so that only the end of the extender is accessible.

Arterial blood gas (ABG)

| **Consent** verbal | **Level** F1 | **Difficulty** 3/5 |

Indications assessment of hypoxia, CO_2 retention, acid–base status, acutely ill patients, DKA.

Contraindications *absolute* competent patient refusal; **radial** AV fistula, poor/absent collateral circulation, bony fractures; **femoral** femoral artery graft; *relative* overlying infection, abnormal clotting.

Site radial artery (usual), femoral artery, ulnar artery, brachial artery (last resort).

Equipment non-sterile gloves, antiseptic swab, heparin-filled syringe and cap, needle (blue for radial, green for femoral), gauze/cotton ball, tape, sharps bin.
Checks note the concentration of O_2 the patient is on and their temperature. Locate the nearest ABG analysis machine. **Radial ABG** check ulnar circulation adequacy by squeezing the hand into a fist, occluding the radial and ulnar arteries in the wrist, holding for 10s then opening the hand and releasing the pressure on the ulnar artery only; looking for reperfusion of the whole hand (modified Allen's test).
Patient position upper limb sit the patient upright, arm and wrist extended, put a pillow under the wrist to hold the position; **femoral ABG** lie patient flat on their back with their groin exposed.

Procedure wash hands and wear non-sterile gloves. Attach needle to syringe and expel excess heparin (if present). Palpate both radial pulses and select the better side. Local anaesthetic can be given intradermally or topically prior to this procedure. Roll your finger back and forth over the artery to assess its width and course. Do not use a tourniquet. Clean the skin using 2% chlorhexidine. Place a finger on the radial pulse, hold the syringe like a pen with the bevel facing upwards and proximally (Fig. 16.4). Warn the patient and insert the syringe at 30° to the skin, aiming for the centre of the artery against the direction of blood flow. Once you hit the artery the blood should pulse into the syringe (best method of assessing whether arterial or venous). If not reassess the positions of the pulse and needle by feeling for the needle tip as you gently press the syringe upwards. Once you have about 1ml of blood apply gentle pressure to the puncture site with cotton wool and withdraw the needle. Ensure firm pressure applied to the site for 3 mins – use an assistant if necessary but not the patient. Remove the needle using a sharps bin and put the cap on the syringe. Label the syringe at the bedside with the patient's details, O_2 concentration and temp and take it to the ABG machine.

Confirmations during procedure pulsatile, bright-red blood fills the syringe automatically; **post-procedure** blood O_2 saturation (SaO_2) is the same as that measured with a sats probe (SpO_2).

Complications bleeding, haematoma, arterial damage and peripheral ischaemia, pain, infection, local tendon/nerve damage.

Safety steady the patient's arm on a pillow to reduce movement and risk of needle-stick injury, dispose of needles into a sharps container immediately, do not resheath them.

Alternatives
- **Femoral blood gas** similar to femoral stab (📖 p516) but aim for the femoral pulse (usually 2 fingers width below the inguinal ligament), with the patient lying flat on their back. Insert the green (21G) needle at 90° to the skin
- **Brachial artery gas** (if unable to get radial or femoral) extend the patient's arm and insert needle at 45° into the brachial artery (medial to the biceps tendon, on the inner aspect of the upper forearm)
- **Arterial cannula** used for repeated arterial samples or direct BP measurement (seek senior/specialist advice).

Hints and tips
- Consider applying topical (📖 p521) or infiltrated local anaesthetic (bleb of 1% lidocaine over the artery using an orange needle)
- If no blood is seen reposition the needle without withdrawing it completely from the skin; ask the patient to dorsiflex the wrist fully
- You may miss the artery which lies superficially and hit the bone (painful); if this happens gently withdraw the needle to just under the skin, reposition the needle in line with the pulse and try again, taking your time
- The ED, ICU, HDU, neonatal, and labour wards often have ABG machines; if you cannot process the ABG within a few minutes put it on ice (remove and dispose of the needle first)
- Expel air bubbles from the syringe before presenting the sample to the analysis machine.

Interpretation see 📖 p584

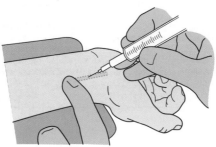

Fig. 16.4 Obtaining an arterial blood sample from the right radial artery.

SC/IM injections

| Consent verbal | Level F1 | Difficulty 1/5 |

Indications preferred route of administration for many drugs; where IV access not possible.

Contraindications *absolute* competent patient refusal, drug allergy; *relative* abnormal clotting.

Site
- **SC** upper arm (tricep/deltoid), anterior abdominal wall, anterior thigh
- **IM** shoulder (deltoid), lateral thigh, superior lateral quadrant of the buttocks (to avoid the sciatic nerve; Fig. 16.5).

Equipment non-sterile gloves, antiseptic swab, drug, syringe, green (21G) and blue (23G) or orange (25G) needle, cotton wool, sharps bin.

Checks patient's name, hospital number, and DoB (ask patient or check ID band), dose and strength prescribed, batch number and expiry date, allergies (ask patient, check allergy bands and drug chart).

Patient position so that target site is exposed and accessible.

Procedure wash hands and wear non-sterile gloves. Draw up the medication into a syringe using a filtered needle (ie one with foam at the base of the needle that prevents glass entering the syringe) and expel any air bubbles:
- **SC** attach an orange needle to the syringe and clean the area for injection with a chlorhexidine swab. Raise the skin and subcutaneous tissue between your fingers by pinching it and insert the needle at 45° into the skin. Pull the syringe back slightly to check you are not in a blood vessel. Inject the medication slowly, watching the patient as you do so, then withdraw the needle and hold cotton wool over the site
- **IM** attach a blue needle to the syringe and clean the area for injection with a chlorhexidine swab. Insert the needle vertically into the skin and pull back slightly to check you are not in a blood vessel. Inject the medication slowly, watching the patient as you do so, then withdraw the needle and hold cotton wool over the site. Depth of needle insertion varies depending on depth of patient's subcutaneous fat layer, but in normal BMI patient insert approximately 2–2.5cm.

Confirmation drug successfully administered, assess the patient and monitor the HR, BP, and RR to ensure there is no acute reaction, remember to write the time given and sign the drug chart. See Table 16.3.

Complications anaphylaxis (📖 p470), drug overdose (📖 p493), local swelling, pain and bruising, bleeding, accidental IV injection.

Safety stay on the ward for at least 5min after giving drugs in case of an acute reaction. Dispose of sharps immediately in a sharps bin at the bedside.

Alternatives consider other routes (PO/IV/PR/SL/IN) or other drugs.

Hints and tips
- Use a longer needle for IM injections in obese patients
- If blood is aspirated, withdraw and repeat the procedure in a different site with a clean needle
- For repeated injections, rotate injection sites to limit local reactions
- Most nurses can give IM/SC injections and are more experienced at it
- Try to avoid IM injections as much as possible as they are fairly painful.

Table 16.3 *Drugs commonly given via SC and IM routes*

Subcutaneous	Intramuscular
• Insulin	• Metoclopramide
• LMWH	• Cyclizine (very painful)
• Diamorphine	• Tramadol/pethidine
• Morphine	• Chlorphenamine
	• Haloperidol

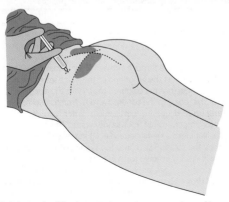

Fig. 16.5 Safe area for IM injection in the upper outer quadrant of buttock: avoid the areas marked in red.

IV injections

Consent verbal	**Level** F1	**Difficulty** 1/5

Indications rapid onset of action needed, to avoid enteral administration, to provide steady plasma concentration from infusion, only route of administration available or tolerated.

Contraindications *absolute* competent patient refusal, drug allergy.

Site via a cannula (see 🕮 p518) or central line (🕮 p534).

Equipment IV fluid/drug/blood, IV cannula *in situ*, syringe, green needle, giving set (tube connecting the bag to the cannula), 0.9% saline flush.

Checks patient's name, hospital number and DoB (ask patient or check ID band), dose and infusion rate prescribed, batch number and expiry date, allergies (ask patient, check allergy bands and drug chart), cannula is sited appropriately and flushing, some drugs need therapeutic monitoring.
- If you are unfamiliar with an IV drug look it up in the *BNF* before giving
- Always follow the *BNF* and manufacturers' instructions.

Patient position sitting up with the cannula exposed.

Procedure flush the cannula to make sure it is working then:
- **IV infusion** hang the bag on a drip stand and puncture the port on the bag of fluids with the sharp plastic end of the giving set. Open the valve and run the fluid through into a sink (or kidney bowl) to remove air bubbles. Connect the other end of the giving set to the horizontal cannula porthole (not the coloured top). Alter the drip speed and tape a loop of the tubing to the patient's arm to limit traction on the cannula
- **Drawing up IV drugs** if the drug is in powder form reconstitute with solvent as directed (often 0.9% saline/water; Appendix 4 of *BNF*). Draw solvent into a syringe and inject it into the drug vial. Shake well then draw the solution back into the syringe with a filter needle. If the drug is already in liquid form in a glass ampoule, use a filter needle to draw up the drug to prevent aspiration of tiny shards of glass
- **Giving IV drugs** tap the syringe to bring air bubbles to the top then expel any air and remove the needle. Attach the syringe to the side port and slowly administer the medication according to the drug manufacturer's instructions or the *BNF*. Flush with 5ml 0.9% saline.

Confirmation infusion running/IV drug successfully administered, assess the patient and monitor the HR, BP and RR to ensure there is no acute reaction, remember to write the time given and sign the drug chart.

Complications anaphylaxis (📖 p470), drug overdose (📖 p493), local irritation/thrombophlebitis, leakage of drug from tissued cannula, haematoma.

Safety if multiple infusions are set up check they can be given through the same cannula. If not, insert a second cannula or give the drugs at different times. Stay on the ward for at least 5min after giving IV drugs in case of an acute adverse reaction.

Alternatives consider other routes of administration (PO, IM, SC, PR, SL, IN). As a last resort fluids (0.9% saline or glucose saline without KCl) can be given very slowly SC (no faster than 1l over 12h). Do not give 5% glucose SC due to infection risk. Blood transfusions (📖 p398) can only be given IV. You may need a central line (📖 p534) for some IV infusions/drugs.

Hints and tips
- Flush the cannula, especially after giving irritant drugs (eg cyclizine, amiodarone)
- If you are unsure of infusion rates, consult the *BNF*
- Some medications must be given at a constant rate using a syringe driver (eg heparin, magnesium, GTN, opioids)
- Keep IV infusions above the level of the patient's heart to prevent blood entering the giving set
- Keep syringe drivers below the level of the patient's heart to prevent drug siphoning (though most modern giving sets contain anti-siphoning valves)
- Most nurses can administer IV infusions or drugs though some IV injections must be given by a doctor; there is usually good reason for this – find out what it is before giving the injection.

ECGs and cardiac monitors

| **Consent** verbal | **Level** F1 | **Difficulty** 1/5 |

Indications
- **ECG** chest/back/abdo pain or suspicion of cardiac ischaemia, unexplained SOB, ↓GCS, ↑K^+, arrhythmias, pre-op
- **Cardiac monitoring** peri- and post-cardiorespiratory arrest, peri- and post-MI, ↑K^+, unstable arrhythmias, cardioversion, administration of certain drugs, administration of anaesthesia.

Contraindications *absolute* competent patient refusal; *relative* patient contaminated with toxic substance or other risk to operator.

Site anterior chest wall and limbs.

Equipment ECG/cardiac monitor, adhesive electrodes.
Checks sufficient ECG paper, paper moving at 25mm/s.
Patient position sitting at 45° for ECG.

Procedure
- **ECG** apply adhesive electrodes and connect, as described in the box and Fig. 16.6, then turn the ECG machine on. Ask the patient to sit back and stay still. Press 'record' (often an ECG picture or '12'). The ECG should print once the machine has collected enough data
- **Cardiac monitoring** apply the leads as follows: **red** right shoulder; **yellow** left shoulder and **green/black** over the apex beat or spleen; see Fig. 16.7. The machine will show the trace of lead 'II' on a standard 12-lead ECG. Other views can be obtained with 3 leads.

Limb leads *red* right shoulder; *yellow* left shoulder; *green* left foot; *black* right foot
Chest leads V1 (red) right sternal edge, 4th intercostal space; V2 (yellow) left sternal edge, 4th intercostal space; V3 (green) between V2 and V4; V4 (brown) mid-clavicular line, 5th intercostal space; V5 (black) anterior-axillary line, horizontal with V4; V6 (purple) mid-axillary line horizontal with V4 (see Fig. 16.6).

Confirmation adequate ECG printout or trace on cardiac monitor.
Complications skin reaction to adhesive electrodes (rare).
Safety caution with electricity and wet/bloody environments.
Alternatives for posterior MIs the ECG is set up with posterior leads; the leads are attached three places further on, ie V1 is connected to V4, V2 to V5, etc. Leads V4–6 are attached round the posterior chest at the same horizontal level as V6 to become V7–9, see Fig. 16.8. Ensure you document this on the ECG trace.
Hints and tips adhesive electrodes do not stick to hairy skin so you may need to shave a small patch. If the patient is sweaty, clean the skin with an alcohol wipe first. In desperation use a pen to hold single leads in place. The limb leads can be placed on the ankles and wrists or over the hips and shoulders, however comparing ECGs taken by different methods can be hard. Consider a chaperone for female patients.

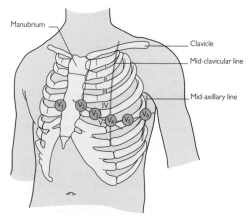

Fig. 16.6 Position of the chest leads for 12-lead ECG.

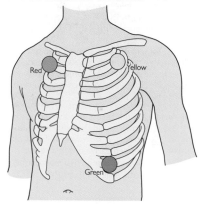

Fig. 16.7 Position of the three leads for cardiac monitoring.

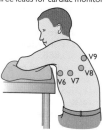

Fig. 16.8 Position of the posterior chest leads; V7–9.

Exercise tolerance test

Consent verbal/written　　　**Level** F2　　　**Difficulty** 4/5

Indications diagnosis of suspected IHD, assess cardiac fitness, prognosis post-MI, evaluation of treatment (eg angioplasty, CABG), assessing exercise-induced arrhythmias.

Contraindications *absolute* competent patient refusal, unstable angina; *relative* severe aortic stenosis, recent (<5d) ST elevation MI, uncontrolled arrhythmia, ↑BP or heart failure, physical inability (eg severe COPD, stroke, arthritis), β-blockade; inability to interpret (paced rhythms, LBBB).

Equipment treadmill, ECG, sphygmomanometer, GTN, arrest trolley.
Checks exclude contraindications, arrest trolley accessible.
Patient position record first ECG with patient lying down, second with patient standing up and serial ECGs as patient walks on the treadmill.

Procedure the technician connects the BP cuff and ECG leads to the patient with a specialised harness; a baseline BP is recorded. The test commences with the treadmill moving slowly then gradually speeding up whilst increasing the gradient; this is pre-programmed and most hospitals use the Bruce protocol (OHCM9 📖 p102). BP is recorded every 3–5min. Real-time ECGs are often shown on a monitor where changes to the ST segment can be observed. The test is complete once the patient reaches ≥90% of their maximal heart rate (220 − age in years) or they complete the protocol (30min). The test is often stopped early (see below). BP and ECG measurement continues for a further 10–15min as the patient rests.

Confirmation deciding if the test is positive or not is difficult, since stopping early (see below) could be either positive or negative depending on the ECG tracing. A senior cardiologist often determines the result. If the test is stopped early consult a senior.

Complications atrial and ventricular arrhythmias (including VF and VT), syncope, shortness of breath, angina, MI, death.

Safety stop the test if:
- Patient has chest pain or severe shortness of breath
- Patient is exhausted, feeling faint, or at risk of falling
- ST segment depression >2mm in any lead
- ST elevation
- Atrial or ventricular arrhythmia (occasional ectopics do not count)
- Systolic BP ≥230mmHg or a fall in systolic BP ≥20mmHg
- Development of AV block or LBBB.

Alternatives the test can be performed on an exercise bicycle, an arm bicycle or induced pharmacologically with an IV β-agonist. Stress echo-cardiography (OHCM9 📖 p106) and nuclear cardiography can also be used to assess cardiac disease.

Hints and tips most hospitals have specific protocols for exercise testing. The technician is usually much more experienced than the junior doctor and if they suggest stopping a test it is worthwhile doing so.

Chemical cardioversion (adenosine)

Consent verbal	**Level** F2	**Difficulty** 4/5

Indications regular narrow complex tachycardia, known SVT with bundle branch block.

Contraindications *absolute* serious adverse event with adenosine in past; *relative* cardiovascular instability (↓GCS, systolic BP <90mmHg, chest pain, heart failure), 2nd- or 3rd-degree heart block, asthma, accessory-pathways (eg WPW), sick-sinus syndrome.

Things to try first vagal manoeuvres: 10s of carotid sinus massage (never both sides together); straining down as if passing a stool; trying to blow the plunger out of a clean 10ml syringe from the narrow end; immersing the face in icy cold water (often difficult to perform on the ward).

Equipment defibrillator with monitoring strip recorder and paper, BP monitoring, pulse oximetry, large-bore venous access (≥green cannula in antecubital fossa), O_2 supplementation, arrest trolley (equipment and drugs), adenosine, saline flushes and drawing-up needles and syringes.

Patient position allow the patient to get themselves into a position where they are comfortable, either laying flat or at 45° in bed.

Patient explanation tell the patient about the procedure including the common symptoms such as facial flushing, lightheadedness, chest tightness and nausea; most symptoms last <60s after administration.

Pre-procedural checks ensure a 12-lead ECG has been undertaken. Check the patient still has a tachycardia. Give the patient supplemental O_2, ensure O_2 sats and BP monitoring are attached to the patient (on the opposite arm to the venous access) and that observations are being noted every few minutes. Attach leads of defibrillator to monitor heart rhythm (select 'leads' on the defibrillator). Have at least one assistant who is ALS trained. Draw up 6mg of adenosine and a 10ml 0.9% saline flush. Check the cannula is patent and flushing painlessly.

Procedure commence rhythm strip recording/printing on the defibrillator (usually press 'record'). Warn the patient you are going to give the drug. Inject 6mg adenosine rapidly, followed immediately by the 10ml flush. Observe the rhythm strip and patient.

Possible outcomes and further management:

- **No effect** on HR or rhythm within 60s; repeat procedure using 12mg of adenosine; if still no response seek senior/specialist advice
- **Transient slowing** of HR, but restoration of original tachycardia; observe underlying rhythm on rhythm strip during slowing; if AF then treat for fast AF (🕮 p248), otherwise treat according to ALS (🕮 p228)
- **Conversion** of tachycardia into sinus rhythm; success
- **Evolution into a more pathological rhythm**, eg VF/VT; follow appropriate ALS algorithm (🕮 p228).

Complications see patient explanation, above.

Safety never perform this procedure for the first time on your own.

Cardioversion and defibrillation

> **Consent** verbal/common law in emergency otherwise verbal/written
> **Level** F2   **Difficulty** 3/5

Indications emergency VF, VT (with or without a pulse), fast AF (new onset or haemodynamically unstable), SVT if other treatments have failed (📖 p248) or patient haemodynamically unstable; **elective** AF.

Contraindications *absolute* competent patient refusal; *relative* wet or bloody environment (moisture and electricity don't mix), if arrhythmia very likely to persist (eg chronic AF with valvular pathology).

Site one electrode to the right of the upper sternum below the clavicle and the other electrode level with the 5th left intercostal space in the anterior axillary line (see Figs 16.9 and 16.10). In refractory VF/VT consider shocking in the anterior/posterior position (Fig. 16.11).

> **Equipment** defibrillator with hands-free electrodes (or paddles and gel-pads where still in use), arrest trolley, ECG machine.
> **Checks** defibrillator working and battery charged; gel-pads and resuscitation drugs available, at least one assistant, patient's cardiac rhythm requires cardioversion, nobody touching the patient/bed, O_2 removed. In elective cases check the patient is starved and adequately anticoagulated with good IV access.
> **Patient position** supine.

> **Procedure**
> - *Emergency* follow ALS (📖 p228)/APLS algorithms. Attach hands-free electrodes. Set defibrillator to required energy, make sure no one is in contact with the patient or bed and the O_2 is removed. **Give a clear verbal warning to stand clear.** Shock. Continue CPR as per ALS/APLS algorithm
> - *Elective* ensure the anaesthetist is available and inform the nursing staff. Attach hands-free electrodes before the patient is anaesthetised. Once anaethetised set the defibrillator to 'synchronised shock' and shock in accordance with ALS/APLS algorithms, checking that no one is in contact with the patient/bed and that O_2 is removed. **Give a clear verbal warning to stand clear.** Shock.

Confirmation restoration of sinus rhythm for elective cases or a cardiac output in the emergency situation; perform 12-lead ECG.

Complications life-threatening arrhythmias, thromboembolism, aspiration, local burning to skin, risks to user and bystanders

Safety users of the manual defibrillator must have passed an ALS or ILS course; caution with electricity and wet/bloody environments.

Alternatives automated external defibrillators (AEDs) are becoming widespread and require no rhythm recognition by the user. Two hands-free electrodes are applied to the patient and the AED determines if a shock is advisable or not; if a shock is advisable the operator just presses the 'shock' button when the AED tells them to. AEDs should not be used for elective cardioversions.

Hints and tips always defibrillate safely; if in doubt contact your resuscitation officer for some extra training.

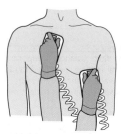

Fig. 16.9 Position of manual defibrillator paddles. Make sure gel-pads are placed on the skin underneath the paddles as these reduce the impedance and limit skin burns.

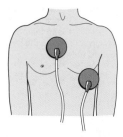

Fig. 16.10 Position of hands-free adhesive defibrillation electrodes. The electrodes for most hands-free systems indicate where they should be placed: to the right of the upper sternum and over the 5th left intercostal space in the anterior axillary line.

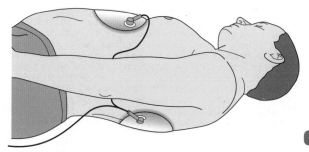

Fig. 16.11 Position of either manual paddles or hands-free electrodes in the AP position. The anterior site is to the left of the lower sternal border and the posterior position is just inferior to the left scapula.

Central lines

| **Consent** verbal/written | **Level** F2+ | **Difficulty** 3–5/5 |

Indications monitoring fluid balance, temporary pacing wires, drug administration, parenteral feeding, permits blood sampling, pulmonary artery catheterisation (Swann–Ganz catheters).
Contraindications *absolute* competent patient refusal; *relative* infection at site, abnormal clotting, shock.
Site internal jugular, subclavian or femoral vein.

Equipment 5ml/10ml syringes, blue (23G) and green (21G) needles, non-absorbable suture, Seldinger central line kit (introducing needle, 5ml syringe, guidewire, dilator, small blade, central line with 2–5 lumens and bungs), 1% lidocaine, sterile gown, hat, mask and gloves, dressing pack, sterile drapes, portable ultrasound, continuous ECG monitoring on patient.
Patient position flat on their back with their head down for internal jugular and subclavian cannulation; flat on their back with head up for femoral cannulation – helps fill the vein.

Procedure using aseptic technique, clean with 2% chlorhexidine and drape the area. Identify landmarks and using ultrasound identify the vein. Anaesthetise the skin and deep layers with 10ml lidocaine. Whilst the anaesthetic takes effect, flush all lumens of the central line with saline and cap all except the green one. Attach 5ml syringe filled with saline to the central line needle and introduce through the skin, directing it towards the vein under ultrasound guidance, visualising the needle tip at all times, aspirating whilst advancing. Once dark red blood is aspirated freely into the syringe, stop advancing. Remove syringe whilst holding the needle firmly in place. If blood spurts out in a pulsatile fashion it is likely to be an arterial cannulation – STOP (see 'What to do if the artery is cannulated'). Once venous flashback obtained, advance the guidewire through the lumen of the needle (should advance without resistance), checking for ectopic beats on ECG. Once about half of the guidewire is inserted, remove the needle, but always holding onto the guidewire. Make a small incision in the skin adjacent to the guidewire with the blade; thread the dilator over the guidewire and firmly advance the dilator through the skin and deep layers, rotating to ease its passage. Stop once half the dilator is through skin and remove it whilst holding on to the guidewire. Pass the central line over the guidewire and advance it through the skin, holding onto the guidewire at all times. Remove the guidewire once the central line is inserted and cap the open lumen. Check blood can be easily aspirated from each lumen and flush with saline. Suture the line to the skin, clean the skin and apply clear sterile dressing.

Confirmation blood aspirated from all lumens, blood O_2 sats <finger O_2 sats (SvO_2<SpO_2), CXR to locate the catheter tip and exclude pneumothorax. Always confirm guidewire removed.
Complications arterial cannulation, bleeding, pneumothorax (subclavian >internal jugular), failure to identify vein, air embolism, infection.
Safety never perform this procedure for the first time on your own.
Hints and tips make sure you and the patient are both comfortable before you start. Use sufficient LA. Ultrasound should be used routinely for internal jugular line placement.

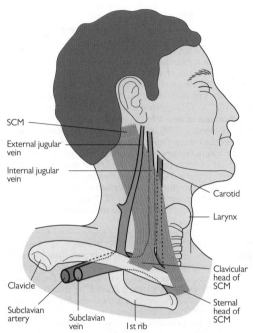

Fig. 16.12 Anatomy of the major vessels in the neck. The internal jugular is the most common site and has fewer acute complications than subclavian cannulation; subclavian lines have lower rates of infection than internal jugular lines, femoral cannulation has the highest rate of infection. The internal jugular lies deep to sternocleidomastoid muscle (SCM). The needle should puncture the skin midway between the mastoid process and the sternoclavicular joint, lateral to the carotid pulse. The needle should then be directed towards the nipple on the same side to hit the vein.

Labels on figure: SCM; External jugular vein; Internal jugular vein; Clavicle; Subclavian artery; Subclavian vein; 1st rib; Carotid; Larynx; Clavicular head of SCM; Sternal head of SCM

Accidental arterial cannulation
Signs of arterial cannulation
- Bright-red blood, rather than dark-red
- Pulsatile blood, rather than constant low flow
- ↑O_2 sats (>95%) of blood compared with finger O_2 sats
- If the left carotid artery is cannulated the central line will cross the midline on the CXR.

What to do if the artery is cannulated
- Identify arterial cannulation
- Remove all needles, guidewires and lines; press firmly over site for 10min
- Seek senior help.

Thrombolysis

Consent verbal/written	**Level** F2	**Difficulty** 3/5

Indications acute myocardial infarction which meets the following criteria: presentation within 12h of onset of symptoms; typical chest pain lasting >30min; >2mm ST elevation in two or more chest leads (V1–V6) or >1mm in two or more limb leads (aVR, aVL, aVF, I, II, III) or >2mm ST segment depression in V1 to V3 (suggesting posterior infarct) or new LBBB.

Contraindications *absolute* ▶▶ PCI available within 2h, competent patient refusal, active bleeding, CNS trauma, neoplasms or arteriovenous malformations, previous intracerebral haemorrhage, ischaemic stroke in previous 6mth, major trauma/surgery within previous 3wk, non-compressible punctures in the last 24 hours (eg liver biopsy, lumbar puncture) *relative*, TIA in previous 6mth, prolonged CPR, known bleeding disorder or current anticoagulation therapy, pregnancy, active dyspepsia or history of GI haemorrhage, sustained hypertension (systolic BP >180mmHg), advanced liver disease, infective endocarditis. Age is not a contraindication.

Site peripheral IV cannulae.

Agent check local policy for choice of thrombolytic agent.

Streptokinase is a naturally occurring thrombolytic derived from streptococcal bacteria and as such will cause an antibody response in the patient so repeat doses can be given within 4d of the first dose but never again after that. The standard dose is 1.5 million units in 50ml 0.9% saline by IV infusion over 1h but check the *BNF*/local guidelines. If streptokinase has been administered more than 4d ago or systolic BP <110mmHg use a recombinant thrombolytic agent.

Alteplase, reteplase, and ***tenecteplase*** are all recombinant tissue plasminogen activators; doses should be determined from the *BNF*/ local guidelines. Alteplase is given as a bolus followed by an infusion. Reteplase is given as two boluses. Tenecteplase is given as a single bolus. Heparin is commenced following administration of all the recombinant thrombolytics (see 📖 p198).

Monitoring during treatment monitor cardiac rhythm continuously and BP every 5min. Reperfusion arrhythmias (including VT) are common and usually self-limiting. Use ALS algorithm if persistent or cause compromise.

Desired outcome eventual normalisation of ST segments and improvement in chest pain. If symptoms and/or ST segment changes persist seek senior cardiology help; a second thrombolysis dose may sometimes be given.

Complications bleeding (intracranial (1%), other major bleed (5%)), reperfusion arrhythmias, hypotension, anaphylaxis. If hypotension occurs during treatment with streptokinase, slow the infusion down.

Safety never perform this procedure for the first time on your own.

Alternatives primary coronary intervention (PCI) (see OHCM9 📖 p808).

Hints and tips only undertake in a well-monitored environment (ED resus, CCU, HDU). Bleeding from cannula sites is common and patients should be warned not to worry about this. In the event of massive life-threatening haemorrhage, antifibrinolytics (eg tranexamic acid) and FFP can be used to reverse the process.

Pleural tap

Consent verbal/written	**Level** F2	**Difficulty** 3/5

Indications diagnosis of effusion, aspiration of small pneumothorax, symptomatic relief.

Contraindications *absolute* competent patient refusal; *relative* local infection, contralateral pneumothorax/effusion, abnormal clotting.

Site simplest and safest sites are shown in Fig. 16.13, directly below the inferior angle of the scapula or in the posterior-axillary line; choose an intercostal space two or three spaces below the top of the effusion. See Fig. 16.14.

Equipment 5, 10, 20, 50ml syringes, orange (25G) and green (21G) needles, ±intravenous cannula (14–16G), 3-way tap, 3 specimen containers and fluoride oxalate blood tube (☐ p517), sterile jug/bowl, 1% lidocaine, sterile gloves, dressing pack, antiseptic swab.
Checks confirm side of the effusion clinically and on CXR; lay equipment out on clean treatment trolley; recruit an assistant.
Patient position see Fig. 16.13.

Procedure wash hands and wear sterile gloves. Clean area thoroughly with Betadine® or chlorhexidine. Infiltrate 5–10ml of LA with orange needle into subcutaneous and then deeper layers towards pleura, avoiding neurovascular bundles (Fig. 16.15). Allow 2min to take effect. Using either a green needle on a 20ml syringe or a cannula, gently advance the needle through the anaesthetised area over the rib directly towards the pleura. Once in the pleural space, fluid is easily drawn into the syringe or a flashback will be seen in the cannula; if using the cannula then remove the needle, leaving the plastic component in place, and attach a syringe. Aspirate volume required and divide into specimen containers. If performing a therapeutic procedure use the cannula and attach a 3-way tap with a 50ml syringe; withdraw and dispose of fluid into a jug. Once complete withdraw needle/cannula and apply plaster to skin.

Confirmation pleural fluid aspirated, always get a CXR (?pneumothorax and reassess the level of the effusion if a therapeutic procedure).

Complications pneumothorax, haemothorax, pain, bleeding, damage to intercostal nerve, local or intrapleural infection, visceral puncture (liver, spleen, kidney).

Safety do not perform this procedure without supervision; take care not to allow air into the pleural space. If aspirating fluid (ie not pneumothorax) ultrasound guidance is strongly recommended. The use of ultrasound to mark a spot for subsequent drainage attempts is not recommended.

Alternatives retry in a different rib space; radiology might perform a diagnostic tap under ultrasound guidance; chest drain for large effusions.

Hints and tips make sure you and the patient are comfortable before you start; try to anaesthetise the skin fully and insert the local anaesthetic needle at right angles to the skin when infiltrating down to the pleura.

Aspiration of pneumothorax tension pneumothorax is a medical emergency and requires immediate treatment (☐ p279). A small spontaneous pneumothorax (<2cm) in a patient who is not breathless can be aspirated using this technique (☐ p279).

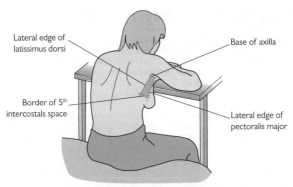

Fig. 16.13 Position of the patient for aspiration of pleural fluid. Get the patient to lean forwards over a table or the back of a chair to open up the rib spaces and prevent excessive movement.

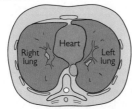

Fig. 16.14 Position of the normal heart within the thorax at level of T6/T7 vertebra. The diaphragm lies between T8/T12. Posterior and lateral approaches for pleural aspiration with standard green (21G) needle or IV cannula are highly unlikely to puncture the heart, even on the left side of the chest.

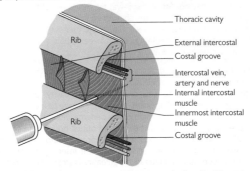

Fig. 16.15 Safe pleural aspiration to avoid neurovascular bundles. The main bundle sits just posterior to the inferior rib edge, though collateral branches are located adjacent to the superior border. The safe approach is to advance the needle above a rib, but not right against its superior edge.

Chest drain (Seldinger method)

| **Consent** verbal/written | **Level** F2+ | **Difficulty** 3-5/5 |

Indications pneumo/haemothorax, pleural effusion, empyema.
Contraindications *absolute* competent patient refusal; *relative* local infection, abnormal clotting.
Site mid-axillary line, 5th intercostal space for a pneumothorax or below fluid level in an effusion.

Equipment 5, 10, 20ml syringes, orange (25G) and green (21G) needles, suture, Seldinger chest drain pack, bottle with underwater seal (400ml sterile water), 1% lidocaine, sterile gloves, hat, mask and gown, dressing pack, antiseptic swab, sharps bin, portable ultrasound.
Checks confirm side of the effusion clinically and on CXR; lay equipment out on clean treatment trolley; recruit an assistant.
Patient position hunched forwards over a table (Fig. 16.16a) or reclining back with their arm behind the head (Fig. 16.16b); choose according to comfort.

Procedure wash hands and wear sterile gloves. Clean area thoroughly with Betadine® or chlorhexidine. Infiltrate 5–10ml of LA with orange then green needle into subcutaneous and then deeper layers towards pleura, avoiding neurovascular bundles (Fig. 16.15, 🕮 p539). Allow 2min to take effect. Attach Seldinger needle onto the syringe and advance through the area of infiltration as for a pleural tap (🕮 p538). Once needle tip is inside the pleural space, remove the syringe and pass the guidewire through the needle. Never let go of the guidewire. Withdraw the needle fully leaving half the guidewire in the chest. Make a small incision with the scalpel alongside the guidewire and pass the dilator along the guidewire to make a tract to the pleural space. Withdraw dilator, but leave the guidewire *in situ*. Pass the chest drain over the guidewire to the required depth then remove the guidewire. Attach the 3-way tap to the end of the chest drain and turn 'off to chest'. Suture the chest drain to the chest wall using more LA if needed. Connect the 3-way tap to the tubing of the chest drain bottle and open the 3-way tap. Fluid drainage/bubbling will commence. Cover wound with clear dressings.

Confirmation fluid or air draining from pleural cavity, CXR (confirmation of position and reduction of effusion/pneumothorax).
Complications failure to site drain in pleural cavity, pneumothorax, haemothorax, pain, bleeding (local/internal), damage to intercostal nerve, local or intrapleural infection, pulmonary oedema, visceral puncture.
Safety chest drains should only be inserted out of hours in an emergency or if patient has significant respiratory compromise. Do not attempt this procedure without direct senior supervision. If inserting a drain for fluid (ie not for pneumothorax) ultrasound guidance is strongly recommended.
Alternatives narrow-bore pigtail chest drains can be inserted under ultrasound guidance by a radiologist, but these block easily if the fluid drained is too viscous. Traditional wide-bore chest drains are predominantly used in trauma cases (see box).
Hints and tips make sure both you and the patient are comfortable before you start; use sufficient LA.

(a)

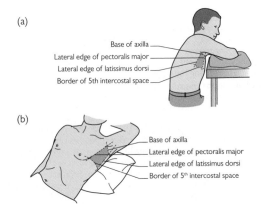

Base of axilla
Lateral edge of pectoralis major
Lateral edge of latissimus dorsi
Border of 5th intercostal space

(b)

Base of axilla
Lateral edge of pectoralis major
Lateral edge of latissimus dorsi
Border of 5th intercostal space

Fig. 16.16 (a) Position of the patient for chest drain insertion. Ask the patient to lean forwards over a table or the back of a chair, since this opens up the rib spaces and prevents them from moving too much. Aim for the safe triangle (see Havelock, T. *et al.* Pleural procedures and thoracic ultrasound: British Thoracic Society pleural disease guideline 2010 *Thorax* 2010 **65**(Suppl 2):ii61 for further information, available at √🖰www.brit-thoracic.org.uk). (b) Alternative position of the patient for chest drain insertion. Position the patient at about 45° with their arm above and behind the head, exposing the axilla.

Removing a chest drain
- Leave the drain unclamped
- Remove dressings from skin
- Clean skin with Betadine® or chlorhexidine
- Remove all sutures
- Gently but firmly remove drain as patient exhales; occlude wound
- Re-suture mattress sutures around drain site (📖 p560)
- Apply sterile dressing. Sutures should stay in for 5d
- CXR to ensure no pneumothorax has developed during drain removal.

> **Surgical chest drain**
> - Used in the management of trauma to drain haemothoraces and pneumothoraces. A wide-bore (32 or 36Ch) chest drain is used. These often come with a metal trochar, which should be discarded before drain insertion
> - Landmarks, local anaesthesia and aseptic technique as per Seldinger drains. Patient is normally lying in position (b) in Fig. 16.16.
> - Skin is incised using a scalpel, followed by blunt dissection to the pleural space using a curved clamp and your finger. Never insert a chest drain into a pre-existing chest wound
> - The tip of the drain is gripped with the curved clamp and advanced into the pleural space. The drain is then secured in place with a mattress suture and connected to the chest drain bottle
> - Confirmation of position as per Seldinger drains.

Decompression of tension pneumothorax see 📖 p279.

Endotracheal intubation (adult)

Consent assumed if unconscious	**Level** F2	**Difficulty** 5/5

Emergency indications securing a definitive airway in the unconscious patient and protecting the lungs from gastric contaminants.

Contraindications *absolute* a conscious or semi-conscious patient, inexperienced operator; *relative* upper airways obstruction from foreign body, known or suspected cervical fractures, laryngeal oedema/trauma.

Equipment endotracheal tube (ETT), 7–8mm internal diameter for a woman, 8–9mm for a man; have smaller tubes available. 10ml syringe and water-based lubricant. Working laryngoscope (commonly size 3 and size 4 Macintosh) and spare laryngoscope in case batteries fail. Bougie and Magill forceps. Stethoscope. Guedel, and nasopharyngeal airways. LMA sizes 3, 4, and 5. Bag and mask for pre-oxygenation. Tape to secure ETT and suction with yanker attached. CO_2 monitor is essential. Gloves.

Patient position laying flat, with single pillow under neck to achieve 'sniffing morning air' position (neck flexed, head extended).

Procedure an IV induction agent and a muscle relaxant must be given in a non-arrest situation, but this should only be undertaken by someone who is experienced and well rehearsed in intubating in an emergency and in the presence of a skilled assistant who can apply cricoid pressure. Check equipment and lubricate the ETT with aqueous gel. Pre-oxygenate the patient for 3min with 15l/min O_2 if time allows using the bag and mask, assisting their ventilation if it is inadequate. Once induction agent and muscle relaxant have worked, remove mask, tilt head backwards (unless there is C-spine injury) and open the mouth. Holding the laryngoscope in your left hand, advance the tip of the laryngoscope blade between the teeth on the right-hand side of the patient's mouth over the top of the tongue. Sweep the tongue to the left of the patient's mouth. Advance the laryngoscope in the midline until the uvula can be seen, then advance further until the epiglottis is visualised (Fig. 16.18). Lift the laryngoscope away from you, do not lever as this will break the patient's teeth. As you lift the laryngoscope, the epiglottis should also be lifted and the vocal cords and the opening into the trachea (the glottis) visualised. Take the ETT in your right hand and pass it through the mouth and observe it passing between the vocal cords. When the ETT is at about 20cm at the lips the assistant should inflate the cuff; gently remove the laryngoscope, holding the ETT securely in place. Attach the CO_2 monitor and re-inflating bag to the ETT and gently squeeze. Once satisfied with the position of the ETT allow assistant to release cricoid pressure and secure ETT in place with tape and continue to ventilate, giving sedatives/hypnotics as required.

Confirmation the chest should rise and fall, the ETT should mist up and the CO_2 monitor should detect CO_2 as the chest falls. Auscultate in both axillae for breath sounds and over the epigastrium to exclude air entering the stomach. Obtain a CXR to check the ETT is not in too far, as it is often past the carina in the right main bronchus. See Fig. 16.18.

Endobronchial intubation can often be detected clinically prior to check X-ray, allowing adjustment of tube position and hopefully decreasing need for repeated imaging.

Complications failure to visualise the vocal cords – revert to bag and mask ventilation ± Guedel/nasopharyngeal airway, or attempt to put in an LMA until expert help arrives. **Oesophageal intubation** – no air entering chest, no CO_2, gurgling in stomach; remove ETT immediately and revert to bag and mask ventilation ± Guedel/nasopharyngeal airway, or attempt to put in an LMA until expert help arrives. **Endobronchial intubation** – difficulty in ventilating the patient, only one side of the chest wall moves and breath sounds only audible on that side; withdraw the ETT a centimetre at a time and re-check.

Safety never undertake this procedure on your own. If in doubt bag and mask ventilate a patient until expert help arrives or insert an LMA if appropriately trained to do so (see 🕮 p544). You will never be criticised for supporting an obtunded patient's breathing with bag and mask ventilation alone with a Guedel airway *in situ*, but you will be if you unsuccessfully undertake a procedure you are unfamiliar with and untrained to perform.

Hints and tips speak to a friendly anaesthetist and ask to go to theatre to watch and help at intubations and other airway skills.

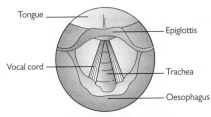

Fig. 16.17 Structures which should be visible at laryngoscopy.

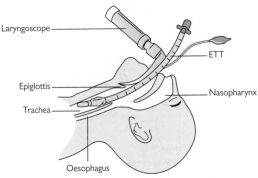

Fig. 16.18 Position of the laryngoscope and ETT once inserted.

Laryngeal mask airway (LMA)

Contraindications, consent, equipment and positioning as for intubation. *Sizes:* women 3 or 4, men 4 or 5.

Procedure as for intubation. Check equipment and check that cuff on LMA works and there is no leak; apply a small amount of lubrication to the top of the LMA around the cuff. Once the patient is adequately pre-oxygenated and sedated, remove mask, tilt head backwards (avoid if C-spine injury), and open mouth. Standing at the patient's head, take the LMA in your right hand holding it like a pen with the black line on the LMA shaft facing you. Slide the LMA along the roof of the mouth firmly and smoothly. Keep advancing until the mask of the LMA disappears from view and it reaches a natural stop. Inflate the cuff with the required volume of air (documented on the LMA itself). Attach the CO_2 monitor and re-inflating bag to the LMA and gently squeeze. Once satisfied with the position of the LMA, secure it in place with tape and continue to ventilate, giving sedatives/hypnotics as required. See Fig. 16.19.

Confirmation the chest should rise and the CO_2 monitor should detect CO_2 as the chest falls (exhalation). Auscultate in both axilla to listen for breath sounds. If unsure, remove, re-oxygenate with a bag and mask and attempt once more.

Complications failure to ventilate the patient revert to bag and mask ventilation ± Guedel/nasopharyngeal airway and reattempt once more. If still unsuccessful revert to bag and mask ventilation ± Guedel/naso-pharyngeal airway until expert help arrives.

Safety never undertake this procedure on your own. If in doubt, bag and mask ventilate a patient until expert help arrives. You will never be criticised for supporting an obtunded patient's breathing with bag and mask ventilation alone, but you will be if you unsuccessfully undertake a procedure you are unfamiliar with and untrained to perform.

Hints and tips speak to a friendly anaesthetist and ask to go to theatre to watch and help at inserting an LMA and other airway skills.

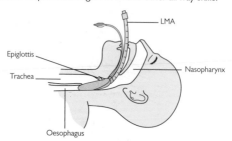

Fig. 16.19 Position of an LMA once inserted.

Urethral catheterisation

Consent verbal   **Level** F1   **Difficulty** 2/5

Indications monitor urine output/fluid balance, urinary retention, incapacitation (eg ↓GCS), incontinence, urological investigations.

Contraindications *absolute* competent patient refusal; *relative* suspected urethral injury, urethral strictures/fistulas, active UTI, prostatic tumour or hypertrophy.

Site via urethra into bladder.

Equipment catheter pack (kidney dish, bowl, cotton balls, sterile towel and gloves), Foley catheter (10–16F), antiseptic solution, gauze, 10ml 1% lidocaine/lubricant gel in pre-filled syringe, 10ml saline-filled syringe, catheter bag.

Checks no latex allergy/UTIs, correct sex catheter.

Patient position lying on back, genitalia exposed (legs apart in women).

Procedure wash hands and wear sterile gloves. Prepare the equipment, using aseptic technique. Ask an assistant to pour antiseptic solution into the sterile bowl.

Male create a hole in the centre of the towel and drape it over the patient with the penis through the hole. Hold the penis with gauze in your non-dominant hand. Retract the foreskin and clean the penis with antiseptic. Hold the penis upright and instil 10ml lidocaine gel into the meatus. Occlude the penile tip to help push the gel along the urethra. Allow 2min for the anaesthetic to take effect, lubricate the tip of the catheter with lubricant. Put the kidney bowl between the patient's thighs and place the draining end of the catheter in it. Using your clean hand insert the catheter tip into the urethra and advance. Continue to advance the catheter to the hilt once urine starts draining to make sure the catheter balloon is within the bladder. Once urine is seen to flow, inflate the balloon with 10ml water via the side port. Stop if there is pain or discomfort. Disconnect the syringe and pull back the catheter until you feel resistance. Attach a draining tube and bag to the free end of the catheter. Clean and redress the patient. Always replace the foreskin.

Female (Fig. 16.20) usually performed by nurses. Drape the sterile towel between the patient's thighs. Separate labial folds with your non-dominant hand and clean with antiseptic solution. The urethra is between the vagina and clitoris. Continue as for a male patient. If the catheter is incorrectly inserted into the vagina, do not reuse it to catheterise the urethra, leave it *in situ* and use a fresh, clean catheter to try again.

Confirmation urine drains freely, no pain on inflating balloon.

Complications pain, infection, local trauma, haematuria, strictures (long-term), retention on removing catheter.

Safety never force the catheter or fill the balloon under force.

Alternatives coude-tip urethral catheter (curved tip to aid insertion past an enlarged prostate), insertion using guidewire ± flexible cystoscopy, or suprapubic catheter – seek senior advice (see 🕮 p548).

Hints and tips

- Double glove on your dominant hand and remove the top glove once you have finished cleaning the genitalia so that you remain sterile when handling the catheter
- Avoid touching the lubricant gel with the hand holding the catheter as this makes the catheter slippery and difficult to grip and insert
- Try not to touch the catheter; it usually comes in a plastic cover which can be shuffled down or torn away as you insert it into the urethra
- If you feel resistance at the prostatic urethra hold the penis vertically and try to advance the catheter
- The urethra is 4–7cm in women so urine should be seen after 8cm; the male urethra is much longer (20cm) so the catheter must be inserted further
- If no urine appears check the catheter is in the correct place and advanced far enough; flush the catheter with saline to make sure it is not blocked with lubricant gel – if you still do not get urine, **do not** inflate the balloon, remove the catheter and seek senior advice
- Urine samples can be taken from a catheter (CSU)
- Start with a 14F silastic catheter if catheterising a patient for the first time. Should urine leak around the catheter once inserted, it will need to be replaced with a wider catheter
- Wider catheters are also advised for patients passing bloody urine, clots, sediment, or particularly thick urine. However, in general, the smallest catheter possible should be used as wide catheters are more likely to cause urethral damage
- Catheters come in 2 lengths, designed for the male and female urethra. The longer male catheters can be used in female catheterisation should shorter catheters be unavailable.

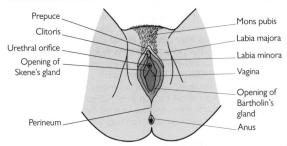

Fig. 16.20 Anatomy of the female genitalia for catheterisation.

Replacing a suprapubic catheter

Consent verbal	**Level** F1	**Difficulty** 1/5

Indications long-term catheter due for change (every 8–10wk) or problem with catheter (blocked, leaking, UTI).

Contraindications *absolute* competent patient refusal; *relative* suprapubic stoma only recently created (<3d), abnormal clotting.

Site suprapubic catheter site, usually midline about 10cm below umbilicus.

Equipment sterile dressing pack, sterile gloves, new long-term catheter (usually 16F) and appropriate syringe with water for inflating balloon, sterile lubricating anaesthetic gel, cleaning solution, new drainage bag, 20ml syringe, disposable gloves and waste bag.

Patient position lying supine, exposing suprapubic catheter site.

Procedure wearing gloves empty current catheter bag. Deflate existing balloon with 20ml syringe, emptying syringe if there is more than 20ml in the balloon. Gently, but firmly, remove the old catheter and put in a waste bag. Clean hands, put on sterile gloves, prepare sterile trolley with dressing pack, and remove perforated end of new catheter. Place sterile drape over insertion site, making a hole in the drape if necessary first. Clean insertion site, then apply some anaesthetic gel over the site and a small amount into the site; wait for 2min for anaesthetic to work. Take the catheter in its plastic cover and pass the tip into catheter site, avoiding touching the rubber directly. Gently feed catheter in all the way. Connect to new drainage bag. Wait for urine to flow out of the catheter before inflating the balloon; volume of water to inflate balloon is stipulated on catheter and its packaging. Withdraw catheter to ensure balloon is working and catheter cannot fall out. Document in patient's records the date and the sizes and types of catheter taken out and then put in.

Confirmation urine flowing freely.

Complications bleeding at catheter site or blood-stained urine after new catheter sited (common and if minor not a concern), patient discomfort, catheter site closes up after removal of old catheter (uncommon with mature catheter sites, but can occur with freshly formed stomas (<3d).

Safety only undertake catheter changes on mature, established stomas as newly created ones (<3d) may close immediately after removing catheter.

Hints and tips if in doubt, speak to a urology nurse or the urology specialist. Sometimes the old balloon won't deflate, or the old catheter won't pull out – there are numerous reasons for this; speak to your senior or the urology nurse specialist/urology StR on-call.

Replacing a PEG feeding tube

Although placing a definitive replacement is usually performed by a gastroenterologist or an endoscopist, if the PEG has just fallen out it is important to attempt to prevent the hole closing up. With the patient lying down, apply gentle pressure to introduce a well lubricated urinary catheter into the hole. This may prevent the need for a repeat endoscopy and hence should always be attempted urgently.

Nasogastric (NG) tubes

| **Consent** verbal | **Level** F1 | **Difficulty** 2/5 |

Indications stomach emptying, eg bowel obstruction (wide-bore or Ryle's tube), nutrition (fine bore).

Contraindications *absolute* basal skull fracture, facial trauma, competent patient refusal.

Site inserted into the stomach via a nostril.

> **Equipment** non-sterile gloves, NG tube, lubricant jelly, glass of water, adhesive tape, drainage bag and bowl (or spigot).
>
> **Checks** make sure patient is alert, with no history of head injury. Use an appropriate sized tube. Gauge the length of tube to insert by measuring the distance from the nostril to angle of the jaw and from angle of the jaw to the xiphisternum. Warn the patient about initial discomfort (which does improve).
>
> **Patient position** sit the patient upright with head against a pillow

> **Procedure** wash hands and wear non-sterile gloves. Ask the patient to take a sip of water and hold it in their mouth. Cover the tip of the NG tube with lubricant gel and insert into the patient's nostril. Aim the tube directly backwards. Once the patient feels the tube at the back of the throat ask them to swallow so you can advance the tube. Continue advancing until you reach the length measured earlier (usually ~50cm). Tape the tube to the nostril. Attach a drainage bag to the free end of the NG tube.

Confirmation see Table 16.4.

Complications pain/irritation, aspiration, oesophagitis, tracheal/duodenal intubation, electrolyte depletion, local tissue necrosis, gastric perforation, tube may curl in mouth or pharynx.

Safety check the tube is in the correct position with a CXR, essential before the tube is used for feeding

Alternatives if you cannot insert the tube, try the other nostril or consider passing it orally (only if patient unconscious); see 📖 p548 for other options

Hints and tips use a chilled NG tube as these are less flexible.

Table 16.4 *Methods of confirming NG tube placement*	
CXR	Essential before a fine-bore feeding tube is used and recommended for a wide-bore tube. Check tip of NG is visible below diaphragm and not in bronchial tree (check local policy if F1s are allowed to check NG position)
NG aspiration	Aspirate fluid and test pH (stomach fluid usually acidic, pH <4, can be raised in those on PPIs, hence may still need CXR to confirm)
Air injection	Listening for air over the stomach as air is injected is not a valid way to confirm position prior to using the tube and should not be performed

Ascitic tap (abdominal paracentesis)

| **Consent** verbal | **Level** F1 | **Difficulty** 3/5 |

Indications diagnosis from ascitic fluid (Table 16.5).
Contraindications *absolute* competent patient refusal; *relative* abnormal clotting, local infection.
Consent verbal; explain why a tap is required.
Site left/right iliac fossa, at the level of the umbilicus and lateral to the mid-inguinal point (see Fig. 16.21). Avoid the suprapubic area with the bladder and inferior epigastric vessels.

> **Equipment** sterile gloves, antiseptic solution in a bowl, 10ml 1% lidocaine, swabs, green (21G) needle, 20ml syringe, sterile adhesive dressing, sharps bin.
> **Checks** PT/INR/APTT, seek advice if abnormal, empty bladder.
> **Patient position** lying on their bed, tilted slightly to one side.

> **Procedure** percuss the abdomen to assess the location and extent of the ascites. Wash hands and wear sterile gloves. Using aseptic technique clean the target area. Infiltrate around the area with 1% lidocaine initially into subcutaneous, then deeper layers towards the peritoneum. Allow 2min, then insert a green needle with a 20ml syringe vertically into the skin. Advance whilst aspirating until fluid flashback is seen (usually straw-coloured; may be bloodstained). Obtain 20ml fluid, then remove the needle and apply a sterile adhesive dressing.
> - **Send fluid for** FBC, bacteriology (M, -C+S, ± ZN stain/TB culture), biochemistry (protein, glucose, LDH, amylase/lipase), cytology.

Confirmation fluid aspirated from abdominal cavity.
Complications pain, bleeding (local or perforated viscus), perforated bowel/bladder, infection (skin or peritonitis), fluid leakage from wound.
Safety do not have repeated attempts, if unsuccessful contact a senior and consider performing under ultrasound guidance.
Alternatives therapeutic paracentesis (see box).
Hints and tips avoid sites close to old surgical scars to avoid going through adhesions; in obese patients use a longer needle. Afterwards lie the patient with the puncture site upwards to minimise fluid leakage.

Table 16.5 *Classification of ascites*

	Transudate ascites	Exudate ascites
Total protein	<30g/l	>30g/l
Aetiology	• Cirrhosis • Nephrotic syndrome • CCF	• Infection (>250 white cells/mm^3) • Pancreatic cause • Malignancy • Budd–Chiari syndrome

Therapeutic paracentesis

Ascites may need to be drained for symptomatic relief, to reduce infection risk and prevent respiratory compromise. Up to 6l of ascitic fluid can be drained. In order to prevent hypotension from removal of this fluid, 100ml salt-poor albumin IV should be given for every 1.5l ascitic fluid drained. The patient's FBC, U+E, LFT, and PT and APTT should be checked before the procedure.

A Seldinger paracentesis set or a dedicated pigtail drain insertion kit may be used. The procedure is similar to an ascitic tap except that a drain is introduced, either over a guidewire or directly from an introducer needle. Unless tunnelled (eg for malignant effusions) the drain should be removed within 6h due to the risk of introducing infection.

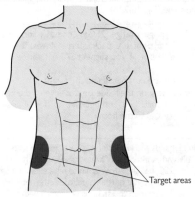

Fig. 16.21 Target areas for ascitic tap at the level of the umbilicus, 3–4cm lateral to the mid-inguinal line.

Lumbar puncture (LP)

| **Consent** verbal | **Level** F2 | **Difficulty** 3–4/5 |

Indications suspected meningitis, encephalitis, subarachnoid haemorrhage (SAH), investigation of other neurological conditions.

Contraindications *absolute* competent patient refusal, ↑intracranial pressure (see 📖 p360, check CT), infection at the site, cardiorespiratory compromise (treat first, including antibiotics); *relative* abnormal clotting, spinal deformity, spinal metalwork.

Consent verbal; explain why the lumbar puncture is required.

Site draw a line between the iliac crests and feel for a gap in the spine where the line crosses it, this is about L3/L4. The cord ends at L1/L2, so never do LPs above the L2/L3 interspace; mark the spaces using arrows away from the spine (Fig. 16.22b).

Equipment 2ml syringe, orange (25G) needle, 1% lidocaine, antiseptic swab, gauze, lumbar puncture pack, sterile gloves, 3 specimen pots labelled 1/2/3 (or 4 pots if you suspect SAH), fluoride oxalate blood tube (📖 p517).

Checks check pots are numbered and the assistant knows this.

Patient position lying on their side on the edge of the bed with their back exposed, legs curled up, and neck flexed (foetal position). Their body should be parallel to the floor.

Procedure wash hands and wear sterile gloves, gown, hat and mask. Clean area thoroughly with antiseptic. Infiltrate subcutaneously with 5–10ml of 1% lidocaine and 25G needle. Allow 2min to take effect during which you should assemble the manometer (thin tube, check the numbers match up). Insert spinal needle between the spinous processes with the bevel facing up and aim for the umbilicus (Fig. 16.22a). You should feel resistance from the supraspinous ligaments then the ligamentum flavum and dura followed by a lack of resistance as you enter the subarachnoid space (Fig. 16.22c). Withdraw the stylet and look for clear fluid (do not panic if you see blood, this is probably a spinal vessel – withdraw and use a lower space). If there is no CSF pull back 2–3cm and realign. If the patient feels pain shooting down their leg you are hitting a nerve root so withdraw, then next time head more towards the midline. Once CSF is seen attach the manometer and measure opening pressure (normal opening pressure is 7–20cm CSF). Use the 3-way tap to drain the manometer fluid into the 3 specimen pots (10 drops in each) and the fluoride tube (6 drops). Withdraw the entire needle and cover the wound with a sterile plaster. Take a blood sample in a fluoride oxalate (📖 p517) tube and send for glucose levels. Advise the patient to lie flat for 1h. Ask the nurses to check neurological obs and BP.

Confirmation CSF fluid seen.

Complications headache post-procedure (worse sitting up, occurs within a week and lasts 3–4d, 🔲 p361), infection, trauma to nerve roots.

Safety never do this procedure for the first time on your own.

Alternatives can be performed under X-ray guidance though this is rare.

Hints and tips position is everything; explain exactly what you want the patient to do, lie the patient on their side, make sure their back is straight in the vertical plane and their legs are tightly curled up. If you are having difficulty finding the midline, ask the patient if it feels to the left, right or middle. Make sure the needle is horizontal.

CSF samples send sample 2 and the fluoride tube for biochemistry (protein, glucose, pH), samples 1 and 3 to microbiology for M, -C+S (consider requesting viral culture/PCR) and the fourth in a brown envelope (away from light) to biochemistry for xanthochromia if SAH suspected.

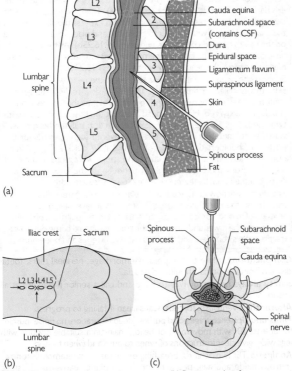

Fig. 16.22 (a) Anatomy of a lumbar puncture. (b) Position and surface anatomy for a lumbar puncture. (c) Cross-section of the spine during a lumbar puncture.

Normal vaginal delivery

| **Consent** verbal | **Level** F1 | **Difficulty** 2/5 |

The first stage of labour often takes many hours. Monitor maternal HR, BP, temp, contractions, and foetal HR every 15min. Second stage begins once the cervix is fully dilated – see box.

Equipment sterile gloves, cord clamp x 2, cord scissors, swabs, Syntometrine® injection (ergometrine 0.5mg and oxytocin 5units given IM into the thigh as the baby's anterior shoulder is delivered), neonatal resuscitaire, name tags for baby.
Patient position usually on her back with legs open and supported.

Procedure wash hands and wear sterile gloves. Stand between the woman's legs slightly to one side with sterile swabs to hand. When the head becomes visible (crowning) it should be facing towards the mother's back with its occiput anterior (Fig. 16.23a). The head will continue to descend and the mother's perineum will stretch; press the skin between the anus and vagina with a swab to protect it and place your other hand on the baby's head to control the descent (Fig. 16.23b). As the top of the head passes the vagina instruct the mother to stop pushing and to pant; meanwhile allow the head to slowly emerge (Fig. 16.23c).
Support the head once it has been delivered; the head will turn to one side, this is called restitution (Fig. 16.23d). Ask a midwife to get the Syntometrine® injection ready and to give to the mother as the anterior shoulder is delivered. Hold the head firmly at the base of the skull with two hands (Fig. 16.23e). On the next contraction pull the head downwards so the anterior shoulder can be delivered then upwards for the posterior shoulder; the whole body will follow quickly (Fig. 16.23f). Place the baby on the mother's chest and apply two clamps to the cord 15–30cm from the baby and cut in between. If the baby is not well crash-call the neonatal team; see 📖 p236 for resuscitation.
The uterus will now contract and the placenta will separate. Keep gentle traction on the cord; after about 2–5min it will give slightly as a small amount of blood comes out of the vagina. Gently pull the cord whilst pressing on the lower abdomen and the placenta should come out. Check the placenta is complete and the cord has two arteries and one vein.

Complications failure to progress, haemorrhage, perineal tears, foetal distress, foetal hypoxia, shoulder dystocia.
Safety always have midwives to hand and call a senior if you are at all unsure at any stage.
Alternatives ventouse, forceps, Caesarean if failing to progress.
Hints and tips encourage good pushes (deep inspiration, no noise, pushing for at least 20s with movement of head), maintain a suitable position with legs wide, give clear instructions of when to push and when to stop.
Analgesia TENS machines, breathing exercises, paracetamol, Entonox® (nitrous oxide and air), pethidine or diamorphine (early–mid 1st stage only), epidural.

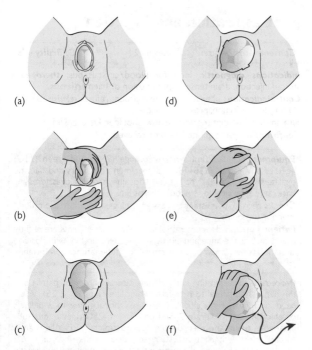

Fig. 16.23 (a–f) Birth from the perspective of the junior doctor.

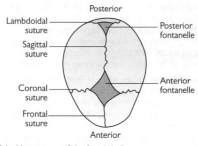

Fig. 16.24 Palpable anatomy of the foetal skull.

Joint aspiration and injection

Consent verbal/written   **Level** F2   **Difficulty** 4/5

Indications diagnostic look for blood/crystals/pus; **therapeutic** steroid injection, drain tense/septic effusion or haemarthrosis.

Contraindications *absolute* competent patient refusal; *relative* abnormal clotting, local infection, prosthetic joint.

Site any synovial joint (eg wrist, elbow, shoulder, knee, ankle).

Confirmation fluid aspirated, tension relieved.

Equipment 2, 10, 20ml syringes, orange (25G) and green (21G) needles ±IV cannula (16–18G), 3 specimen containers and fluoride oxalate blood tube (📖 p517), 1% lidocaine, sterile gloves, dressing pack, antiseptic cleaning solution, sharps bin.

Checks recruit an assistant to pass you things, make sure aspiration/ injection is required.

Patient position depends on joint; easier if larger joints are slightly flexed such as the knee and elbow as this opens up the joint. Position larger joints over a few pillows to make the patient more comfortable.

Procedure for aspirating knee identify lateral border of patella and the depression lateral to it over the joint line (see Fig. 16.25). Wash hands and wear sterile gloves. Clean area thoroughly with Betadine® or chlorhexidine. Infiltrate 2–5ml of LA with 25G needle into sub-cutaneous tissue and then deeper towards joint space. Allow 2min to take effect. Either attach 21G needle to a 10ml syringe or a 16G cannula; advance the needle through the area of LA infiltration directly towards the joint space. A slight 'pop' might be felt as the synovium is punctured. Once in the joint space fluid will be easily drawn into the syringe, or a flashback in the cannula will be seen; if using a cannula then remove the needle, leave the plastic component in place, and attach a syringe. Aspirate as much as needed and divide into specimen pots. Once complete withdraw needle/cannula and apply plaster to skin. Medial approaches are also described (OHCS8 📖 p708).

Complications failure to tap synovial fluid, pain, bleeding, subsequent infection of subcutaneous tissues or within joint.

Safety never perform this for the first time on your own; always perform aspiration aseptically, as an iatrogenically infected joint is disastrous; avoid advancing needle through infected skin.

Alternatives seek help from orthopaedic surgeon/rheumatologist; some radiologists perform this under ultrasound guidance.

Hints and tips thick viscous effusions are difficult to draw up through small needles, so use a larger needle or cannula. Always speak to the relevant laboratory beforehand and enquire what volume and in which container they need their sample.

Joint injection

Steroid injections are used for a number of inflammatory disorders, but should be performed by an expert. If there is doubt whether a joint is infected or not, then steroids must not be injected into that joint (OHCS8 📖 p708).

Table 16.6 *Synovial fluid in health and disease*

Aspiration of synovial fluid is used primarily to look for infectious or crystal (gout and pseudogout) arthropathies.

	Appearance	Viscosity	WBC/mm³	NØ
Normal	Clear, colourless	High	<200	<25%
Non-inflammatory[1]	Clear, straw	High	<5000	<25%
Haemorrhagic[2]	Bloody, xanthochromic	Variable	<10,000	<50%
Acute inflammatory[3]	Turbid, yellow	Reduced		
● Acute gout			2,000–5,000	~80%
● Rheumatoid arthritis			5,000–10,000	~65%
Septic	Turbid, purulent	Reduced		
● TB			10,000–30,000	~70%
● Gonorrhoeal			10,000–30,000	~60%
● Septic (other)[4]			10,000–100,000	~95%

[1] eg degenerative joint disease, trauma.
[2] eg tumour, haemophilia, trauma.
[3] Includes eg Reiter's, pseudogout, SLE etc.
[4] Includes staphs, streps, Lyme disease, and pseudomonas (eg post-op).

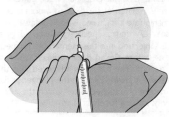

Fig. 16.25 Aspirating a left knee joint using a lateral approach; rest the flexed knee on a pillow.

Local anaesthetic (LA)

Consent verbal	**Level** F1	**Difficulty** 2/5

Local anaesthetics (LAs) should not be used without knowledge of their side effects, toxic doses, and properties. A basic understanding about this drug class is essential as it will improve the patient's outcome.

Indications suturing, wound cleaning, FB removal, cannulation, cardiac arrhythmias, minor and major surgery (cataracts/hip replacement); topical preparations for cannulation, catheterisation, corneal anaesthesia.

Which LA to use most wards will stock lidocaine (formerly lignocaine); 1% lidocaine solutions are usually sufficient. Other LAs are more likely to be used in the operating theatre or the ED. Different LAs vary in their speed of onset and duration of action. Table 16.7 shows properties of commonly used LAs. See also Tables 16.8. and 16.9.

LAs with adrenaline (epinephrine) the vasoconstricting action of adrenaline prevents the LA from being rapidly redistributed by the circulation, prolonging its action at the injection site and allowing a larger dose to be administered. It is especially useful for scalp and facial anaesthesia. There is debate as to whether one should avoid using LAs with adrenaline near end arteries, (fingers, toes, penis, nose, ears) as this may lead to ischaemia/gangrene.

Types of block a *field block* is infiltration of LA into the tissue around a wound; this numbs small cutaneous nerves. In a **peripheral nerve block** a specific nerve is anaesthetised (eg digital, median) with subsequent anaesthesia in the region supplied by that nerve. A **spinal anaesthetic** blocks motor and sensory nerves below the level at which it is injected (often L3/L4). For full descriptions see OHCS8 ☐ p634.

Bier's block an IV injection of LA distal to a double-cuffed tourniquet, often used to manipulate a fractured wrist in an awake patient (OHCS8 ☐ p744). IV use of LA requires specialist training with close supervision.

Haematoma LA injection into the haematoma formed around a long bone fracture, eg before closed distal radius fracture manipulation in the conscious patient. The needle is advanced into the 'step' felt at the fracture site whilst pulling back on the plunger. A flashback is seen when the haematoma is reached, after which the anaesthetic should be injected slowly, looking for signs of toxicity.

LA toxicity Always observe for the symptoms and signs of toxicity shown in Table 16.10. This usually occurs when serum concentrations peak (usually 45–60min after use). The toxic dose of LAs represents the maximum dose that should be injected into the tissues.

Management of LA toxicity if suspected, stop any further injection or infusion of LA, check ABC and give 15l/min O_2; call for senior help; midazolam 1–4mg/STAT IV increases the convulsion threshold and may prevent seizures; consider:
- *Intubation* if conscious level falls or seizures are resistant to therapy (☐ p542).
- *CPR* if there is no palpable pulse or signs of life (☐ p228).
- *IV lipid emulsion* will create a 'sink' for lipophilic drugs.

Allergy to LAs this is rare but more likely with the ester group of LAs (cocaine, tetracaine (formerly amethocaine)) than the amide group of LAs (lidocaine, bupivacaine, prilocaine); treat as for anaphylaxis (📖 p470).

Alternatives Entonox®, sedation ± LA, general anaesthesia ± LA.

Hints and tips LAs sting as they are injected; lidocaine is less painful if it is warmed and injected slowly. LAs are 'activated' by alkaline conditions and so are much less effective when injected into inflamed/infected tissues which have a lower (acidic) pH.

Table 16.7 *Commonly used local anaesthetics and their properties*

Local anaesthetic	Onset	Duration	Maximum dose
Bupivacaine (Marcain®)	Medium	Long	2mg/kg
Levobupivicaine (Chirocaine®)	Medium	Long	2mg/kg (data lacking)
Lidocaine	Fast	Medium	3mg/kg
Lidocaine (with adrenaline)	Fast	Medium	7mg/kg
Prilocaine (Citanest®)	Fast	Medium	6mg/kg
Ropivacaine (Naropin®)	Medium	Long	3–4mg/kg

Table 16.8 *Calculating LA concentrations*
Multiply the percentage solution by 10 to give the concentration in mg/ml

% solution	mg/ml	% solution	mg/ml
0.25%	2.5mg/ml	1%	10mg/ml
0.5%	5mg/ml	2%	20mg/ml
0.75%	7.5mg/ml	4%	40mg/ml

Table 16.9 *Maximum doses of lidocaine without adrenaline /kg*
Volume in brackets represents ml of 1% lidocaine solution

Weight (kg)	Maximum dose	Weight (kg)	Maximum dose
50	150mg (15ml)	80	240mg (24ml)
60	180mg (18ml)	90	270mg (27ml)
70	210mg (21ml)	100	300mg (30ml)

Table 16.10 *Symptoms and signs of systemic local anaesthetic toxicity*

Mild toxicity	• Tingling around the mouth • Metallic taste • Tinnitus	• Visual disturbance • Slurred speech
Moderate toxicity	• Altered consciousness • Convulsions	• Coma
▶▶ Potentially fatal toxicity	• Respiratory arrest • Cardiac arrhythmias	• Cardiovascular collapse

Suturing

Consent verbal (in the ED), written (elective surgery), common law (emergency surgery)   **Level** F2   **Difficulty** 3/5

Indications the two main indications for skin suturing are:
- Wound closure
- Keeping drains and lines in place.

Contraindications *absolute* competent patient refusal, foreign body in wound, dirty or infected wound, old wound (>12h except on face), bite.
Site appropriate to wound/drain/line site.

Equipment sterile drape, sterile gloves, sterile water, 10ml syringe, green (21G) needle, orange (25G) needle, LA, appropriate suture material, suture pack (toothed forceps, needle-holder, scissors, gauze), assistant to hold the local anaesthetic, sharps bin.
Checks tetanus status (📖 p436), no infection or foreign bodies, no neurovascular deficit requiring referral, no damage to the underlying structures (eg tendons); if in doubt ask for senior opinion.
Patient position patient lying comfortably with wound site exposed.

Anaesthetic perform a field block as follows. Prepare the sterile pack on the trolley with sterile gloves open and antiseptic solution in the receiver. Wash hands and put on sterile gloves. Draw up LA using a green needle and a 10ml syringe. Change to an orange needle for infiltration. Clean the skin with antiseptic solution and use the sterile drape to cover the area except for the wound. Warn the patient and insert the LA needle (it is less painful to go through the walls of the wound than through the skin). Draw back to check you are not in a blood vessel then infiltrate superficially. Allow 2–5min for the LA to work. Use this time to prepare your suture material and hold it with the needle facing upwards in the needle-holder. Before starting to suture, ensure the skin is numb.
Suturing starting at the middle of the wound, pick up the skin edge with the toothed forceps and pass the needle perpendicularly through the skin 5mm from the wound edge and into the wound just under the dermis. Grasp the needle point with the needle holder and pull it through gently. Hold the other skin edge with toothed forceps and again pass the needle through the skin, this time through the dermis first, up to the surface about 5mm from the wound edge. Pull most of the suture through then grasp both ends of the suture, tighten and oppose the skin edge so the edges are slightly everted but without tension. Hold the free end of the suture with the needle-holding forceps and make 3 knots around the forceps (anticlockwise, clockwise, anticlockwise). Make sure you 'lock' each knot by pulling the knot initially in the direction of the wound and then perpendicular to it. Cut the ends of the knot about 1cm long. The knots should lie to the side of the wound not on top of it. Repeat the procedure with sutures 5–10mm apart, depending on the area being sutured. When you have finished, clean the wound, apply a dry dressing, and tell them when the sutures will need to be removed (Tables 16.11 and 16.12).

Confirmation stitches apposing wound edges but not under tension.

Complications infection, poor healing, hypertrophic/keloid scarring, wound breakdown.

Safety avoid touching the needle by using the needle-holder; when you do not need the needle keep it back to front in the needle-holder, with the point covered by the needle holder.

Alternatives steristrips™ and glue (📖 p436); staples have a lower infection rate, but can cause prominent hypertrophic scarring and require staple removers to take them out (may need to attend ward).

Hints and tips

- Make sure you and the patient are in comfortable position with good lighting before you start
- Use toothed forceps on skin as blunt forceps crush the tissue
- LA can be dangerous, see 📖 p558; adrenaline helps haemostasis, but should be used with caution on extremities
- Avoid nylon sutures for drains as this is often uncomfortable
- Consult a senior if the edges need a lot of tension to meet; you may need to use deep or subcutaneous sutures
- See 📖 p436 for treatment of wounds
- Get senior help early; if the sutures do not look right the patient will have the scar for life and it is often better to start again
- Operations are judged by the scars; take time to make them look good.

Table 16.11 *Suture size and suggested dates for removal of sutures (ROS)*

Location	Absorbable?	Suture size	ROS at day
Face and neck	No	6/0	3–4
Lips/mouth/tongue	Yes	6/0 vicryl	N/A
Chest/abdomen	No	3/0	7–10
Limbs	No	4/0	5–7

Table 16.12 *Types of suture material*

Non-absorbable sutures	Absorbable sutures
Nylon (ethylon)	Vicryl
Prolene	PDS
Silk	Monocryl

Wound care advice for patients

- Keep the wound area clean and dry for at least 48h
- Seek medical help if the wound looks infected, ie redness, swelling, tenderness
- Avoid heavy lifting for at least 6wk (except for scalp or face wounds)
- Drive when you can perform an emergency stop and check the view over your shoulder (see 📖 p605).

Reduction of fractures and dislocations

Consent verbal　　　　　**Level** F1　　　　　**Difficulty** 3/5

Indication traumatic injury resulting in a fracture or dislocation.

Contraindications *relative* neurological or vascular deficit (get senior help immediately), open fracture.

Closed Colles' fracture reduction

Equipment three personnel (two to manipulate the fracture, one to apply backslab plaster), plaster, crepe bandage, tube stocking, water, sling and equipment for Bier's block or haematoma block (📖 p558).

Checks X-rays of fracture from two views showing displacement; no neurovascular deficit; adequate analgesia.

Patient position: sitting up with upper limb held at side at roughly 90°.

Procedure: Your assistant applies traction backwards distal to the elbow whilst you apply forward traction gently to unlock the two bone fragments. You may also apply downwards pressure to the bone fragments in order to help them come into alignment. When aligned, flex and deviate the wrist towards the ulna. In this position, the plaster is applied. Only once the cast has set can traction on the limb be released. Neurovascular status should be re-checked and a check X-ray performed. If position is not satisfactory on X-ray, a further attempt at closed reduction can be made. If this fails surgery may be required.

Slings, crutches and analgesia should be provided as appropriate for patients being discharged home. All fractures require orthopaedic follow-up to ensure adequate union of bone, either as an in-patient or via out-patient fracture clinics.

Shoulder dislocations

Around 96% of shoulder dislocations are anterior dislocations and there are many methods that can be used to reduce them. The technique employed should reduce the dislocation without causing additional trauma. The method used depends on patient condition, deepness of sedation, and your competence at the technique. Two of the most commonly used methods are outlined here. Posterior and inferior dislocations frequently require reduction under general anaesthetic, so techniques to reduce these are not covered here.

Never attempt a technique you are not fully familiar with.

Dislocations of the shoulder are diagnosed clinically and on X-ray. Anterior dislocations are normally obvious on AP shoulder views, and confirmed on scapular 'Y'-view (the humeral head sits anterior to the glenoid). Posterior dislocations can look normal or show the 'lightbulb sign' (due to internal rotation of the humerus) on AP view. They are confirmed on 'Y'-view (the humeral head sits posterior to the glenoid).

Equipment 2–3 personnel, one to perform and monitor sedation if used (eg midazolam) and 1 or 2 to perform the reduction, sling.

Checks X-rays (2 views minimum) to diagnose dislocation and check for associated fractures, except in patients with a history of recurrent atraumatic dislocation, no neurovascular deficit, and specifically axillary nerve function (see 'Complications'), adequate analgesia/sedation.

Patient position lying flat on their back.

External rotation technique (single-person technique). The arm is slightly abducted and bent at the elbow to 90°. Support the elbow with one hand and the patient's wrist with the other. Slowly ask the patient to allow their forearm to rotate away from their body (externally rotate), stopping whenever pain or muscle spasm is felt. Support their arm in that position until pain/spasm resolves and then ask them to allow their hand to fall to the side again. Repeat as many times as required, with the hand moving further each time. When externally rotated to between 70° and 110°, the shoulder should click back into position.

Traction-countertraction technique (two-person technique). With the patient relaxed, abduct the arm and apply traction at the distal forearm through the length of the arm whilst your assistant applies counter-traction using a sheet wrapped around the patient's axilla. Apply traction steadily until rotator cuff muscles relax enough to allow the shoulder to click back into position.

For any reduction method, neurovascular status should be documented before and after the procedure and a shoulder X-ray must be performed after reduction. The patient should have a broad arm sling applied, be given adequate analgesia and have orthopaedic follow-up.

Complications axillary nerve and blood vessel injury (ensure the 'badge-patch' area on the lateral side of the upper arm over the deltoid muscle, is checked for sensation and this is documented pre- and post-procedure); Bankart lesions and Hill–Sachs deformities in recurrent dislocations, requiring elective surgery; failure of reduction leading to emergency reduction in theatre.

Alternatives other techniques exist for anterior dislocation reduction. These include the Spaso, modified-Milch, chairback and scapular manipulation techniques (single operator techniques that are relatively atraumatic). Older techniques include Kocher's method and the Hippocratic method; however these techniques have higher levels of associated injury and are not generally used in the UK.

Interpreting results

Full blood count (FBC)

There are three main components: red cells (measured by haemoglobin or Hb), white cells (leucocytes or WCC), and platelets (plts). Remember these components represent the three cell lines from bone marrow.

Main FBC abnormalities		
Anaemia	↓ Hb	📖 p392
Acute blood loss	FBC often initially normal	📖 p478
Infection/inflammation	↑ WCC, ↑ plts	📖 p482
Haematological malignancies	↑↑ WCC	📖 p396
Bone marrow disorders	Persistent change in ≥1 cell line	📖 p396

Hb – red bloods cells (male: 130–180g/L: female: 115–160g/L)
- **↓Hb** Anaemia, classified according to MCV, see 📖 p392 for causes, investigations, and management
- **↑Hb** Dehydration (📖 p378), secondary polycythaemia, eg heart/ lung disease, polycythaemia vera (📖 p396). Consider prophylactic LMWH (📖 p406) due to the increased thrombosis risk.

Reticulocytes (50–100 × 10⁹/l or 0.5–2.5%) these are immature red cells released from bone marrow in response to haemolysis or blood loss (response detectable after a few hours, not hyperacutely). They are also raised secondary to inflammation and infection.

WCC – white blood cells (4–11 × 10⁹/l; Table 17.1)

Table 17.1 *Causes of abnormal white cell differentials*

Cell	Causes
Neutrophils (2.0–7.5 × 10⁹/l)	↑ Bacterial infection, inflammation, acute illness, myeloid leukaemia, steroid therapy
	↓ Viral infection, sepsis, drugs (chemotherapy, steroids, carbimazole), splenomegaly, bone marrow failure, ↓ B₁₂ or folate, autoimmune disease
Lymphocytes (1.3–3.5 × 10⁹/l)	↑ Viral infection, inflammation, lymphocytic leukaemia
	↓ Steroids, chemotherapy, HIV, autoimmune disease, bone marrow failure
Eosinophils (0.04–0.44 × 10⁹/l)	↑ Parasitic/fungal infection, asthma, atopy, lymphoma
	↓ Rarely pathological

Plts – platelets (150–400 × 10⁹/l; Table 17.2)

Table 17.2 *Causes of abnormal platelet counts*

↑	Inflammation, infection, acute illness, recovery from splenectomy, essential thrombocytosis, polycythaemia [rubra] vera (see 📖 p396)
↓	HIT (📖 p406), idiopathic thrombopenic purpura (ITP) (📖 p405), chronic alcoholism, bone marrow failure, DIC (📖 p405), viral infections, splenomegaly, HELLP (📖 p505)

Clotting

Clotting is often measured before procedures and surgery if there is suspicion of an abnormality (eg liver failure). It is also measured to allow correct dosing of warfarin and IV heparin. Prothrombin time (PT) is a measure of the **extrinsic pathway** and should be quoted unless the patient is on warfarin therapy when the international normalised ratio (INR) is used; activated partial thromboplastin time (APTT) is a measure of the **intrinsic pathway** and should be quoted unless the patient is on IV heparin therapy when the APTT ratio (APTTr) is used (Table 17.3). See 🕮 p405 for clotting defects.

Table 17.3 *Causes of abnormal clotting*

Test	Causes
PT (11–16s) [INR 0.8–1.2]	↑ Warfarin, liver disease, DIC, sepsis, deficiency of factors II, V, VII or X, heparin
	↓ Rarely pathological
APTT (35–45s) [APTTr 0.8–1.2]	↑ Heparin, haemophilia A+B, von Willebrand disease, DIC, sepsis, deficiency of factors II, V, VII, IX, X, XI, or XII, liver disease, warfarin
	↓ Rarely pathological
PT and APTT	↑ DIC, sepsis, liver disease, warfarin, heparin

Cardiac markers

These tests are used to diagnose MI, and to distinguish MI from stable and unstable angina (🕮 p241). Assays for cardiac troponins (either I or T) differ between hospitals. Due to different kinetics of release and excretion, measurement of creatine kinase (CK or CK-MB) can also be useful in patients with ongoing chest pain after a recent MI (see 🕮 p243). See Table 17.4.

Table 17.4 *Causes of abnormal cardiac markers*

Test	Causes
Troponin (upper limit of normal depends on assay used – check local advice)	↑ MI (raised after 6–12h), small rise may be seen with CRF, PE, septicaemia, blunt chest trauma
CK (25–195units/l)	↑ MI, rhabdomyolysis (muscle breakdown – check renal function), exercise, recent surgery, hypothyroidism, blunt chest trauma

Inflammatory response

Acute or chronic inflammation can affect a wide range of blood results, including:

- ↑ ESR
- ↑ CRP
- ↑ Ferritin
- ↑ Plts
- ↑ WCC
- ↓ Albumin.

A very high ESR (>100mm/h) should raise suspicions of giant-cell arteritis (🕮 p429), polymyalgia rheumatica (🕮 p454), or myeloma (🕮 p389).

Urea and electrolytes (U+E)

These are measured to assess renal function and the concentration of the two main electrolytes in the blood.

Main urea and electrolyte abnormalities		
Dehydration	↑urea, ± ↑Cr	📖 p378
Acute renal failure	↑K⁺, ↑↑urea, ↑Cr	📖 p372
Chronic renal failure	↑urea, ↑↑Cr, ↓Hb	📖 p373
Upper GI bleed	↑↑urea, others normal	📖 p299
Addison's disease	↓Na⁺, ↑K⁺, ↑urea, ↑Cr	📖 p332

Urea and creatinine (Table 17.5)

Urea and creatinine (Cr) are metabolic waste products which are excreted by the kidney. An increase in either test suggests a degree of renal dysfunction. If both urea and creatinine are raised the patient has renal failure. Check previous U+E results to distinguish between chronic and acute renal failure. Acute renal failure is an emergency, see 📖 p372.

Table 17.5 *Causes of abnormal urea and creatinine*

Test	Causes
Urea (2.5–7.8mmol/l)	↑ Dehydration, upper GI bleed, acute illness, pre-renal failure
	↓ Rarely pathological, can be caused by pregnancy or a lack of protein, eg alcoholism, anorexia, liver failure, malnutrition
Creatinine (Cr) (70–150micromol/l)	↑ Renal failure, may be acute, chronic or acute on chronic; muscle injury
	↓ Rarely pathological, can be seen in pregnancy or ↓BMI
Urea and creatinine	↑ Renal failure, check K⁺ and ECG

Sodium and potassium (Table 17.6)

Numerous diseases can affect electrolyte levels, these are discussed in the section on electrolyte imbalance (📖 p385). Small changes in K⁺ can induce fatal arrhythmias in the heart so abnormal K⁺ levels should be treated as an emergency (📖 p384).

Table 17.6 *Causes of abnormal sodium and potassium*

Electrolyte	Causes
Na⁺ – sodium (133–146mmol/l)	↑ See 📖 p387
	↓ See 📖 p386
K⁺ – potassium (3.5–5.3mmol/l)	↑ Urgent ECG, inform senior, see 📖 p385
	↓ Urgent ECG, inform senior, see 📖 p385

Liver function tests (LFT) and amylase

These are measured to detect jaundice, liver disease, biliary disease and pancreatitis. Liver dysfunction may affect clotting, particularly PT.

Main liver function abnormalities		
Pre-hepatic jaundice	↑bilirubin (unconjugated), ↓Hb, ↑reticulocytes, ↓ haptoglobin	📖 p318
Hepatic jaundice	↑bilirubin (mixed), ↑↑ALT/AST, ↑γGT	📖 p318
Cholestatic jaundice	↑bilirubin (conjugated), ↑↑ALP, ↑γGT	📖 p318
Hepatocellular damage	↑↑ AST/ALT, ↑ γGT, ↑ALP	📖 p313
Liver failure	↑bilirubin, ↑PT, ↓albumin	📖 p313
Alcoholism	↑γGT, ↑MCV, ↓plts	📖 p395
Pancreatitis	↑↑amylase/lipase, ↓Ca²⁺, ↑glucose, ↑↑CRP	📖 p296
HELLP (pregnant)	↑AST/ALT, ↑γGT, ↓Hb, ↓plts	📖 p505

Liver function tests (Table 17.7)
See 📖 p312–319 for the investigation and management of liver disease.

Table 17.7 *Causes of abnormal liver function tests*

Test		Causes
ALT or AST (3–35units/l)	↑	Hepatocellular damage, biliary disease, alcohol, muscle damage, MI, pancreatitis
	↓	Rarely pathological, consider ↓vitamin B_6
ALP (30–130units/l)	↑	Biliary disease/damage, liver disease, alcohol, bone disease (especially Paget's), pregnancy, bony metastases
	↓	Rarely pathological
γ GT(10–55units/l)	↑	Biliary or liver disease, alcohol
	↓	Rarely pathological
Bilirubin (3–21micromol/l)	↑	Jaundice (📖 p318 – haemolysis, liver disease, obstruction of biliary system), Gilbert's syndrome
	↓	Rarely pathological
Albumin (35–50g/l)	↑	Dehydration
	↓	Inflammation, cirrhosis, pregnancy, chronic disease

Amylase and lipase (Table 17.8)

Table 17.8 *Causes of abnormal amylase and lipase*

Test		Cause
Amylase (0–120units/l)	↑	Acute or chronic pancreatitis, abdominal disease (eg perforation), burns, anorexia, salivary adenitis, renal disease
Lipase (5.0–65units/l)	↑↑↑	Acute pancreatitis (eg 3× upper limit of normal)

Depending on the laboratory and the patient population, lipase tends to be slightly more specific for pancreatic pathology than amylase. There is no indication for requesting both.

Calcium and phosphate

Calcium and phosphate are electrolytes predominantly stored in bones. Blood levels are affected by many diseases including parathyroid and bone abnormalities. See Tables 17.9 and 17.10.

Main calcium and phosphate abnormalities		
Bone metastases	↑Ca^{2+}, ↑ALP	📖 p389
Hypoparathyroidism	↓Ca^{2+}, ↑PO_4^{3-}, ↓PTH	📖 p388
Primary hyperparathyroidism	↑Ca^{2+}, ↓PO_4^{3-}, ↑ALP, ↑PTH	📖 p389
Myeloma	↑Ca^{2+}, ↑urea, ↑Cr, ↓Hb, ↑ESR	📖 p389
Paget's	↑↑ALP, ↔Ca^{2+}, ↔PO_4^{3-}	📖 p389

Table 17.9 *Causes of abnormal calcium and phosphate*

Test	Causes
Ca^{2+} – calcium (2.2–2.6mmol/l)	↑ Primary/tertiary hyperparathyroidism, malignancy (myeloma, bone metastases, PTH-related peptide secreting tumours), excess vitamin D supplements, sarcoidosis
	↓ Vitamin D deficiency (Asians, Africans, chronic renal failure), hypoparathyroid, acute pancreatitis, alkalosis, magnesium deficiency
PO_4^{3-} – phosphate (0.8–1.5mmol/l)	↑ Chronic renal failure, ↓PTH, myeloma, excess vitamin D, rhabdomyolysis, cell lysis (eg post-chemo), acidosis
	↓ Malabsorption/malnutrition, alcohol, ↑PTH, burns, alkalosis, post-DKA treatment

Table 17.10 *Effects of parathyroid hormone disease on blood tests*

Disease	Ca^{2+}	PO_4^{3-}	PTH
Primary hyperparathyroidism	↑	↓	↑
Secondary hyperparathyroidism	↓	↓	↑
Tertiary hyperparathyroidism[1]	↑	↑	↑
Hypoparathyroidism	↓	↑	↓

[1] The hyperphosphataemia in tertiary hyperparathyroidism results from the inability of the diseased kidneys to excrete it rather than as a function of the high levels of PTH, per se.

Endocrine tests

Cortisol (□ p332)

Short Synacthen® test

- Take blood for cortisol ideally at 9am. Occasionally ACTH is also tested; it needs to be transported on ice. Call biochemistry to check which bottle to use
- Give 250micrograms Synacthen® IM/IV
- Take blood for cortisol 30min later
- A baseline or 30min cortisol level above 550nmol/l is normal and excludes primary adrenal insufficiency
- If 30min cortisol <550nmol/l and ↓ACTH → ACTH deficiency
- If 30min cortisol <550nmol/l and ↑ACTH →Addison's disease (□ p332).

Glucose

This test is performed when the patient is not acutely unwell and on a normal diet. The patient is fasted overnight. 75g glucose in 300ml water is given after the baseline fasting glucose blood sample has been taken. A 2h plasma glucose sample is also taken. See Table 17.11.

Table 17.11 *Interpretation of oral glucose tolerance test*

Fasting glucose	Glucose after 2h	Diagnosis
Any value	≥11.1mmol/l	Diabetes mellitus
≥7mmol/l	Any value	Diabetes mellitus
<7mmol/l	7.8–11.0mmol/l	Impaired glucose tolerance (IGT)
6.1–6.9mmol/l	≤7.7mmol/l	Impaired fasting glucose (IFG)
<6.1mmol/l	≤7.7mmol/l	Normal

Thyroid function (Table 17.12; □ p334)

Table 17.12 *Thyroid function*

	T_4	T_3	TSH
Hyperthyroidism	↑	↑	↓↓
T_3 hyperthyroidism	normal	↑	↓↓
Subclinical hyperthyroidism	normal	normal	↓
1° hypothyroidism (thyroid disease)	↓	↓	↑↑
2° hypothyroidism (pituitary disease)	↓	↓	↓ or normal
Subclinical hypothyroidism	normal	normal	↑

Electrocardiogram (ECG)

Examine all ECGs in a systematic manner to avoid missing the basics. Never be tempted to trust the automated interpretation: these are rarely accurate.
Check patient details, date and time of ECG, speed of paper (25mm/s).
Rate at 25mm/s each large square represents 0.2s and each small square 0.04s. To calculate rate divide 300 by the number of large squares between one R wave and the next R wave (see Table 17.13).

Table 17.13 *Calculating heart rate from the ECG*

Large squares	Heart rate (bpm)	Large squares	Heart rate (bpm)
1	300	2 3/5	115
1 3/5	188	2 4/5	107
2	150	3	100
2 1/5	136	4	75
2 2/5	125	5	60

Rhythm *Sinus rhythm* each QRS has a P wave before it. *Atrial fibrillation* no P wave and the QRS complexes are irregularly irregular. *Atrial flutter* the baseline is described as saw-tooth and the QRS are often regularly spaced. *Ventricular rhythm* QRS is wide (>0.12s or >3 small squares) and has no association with P waves. *Nodal rhythm* P wave may be absent or part of the QRS complex, but rhythm is regular. *Regularly irregular* rhythms suggest a degree of heart block (📖 p258).
Axis Look at lead I and count the number of small squares that make up the height of the R wave (positive deflection). Next count the number of small squares that make up the Q and/or S wave (negative deflections). Work out the difference between the R and Q/S wave (ie R wave squares – Q/S wave squares). Do the same for lead aVF.
Draw a large cross (Fig. 17.1a) and plot the numbers for lead I and aVF. The line between where they meet and the middle is the cardiac axis. An example is shown where lead I has a 10 square R wave and 7 square S wave (10 − 7 = 3) and lead aVF has an 8 square R wave and 1 square S wave (8 − 1 = 7). The normal axis is from −30° to +90° (Fig. 17.1b).

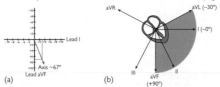

Fig. 17.1 (a) Calculating the cardiac axis; (b) the normal cardiac axis.

Table 17.14 shows a quick way of working out the rough position of the axis by comparing the size of the R wave to the size of the Q wave.

Table 17.14 *Calculating the cardiac axis from the ECG*

		Lead I	
		R > Q/S	R < Q/S
Lead aVF	R > Q/S	0 to 90°	90 to 180°
	R < Q/S	0 to −90°	−90 to 180°

P wave absent in AF (☐ p252) and atrial flutter (☐ p253). Bifid P wave suggests left atrial hypertrophy. Peaked P waves are seen in right atrial hypertension (eg pulmonary hypertension) and transiently in ↓K⁺.

PR interval normally 0.12–0.2s (3–5 small squares). Longer in heart block (☐ p258) and shorter in WPW (☐ p253). See Fig. 17.2.

QRS complex normally <0.12s (<3 small squares). Wider QRS implies ventricular rhythm (eg 3ʳᵈ-degree heart block) or bundle branch block (causes in Table 17.15). Paced rhythms may also have wide QRS complexes.

Hypertrophy *left (LVH):* sum of S wave in V3 and R wave in aVL >28mm (men) or >20mm (women)[1] is suggestive of LVH (not diagnostic); *right (RVH):* R>Q or S wave in V1, deep S wave in V6, T wave inversion in V2, ± V3, ± V4, right axis deviation.

ST segment usually level with baseline; elevation >1mm (for causes see Table 17.15, infarction ☐ p244); depression >0.5mm suggests ischaemia (☐ p245–246).

T wave inversion (pointing down) in leads I, II or V4–V6 suggests ischaemia. Often peaked in ↑K⁺ and acute MI, flattened in ↓K⁺.

Other components of the ECG

- *QT interval* is dependent on heart rate. The QTc (QT interval corrected for heart rate) is calculated by most ECG machines. An abnormal QTc is >450ms (♂) and >470ms (♀) (☐ p254). QTc prolongation is associated with increased risk of ventricular arrhythmias
- *U wave* (positive in most leads) follows the T wave and precedes the P wave; if present it implies ↓ K⁺ though can be a normal finding
- *Δ wave* a slurred upstroke to the QRS complex found in conduction defects eg WPW ☐ p253
- *J wave* an upwards wave seen immediately after the QRS complex and before the T wave in hypothermia.

Hints and tips being able to read an ECG systematically is much more important than a spot ECG diagnosis. The common ECG abnormalities which should not be missed are: AF, MI or ischaemia, LBBB/RBBB, 3ʳᵈ-degree heart block and ventricular tachycardia.

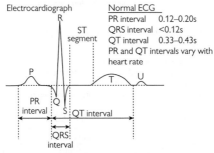

Fig. 17.2 The normal QRS complex and normal ECG intervals.

---

[1] Cornell voltage criteria for LVH, from Casale *et al.* Improved sex specific criteria of left ventricular hypertrophy for clinical and computer interpretation of electrocardiograms: validation with autopsy findings. *Circulation.* 2010 **75**(3):565–72.

Table 17.15 *Causes of ...*

ST elevation	STEMI, pericarditis, ventricular aneurysm, LBBB, hypothermia, coronary artery spasm (Prinzmetal's angina), early repolarisation (high takeoff)
LBBB	Acute MI, ischaemic heart disease, hypertensive heart disease, cardiomyopathy, aortic valve disease
RBBB	Normal, heart failure, PE, pulmonary hypertension
Left axis deviation	Left ventricular hypertrophy, inferior MI, left anterior hemiblock, hyperkalaemia
Right axis deviation	Right ventricular hypertrophy, chronic lung disease, normal in children, left posterior hemiblock

Coronary artery territories and the ECG (Fig. 17.3 and Table 17.16)

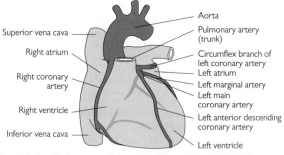

Fig. 17.3 Simplified structure of the heart and its coronary blood supply.

Left anterior descending artery (LAD) and its many branches supply the anterior and anteriolateral walls of the left ventricle, and the anterior two-thirds of the septum.

Left circumflex artery (LCX) and its branches supply the posterolateral wall of the left ventricle.

Right coronary artery (RCA) supplies the right ventricle, the inferior and posterior walls of the left ventricle and the posterior third of the septum; the RCA also gives off the AV nodal coronary artery in ~85% of individuals, with the LCX supplying this in the remaining 15% of people.

Table 17.16 *Territories of the heart on the ECG*

I Lateral	aVR Multiple	V1 Septal	V4 Anterior
II Inferior	aVL Lateral	V2 Septal	V5 Lateral
III Inferior	aVF Inferior	V3 Anterior	V6 Lateral

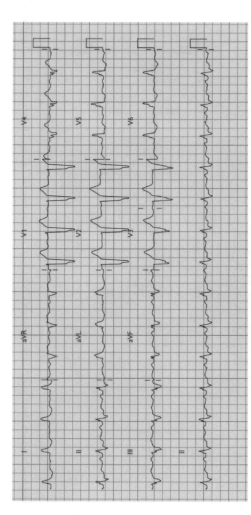

Fig. 17.4 Left bundle branch block: Note W pattern in V1 and M pattern in V5/V6, also no Q wave in V5/V6 and inverted T wave in I and aVL. Remember 'WiLLiaM and MaRRoW'.

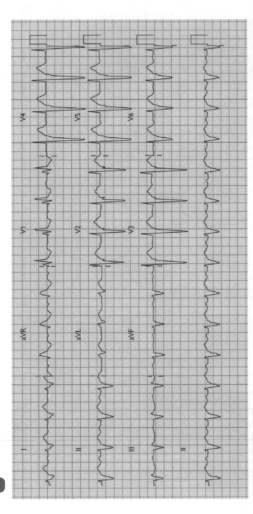

Fig. 17.5 Right bundle branch block: Note M pattern (RSR) in V1, W pattern in V5/V6 and inverted T wave in V1. Remember' WiL*Li*aM and Ma*RR*oW'.

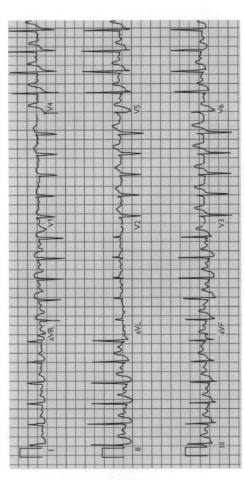

Fig. 17.6 Acute inferolateral ischaemia: Note ST depression in leads I, II, III, aVF and V3 to V6, also T wave inversion in aVR (normal variant) and aVL.

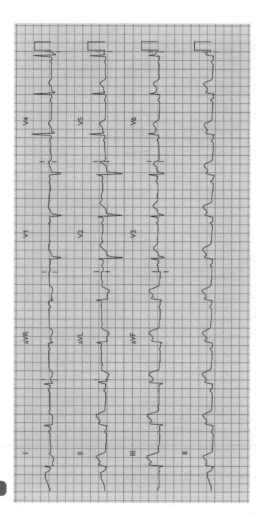

Fig. 17.7 Acute inferolateral myocardial infarction: Note ST elevation in leads II, III and aVF (inferior leads) and also in V5 and V6 (lateral leads). The ST depression in I, aVL and V2 are reciprocal changes and often seen with large infarcts.

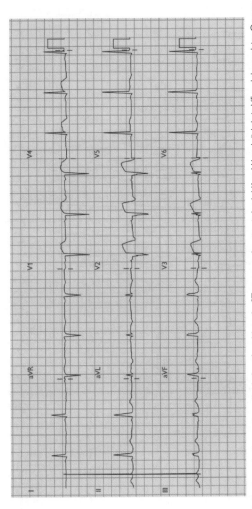

Fig. 17.8 Acute anterior myocardial infarction: Note the ST segment elevation in leads V1 to V4 and slightly in V5 and the evolving Q wave.

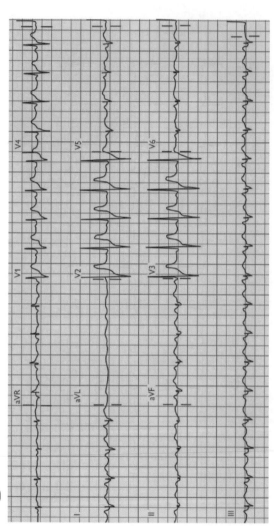

Fig. 17.9 Acute posterior myocardial infarction: Note dominant R wave and ST depression in V1–V3 (often seen with ST elevation in V5/V6 reflecting posterolateral infarction).

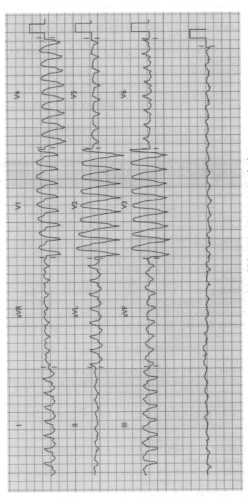

Fig. 17.10 Ventricular tachycardia: Note the broad nature of the QRS and regular repeating rhythm.

Chest X-ray (CXR)

The main patterns of acute disease are:

- *Pneumonia* (📖 p276) asymmetrical shadowing (consolidation), blunting of angles, blurring of heart and diaphragm borders, air bronchograms
- *Pulmonary oedema* (📖 p282) enlarged heart, symmetrical hazy/reticular shadowing, blunted costophrenic angles or pleural effusions, indistinct hilar vessels, enlarged upper lobe vessels, Kerley B lines, distinct septa
- *Pleural effusion* (📖 p279) featureless white area at the base with loss of costophrenic and/or costocardiac angles on the affected side ± meniscus (upper surface sloping up to the chest wall)
- *Asthma/COPD* (📖 p273–274) hyperinflated, flattened diaphragm, barrel chested
- *Pneumothorax* (📖 p279) line of separated pleura with peripheries lacking lung markings – may be large and deviating mediastinum (eg tension).

> ### Adequacy of a CXR – interpret cautiously unless the following are normal
>
> - **Rotation** heads of the clavicles should be the same distance from the vertebral bodies on each side; the spinous processes should be in the middle of the vertebral bodies
> - **Penetration** intervertebral discs should be visible behind the heart and the lung fields should have markings
> - **Inspiration** ≥7 posterior ribs should be visible.

Develop a routine so you spot all the abnormalities:

- Lung outline:
    - **blunting/loss** of costophrenic and cardiophrenic angles
    - **indistinct heart border**, lung border or diaphragm edges
    - **pneumothorax** best seen by inverting the image or rotating by 90°
    - **Kerley B lines** 1–2cm horizontal lines at the edges, extending to the plerural margin
    - **pleural plaques/thickening** does the edge look whiter in some areas?
- Lung fields:
    - **colour** too dark suggests pneumothorax, emphysema or high penetration, while white shadowing suggests pulmonary oedema, pneumonia, effusion or under-penetration. Describe shadowing as nodular (lumpy), reticular (fine lines eg pulmonary oedema) or alveolar (fluffy eg consolidation). Air bronchograms may be seen (air filled bronchus seen against surrounding opacified alveoli) suggesting an airspace process (eg oedema, consolidation)
    - **vascular markings** the upper lobe vessels should be thinner than lower lobe ones
    - **cavities** ie dark circles, consider bronchiectasis, bullae or abscesses (may have an air/fluid level)
    - **localised white lesions** eg carcinoma or abscess
- Lung size there should be ≥7 posterior ribs (see Figs 17.11 and 17.12), ≥10 hyperinflated, ≤6 poor inspiratory effort; for anterior ribs the numbers are two lower

- *Diaphragm:*
  - Is there a pneumoperitoneum (eg perforated bowel), thin black line under the diaphragm?
  - Is the right side slightly higher than the left? If not consider pressure from within abdomen or diaphragmatic paralysis as causes
  - Are the domes convex? Flat suggests hyperexpansion
- *Mediastinum:*
  - This should be <8cm wide at the aortic arch, wider suggests abnormal tissue eg aortic dissection or lymphadenopathy
  - The heart should be <50% the width of the chest on a PA film, larger suggests cardiomegaly (difficult to interpret on AP films)
  - Is there collapse or consolidation behind the heart?
- *Trachea* should be central and uncompressed
- *Hila* these should have a concave shape with distinct vessels
- *Bones* look at the spine, clavicles, scapulae, shoulder and ribs. Look for fractures, osteolytic and osteosclerotic lesions. Is the spine straight?
- *Soft tissues* surgical emphysema (pneumothorax), breast lesions.

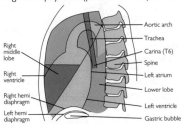

Fig. 17.11 Major features of a lateral CXR.

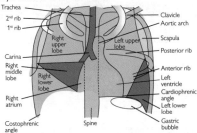

Fig. 17.12 Major features on an anteroposterior CXR.

Central lines (📖 p534) check for pneumothorax and haemothorax; note the position of the end of the line, it should be at the level of the carina.

Feeding NG tubes (📖 p549) the end of the tube should be seen below the diaphragm; if not advance the tube 5cm and repeat CXR. If tube in bronchus, remove completely and resite.

Chest drains (📖 p540) the end should be within the ribcage, ideally angled downwards for effusions and up for pneumothoraces; note the size of pneumothorax or effusion and any surgical emphysema.

Arterial blood gases (ABGs)

ABG analysis measures PaO_2 and $PaCO_2$, and calculates HCO_3^- in a heparinised specimen (can also be undertaken on venous or capillary blood or on fluid aspirated from the chest or abdomen). Base excess and anion gap are also calculated. In addition, pH, O_2 saturation, and concentrations of Na^+, K^+, Ca^{2+}, Cl^- and lactate are measured. For advice on how to perform an ABG see 📖 p522. See Table 17.17.

Table 17.17 *Normal ranges (patient breathing room air)*

Parameter	Value	Parameter	Value
pH	7.35–7.45	HCO_3^-	22–28mmol/l
PaO_2	10.6–13.3kPa	Base excess (BE)	−2 to +2
$PaCO_2$	4.7–6.0kPa	O_2 saturation	95–100%

NB Note that a low or normal PaO_2 in a patient on a high concentration of inspired O_2 is very worrying and suggests significantly impaired gas exchange.

First look at the pH:
• pH <7.35 = acidaemia
• pH 7.35 to 7.45 = normal pH
• pH >7.45 = alkalaemia.

Next look at the $PaCO_2$ and bicarbonate (HCO_3^-) (Tables 17.18 and 17.19):

Table 17.18 *Types of acidaemia*

	$\downarrow HCO_3^-$	$\leftrightarrow HCO_3^-$	$\uparrow HCO_3^-$
$\downarrow PaCO_2$	Metabolic acidosis	X	X
$\leftrightarrow PaCO_2$	Mixed acidosis	X	X
$\uparrow PaCO_2$	Mixed acidosis	Acute respiratory acidosis	Chronic respiratory acidosis

X – incompatible

Table 17.19 *Types of alkalaemia*

	$\downarrow HCO_3^-$	$\leftrightarrow HCO_3^-$	$\uparrow HCO_3^-$
$\downarrow PaCO_2$	Chronic respiratory alkalosis	Acute respiratory alkalosis	Mixed alkalosis
$\leftrightarrow PaCO_2$	X	X	Mixed alkalosis
$\uparrow PaCO_2$	X	X	Metabolic alkalosis

X – incompatible

Base excess

This is the amount of 'base' needed to restore pH to the normal range (Table 17.20):
- Base excess >+2, patient has excess base present (ie alkalosis)
- Base excess <−2, patient has insufficient base present (ie acidosis).

Table 17.20 *Causes of acid–base disturbance*

	Acidosis	**Alkalosis**
Metabolic	Shock	Vomiting
	DKA	Diarrhoea
	Renal/liver failure	Hypokalaemia
	Drug overdose (eg TCA)	
	Renal tubular acidosis	
	Lactate (📖 p477)	
	Refer to 'anion gap' box	
Respiratory	Severe asthma/COPD	Cranial lesions (eg stroke)
	Severe pneumonia	Anxiety/hyperventilation
	Severe pulmonary oedema	
	Myasthenia gravis	
	Drugs (eg sedatives, opioids)	
	Chest trauma/scoliosis	
	Obesity	

If all else fails calculate the anion gap or speak to a biochemist

If the differentials for a metabolic acidosis are still unclear then calculate the anion gap which should answer any remaining problems (see box); alternatively ask a senior or speak directly to the clinical biochemist in the laboratory.

The anion gap

This is calculated by $([Na^+] + [K^+]) - ([Cl^-] + [HCO_3^-])$.
Normal value is 6–16mmol/l.
It helps to distinguish the different causes of a metabolic acidosis:
- Raised anion gap (>16mmol/l):
  - lactic acidosis (📖 p477 shock, sepsis/infection)
  - urate (renal failure)
  - ketones (DKA, alcohol, starvation)
  - drugs/toxins (salicylates, biguanides, ethylene glycol, methanol)
- Normal anion gap (6–16mmol/l):
  - renal tubular acidosis
  - diarrhoea
  - drugs (acetazolamide)
  - Addison's disease
  - pancreatic fistula
  - ammonium chloride ingestion.

Respiratory function tests

Peak expiratory flow rate (PEFR)

Indications used for the diagnosis, monitoring (eg daily diary/obs) and severity assessment of asthma (Table 17.21).

Method reset the tab and fit a clean mouthpiece. Ask the patient to stand up and hold it in their hands (not covering the scale), breathe in deeply and blow as hard and fast as they can (with encouragement). Use the best reading of three attempts.

Table 17.21 *PEFR in asthma (exacerbation severity)*

PEFR[1]	>80%	80–50%	55–33%	<33%
Asthma severity	Normal	Mild–moderate	Severe	Life-threatening

[1] Compared with best or predicted (see Fig. 17.14).

Spirometry

Indication diagnosis and monitoring of respiratory disease.

Before testing omit morning inhalers or nebulisers (unless severely ill) to allow reversibility assessment.

Method can be performed by technicians in a respiratory function laboratory or by you at the patient's bedside. The patient must inhale as deeply as they can then exhale as fast and as long as they can manage. The following measurements are made (Table 17.22):

- Forced expiratory volume in 1s (FEV_1), the volume exhaled in the first second after deep inspiration and forced expiration, similar to PEFR
- Forced vital capacity (FVC), the total volume exhaled from maximal inspiration to maximal exhalation.

Beyond spirometry respiratory function laboratories can also measure:

Residual volume (RV), the volume of gas remaining in the lungs after a maximum expiration

Total lung capacity (TLC) is the combination of FVC and RV.

Table 17.22 *Spirometry findings in lung disease*

	Obstructive	Normal	Restrictive
FEV_1	↓↓	↔	↓
FVC	↓	↔	↓↓
FEV_1/FVC	<75%	75–80%	>80%
RV	↑	↔	↓
TLC	↑	↔	↓

Obstructive asthma, COPD, emphysema.

Restrictive interstitial lung disease, sarcoid, connective tissue disorders, neuromuscular disease (including myasthenia gravis and Guillain–Barré).

Other spirometry measurements

Reversibility asthma (a reversible obstruction) is diagnosed if there is ≥250ml and ≥15% improvement in PEFR or FEV$_1$ with bronchodilators. Asthma can coexist with COPD (non-reversible obstruction).

Gas transfer also called transfer factor; is measured using carbon monoxide. It is reduced in emphysema, acute asthma, anaemia and interstitial lung disease and increased with chronic asthma, left heart failure, polycythaemia and exercise.

Flow volume loops graphical representations of the results with volume on the x-axis and flow rate on the y-axis. Exhalation is above the line and inhalation below the line. There are four main patterns (Fig. 17.13).

Upper airway obstruction lesion occluding the bronchi, trachea or larynx associated with stridor, see 📖 p284.

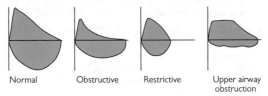

Normal   Obstructive   Restrictive   Upper airway
                                                          obstruction

Fig. 17.13 Flow volume loops (flow on y-axis, volume on x-axis).

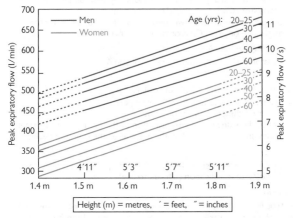

Fig. 17.14 Normal peak expiratory flow values.

Abdomen X-ray (AXR)

The main patterns of disease are:

- *Bowel perforation* free gas seen on lateral decubitus AXR (ie patient lying on one side) abdominal film or erect CXR underneath the diaphragm
- *Dilated loops* of small bowel >2.5cm or large bowel >6cm (see Table 17.23)
- *Sigmoid volvulus* grossly dilated loop of bowel ('coffee bean'-shaped)
- *Constipation* faecal loading in the large bowel, often starting from the rectum. If faeces seen, the colon is unlikely to be inflamed
- *Gallstones/renal stones* calcifications in the RUQ or along the urinary tract; 10% of gallstones and 60% of renal stones are visible on AXR
- *Chronic pancreatitis* calcified specks in the epigastric/pancreatic area
- *Chronic renal failure* small kidneys
- *Abdominal aortic aneurysm* wide aorta on the left hand side of the spine; may see a calcified outline of the aortic walls (📖 p474).

Develop a routine so you spot all the abnormalities (Figs 17.5 and 17.16):

Bowel pathology

- *Bowel wall oedema* can be seen on plain AXR
- *Bowel gas* (best seen in a supine film) dilated loops of bowel due to mechanical obstruction or paralytic ileus
- *Fluid level* obstruction, ileus, gastroenteritis
- *Stomach* dilated in pyloric stenosis; look for linitis plastica ('leather bottle stomach') in advanced stomach cancer
- *Gas outside the lumen* bowel perforation (look for air under the diaphragm on erect CXR or lateral decubitus AXR).

Biliary tree look for:

- Gallstones (NB only 10% are radio-opaque)
- Is there a stent *in situ*?

Urinary tract and bladder look for:

- Renal and ureteric stones (60% are visible)
- Urinary catheters or ureteric stents
- Size of the kidneys, obvious dilatation of the pelvicalyces; the right kidney should be lower than the left one, as the liver is above it.

Pelvis

- *Uterus/ovaries* foreign bodies (eg IUCD, ring pessary), fibroids, cysts
- *Prostate* size, calcification (difficult to see).

Bones

- *Lytic lesions (dark)* think bronchial/breast/renal carcinoma, myeloma
- *Sclerotic lesions* think prostate/breast carcinoma, Paget's disease
- *Fusion of the vertebrae/sacroiliac joints, curving of the spine* degenerative disease, scoliosis, ankylosing spondylosis.

Other soft tissues

- *Psoas muscle* if absent, think of ascites, haematoma or retroperitoneal mass.

Hints and tips

- AXRs are daunting to interpret initially, so it's important to keep in mind what you are trying to confirm/exclude on them
- Stand back and approach things in a systematic manner
- Take the findings on AXR together with the clinical picture and discuss what management is necessary with the rest of your team.

Table 17.23 *Large bowel vs. small bowel obstruction*

	Small intestine	Large intestine
Number of loops	Lots	Few
Distribution of loops	Central	Peripheral
Diameter of loops	>2.5cm	>6cm
Haustrae[1]	No	Yes
Valvulae conniventes[2]	Yes	No
Faeces present	No	Yes

[1] *Haustra*: folds which do not completely cross the bowel lumen wall.
[2] *Valvulae conniventes*: folds which completely cross the bowel lumen wall.

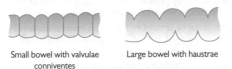

Small bowel with valvulae
conniventes

Large bowel with haustrae

Fig. 17.15 Radiological differences between small bowel and large bowel.

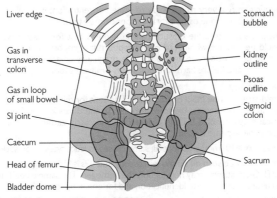

Liver edge — Stomach bubble
Gas in transverse colon — Kidney outline
— Psoas outline
Gas in loop of small bowel — Sigmoid colon
SI joint —
Caecum —
— Sacrum
Head of femur —
Bladder dome —

Fig. 17.16 Features of the abdominal X-ray.

Urine tests

Urine samples should be 'mid-stream' (MSU) to limit urethral contamination, alternatively they can be taken from a catheter (CSU).

Dipstick

UTIs can be asymptomatic and urinary symptoms (dysuria, frequency, urgency) can be present without a UTI. See box on ☐ p484 for information regarding the sensitivity of urine dipsticks for detecting UTIs.

Nitrites are produced by Gram-negative bacteria (eg *E. coli*) and suggest urinary tract infection (UTI).

Leucocytes (white cells) arise from inflammation of the kidneys and urinary tract, most commonly UTIs, but also stones, trauma, neoplasia, infection of related structures (eg prostate, appendix) and renal disease.

Blood dipsticks detect haemoglobin and may distinguish this from blood cells. Send the urine for microscopy if either are seen. A positive dipstick with no red cells on microscopy suggests myoglobinuria or haemoglobinuria. See ☐ p374 for the causes of haematuria.

Protein dipsticks detect albumin which should not be present in urine. If protein is persistently positive then see ☐ p375. Bence Jones protein (seen in myeloma) is not detected by dipsticks.

Glucose should not be present in urine but is common with increasing age; its presence may suggest, but cannot diagnose, DM (☐ p328).

Ketones are raised in DKA (along with glucose). They can also be raised after fasting, low carbohydrate diets and acute illness.

pH normal range 4.5–8; urine pH can be affected by systemic acidosis and alkalosis. Acid pH suggests systemic acidosis and vice versa.

Specific gravity a very rough guide to urine concentration; it should not be relied upon (urine osmolality is a superior measure).

β-hCG a separate urine dipstick can be used to test for pregnancy; it should be positive within 12d of conception. It is important to test all women of reproductive age to exclude pregnancy as a cause of their symptoms and before harmful medications or investigations (eg X-ray).

Microscopy

A mid-stream urine MSU or CSU should be sent for microscopy if there are nitrites, leucocytes, blood or protein on the dipstick or if there is clinical suspicion of a UTI. In children a clean catch, catheter urine or suprapubic aspirate is used.

White cells >10/mm^3 is abnormal; same causes as leucocytes on dipstick.

Bacteria may be seen on simple microscopy and this is highly suggestive of a UTI; Gram staining may help identify the pathogen. The sample needs to be cultured for complete identification and for antibiotic sensitivities.

Red cells >2/mm^3 is abnormal; see ☐ p374 for management of haematuria.

Casts hyaline and fine granular casts are not significant; dense granular, red-cell and epithelial casts suggest renal disease; white-cell casts are found with pyelonephritis.

Culture and sensitivity

Samples sent for microscopy are routinely cultured over 48h. The culture is said to be positive if >100,000 colony forming units/ml are present. The sample is recultured in different mediums to determine the bacteria present and their sensitivity to antibiotics. A mixed culture (more than one organism present) suggests a contaminated sample. Urine culture is not 100% sensitive or specific – it can be wrong and require repeating. CSU obtained from long-term catheters are frequently positive. Only treat if the patient is symptomatic.

Biochemistry

Sodium concentration is a useful test in acute renal failure. A low urine sodium (<20mmol/l) suggests hypoperfusion, eg hypovolaemia, while a raised concentration (>40mmol/l) suggests acute tubular necrosis. It is also used in the assessment of hyponatraemia ([] p386).

Urine osmolality is a measure of the concentration of the urine; the normal range is 500–800mOsmol/kg. It is used in the investigation of renal disease and diagnosis of diabetes insipidus. In acute renal failure it can help distinguish between prerenal failure (>500mOsmol/kg) and acute tubular necrosis (<350mOsmol/kg).

24h urine protein total protein and microalbumin can be measured, total protein is the more common test; microalbumin is used to detect developing renal failure in diabetics and a value of >30mg/24h is abnormal. Urine creatinine should also be measured to determine GFR. See Table 17.24.

Table 17.24 *Proteinuria*

24h protein	Significance
<150mg	Normal
150mg–3g	Proteinuria, likely renal losses if >2g ([] p375)
>3g	Nephrotic syndrome ([] p376)

Creatinine clearance the excretion of creatinine per minute can be calculated from a 24h urine collection and this gives an estimation of the glomerular filtration rate (GFR), [] p373.

Catecholamines/VMA if a phaeochromocytoma is suspected a 24h urine sample is analysed for total catecholamines, vanillylmandelic acid (VMA), metanephrines and creatinine.

Toxicology urine can be screened for a wide range of recreational and medical drugs. Dipsticks give results in <10min while lab-based tests can often take several days.

CSF

Microscopy

Red cells (normal 0 per mm^3) these are raised from a bloody tap (more in the first bottle than the third) or from a subarachnoid haemorrhage (same in first and third bottles), however the two can only be distinguished reliably by measuring for xanthochromia (subarachnoid only). High levels of blood cells will disrupt the measurement of WBC and protein. The following calculations may help:

- True CSF WBC = CSF WBC − (bld WBC × CSF RBC ÷ bld RBC)
- True CSF protein = CSF protein − (RBC ÷ 100).

White cells (normal <4 per mm^3) raised levels in infection or post-sub-arachnoid, levels tend to be higher in bacterial meningitis (Table 17.25). The main type of white cell suggests the infectious agent:

- Neutrophils/polymorphs (normal 0 per mm^3) bacterial infection
- Lymphocytes/mononuclear (normal <4 per mm^3) viral infection or TB.

Bacteria a Gram stain may show bacteria in the sample; this is always pathological. Talk to a microbiologist about treatment.

Biochemistry

Protein (normal <0.4g/l); levels >1.0g/l are usually only seen in bacterial or TB meningitis (Table 17.24). Less dramatic rises can occur in all types of meningitis and also multiple sclerosis or Guillain–Barré.

Glucose (>2.2mmol/l or >70% plasma) reduced in meningitis, especially bacterial meningitis (Table 17.25).

Xanthochromia is a yellowing of the CSF caused by the breakdown of blood; it is present 4–12h following a subarachnoid haemorrhage.

Table 17.25 *CSF in different forms of meningitis*

	Normal	**Bacterial**	**TB**	**Viral**
Appearance	Clear	Cloudy	Clear	Clear
White cells	<4 × 10^6/l	5–2000 × 10^6/l	5–500 × 10^6/l	5–1000 × 10^6/l
Type of cell	Lymphocytes	Neutrophils	Lymphocytes	Lymphocytes
Glucose	>70% plasma	Very low	<50% plasma	>70% plasma
Protein	<0.4g/l	>1g/l	>1g/l	0.5–0.9g/l

Culture and PCR

Bacteria it can take several days for bacteria to grow but the majority are positive within 48h. It may take a further 24–48h to identify the type of bacteria and its sensitivity to antibiotics. Liaise with a microbiologist.

TB culture can take weeks because it is a slow growing bacteria. It may be possible to detect TB sooner using PCR. Talk to the laboratory technicians and microbiologists.

Viral PCR should be requested at the time of submitting a sample, if viral meningitis or encephalitis is suspected

Autoantibodies and associated diseases

Table 17.26 *Autoantibodies and associated diseases*

Autoantibody	Disease (% frequency where known)
Acetylcholine receptor	Myasthenia gravis (80%)
Antinuclear (ANA)	SLE (95%), RA (32%), JIA (76%), chronic active hepatitis (75%), Sjögren's syndrome (70%), systemic sclerosis (64%), normal 'controls' (0–2%)
Anticardiolipin	Primary antiphospholipid syndrome
Anticentromere	Limited systemic sclerosis (70%)
Anti-Ro	Sjögren's syndrome, subacute cutaneous lupus, SLE (30%), systemic sclerosis (60%), interstitial pneumonitis
Anti-La	Sjögren's syndrome (65%), SLE (15%)
c-ANCA/Anti-MPO	Wegener's granulomatosis (90%), MPA (11%), Churg–Strauss syndrome
p-ANCA/Anti-PR3	Churg–Strauss syndrome (60%)
dsDNA	SLE (60%)
ssDNA	SLE (70%), autoimmune rheumatic disease, inflammation
ENA	Includes: Anti-Ro, Anti-La, Anti-Jo-1, RNP, Scl-70, Anti-Sm
Gastric parietal cell	Autoimmune gastritis, pernicious anaemia
Glycolipid	Multi-focal motor neuropathy, Guillain–Barré syndrome, Miller–Fisher syndrome
Glomerular basement membrane	Goodpasture's syndrome
IgA-endomysial	Coeliac disease
Anti-Jo-1	Myositis
Mitochondrial (AMA)	Primary biliary cirrhosis (>95%)
Rheumatoid factor	RA (50–90%), SLE (15–35%), systemic sclerosis (20–30%), juvenile RA (7–10%), polymyositis (5–10%), infection (0–50%)
RNP	SLE and MCTD
Anti-Scl-70	Diffuse systemic sclerosis (30%)
Anti-Sm	SLE (30–40%)
Smooth muscle (SMA)	Chronic active hepatitis (40–90%), primary biliary cirrhosis (30–70%), idiopathic cirrhosis (25–30%), viral infections (80%), 'controls' (3–12%), autoimmune sclerosing cholangitis
Thyroid peroxidase	Hashimoto's thyroiditis (>80%), Graves' disease (50%)
Thyrotropin receptor	Graves' disease (50–80%)

Cervical spine radiographs

Cervical spine (C-spine) radiographs are mainly taken in trauma patients to exclude bony injury to this area that could result in high spinal cord damage and major disability. The patient normally has their neck immobilised with blocks, stiff-neck collar, and tape when the images are taken, which can make obtaining adequate views more difficult.

> If the patient's history suggests a fracture you must proceed with caution. Significant neck injury can be present even when plain C-spine x-rays appear normal. If in any doubt, discuss with your senior or a radiologist as CT imaging may be necessary. Spinal cord injury can still be present despite a normal CT (SCIWORA – spinal cord injury without radiological abnormality). This is due to non-bony injury causing instability (eg injury to cartilage, or ligaments). See ☐ p441 for a selection of patients for imaging.

The standard images taken in a C-spine series are:
- Lateral view – an X-ray taken from the side
- Long AP view – an X-ray taken from the front
- Peg view – an open mouth AP view, which shows C1/C2 articulation and the odontoid peg.

Identification Check the radiograph for the name of the patient and when the image was taken.

Interpreting the lateral view – ABCDE approach

Adequacy Is the X-ray penetration appropriate; can you see the vertebral bodies, spinous processes and soft tissues clearly? Can the whole of the C-spine be seen from C1 to the top of the T1 vertebral body? Is any part of the view obscured by a radio-opaque item such as jewellery?

Bodies Check all vertebral bodies have smooth outlines and attached spinous processes. All bodies below the level of C2 should be of similar size and shape. Check for any fragments of bone that have become detached (avulsed); this could suggest ligament injury.

Curves (alignment) Follow the three curves in Fig. 17.17 and ensure they are smooth. Ligament injury or fractures can cause disruption of these arcs.

Disc spaces Should be roughly equal between each vertebral body. Widening suggests serious injury.

Everything else (soft tissues) Abnormal widening of the prevertebral soft tissue or a localised bulge suggests a serious neck injury. Revisit the bodies, curves and disc spaces if there is widening.

Maximum normal width of prevertebral soft tissues	
C1–4	7mm
C5–7	22mm (roughly equal to the width of the vertebral bodies)

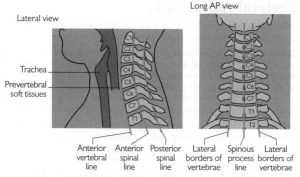

Fig. 17.17 Lateral (left) and long AP (right) views of the cervical spine.

Interpreting the anteroposterior (AP) view

- Check the spinous processes are in a straight line and the distance between the spinous processes is equal
- Check each vertebral body for any obvious bony injury.

Interpreting the peg view

- Check that the lateral margins of C1 and C2 line up
- Check the distance between the odontoid peg and the inner aspect of C1 is equal on both sides (Fig. 17.18). (This may not be the case due to injury or if the neck is rotated. If lateral C1 and C2 margins line up, this is more likely to be due to rotation.)
- Check there are no obvious fractures of C1 or C2. Look closely to ensure the odontoid peg is not fractured at its base.

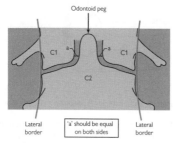

Fig. 17.18 Peg view showing central location of the odontoid peg.

Skeletal radiographs

Identification Check the radiograph for the name of the patient and when the image was taken; check if the image is of the left or right side.

Bones For each bone follow the edge of the cortex around the whole circumference, looking for steps, or cracks; does the bone look normal, or clearly very bowed or angulated around a fracture? Check the consistency of the bone matrix itself; is it uniformly pale and very opaque (osteopenic) or dense and very mineralised (sclerotic); are there cysts (lytic lesions) or patches of more dense bone (sclerotic lesions or callus)? See Table 17.27.

Joints Always check the joint above and below the bone in question, eg elbow and wrist when looking at the radius or ulna. Does the joint look normal, are the bones involved in the articulation in their normal position, is the distance between these bones increased or decreased? Re-check for breaks in the cortex of the bones within the joint (intra-articular fractures).

Soft tissue signs Soft-tissue oedema is often subtly seen on some radiographs, suggesting there is overlying swelling; this is especially seen around peripheral bones/joints (wrists, hands, ankles, feet, etc). Very occasionally gas can be seen on radiographs, and appears black; this can arise from gas-forming bacteria (classically *Clostridium* species), but also from open wounds. Bleeding and oedema adjacent to some joints gives rise to specific features; one of the best examples of these is the anterior fat pad sign of the elbow (Fig. 17.19). Small amounts of intra-articular haemorrhage force a normally hidden fat pad to appear on the lateral elbow radiograph, anterior to the distal humerus. The presence of this sign strongly suggests there is a peri-articular fracture. The posterior fat pad is often seen even in the absence of trauma/injury.

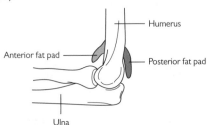

Fig. 17.19 The anterior and posterior fat pads on a lateral elbow X-ray.

If all else fails Sometimes it is difficult to see a radiological cause of the patient's complaint. Always ask a senior to review the radiograph or show it to a senior radiographer or the radiologist who is 'hot reporting'.

PACS Picture **A**rchiving and **C**ommunication **S**ystem is the electronic system on which hospitals store their radiology images. Viewing the images is undertaken on-screen and various manipulations of the image can be performed by the user such as inverting, rotating, magnifying, and altering the contrast – this makes finding fractures much easier.

Table 17.27 *Describing fractures*

Side	Right or left, dominant or not
Bone	Clavicle, radius, tibia etc
Location	Proximal, midshaft, distal
Type	Simple (2 bits), comminuted (≥3 bits), oblique, spiral
Shape	Displaced, angulated, impacted, rotated
Joint surface	Intra-articular fracture or not, dislocation
Complications	Compound (open fracture, 📖 p435), neurovascular involvement

Fractures in children Children's bones are still growing and generally softer and more malleable than adult bones. The greenstick fracture is a fracture of the shaft of a long bone, but like a green twig, snapping it often only breaks just one cortex rather than both (the classical definition of a fracture is a break to both cortices). Greenstick fractures are most common in the forearm. Fractures at the growing ends of bones usually take on one of five forms (see Salter–Harris classification – Fig. 17.20) and must be managed carefully to ensure the bone continues to develop/grow normally.

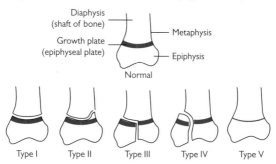

Fig. 17.20 Long bone nomenclature (top) and the Salter–Harris classification of growth plate fractures (bottom).

Pathological fractures are fractures at a site where the bone is weakened, usually where there is a cyst, metastatic lesion or inherited defect.

For specific bones/joints covered elsewhere			
Hip	📖 p147	Elbow	📖 p151
Knee	📖 p147	Wrist	📖 p151
Ankle	📖 p148	Hand	📖 p152
Foot	📖 p148	Back	📖 p149
Shoulder	📖 p150	C-spine	📖 p440

Table 17.27 Comparing fractures

Fractures in children

Pathological fractures

Appendices

Useful numbers and websites

Medical organisations
General Medical Council (GMC)
- 0161 923 6602 ⌂www.gmc-uk.org

British Medical Association (BMA)
- 020 7387 4499 ⌂bma.org.uk

Medical Defence Union (MDU)
- 0800 716 376 ⌂www.the-mdu.com
- 24h help 0800 716 646

Medical Protection Society (MPS)
- 08457 187 187 ⌂www.medicalprotection.org
- 24h help 0845 605 4000

Medical and Dental Defence Union of Scotland (MDDUS)
- 0845 270 2034 ⌂www.mddus.com
- 24h help 0845 270 2034

Counselling lines
BMA Counselling Service
- 08459 200 169 or 01455 254 189

Doctors' Support Network (mental illness)
- 0844 395 3010 ⌂www.dsn.org.uk

Sick Doctor's Trust (alcohol and drug addiction)
- 0370 444 5163 ⌂www.sick-doctors-trust.co.uk

Financial organisations
BMA Services
- 0845 609 2008 ⌂www.bmas.co.uk

Other
Gay and Lesbian Association of Doctors and Dentists (GLADD)
- ⌂www.gladd.co.uk

National Confidential Enquiry into Patient Outcome and Death (NCEPOD)
- ⌂www.ncepod.org.uk

Medical Research Council (MRC)
- 01793 416 200 ⌂www.mrc.ac.uk

Medical Women's Federation
- 0207 387 7765 ⌂www.medicalwomensfederation.org.uk

Médecins Sans Frontières (MSF)
- 0207 404 6600 ⌂www.msf.org

Voluntary Services Overseas
- 0208 780 7500 ⌂www.vso.org.uk

Wellcome Trust
- 0207 611 8888 ⌂www.wellcome.ac.uk

(Royal) College of

Anaesthetists	020 7092 1500	www.rcoa.ac.uk
Emergency Medicine	020 7404 1999	www.collemergencymed.ac.uk
General Practitioners	020 3188 7400	www.rcgp.org.uk
Obstetricians and Gynaecologists	020 7772 6200	www.rcog.org.uk
Ophthalmologists	020 7935 0702	www.rcophth.ac.uk
Paediatrics and Child Health	020 7092 6000	www.rcpch.ac.uk
Pathologists	020 7451 6700	www.rcpath.org
Physicians of London	020 7935 1174	www.rcplondon.ac.uk
Physicians of Edinburgh	0131 225 7324	www.rcpe.ac.uk
Physicians of Ireland	0035318639700	www.rcpi.ie
Physicians and Surgeons of Glasgow	0141 221 6072	www.rcpsg.ac.uk
Psychiatrists	020 7235 2351	www.rcpsych.ac.uk
Radiologists	020 7636 4432	www.rcr.ac.uk
Surgeons of Edinburgh	0131 527 1600	www.rcsed.ac.uk
Surgeons of England	020 7405 3474	www.rcseng.ac.uk
Surgeons of Ireland	0035314022100	www.rcsi.ie

Selected learned bodies

Academy of Medical Royal Colleges	www.aomrc.org.uk
Academy of Medical Sciences	www.acmedsci.ac.uk
Anatomical Society of Great Britain	www.anatsoc.org.uk
Association for Palliative Medicine	www.palliative-medicine.org
Association for Study of Medical Education	www.asme.org.uk
Association of Anaesthetists	www.aagbi.org
Association of British Neurologists	www.theabn.org
British Association of Dermatologists	www.bad.org.uk
British Association of Paediatric Surgeons	www.baps.org.uk
British Cardiac Society	www.cardiac.org.uk
British Geriatrics Society	www.bgs.org.uk
British Society for Rheumatology	www.rheumatology.org.uk
British Society of Gastroenterology	www.bsg.org.uk
British Thoracic Society	www.brit-thoracic.org.uk
Resuscitation Council	www.resus.org.uk
Royal Society of Medicine	www.roysocmed.ac.uk

Online reference sources

British National Formulary	www.bnf.org
Cochrane Library	www.thecochranelibrary.com
NHS Clinical Knowledge Summaries	www.cks.nhs.uk
NICE Evidence Search	www.evidence.nhs.uk
NICE Clinical Knowledge Summaries	cks.nice.org.uk
NICE Pathways	pathways.nice.org.uk
NICE Guidance	guidance.nice.org.uk

Height conversion

Metres (m) to inches (inch), multiply by 39.37 (12 inches to the foot)
Inches to metres, multiply by 0.0254.

m	inch	feet	inch	m	inch	feet	inch
1.36	53.5	4	5.5	1.67	66	5	6
1.37	54	4	6	1.69	66.5	5	6.5
1.38	54.5	4	6.5	1.70	67	5	7
1.40	55	4	7	1.71	67.5	5	7.5
1.41	55.5	4	7.5	1.73	68	5	8
1.42	56	4	8	1.74	68.5	5	8.5
1.43	56.5	4	8.5	1.75	69	5	9
1.45	57	4	9	1.76	69.5	5	9.5
1.46	57.5	4	9.5	1.78	70	5	10
1.47	58	4	10	1.79	70.5	5	10.5
1.48	58.5	4	10.5	1.80	71	5	11
1.50	59	4	11	1.81	71.5	5	11.5
1.51	59.5	4	11.5	1.83	72	6	0
1.52	60	5	0	1.84	72.5	6	0.5
1.54	60.5	5	0.5	1.85	73	6	1
1.55	61	5	1	1.87	73.5	6	1.5
1.56	61.5	5	1.5	1.88	74	6	2
1.57	62	5	2	1.89	74.5	6	2.5
1.59	62.5	5	2.5	1.90	75	6	3
1.60	63	5	3	1.92	75.5	6	3.5
1.61	63.5	5	3.5	1.93	76	6	4
1.62	64	5	4	1.94	76.5	6	4.5
1.64	64.5	5	4.5	1.95	77	6	5
1.65	65	5	5	1.97	77.5	6	5.5
1.66	65.5	5	5.5	1.98	78	6	6

Temperature

Degrees Fahrenheit (°F) to degrees Celsius (centigrade °C)
$$°C = (°F - 32) \times 0.56$$
Degrees Celsius (centigrade °C) to degrees Fahrenheit (°F)
$$°F = (°C \times 1.8) + 32$$

Pressure

Millimetres of mercury (mmHg) to kilopascals (kPa)
$$kPa = mmHg \times 0.113$$
Kilopascals (kPa) to millimetres of mercury (mmHg)
$$mmHg = kPa \times 7.519$$

Weight conversion

kg to pounds (lbs), multiply by 2.2046 (14lb to the stone; 16oz per lb)
Pounds to kg, multiply by 0.4536.

kg	St	lbs	kg	St	lbs	kg	St	lbs
1	0	2lb 3oz	43	6	11	85	13	5
2	0	4lb 7oz	44	6	13	86	13	8
3	0	6lb 10oz	45	7	1	87	13	10
4	0	8lb 13oz	46	7	3	88	13	12
5	0	11	47	7	6	89	14	0
6	0	13	48	7	8	90	14	2
7	1	1	49	7	10	91	14	5
8	1	4	50	7	12	92	14	7
9	1	6	51	8	0	93	14	9
10	1	8	52	8	3	94	14	11
11	1	10	53	8	5	95	14	13
12	1	12	54	8	7	96	15	2
13	2	1	55	8	9	97	15	4
14	2	3	56	8	11	98	15	6
15	2	5	57	9	0	99	15	8
16	2	7	58	9	2	100	15	10
17	2	9	59	9	4	101	15	13
18	2	12	60	9	6	102	16	1
19	3	0	61	9	8	103	16	3
20	3	2	62	9	11	104	16	5
21	3	4	63	9	13	105	16	7
22	3	7	64	10	1	106	16	10
23	3	9	65	10	3	107	16	12
24	3	11	66	10	6	108	17	0
25	3	13	67	10	8	109	17	2
26	4	1	68	10	10	110	17	5
27	4	4	69	10	12	111	17	7
28	4	6	70	11	0	112	17	9
29	4	8	71	11	3	113	17	11
30	4	10	72	11	5	114	17	13
31	4	12	73	11	7	115	18	2
32	5	1	74	11	9	116	18	4
33	5	3	75	11	11	117	18	6
34	5	5	76	12	0	118	18	8
35	5	7	77	12	2	119	18	10
36	5	9	78	12	4	120	18	13
37	5	12	79	12	6	125	19	10
38	6	0	80	12	8	130	20	7
39	6	2	81	12	11	135	21	4
40	6	4	82	12	13	140	22	1
41	6	6	83	13	1	145	22	12
42	6	9	84	13	3	150	23	9

Body mass index (BMI)

BMI calculation	BMI	Weight status
BMI = weight (kg)/height² (m²) eg: 77kg, 1.83m **77/(1.83 x 1.83) = 23 (normal)**	<18.5	Underweight
	18.5–24.9	Normal
	25.0–29.9	Overweight
	≥30	Obese
	≥40	Morbidly obese

Body mass index chart for adults

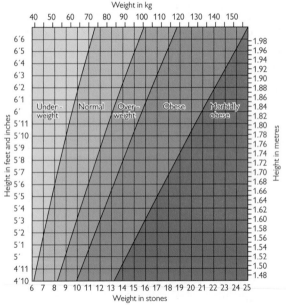

Fig. A1 Body mass index. Plotting weight against height estimates BMI.

Driving regulations (August 2013)

The DVLA issues strict regulations about which medical conditions affect your ability to drive. A summary of this information for holders of standard Group 1 licences is shown here; the full guidelines are available on the DVLA website (www.dvla.gov.uk). This list is not exhaustive and a patient should stop driving if they, or their doctor, believe they are incapacitated.

Neurology	
Stroke	Cease for 1mth; resume only if minimal residual deficit
TIA	Cease for 1mth
Chronic neuro disorder	Variable*
Meningitis	Drive if well
First seizure (or suspected)	Cease for 6mth*
Epilepsy	Cease until 1yr since last seizure (continue if seizures during sleep only for >3yr)*
Severe head injury/intra-cranial bleed	Cease for 6–12mth*
Brain tumours and mets	Variable*
Neurosurgery	Variable*
Visual field defects and diplopia	Cease driving (may be allowed if stable)
Visual acuity	Better than 6/12 corrected with both eyes
Unexplained syncope	Cease 4wk if low risk or cause found; else cease for 6mth*
Recurrent severe vertigo	Once attacks controlled*

Diabetes	
Diabetes on insulin or oral hypoglycaemic agents	Must be able to recognise hypo and not had >1 hypo requiring assistance in past 12mth*
Diabetes on diet only	Drive if well
Recurrent hypoglycaemia	Cease until controlled

Cardiovascular	
Angina	If symptoms at rest, at wheel or with emotion, cease until stabilised
MI/ACS	Cease for 1wk if successful angioplasty, else cease for 4wk
Angioplasty	Cease for 1wk
Pacemaker	Cease for 1wk*
ICD (if inserted for incapacitation)	Cease 6mth after insertion/shock*
ICD (if inserted prophylatically)	Cease for 1mth
CABG	Cease for 4wk*
Incapacitating arrhythmia	Cease for 4wk after controlled*
Stable arrhythmia	Drive if well
AAA ≥6cm	Annual review required if 6–6.5cm; if ≥6.5cm, cease until repaired*
Aortic stenosis	Cease if symptomatic*

Psychiatry and substance abuse	
Severe psychiatric illness	Cease until stable for 3mth*
Alcohol dependence	Cease until 1yr abstinence*
Opioid, benzo + cocaine dependence	Cease for 1yr after previous use*
Other recreational drugs	Cease 6mth after previous use*

Other	
COPD	Drive if well
Sleep apnoea + narcolepsy	Cease until symptoms controlled*
Chronic renal failure	Drive if well
HIV	Drive if well

*Patient must notify the DVLA.

If a patient refuses to notify the DVLA about a medical condition you have a duty to break confidentiality and inform the DVLA on their behalf. Seek advice from senior colleagues.

Interesting cases

Note down any interesting or unusual cases which could be used for a teaching or a Grand Round case presentation. Do not include personally identifiable patient information.

Hospital number

Details

Hospital number

Details

Hospital number

Details

Hospital number

Details

Hospital number

Details

Hospital number

Details

Hospital number

Details

Hospital number

Details

Telephone numbers 1

Hospital:	Telephone:	
	Extension	Bleep

Your firm's timetable 1

Time	Monday	Tuesday	Wednesday	Thursday	Friday

Telephone numbers 2

Hospital:	Telephone:	
	Extension	Bleep

Your firm's timetable 2

Time	Monday	Tuesday	Wednesday	Thursday	Friday

Telephone numbers 3

Hospital:	Telephone:	
	Extension	Bleep

Your firm's timetable 3

Time	Monday	Tuesday	Wednesday	Thursday	Friday

Index

Bold type indicates main references

Common adult drug doses

Typical doses for common indications for adults with normal BMI and renal function are given. For more details and other indications see Chapter 5. **Users are advised to always check local prescribing guidelines and formularies and to consult the *BNF* when prescribing drugs.**

Analgesia *BNF* 4.7	
Amitriptyline (neuropathic)	10mg PO nocte (titrated up to 75mg)
Codeine (weak opioid)	30–60mg/4h PO/IM (max 240mg/24h)
Ibuprofen (NSAID)	200–400mg/6–8h PO (max 2.4g/24h)
Paracetamol	1g/4–6h PO/IV (max 4g/24h)
Morphine (strong opioid)	2.5–5mg/4h IV or 5–10mg/4h IM/SC or eg Oramorph® 5–10mg/4h PO
Tramadol (moderate opioid)	50–100mg/4h PO/ IM/IV (max 600mg/24h)

Antiemetics *BNF* 4.6	
Cyclizine (antihistamine)	50mg/8h PO/IV/IM
Metoclopramide (antidopaminergic)	10mg/8h PO/IV/IM
Ondansetron (5HT₃ antagonist)	4–8mg/8h PO/ IV/IM
Prochlorperazine (phenothiazine)	10mg/8h PO/IV/IM

Cardiovascular *BNF* 2	
Amlodipine (Ca²⁺-channel blocker)	*for HTN:* 5–10mg/24h PO
Aspirin (antiplatelet)	*long-term prophylaxis:* 75mg/24h PO
Atenolol (β-blocker)	*for AF or angina:* 50–100mg/24h PO
Bisoprolol (β-blocker)	*for heart failure:* 1.25mg/24h PO initially (max 10mg/24h)
Clopidogrel (antiplatelet)	*long term prophylaxis:* 75mg/24h PO
Furosemide (loop diuretic)	*for heart failure:* 40mg/24 PO initially (max 80–120mg/24h)
Ramipril (ACEi)	*for failure or HTN:* 1.25mg/24h PO initially (max 10mg/24h)
Verapamil (Ca²⁺-channel blocker)	*for AF or angina:* 40–120mg/8h PO
Simvastatin (statin)	20–40mg PO nocte

Respiratory *BNF* 3	
Salbutamol (short acting β-agonist)	1–2 puffs INH PRN (metered dose inhalers)
Salmeterol (long acting β-agonist)	2 puffs/12h INH (metered dose inhalers)
Steroid and combination inhalers	Multiple, non-interchangeable formulations – see chapter 5 and *BNF 3.2*
Tiotropium (long acting anticholinergic)	18micrograms/24h INH

Gastroenterology *BNF* 1	
Bisacodyl (stimulant laxative)	5–10mg/nocte PO or 10mg/mane PR
Gaviscon® (antacid)	10–20ml PRN PO (eg after meals)
Fybogel® (bulk forming laxative)	1 sachet/12h PO
Glycerin (stimulant laxative)	1 suppository/PRN PR (max 4/24h)
Hyoscine butylbromide (antimuscarinic)	eg Buscopan® 20mg/6h PO
Lactulose (osmotic laxative)	10–15ml/12h PO
Movicol® (osmotic laxative)	1–3 sachets/24h PO
Omeprazole (PPI)	20–40mg/24h PO
Phosphate enema (stimulant laxative)	1/PRN PR
Ranitidine (H₂-antagonist)	150mg/12h PO
Senna (stimulant laxative)	2 tablets/nocte PO

Miscellaneous	
Chlorphenamine (sedating antihistamine)	4mg/4–6h PO (max 24mg/24h)
Zopiclone (hypnotic)	3.75–7.5mg/24h PO

Empirical antibiotic choices *BNF* 5.1

Choices suitable for patients with penicillin allergies are given in italics. For MRSA colonised patients alternative regimens may be required. **Always consult local guidelines and the BNF.**

Respiratory infections

Community acquired pneumonia: CURB65=0–1	Amoxicillin 500mg–1g/8h PO *or: doxycycline 200mg PO STAT then 100mg/24h PO*
Community acquired pneumonia: CURB65=2	Amoxicillin 1g/8h PO/IV + clarithromycin 500mg/12h PO/IV *or: doxycycline 200mg PO STAT then 100mg/24h PO*
Community acquired pneumonia: CURB65≥3	Co-amoxiclav 1.2g/8h IV + clarithromycin 500mg/12h IV *or: vancomycin 1g/12h IV + ciprofloxacin 200mg/12h IV*
Hospital acquired pneumonia (non-severe)[1]	Co-amoxiclav 1.2g/8h IV *or: clarithromycin 500mg/12h PO/IV*
Hospital acquired pneumonia (severe)[1]	Tazocin® 4.5g/8h IV *or: vancomycin 1g/12h IV + ciprofloxacin 200mg/12h IV*
COPD (PO therapy)	Amoxicillin 500mg/8h PO *or: doxycycline 200mg PO STAT then 100mg/24h PO*
COPD (IV therapy)	Co-amoxiclav 1.2g/8h IV + clarithromycin 500mg/12h IV *or: vancomycin 1g/12h IV + ciprofloxacin 200mg/12h IV*

Bone + joint infections

Acute osteomyelitis or septic arthritis[2]	Co-amoxiclav 1.2g/8h IV *or: vancomycin 1g/12h IV + ciprofloxacin 400mg/12h IV*

CNS infections

Community acquired meningitis	Ceftriaxone 2g/12h IV + vancomycin 1g/12h IV[3] *or: chloramphenicol 25mg/kg/6h IV + vancomycin 1g/12h IV*

Skin and soft tissue infections

Cellulitis, infected eczema and simple wound infections (MRSA⁻ᵛᵉ)	Flucloxacillin 1g/6h PO/IV[4] *or: clarithromycin 500mg/12h PO/IV*
Cellulitis, infected eczema and simple wound infections (MRSA⁺ᵛᵉ)	doxycycline 200mg PO STAT then 100mg/24h PO or if severe: vancomycin 1g/12h IV
Cellulitis around IV cannula sites or other prosthesis	As for MRSA⁻ᵛᵉ cellulitis if non-severe. If severe: vancomycin 1g/12h IV + Tazocin® 4.5g/8h IV *or: vancomycin 1g/12h IV + ciprofloxacin 200mg/12h IV*
Cellulitis in diabetics and wound infections following 'dirty' surgery	Co-amoxiclav 625mg PO or co-amoxiclav 1.2g/8h IV *or: clarithromycin 500mg/12h PO + ciprofloxacin 500mg/12h PO + metronidazole 400mg/8h PO*
Infected animal bites	Co-amoxiclav 625mg/8h PO *or: metronidazole 400 mg/8h PO + doxycycline 200mg/24h PO*
Wound infections following trauma surgery or cellulitis around diabetic ulcers	Co-amoxiclav 1.2g/8h IV[4] *or: clarithromycin 500mg/12h IV + ciprofloxacin 200mg/12h IV + metronidazole 500mg/8h IV*

Urinary tract infections

UTI (PO therapy) including pyelonephritis	Co-amoxiclav 625mg/8h PO *or: ciprofloxacin 500mg/12h PO*
UTI (IV therapy) including pyelonephritis	Co-amoxiclav 1.2g/8h IV *or: gentamicin 5mg/kg/24h IV*

[1] Where aspiration likely, add in metronidazole 400mg/8h PO or 500mg/8h IV.
[2] Hospital acquired cases and prosthetic joints will require more aggressive initial regimens.
[3] Add amoxicillin 2g/4h IV if pregnant or immunocompromised or age>50yr to cover listeriosis (*or: co-trimoxazole 15mg/kg/6h IV if penicillin allergy*).
[4] If MRSA suspected, add doxycycline 200mg/24h PO or vancomycin 1g/12h IV.

Emergency adult drug doses

Only use this page if you are ALS/ILS trained; otherwise contact a senior and turn to the appropriate emergency page.

Doses are appropriate for an otherwise healthy 70kg adult. 'Max freq' shows maximum frequency drugs should be used in an emergency.

	Dose	Max freq	Route
Cardiac and shock			
Adenosine	6, 12, 12mg	5min	Fast IV
Adrenaline, anaphylaxis	0.5ml 1:1000 (0.5mg)	5min	IM
Adrenaline, arrest	10ml 1:10,000 (1mg)	~3min	IV
Atropine, bradycardia	0.5mg, 3mg max	1min	IV
Atropine, arrest	3mg (no longer recommended)	Once	IV
Aspirin	300mg	Once	PO
Calcium gluconate 10%	10ml in 2min, 50ml max	15min	IV
Clopidogrel	300mg	Once	PO
Diamorphine	2.5mg	5min	IV
Digoxin infusion	500micrograms in 30min (📖 p196)	Once	IV
Morphine	5mg	5min	IV
Verapamil	5mg in 2min, 15mg max	5min	IV
Respiratory			
Aminophylline[1]	5mg/kg in 20 min	Once	IV
Furosemide	40–120mg (1mg/kg)	Once	IV
GTN infusion	10–200micrograms/min Systolic >90	Infusion	IV
Isosorbide dinitrate	2–10mg/h Systolic >90	Infusion	IV
Hydrocortisone	200mg	Once	IV
Ipratropium	500mcg	4h	Neb
Magnesium	2g (8mmol) over 15 min	Once	IV
Salbutamol, infusion	250micrograms over 10 min	Once	IV
Salbutamol, neb	5mg	Continuous	Neb
Neuro and epilepsy			
Glucose 10%, 20%, 50%	200, 100, 50ml respectively	Check glucose	IV
Diazepam	10mg, 30mg max	5min	IV/PR
Lorazepam	4mg, 12mg max	5min	IV
Naloxone	0.4mg, 10mg max	3min	IV
Phenytoin infusion	20mg/kg at <50mg/min	Once	IV

[1] Do not give loading dose of IV aminophylline if patient taking oral theophylline (unless plasma levels known).